# Orthopedic Manual Therapy
## An Evidence-Based Approach

### Chad Cook, PT, PhD, MBA, OCS, COMT

*Assistant Clinical Professor*
*Department of Community and Family Medicine*
*Division of Physical Therapy*
*Duke University*

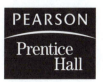

PEARSON
Prentice
Hall

Upper Saddle River, New Jersey 07458

**Library of Congress Cataloging-in-Publication Data**

Cook, Chad.
    Orthopedic manual therapy : an evidence based approach / Chad Cook.
        p. ; cm.
    Includes bibliographical references and index.
    ISBN 0-13-171766-9
1.  Manipulation (Therapeutics)    2.  Orthopedics.    3.  Medicine, Physical.    I.  Title.
    [DNLM: 1.  Manipulation, Orthopedic—methods—Handbooks.    WB 39 C771o 2007]
    RM724.C66 2007
    615.8'2—dc22

                                                                    2006015857

**Publisher:** Julie Levin Alexander
**Assistant to Publisher:** Regina Bruno
**Executive Editor:** Mark Cohen
**Associate Editor:** Melissa Kerian
**Editorial Assistant:** Nicole Ragonese
**Director of Production and Manufacturing:** Bruce Johnson
**Managing Production Editor:** Patrick Walsh
**Production Liaison:** Christina Zingone
**Production Editor:** Karen Berry, Pine Tree Composition
**Manufacturing Manager:** Ilene Sanford
**Manufacturing Buyer:** Pat Brown
**Senior Design Coordinator:** Maria Guglielmo
**Director of Marketing:** Karen Allman
**Senior Marketing Manager:** Harper Coles
**Composition:** Pine Tree Composition, Inc.
**Printer and Binder:** Courier Westford
**Cover Printer:** Phoenix Color

**Notice:** The authors and the publisher of this volume have taken care that the information and technical recommendations contained herein are based on research and expert consultation, and are accurate and compatible with the standards generally accepted at the time of publication. Nevertheless, as new information becomes available, changes in clinical and technical practices become necessary. The reader is advised to carefully consult manufacturers' instructions and information material for all supplies and equipment before use, and to consult with a health care professional as necessary. This advice is especially important when using new supplies or equipment for clinical purposes. The authors and publisher disclaim all responsibility for any liability, loss, injury, or damage incurred as a consequence, directly or indirectly, of the use and application of any of the contents of this volume.

Pearson Education LTD., *London*
Pearson Education Australia PTY, Limited, *Sydney*
Pearson Education Singapore, Pte. Ltd
Pearson Education North Asia Ltd., *Hong Kong*
Pearson Education, Canada, Ltd., *Toronto*

Pearson Educación de Mexico, S.A. de C.V.
Pearson Education–Japan, *Tokyo*
Pearson Education Malaysia, Pte. Ltd
Pearson Education, Upper Saddle River, New Jersey.

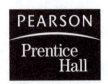

10   9   8   7   6   5   4   3   2   1
ISBN 0-13-171766-9

# Contents

# Acknowledgments

I would like to acknowledge several individuals who have influenced my completion of this project.

- Robert Sprague, PT, PhD, FAAOMPT, who mentored me and many of my colleagues.
- Christopher Showalter, PT, OCS, FAAOMPT, who has provided me with opportunities to grow and excel as a clinician and as a teacher.
- Philip Sizer, PT, PhD, FAAOMPT, who has functioned as a sounding board, research collaborator, and advisor.
- Ron Peyton, PT, ATC, who inspired and provided me with many opportunities.
- The Pioneers and Clinical Masters of Manual Therapy. Without them, we'd have nothing to follow.
- The work of G.D. Maitland. Quite simply, a clinical genius.

# Preface

The *International Federation of Orthopaedic Manipulative Therapists* (IFOMT)[1], a multinational organization of physiotherapists who specialize in manual therapy, classify orthopaedic manual therapy as "... a specialized area of physiotherapy/ physical therapy for the management of neuro-musculoskeletal conditions, based on clinical reasoning, using highly specific treatment approaches including manual techniques and therapeutic exercises." Historically, orthopedic manual therapy has enveloped treatment methods such as manipulation, mobilization, neuromuscular mobilization, and massage/soft tissue therapies.[2]

IFOMT recognizes the necessity for evidence-based applications, stating: "orthopaedic manual therapy also encompasses, and is driven by, the available scientific and clinical evidence and the bio-psychosocial framework of each individual patient."[1] Organizations such as IFOMT have dedicated website support services providing methods for critical evaluation of manual therapy techniques, assessment procedures, and research. Refereed journals such as *Manual Therapy*, *Manual Medicine*, the *Journal of Manipulative and Physiological Therapeutics*, and the *Journal of Manual and Manipulative Therapy* have committed to publishing research in the field of orthopedic manual therapy. Contributions within these and other journals have improved clinicians' selection of effective treatment techniques supported by clinical "evidence."

Literature describing and measuring "evidence-based" care has grown significantly over the last decade.[3] The core components of this concept were developed in the 1970s and 1980s with the application of epidemiological principles of patient care.[4,5] These epidemiological principles advocate that using evidence-based care allows clinicians to apply the current best evidence from research to the clinical care of the individual patient.[4,6]

In the early 1990s, Sackett defined evidence-based medicine as "the integration of best research evidence with clinical expertise and patient values."[7] Furthermore, Sackett suggested that the definition requires a clinician to base clinical decision making on three components: (1) research, (2) clinical expertise, and (3) patient centeredness. Sackett acknowledged that evidence-based principles drive clinical practice and, in turn, clinical practice drives the need for investigation of evidence. This does not connote that the use of specific uninvestigated clinical methods are inappropriate. However, this does imply that previously measured treatment methods, created with a poor empirical construct or that have demonstrated a lack of effectiveness and reliability among clinicians, may not be appropriate for care.

Often, agreement upon what constitutes evidence-based practice is a significant point of contention. Some argue that evidence-based care is wholly a matter of opinion and purely within the eye of the beholder.[8] Others steadfastly advocate their own philosophies and fail to recognize methods outside their own practice pattern. It is imperative to acknowledge that many treatment techniques based on habit, custom, guru-based promotion, or protocol are potentially not applicable for care.[4] Furthermore, extrapolation of complex theoretical anatomical or biomechanical constructs that lack a measurable carryover to clinical care are not considered "evidence-based."[9]

How does one apply and measure Sackett's definition during clinical practice? Essentially, there are two ways. The first requires the application of treatment techniques extracted from clinical trials. Comparative randomized clinical trials represent the highest form of validation for selected treatment techniques. Second, the use of outcome scales to measure improvements during patient care application is essential.[6,9] By measuring the outcomes of a patient care approach, we ensure that current treatments are as applicable today as yesterday.

After an assiduous investigation of the literature, I have outlined the examination and treatment methods that have demonstrated evidence-based success during clinical trials. When information from clinical trials was lacking, I provided evidence supported by case controls or case series designs. When information was absent, selected patient-response philosophies from Maitland, McKenzie, and others were integrated within the examination and treatment process. In essence, the assessment, treatment, and clinical reasoning methods are grounded in evidence-based principles and serve to expand a growing field of orthopedic manual therapy literature.

# *References*

1. International Federation of Orthopaedic Manual Therapists. Accessed January 6, 2005, at: http://www.omt.org/homepage/ifomt/ifomt.htm

2. Gross A, Kay T, Hondras M, Goldsmith C, Haines T, Peloso P, Kennedy C, Hoving J. Manual therapy for mechanical neck disorders: a systematic review. *Man Ther.* 2002;7:131–149.

3. Nieuwboer A. How self evident is evidence based practice in physiotherapy? *Physiother Res Int.* 2004;9:iii–iv.

4. Cohen AM, Stavri PZ, Hersh WR. A categorization and analysis of the criticisms of evidence based medicine. *Int J Med Informatics.* 2004;73:35–43.

5. Sackett DL. The fall of clinical research and the rise of clinical practice research. *Clin Invest Med.* 2000;23:331–333.

6. Buetow MA, Kenealy T. Evidence based medicine: the need for new definition. *J Evaluation Clin Pract.* 2000;6:85–92.

7. Sackett DL, Strauss SE, Richardson WS, Rosenberg W, Haynes RB. Evidence-based medicine. *How to practice and teach EBM.* Edinburgh; Churchill Livingstone: 2000.

8. Driever M. Are evidence based practice and best practice the same? *Western J Nursing Res.* 2002;24:591–597.

9. Bialocerkowski A, Grimmer K, Milanese S, Kumar S. Application of current research evidence to clinical physiotherapy practice. *J Allied Health.* 2003;33:230–237.

# Reviewers

**Stephania Bell, MS, PT, OCS, CSCS**
Kaiser Hayward Orthopedic Manual Therapy Fellowship
Union City, California

**Robert E. Boyles, PT, DSc, OCS, FAAOMPT**
Assistant Professor, Physical Therapy
U.S. Army–Baylor University
Fort Sam Houston, Texas

**Jean-Michel Brismee, ScD, PT, OCS, FAAOMPT**
Assistant Professor, Physical Therapy
Texas Tech University Health Sciences Center
Odessa, Texas

**Joshua Cleland, DPT, PhD, OCS**
Assistant Professor, Physical Therapy
Franklin Pierce College
Concord, New Hampshire

**Evan Johnson, PT, MS, OCS, MTC**
Assistant Professor, Clinical Physical Therapy
Columbia University
New York, New York

**Kenneth E. Learman, MEd, PT, OCS, COMT, FAAOMPT**
Assistant Professor, Physical Therapy
Youngstown State University
Youngstown, Ohio

**Kevin Ramey, MS, PT**
Program Director, Rehabilitation Sciences
Texas Tech University Health Sciences Center
Odessa, Texas

**Christopher R. Showalter, LPT, OCS, FAAOMPT**
Clinical Director
Maitland-Australian Physiotherapy Seminars
Cutchogue, New York

**Andrea P. Simmons, CMT, CNMT**
Program Chair, Massage Therapy
Medical Careers Institute
Richmond, Virginia

# 1

# Orthopedic Manual Therapy

## Objectives

- Outline the mechanical changes associated with manual therapy intervention.
- Compare and contrast the effects of static stretching, manually assisted movements, mobilization, and manipulation.
- Outline the neurophysiologic changes associated with manual therapy intervention.
- Outline the proposed psychological changes associated with manual therapy intervention.

## THE SCIENCE OF ORTHOPEDIC MANUAL THERAPY

The precise nature of why manual therapy benefits various conditions has given rise to conflicting theories and heated debate.[1] Explanations outlining the reasons why manual therapy is beneficial have ranged from the scientifically pertinent to the inexplicably strange. To date, most theories remain hypothetical, have involved investigations that were poorly designed, or were predominantly promoted by personal opinion. There are no shortages of hypotheses driven primarily by researchers and theoreticians in chiropractic, physical therapy, osteopathic, and massage-based fields. Hypotheses include: movement of the nucleus pulposus[2,3], activation of the gate-control mechanism[4], neuromechanical and biomechanical responses[5,6], and reductions in paraspinal muscle hypertonicity.[7,8]

The constructs behind the use of mobilization and manipulation are similar and both share comparable indications and contraindications for use. Most importantly, the application of each treatment method results in similar functional outcomes and similar hypothesized effects.[9] These hypothesized effects are frequently categorized as biomechanical, muscular reflexogenic, or neurophysiologic.[5,10] Additionally, manual therapy may provide measurable psychological changes. The remainder of this chapter is dedicated to analysis of these four areas.

## BIOMECHANICAL CHANGES

### Joint Displacement

It is suggested that restricted tissue mobility may have a physiological origin within the joint segment and surrounding tissues.[11] These physiological changes are often termed a "hypomobility" during joint assessment. **Hypomobility** may lead to a lower volume of synovial fluid within the joint cavity, which results in an increase in intra-articular pressure during movement.[11] Consequently, the distance between articular surfaces declines and reduces the lubricating properties of the joint and increasing irregular collagen cross-links.[12,13] Cross-links between collagen-based fibers inhibit normal connective tissue gliding, which leads to restricted joint movement[14] and corresponding range of motion loss and impairment. Additional contributors such as intra-articular meniscoids[15], entrapment of a fragment of posterior annular material from the intervertebral disc[16], and excessive spasm or **hypertonicity** of the deep intrinsic musculature[17,18] may further the impairment of joint mobility. Consequential debilitating changes include impaired strength, endurance, coordination, and alterations in the autonomic nervous system.[19]

Some evidence exists that mobilization and/or manipulation techniques solicit joint displacement.[20] In theory, this joint displacement solicits a temporary increased in the degree of displacement that is produced with force due to hysteresis effects.[21] Chiropractors suggest that when joint structures are rapidly stretched, cavitation internally occurs and an audible "pop" may be heard. Mierau[22] reported an increased range of motion after cavitation. Nonetheless, it is important to note that the "pop" is not necessary for pain reduction. Flynn et al.[23] recently reported that the outcome of a cohort of patients who received spine manipulation was not altered by whether or not a pop occurred during the manipulative procedure.

The amount of movement necessary for reduction of symptoms is unknown. Overall, most studies have either been poorly performed[24,25], have used spine cadavers for the experimental analysis[26], or have reported the effect of manipulation on the spine of a canine.[27] Additionally, one well-cited study used surface markers during assessment of joint-related movements.[24] The use of surface markers is associated with a high degree of error since the measurement of skin displacement is a component of the movement. Subsequently, the findings of translational and sagittal rotational movement by Lee and Evans[24] are misleading, since relatively large quantities of soft tissue displacement was included in the overall value.

Several studies have investigated the mechanical effect of manual therapy on range of motion, most of which have included only fair methodology. In an **in-vivo analysis,** Keller et al.[28] reported peak shear movements of 0.3 mm, axial movements of 1 mm, and sagittal rotation of 1 degree during manipulation forces. Mean movements of around half a millimeter for medial to lateral, anterior to posterior, and axial displacement were recorded and are likely to accurately represent true manipulative displacement.[28] The authors imbedded pins in the spine of surgical patients and performed manipulation using various forces.

## Passive Movements Lead to Range-of-Motion Gains

The majority of manual therapy treatment approaches use methods that are passive in nature and are designed to increase the mobility of restricted joint and surrounding tissues. Passive manual therapy techniques are designed to increase range of motion of a targeted, specific region and normalize **arthrokinematic** gliding and rolling movement. It is suggested that the improvement in arthrokinematic gliding and rolling will normalize osteokinematic rotation and enable the normalization of active movements.[29] Notionally, to accomplish the arthrokinematic movements, a favorable passive force is required to improve the consequences of the negative changes.[30,31] These passive forces have the capacity to target tissue that is not placed under tension during active movements. Four forms of passive movements include (1) static stretching, (2) manually assisted movement, (3) mobilization, and (4) manipulation.

### Static Stretching

**Static stretching** has received a fair amount of experiential investigation. An overwhelming majority identify

that static stretching does lead to mechanical changes in range of motion. Regardless if stretching was performed against a control that received no treatment or a pragmatic control that received a comparative treatment, static stretching yielded positive results.

It has been suggested that passive static stretching does lengthen muscle fibers[32] and can assist in prevention of muscular atrophy secondary to immobilization.[33] However, less is known about the long-term benefit of static stretching on range of motion. The majority of these studies used measurements that were limited to pre- and post-analysis, which hampers the ability to determine the lasting effects of static stretching.

Table 1.1 outlines a summary of the static stretching studies analyzed. Within the study, the region tested corresponds to the isolated physiological area. The second column *demonstrated range-of-motion (ROM) benefit with stretching* was recorded as a "yes" or a "no." Each study was also evaluated to determine if a randomized comparison was performed. Three possible choices in "yes" control, in which the control group received no intervention; "yes" pragmatic, in which the control group received a comparable treatment; or "no," in which no control comparison was used. The column *stretch was mutually exclusive* relates to whether the static stretch was performed in isolation, or whether it was performed with other interventions. The next heading, *symptomatic subjects*, is a report of whether the subjects used in the trial were asymptomatic or exhibited impairment or impaired function. Lastly, the final column records the strength of evidence. Each study

## Summary

- Although very limited in gross amount, joint displacement does occur during manipulation and mobilization.
- Joint displacement is associated with an audible pop.
- An audible pop is not necessary for neurophysiologic changes.
- Joint displacement may be associated with passive movement to mechanoreceptors and may be a reason behind neurophysiologic change. Static stretching does improve range of motion in asymptomatic subjects.
- Structural changes can occur with as little as 15 minutes of stretching a day.
- Static stretching does lead to temporary improvements in tissue mobility.
- Whether static stretching leads to long-term or permanent changes beyond the application data is unknown.

is evaluated using a modification of the method described by Moseley et al.[34] If a study qualified as a very well-designed, randomized controlled trial it was classified as "Level 1"; a fairly well-designed, randomized pragmatic controlled trial, a "Level II"; and a pseudo-randomized trial, a "Level III."

Within these studies, variations in static hold associated with the length of time required to obtain optimal results has been presented. Although there is no consensus on a single specific time, it is apparent that a static hold of 15–30 seconds provides the most significant gains when compared to shorter or longer time periods.

Collectively, there are weaknesses in the methodology of static stretching studies. Although a preponderance of investigations have shown that static stretching does lead to increases in range of motion, an overwhelming majority used asymptomatic subjects and most limited investigation to outcomes associated with hamstring stretching. One other consideration was the small sample sizes. This aspect and the failure to use comparable controls prevented most studies from demonstrating high quality. Lastly, only one study was found that included subjects age 65 and older. Generalizing results to asymptomatic subjects or older individuals at this point may be injudicious.

**TABLE 1.1**    Tabulated Results of Experimentally Investigated Static Stretching Studies

| | Region Tested | Demonstrated ROM Benefit with Stretching | Randomized Comparison | Stretch was Mutually Exclusive | Symptomatic Subjects? | Level of Evidence |
|---|---|---|---|---|---|---|
| Bandy et al.[35] | Hamstring Length | Yes | Yes (control) | Yes | No | II |
| Bandy et al.[36] | Hamstring Length | Yes | Yes (control) | Yes | No | II |
| Bandy & Irion[37] | Hamstring Length | Yes | Yes (control) | Yes | No | II |
| Bohannon[38] | Hamstrings | Yes | Yes (control) | Yes | No | II |
| Godges et al.[39] | Hip Extension | Yes | Yes (pragmatic and control) | Yes | No | II |
| Halbertsma & Goeken[40] | Hamstring Length | No | Yes (control) | Yes | No | II |
| Leivseth et al.[41] | Hip | Yes | No | Yes | Yes | III |
| Magnusson et al.[42] | Hamstring Length | Yes | Yes (control) | Yes | No | II |
| McCarthy et al.[43] | Hamstring Length | Yes | Yes (control) | No | No | II |
| Pollard & Ward[44] | Hip | Yes (at the cervical spine) | Yes (control) | Yes | No | III |
| Reid & McNair[45] | Hamstring Flexibility | Yes | Yes (control) | Yes | No | II |
| Roberts & Wilson[46] | Hip Flexion, Knee Flexion, & Extension | Yes | Yes (control) | Yes | No | II |
| Starring et al.[47] | Hamstring Length | Yes | Yes (control) | Yes | No | II |
| Steffen & Molllinger[47] | Knee Flexion Contracture | No | Yes (pragmatic) | Yes | Yes | II |
| Tanigawa et al.[49] | Hamstrings | Yes | Yes (control) | Yes | No | II |

**TABLE 1.2**    Tabulated Results of Experimentally Investigated Manually Assisted Methods of Stretching/Mobilization

| | Region Tested | Demonstrated ROM Benefit with Manually Assisted Movements | Randomized Comparison | Manually Assisted Movement Method was Mutually Exclusive | Symptomatic Subjects? | Level of Evidence |
|---|---|---|---|---|---|---|
| Ballantyne et al.[53] | Hamstring Flexibility (Passive Knee Extension) | Yes | Yes (pragmatic) | Yes | No | II |
| Etnyre & Abraham[51] | Ankle Dorsiflexion | Yes | Yes (pragmatic) | No (repeated measures) | No | III |
| Ferber et al.[54] | Knee Extension | Yes | No | Yes (several types) | No (older) | III |
| Lenehan et al.[55] | Thoracic Trunk Rotation | Yes | Yes (control) | Yes | No | II |
| McCarthy et al.[43] | Cervical Range of Motion | Yes | Yes (control) | No | No | III |
| Schenk et al.[56] | Lumbar Extension | Yes | Yes (control) | Yes | Yes | II |
| Schenk et al.[57] | Cervical Range of Motion | Yes | Yes (control) | Yes | Yes | II |
| Winters et al.[58] | Hip Extension | Yes (same as static stretch) | Yes (pragmatic) | Yes | Yes | II |

### Manually Assisted Movement (PNF Stretching)

Manually assisted movements are another variation of stretching. This method requires variations in active contraction by the subject against passive application of a stress by the clinician. Often, these methods are described as **proprioceptive neuromuscular facilitation** (PNF). PNF exercises are designed to "hasten the response of the neuromuscular mechanism though stimulation of the proprioceptors."[50] Although PNF techniques were theoretical when created, the basis of the theory is fairly well substantiated.[51]

A **muscle energy technique** (MET) is another manually assisted method of stretching/mobilization. METs are performed when the patient actively uses their muscles, on request, while maintaining a targeted preposition against a distinctly executed counterforce.[52] METs may be classified as isotonic or isometric contractions, each with opposite desired outcomes. In an isometric contraction, the overall muscle belly length (of the activated muscle) shortens (the tendon lengthens), while during an isotonic contraction the muscle may lengthen or shorten.

The nine studies in Table 1.2 enlisted a mixed set of subjects, some symptomatic, others not. Additionally, a minority did not perform mutually exclusive stretching nor did they compare the methods to a control group. Nonetheless,

manually assisted movements appear to provide similar outcomes as static stretching with all but one exhibiting mechanical range-of-motion gains versus controls.

## *Summary*

- PNF stretching methods have been demonstrated to be as effective as other pragmatic models and significantly effective when compared to placebo.
- METs have demonstrated effectiveness when compared to controls and does lead to increases in spine mobility.
- There is fair evidence that manually assisted techniques lead to ROM increases in both symptomatic and asymptomatic subjects.

### Manipulation

**Manipulation** is an accurately localized or globally applied, single, quick, and decisive movement of small amplitude, following careful positioning of the patient.[59] According to Shekelle, there are four primary lesions that may respond to manipulative treatment.[60] These lesions include (1) entrapped synovial folds or plica, (2) hypertonic muscle, (3) articular or periarticular adhesions, and (4) segmental displacement. Many of the studies associated with manipulation (Table 1.3) involved trials that were either fairly or poorly designed.[60] The majority demonstrated mechanical ROM changes directly after a manipulative treatment, or a large effect size associated with the manipulation.

Cramer et al.[20] demonstrated an increase in facet joint space after high-velocity manipulation to the lumbar spine. However, the subjects within the study had no history of low back pain, thus extrapolation to pathological conditions is questionable. Other studies have investigated range-of-motion gains after manipulative treatment. Five studies examined improvement of cervical spine movements in patients with pathology. Of the five, the strongest study was designed by Whittingham and Nilsson.[61] Their comparison versus sham manipulation demonstrated significant ROM changes in the cervical spine. Some evidence suggests that both rotation and side bend manipulation increased ROM upon application. In the studies that compared against pragmatic controls such as muscle energy techniques, manipulation proved to be similar to the pragmatic control, but substantially better than the baseline measure. Additionally, although manipulation appears to significantly improve range of motion, these studies fail to measure the long-term effects.

## Summary

- The majority of manipulation studies measuring mechanical ROM changes demonstrate only fair design.
- The majority of manipulation studies measuring mechanical ROM changes did demonstrate direct ROM improvements after application.
- Most studies that measure mechanical ROM changes during manipulation demonstrated significant improvement over baseline and similar improvements when compared to pragmatic controls.
- Manipulation appears to provide short-term mechanical ROM changes in both symptomatic and asymptomatic patients.

### Mobilization

**Mobilization** techniques are designed to restore a full, painless joint function by rhythmic, repetitive passive movements to the patients' tolerance, in voluntary and/or accessory ranges.[60] Several studies (Table 1.4) have analyzed range-of-motion changes concurrently during outcome

**TABLE 1.3    Tabulated Results of Experimentally Investigated Manipulation Studies**

| | Region Tested | Demonstrated ROM Benefit with Manipulation | Randomized Comparison | Manipulation was Mutually Exclusive | Symptomatic Subjects? | Strength of Evidence |
|---|---|---|---|---|---|---|
| Andersen et al.[62] | Ankle Dorsiflexion | No (but large effect size) | Yes (control) | Yes | Yes | II |
| Brantingham et al.[63] | Hip Range of Motion | No | Yes (sham manip) | Yes | Yes | III |
| Cassidy, Lopes & Yong-Hing[64] | Cervical Range of Motion | Yes | Yes (muscle energy technique) | Yes | Yes | II |
| Fryer et al.[65] | Ankle Dorsiflexion | No | Yes (control) | Yes | No | III |
| Pollard & Ward[66] | Hip Flexion Range of Motion | Yes | Yes (pragmatic and control) | Yes | No | II |
| Whittingham & Nilsson[61] | Cervical Spine Range of Motion | Yes | Yes (sham manip) | Yes | Yes | I |
| Wood et al.[67] | Cervical Spine Range of Motion | Yes (vs. baseline only) | Yes (pragmatic) | Yes | Yes | II |

**TABLE 1.4**    Tabulated Results of Experimentally Investigated Manually Assisted Methods of Stretching/Mobilization

| | Region Tested | Demonstrated ROM Benefit with Mobilization | Randomized Comparison | Mobilization was Mutually Exclusive | Symptomatic Subjects? | Strength of Evidence |
|---|---|---|---|---|---|---|
| Angstrom and Lindstrom[68] | Hip | Yes | Yes (pragmatic) | No | Yes | II |
| Collins et al.[69] | Ankle Dorsiflexion | Yes | Yes (repeated measures) | Yes | Yes | II |
| Conroy and Hayes[70] | Shoulder ROM | Yes | Yes (pragmatic) | No | Yes | II |
| Gibson et al.[71] | Sagittal Movement of the Lumbar Spine | Yes | Yes (control) | Yes | Unclear | II |
| Ginn et al.[72] | Shoulder | Yes | No | No | Yes | III |
| Green et al.[73] | Ankle Dorsiflexion | Yes | Yes (pragmatic) | No | Yes | II |
| Hjelm et al.[74] | Shoulder ROM | Yes | No | Yes | Yes | III |
| Hoeksma et al.[75] | Hip ROM | Yes | Yes (pragmatic) | No | Yes | II |
| Randall et al.[76] | Metacarpal Joint | Yes | Yes (pragmatic) | Yes | Yes | II |
| Shamus et al.[77] | Metatarso-phalangeal | Yes | Yes (pragmatic) | No | Yes | II |

analyses and have supported the benefit of mobilization for mechanical range-of-motion improvement.

The majority of studies are Level II, with some achieving Level III. Most were performed using asymptomatic subjects using a variety of forms of mobilization methods. Methods such as isolated joint mobilization using oscillations, passive physiological movements, traction, and passive mobilizations with passive movements were equally effective.

Unfortunately, the majority of studies used mobilization with other methods and did not achieve mutual exclusivity. Although most studies used multiple bouts and measured range-of-motion change over time, some did find ROM changes with a single bout or repeated bouts. Hoeksma et al.[75] reported that the addition of manual therapy during treatment of hip osteoarthritis lead to significant improvements in range of motion. The differences peaked at 5 weeks from initiation of treatment. The manual therapy mobilizations consisted of static stretching, traction, and distraction manipulation.

Lastly, it does appear that the disorder may contribute to the likelihood of success. For example, Conroy and Hayes[70] found no differences between the control and mobilization group in population of shoulder impingement, yet Randall et al.[76] found that joint mobilization significantly counteracts the effect of immobilization after metacarpal fractures.

## Summary

- Most studies that have analyzed mechanical changes using mobilization demonstrated fair design.
- Mobilization appears to lead to mechanical ROM changes during single and repeated applications.
- Mobilization is as effective as other pragmatic methods during mechanical ROM intervention.

# Muscle Reflexogenic Changes

For many years, practitioners of manual therapy have purported reflexogenic benefits with selected directed manual therapy techniques.[5,78,82,83] The thrust-like forces incurred during a manipulation[6,76,77,79–81,84,85] or repeated oscillatory forces used during mobilization[76,77,82] are hypothesized to reduce pain through inducing reflex inhibition of spastic muscles. Muscle reflexogenic inhibition is a consequence of stimulation to the skin, muscle, and articular joint receptors.

The primary role of skin, muscle, and articular joint receptors is to detect the presence of movement or energy input and provide the central nervous system with proprioceptive or nociceptive information. The location and the design of the receptor outline the role it plays in proprioception or pain response. Although there is conflicting current literature associated with the proposed benefits of modulating spinal stretch reflexes, much of the work is traced to the pioneering work of Barry Wyke. Within this textbook, the role and function of the articular receptors is briefly outlined.

In the 1970s and 1980s, Wyke[89,90] outlined the contribution of the four forms of articular **mechanoreceptors** found in joint capsule and surrounding tissue. He described Type One mechanoreceptors as small myelinated fibers, consisting of a low threshold and responding to very small increments of tension in the part of the joint capsule in which they lie. Type One mechanoreceptors are triggered by both static and dynamic stimuli but do not respond as quickly as Type Two receptors. These receptors are active during all ranges of movement and during periods of immobility.[91]

Type Two mechanoreceptors are also imbedded in fibrous joint capsules and additionally in the layers of subsynovial tissue. Type Two receptors are thick, multilaminated connective tissue capsules, which enclose a single (occasionally multistranded) unmyelinated nerve terminal that attaches near the apex of a corpuscle.[91] These fibers lie deeper than Type One mechanoreceptors and often run parallel to blood vessels. Type Two mechanoreceptors also display a low threshold but rapidly adapt and are dynamically stimulated. The fibers have a high-velocity discharge and signal joint acceleration and deceleration. It has been suggested that Type Two mechanoreceptors assist in rebiasing the spindle during movements that involve range-of-motion extremes.

Type Three are large, thinly encapsulated corpuscles that are confined within the surface of joint ligaments and vertebral columns.[91] Type Three mechanoreceptors are the largest of the articular corpuscles and are identical structurally to the tendon organs of Golgi.[91] These fibers are responsible for firing when high, quick tension such as long static stretches are used, especially when forces are placed on

ligaments. These mechanoreceptors are slow responding and also may function to bias the muscle spindle.

Type Four mechanoreceptors are lattice-like plexuses and free-nerve endings and are unmyelinated. Type Four mechanoreceptors are not stimulated as much by tissue tension but by capsule tightness or imbalance. Type Four mechanoreceptors often fire a painful noxious stimulus when there is swelling, or an imbalance on the joint capsule. Positional changes such as prolonged posture may affect the responsiveness of the receptors. Type Four mechanoreceptors are inactive under normal situations but will activate under selected situations (prolonged posture or joint-related stiffness) and stimulate pain.

Oddly, not all articular regions have equal representation of mechanoreceptor types. Type One through Four mechanoreceptors have been identified in the cervical spine zygopophyseal joints. However, only Type One through Three mechanoreceptors have been found in the lumbar and thoracic spine but no Type Four mechanoreceptors.[92] This suggests that the current mechanoreceptor system within the lumbar and thoracic spine will respond to extreme rather than midrange joint movements.[92] Mechanoreceptors have been found in varying levels of density throughout other tissues of the spine as well. There are fewer Type One through Three receptors identified in the thoracic and lumbar spines, which may indicate either that their importance is reduced in these regions or that their receptor fields are relatively large in area in these facet joints.[92] Type Three and Four mechanoceptors, identified as nociceptors, have been found within the sacroiliac joint and surrounding support muscular–ligamentous structures.[93] This indicates that the mechanoreceptor system within the sacroiliac joint has a greater role in pain generation than proprioception.

Hypothetically, this small amount of movement of mobilization and manipulation is enough to stimulate neurophysiologic responses that lead to increased range of motion. The increase of range of motion through neurophysiologic mechanisms, proposed by Wyke[4], involves the relationship of mechanoreceptor pain and capsular– tendon changes. Wyke suggested that the effects associated with passive stimulation of the mechanoreceptors were plausible reasons for pain relief and normalization of joint function. The mechanoreceptor theory states that stimulation of the joint receptors reduces overall pain, and may cause tonic reflexogenic effects on the postural, limb, jaw, and eye muscles.

Each of the four articular mechanoreceptors responds to different stimuli and gives disparate yet specific afferent information that modifies neuromuscular function. When the stimulus triggers a response an action potential travels to the central nervous system where it is analyzed and identified. Three (I–III) of the four mechanoreceptors are stimulated by muscle-length change and/or deformation, the fourth (IV) by chemical irritation and/or tension. The nociceptive afferent impulses from the fourth form of mechanoreceptor are transmitted polysynaptically to the responsive aspects of the muscles localized at the region of the irritation (causing a response spasm), which correspondingly produces abnormal reflex activity when irritated. This abnormal reflex activity can further lead to pain and joint restriction.

There are several purported mechanisms that outline the benefit of manual therapy stimulation of joint receptors. One theory is that manual therapy techniques could potentially "reset" the reflex activity by stimulating the muscle spindles and Golgi tendon organs.[7] This theory is expounded by Korr[94], who reported that manipulation increases joint mobility by producing a barrage of impulses stimulating Group Ia and possibly Group II afferents. Zusman[95] hypothesized related changes with mobilization following sustained or repetitive passive movements, although not all authors agree. Recently, Sung and colleagues[96] demonstrated that manipulative techniques applied at a rate of 200 milliseconds in duration lead to higher reflexogenic responses (i.e., Golgi tendon and muscle spindle discharge) than slower techniques that are similar to mobilization.

Others have suggested that muscle activity inhibition through transient reduction in alpha motor neuron activity (H reflex), a decrease in EMG activity, and a reduction of excitatory Type III and IV nociceptors are all consequences of direct spinal manipulation.[28,97] Measurable alterations in electromyographical (EMG) activity in local and distant spinal muscles[7] and depression of the **H reflex** have been documented after use of mobilization and/or manipulation methods.[97,98] Although these effects yield unknown pain inhibition responses, it is theorized that these physiological consequences may reduce the nociceptive afferent barrage to the dorsal horn.[80,84,95] There also appears to be a reduction of afferent nociceptive input into the central nervous system, thus evoking descending pain inhibitory systems[97,100], consequently resulting in analgesia. The reduction of pain through descending mechanisms appears to happen by two separate pathways. The primary (rapid onset) analgesic effect is from the dorsal periaqueductal gray (PAG) area and is sympathoexcitatory in nature.[101,102] This is a nonopioid mechanism since it is unaffected by the administration of naloxone.[103] The secondary mechanism is from the ventral PAG and is sympathoinhibitory in nature and is referred to as an opioid mechanism.[102] It is described as opioid because administration of naloxone will attenuate the effect.[103] The preceding mechanisms of pain control have been clearly linked to spinal manipulation but not as strongly linked to spinal mobilization, according to Wright's review article.[100] There is moderate evidence to support that spinal manual therapy has a hypoanalgesic effect specific to mechanical nociception.[87,104–106] However, the majority of studies were poorly designed or resulted in conflicting findings among authors.[5]

## Summary

- The primary role of skin, muscle, and articular joint receptors is to detect the presence of movement or energy input and provide the central nervous system with proprioceptive or nociceptive information.
- There are four primary articular receptors.
- There are theories dictating why reflexogenic changes occur, including stimulation of mechanoreceptors, resetting reflex responses, and the gate control theory.
- One theory is that manual therapy techniques "reset" the reflex activity by stimulating the muscle spindles and Golgi tendon organs.
- Measurable alterations in electromyographical (EMG) activity in local and distant spinal muscles and depression of the **H reflex** have been documented after use of mobilization and/or manipulation methods.

# NEUROPHYSIOLOGICAL CHANGES

## Pain Inhibition and Analgesia

**Central facilitation** occurs when the dorsal horn is hyperresponsive to afferent input.[107] This process may cause a lowering of the pain threshold and results in lower levels of pain-producing stimuli. Central facilitation may occur regionally at the injured site or in the brain's pain processing centers. During an injury, a chemical reaction occurs that produces a cascade of chemically-related pain. Injury may stimulate the release of proteoglycans, metalo-matrix protease inhibitors, and other factors that trigger an autoimmune reaction and the influx of spinal cord mediators such as bradykinin, serotonin, histamines, and prostaglandins that irritate surrounding type C nerve endings. The result is a diffuse pain that is activated during "normal" activity that usually would not stimulate pain.[108] There is laboratory evidence that exercise and activity (movement) reduces the lactate concentration and reduces the pH change within the tissue.[3] The passive movement associated with mobilization and manipulation may change the pH structure of the area, thus resulting in decreased pain, although further study is needed for substantiation.

As discussed previously, passive mobilization forces arouse descending inhibitory systems that originate in the lateral peri-aqueductal gray matter of the brainstem[104] and exertion of segmental postsynaptic inhibition on the dorsal horn pain pathway neurons.[104] Glover et al.[80] report a reduction of pain 15 minutes after performing a manipulation. They hypothesized that the spine manipulation altered the central processing of innocuous mechanical stimuli, which correspondingly increased the pain threshold levels. Others have found similar short-term affects with manipulation[84,85] and mobilization forces.[109,110] Although it is unsuitable to identify these responses as "short term," it does appear that this response decreases incrementally over 1 to 6 days. At 6 days, the threshold changes were no longer reported.[29]

### Increased Sympathetic Activity

There is also moderate evidence to support that manual therapy provides an excitatory effect on sympathetic nervous system activity.[87,104,105] Particularly the manual therapy mobilization techniques associated with an anteroposterior glide and a lateral glide has been well documented.[19] An excitatory effect on the sympathetic nervous system occurs concurrently with a reduction of hypoanalgesia and may parallel the effects of stimulation of the dorsal periaqueductal gray area of the midbrain, a process that has occurred in animal research.[102] Documented evidence supports the benefit of modulation of pain and remarkably has a nonlocalized effect. Stimulation of the cervical spine has demonstrated upper extremity changes in pain response (pressure-pain), and a measurable **sympathoexcitatory effect.**[106,111]

It may seem counterintuitive to consider the onset of sympathoexcitatory activity beneficial for pain reduction. Nonetheless, Wright[100] outlines that hypoalgesia and sympathoexcitation are correlated, suggesting that individuals who exhibit the most change in pain perception also exhibit the most change in sympathetic nervous system function.

### Pain Gate Mechanism

Other explanations have included the activation of the gate-control mechanism proposed by Melzack and Wall[112], neural hysteresis, and release of endogenous opioids. Small diameter nociceptors tend to open the "gate," thus facilitating perception of pain whereas larger diameter fibers tend to close the gate of pain. Gating pain is a mechanism in which afferent and descending pathways modulate sensory transmission by inhibitory mechanisms within the central nervous system. Some have suggested that manual therapy movements may stimulate afferent fibers in the joint, muscle, skin, and ligaments, potentially providing an effective overstimulation response[113,114], although further work is needed to confirm this theory.

# Psychological Changes

### Placebo

Because orthopedic manual therapy is a mechanical intervention it is very prone to a phenomenon called the placebo effect. The effects are found in drugs, surgery, biofeedback, psychiatric interventions, and diagnostic tests. They include some form of sham treatment, and are not the same as an untreated controlled group.[115] The **placebo** effect is generally qualitative in nature (it is based on patient perception) but can lead to quantitative changes, especially if an individual's stress levels are reduced.

The placebo effect is the measurable or observable after-effect target to a person or group of participants that have been given some form of expectant care. The expectation that they will improve is often the driving force behind any and all aspects of newfound well-being.[116] The common fallacy associated with the placebo effect is the credit of improvement to a specific treatment, just because the improvement followed the treatment.[116] Selected authors have suggested that manual therapy elicits a powerful, short-term placebo effect that in some respect explains the perceived benefit.[105] The ability to design a well-performed sham study, using a sham mobilization or manipulation, is very difficult; therefore, the likelihood of an unadulterated measurement of placebo in a manual therapy study is very low. It is worth mentioning that some of the previously discussed studies found ROM changes that were significantly greater than placebo or sham care. Nevertheless, a study that measures alterations in pain perception has yet to be performed and would most likely yield the most information of the power of placebo during manual therapy intervention.

### Patient Satisfaction and Expectation

Although it is intuitive to consider patient satisfaction is directly related to the outcome of care, it appears this

## Summary

- It is suggested that manual therapy demonstrates pain reduction through inhibition of nociceptors, dorsal horn, and inhibitory descending pathways of the spinal cord.
- Manual therapy may improve chemical alterations secondary to injury and central nervous system thresholds.
- Both manipulation and mobilization forces have demonstrated neurophysiologic changes in discriminatory analysis.
- Manual therapy may improve altered pain thresholds.
- Manual therapy, specifically mobilization, has been shown to demonstrate a sympathoexcitatory effect.
- Sympathoexcitatory activity and hypoalgesia appear to function concurrently and are considered positively responsive during an application of manual therapy.

concept is actually more complicated than one may expect.[117] Some studies have found a significant relationship between the two variables[118,119], while others have shown only tentative or poor relationships.[117] Treatments that consist of manual therapy techniques routinely display better patient satisfaction scores than other nonmanual therapy–related methods[117,118], regardless of whether a benefit occurred during the intervention. Selected authors[117,120] suggest that meeting patient expectations is more likely associated with patient satisfaction (than pure patient outcomes), and manual therapists have a greater capacity of doing so through mechanical methods of patient care administration. Satisfaction differs from expectations because it fails to consider what the patient anticipated to gain from the form of intervention.

Williams et al.[121] report that the most desired aspect of patient expectation is an explanation of the problem and a mechanism in which to adapt to the problem. It is possible that a manual therapist has the potential to reorient a patient's pain experience into a more positive framework[122] that contributes in some part to overall patient satisfaction.[123] By nature, manual therapy provides a mechanical method of treatment that may have significant carryover to home programs and self-treatment. Additionally, by placing a mechanical identifier on a particular disorder, a reduction in esoteric aspects of pain perception and demonstration may improve the communication of symptoms from clinician to patient.

Main and Watson[124] elaborate on the failure to meet patient expectations and report that "failed treatment can have a profoundly demoralizing affect" and may become "significantly disaffected with healthcare professionals, particularly if they feel they have been misled in terms of likely benefit from treatment." This emphasizes the necessity to build a relationship of trust between the clinician and the patient and to explore common goals among the partnership. Curtis et al.[118] reported that patients who had earlier experience with manual therapy treatment demonstrated quicker recovery than subjects with no prior experience.

The likelihood of recognizing those who will "buy in" to a manual therapy treatment plan may improve the development of trust. Axen et al.[125] found that chiropractors had the capacity to predict those with good prognoses over bad prognoses based on the reaction to a first, single manual therapy treatment. This finding, and the discovery in the Curtis et al.[118] study, suggest that certain patients are more apt to benefit from manual therapy than others.

### The Role of Psychological Covariates

Melzack and Casey[126] suggested that an individual's pain perception depends on complex neural interactions in the nervous system. The complexities include impulses generated by tissue damage that are modified both by ascending pathways to the brain and by descending pain-suppressing systems. Nonetheless, pain perception is not limited solely to physiological criteria; pain perception is conspicuously influenced by various environmental and psychological factors. Thus, perception of pain is the result of a dynamic process of perception and interpretation of a wide range of incoming stimuli. The interpretation of the stimuli dictates the description of the pain, regardless of whether the stimuli are associated with truly substantial pain-generating agents. Furthermore, it has been suggested that the risk of progressing from an acute impairment to chronic pain syndrome is unrelated to actual pain intensity[127] and is more directly related to psychosocial factors.[128]

Several psychosocial factors that have been investigated may contribute to perception and chronicity of pain. Development of a chronic pain syndrome appears to reflect a failure to adapt to the change in condition.[128] In many cases, perceived pain does not have to worsen for the patient to regress, although often patients perceive that to be the case. Instead of true pain-related changes, most individuals fail to cope with the unimproved symptoms and the decrease in function. The presence of selected psychosocial factors that interfere with adaptation may promote the development of pain syndromes. These factors include the derivatives of emotion, beliefs, and coping strategies.

#### Emotions

Main and Watson[124] identify anxiety, fear, depression, and anger as the four emotions that best characterize the distress of chronic pain sufferers. Much of patient anxiety may be traced to unmet expectations. Anxiety is often present in patients who have not received a clear explanation for the origin or cause methods to manage pain.[124]

Fear is an emotional response that stems from a belief that selected movements or interventions may damage one's present condition.[124] Fear has been associated with catastrophizing behavior and may increase patient's self-report of pain intensity.[129] Most notably, fear of movement may reduce a patient's buy-in to a particular treatment, specifically if pain is reproduced within the treatment process. Fear of movement or reinjury and subsequent hypokinesis is highly correlated with an increase pain report.[130]

Depression is more difficult to acknowledge. Main and Watson[124] suggest that it is important to distinguish between dysphoric moods from depressive illness. Dysphoric behavior is common in patients who have experienced long-term pain but will most likely be absent of the debilitating effects of depression. Depression often leads to a learned helplessness, dependency on pharmaceuticals, and other debilitating behaviors.

The complex relationship between anger and frustration is not well understood[124] but is believed to alter judgment and may reduce the internal commitment the patient has to improving their own condition. Recent evidence suggests that an expressive anger style is associated with elevated pain sensitivity secondary to dysfunction within the body's antinociceptive system.[131]

### *Coping Strategies*

During their discussion of coping strategies, DeGood and Shutty[132] distinguish three distinct fields of inquiry. These include (1) specific beliefs about pain and treatment; (2) the thought processes involved in judgment or appraisal; and (3) coping styles or strategies. Schultz et al.[133] report that effective treatment to improve coping strategies requires accurate distinction between chronic pain and a chronic pain syndrome. Theoretically, the most effective treatments designed to improve coping strategies should incorporate both psychological and physical components and require intervention by an interdisciplinary team. Generally, early treatment of pain syndromes may improve employment-related outcomes, but even those with longstanding syndromes generally improve dramatically.[134] Improvements in coping include the use of a biopsychosocial model. A biopsychosocial model assumes an interaction between mental and physical aspects of disability, assumes that the relationship between impairment and disability is mediated by psychosocial factors, and that beliefs about illness/disability are as important as illness. Presence of a chronic pain syndrome strongly suggests that medical interventions (including surgery) may not be effective.[134] Prior to physical improvements, separate psychological interventions may be necessary for reducing back pain incidence.[135]

## SUMMARY OF BENEFIT FROM MANUAL THERAPY

Methodology designed to measure the strength of evidence of selected interventions is essential to determine the strength of a study. Subsequently, the "Levels of Evidence" outlined by the U.S. Clinical Practice Guideline for Acute Low Back Problems in Adults.[136] Table 1.5 outlines the parameters to determine the "Levels of Evidence" used within this chapter.

## *Summary*

- The placebo effect could potentially explain some of the pain reduction benefit associated with manual therapy.
- It is difficult to design a study in which an effective and comparable placebo sham is used during manual therapy intervention.
- Treatments that consist of manual therapy techniques routinely display better patient satisfaction scores than other non-manual therapy related methods.
- Manual therapists may improve the likelihood of meeting patient expectations secondary to the nature of the physical intervention.
- Failure to meet patient expectations is associated with poor patient satisfaction.
- Anxiety, fear, depression and anger are common emotional components that may alter a manual therapist's outcome.
- A manual therapist may reduce the anxiety associated with unknown symptoms.
- Fear is commonly associated with decreased movement and trepidation of re-injury.
- Depression co-exists with numerous other variables; all which can lead to poor patient outcomes.
- Anger and outcome are poorly understood, yet there does appear to be a relationship between higher report of pain and increased anger.
- Coping strategy is reportedly a reason why some disorders progress to chronic pain syndrome.
- There is little evidence to suggest that manual therapy intervention will decrease the progression to chronic pain syndrome.
- Purportedly, a biopsychosocial model should demonstrate effectiveness in treating patients with chronic pain syndrome.

**TABLE 1.5** Methodological Guidelines Outlined by the U.S. Clinical Practice Guideline for Acute Low Back Problems in Adults

| Category | Description |
| --- | --- |
| 1. Strong evidence: Level A | Includes interventions deemed either *effective* or *ineffective* with strong support in the literature as determined by consistent findings/results in several high-quality randomized controlled trials or in at least one meta-analysis. |
| 2. Moderate evidence: Level B | Includes interventions deemed either *effective* or *ineffective* with moderate support in the literature as determined by consistent findings/results in one high-quality randomized controlled trial and one or several low-quality randomized controlled trials. |
| 3. Limited/contradictory evidence: Level C | Includes interventions with weak or conflicting support in the literature as determined by one randomized controlled trial (high or low quality), or inconsistent findings between several randomized controlled trials. |
| 4. No known evidence: Level D | Includes interventions that have not been sufficiently studied in the literature in terms of effectiveness and no randomized controlled trials have been done in this area. |

**TABLE 1.6**   An Overview of the Effectiveness of Selected Manual Therapy Methods Using the Methodological Guidelines Outlined by the U.S. Clinical Practice Guideline for Acute Low Back Problems in Adults

|  | Strong Evidence | Moderate Evidence | Limited/ Contradictory Evidence | No Known Evidence |
|---|---|---|---|---|
| Static stretching for temporary increase in ROM in symptomatic subjects | | | ✓ | |
| Manipulation for temporary increase in ROM in symptomatic subjects | | | ✓ | |
| Mobilization for temporary increase in ROM in symptomatic subjects | | ✓ | | |
| Manually assisted movements for temporary increase in ROM in symptomatic subjects | | ✓ | | |
| Mobilization leads to a neurophysiologic change associated with joint-related movement | | ✓ | | |
| Manipulation leads to a neurophysiologic change associated with joint-related movement | | ✓ | | |
| Mobilization or manipulation has the capacity to alter pH levels and alter central sensitization properties | | | ✓ | |
| Manual therapy methods have the capacity to alter psychologically-oriented conditions such as fear, anger, anxiety, or depression | | | | ✓ |
| Manual therapy methods improve the coping capacity of the chronic pain sufferer | | | | ✓ |

Table 1.6 outlines the cumulative findings behind the science of manual therapy. Each conclusion is based on the strength of the studies, whether the findings were positive or negative, and whether any evidence exists to support potential use.

Static stretching yields strong evidence of benefit for asymptomatic subjects but limited evidence for symptomatic patients. It is worth noting that the word "temporary" is used, since most studies, mobilization and manipulation included, only investigate short-term findings. Manipula-tion and mobilization both present moderate beneficial evidence for ROM gains and neurophysiologic changes. The studies fail to provide strong evidence based solely on the strengths of the individual studies. Whether manual therapy provides pH or central sensitization changes or psychological alterations is essentially unknown. Overall, the science behind manual therapy is promising. As research improves we will have the opportunity to better decide which methods and what type of patient impairment are best associated with positive outcomes.

## *Chapter Questions*

1. Identify the three hypothesized effects of manual therapy and describe the scientific evidence that supports their suppositions.
2. Compare and contrast the cumulative findings associated with static stretching, manually assisted movement, mobilization, and manipulation. Outline the weaknesses of the research and areas that would strengthen the aggregate findings.
3. Outline the different forms of neurophysiologic effects of manual therapy.
4. Describe why meeting patient expectations is often considered as important as patient outcome when addressing patient satisfaction.

# *References*

1. Bourdillon J, Day E. *Spinal manipulation.* 4th ed. London; Appleton & Lange: 1987.
2. Haldeman S. The clinical basis for discussion of mechanics in manipulative therapy. In: Korr I (ed) *The neurobiologic mechanisms in manipulative therapy.* London; Plenum Press: 1978.
3. Holm S, Nachemson A. Variations in the nutrition of the canine intervertebral disc induced by motion. *Spine.* 1983;8:866–873.
4. Wyke BD. Articular neurology and manipulative therapy. In Glasgow EF, Twomey LT, ed. *Aspects of manipulative therapy.* 2nd ed. Melbourne; Churchill Livingstone: 1985:81–96.
5. Potter L, McCarthy C, Oldham J. Physiological effects of spinal manipulation: A review of proposed theories. *Phys Ther Reviews.* 2005;10:163–170.
6. Collaca C, Keller T, Gunzberg R. Neuromechanical characterization of in vivo lumbar spinal manipulation. Part 2. Neurophysiologic response. *J Manipulative Physiol Ther.* 2003;26:579–591.
7. Herzog W, Scheele D, Conway P. Electromyographic responses of back and limb muscles associated with spinal manipulative therapy. *Spine.* 1999;24:146–153.
8. Vernon H. Qualitative review of studies of manipulation-induced hypalgesia. *J Manipulative Physiol Ther.* 2000;23:134–138.
9. Hurwitz EL, Morgenstern H, Harber P, Kominski GF, Belin TR, Yu F, Adams AH; University of California-Los Angeles. A randomized trial of medical care with and without physical therapy and chiropractic care with and without physical modalities for patients with low back pain: 6-month follow-up outcomes from the UCLA low back pain study. *Spine.* 2002;27(20):2193–2204.
10. Arkuszewski Z. (abstract). Joint blockage: a disease, a syndrome or a sign. *Man Med.* 1988;3:132–134.
11. Schollmeier G, Sarkar K, Fukuhara K, Uhthoff HK. Structural and functional changes in the canine shoulder after cessation of immobilization. *Clin Orthop.* 1996;(323):310–315.
12. Akeson WH, Amiel D, Mechanic GL, Woo SL, Harwood FL, Hamer ML. Collagen cross-linking alternations in joint contractures: changes in reducible cross-links in periarticular connective tissue collage after nine weeks of immobilization. *Connect Tissue Res.* 1977;5(1):15–19.
13. Amiel D, Frey C, Woo SL, Harwood F, Akeson W. Value of hyaluronic acid in the prevention of contracture formation. *Clin Othop.* 1985;196:306–311.
14. Donatelli R, Owens-Burkhart H. Effects of immobilization on the extensibility of periarticular connective tissue. *J Orthop Sports Phys Ther.* 1981;3:67–72.
15. Mercer S, Bogduk N. Intra-articular inclusions of the cervical synovial joints. *British Journal of Rheumatology.* 1993;32:705–710.
16. Bogduk N, Twomey LT. *Clinical anatomy of the lumbar spine.* London; Churchill Livingstone: 1997.
17. Blunt KL, Gatterman MI, Bereznick DE. Kinesiology: An essential approach toward understanding chiropractic subluxation. In Gatterman MI (ed). *Foundations of Chiropractic: subluxation.* St. Louis, MO; Mosby: 1995.
18. Norlander S, Astc-Norlander U, Nordgren B, Sahlstedt B. Mobility in the cervico-thoracic motion segment: an indicative factor of musculoskeletal neck-shoulder pain. *Scand J Rehabil Med.* 1996;28(4):183–192.
19. Wright A. Pain-relieving effects of cervical manual therapy. In Grant R. *Physical therapy of the cervical and thoracic spine.* 3rd ed. New York; Churchill Livingston: 2002.
20. Cramer G, Tuck N, Knudsen J. et al. Effects of side-posture positioning and side-posture adjusting on the lumbar zygopophyseal joints as evaluated by magnetic resonance imaging: a before and after study with randomization. *J Manipulative Physiol Ther.* 2000;23:380–394.
21. Herzog W. *Clinical biomechanics of spinal manipulation.* London; Churchill Livingstone: 2000.
22. Mierau D, Cassidy JD, Bowen V. Manipulation and mobilization of the third metacarpophalangeal joint. *Man Med.* 1988;3:135–140.
23. Flynn TW, Fritz JM, Wainner RS, Whitman JM. The audible pop is not necessary for successful spinal high-velocity thrust manipulation in individuals with low back pain. *Arch Phys Med Rehabil.* 2003;84(7):1057–1060.
24. Lee R, Evans J. Load-displacement time characteristics of the spine under posteroanterior mobilization. *Aust J Physiotherapy.* 1992;38:115–123.
25. Lee M, Svensson N. Effect of loading frequency on response of the spine to lumbar posteroanterior forces. *J Manipulative Physiol Ther.* 1993;16:439–446.
26. Gal JM, Herzog W, Kawchuk GN, Conway PJ, Zhang Y-T. Forces and relative vertebral movements during SMT to unembalmed post-rigor human cadavers: peculiarities associated with joint cavitation. *J Manipulative Physiol Ther.* 1995;18:4–9.
27. Smith D, Fuhr A, Davis B. Skin accelerometer displacement and relative bone movement of adjacent vertebrae in response to chiropractic percussion thrusts. *J Manipulative Physiol Ther.* 1989;12:26–37.
28. Keller T, Collaca C, Guzburg R. Neuromechanical characterization of in vivo lumbar spinal manipulation. Part 1. Vertebral motion. *J Manipulative Physiol Ther.* 2003;26:567–578.

29. Riddle D. Measurement of accessory motion: critical issues and related concepts. *Phys Ther.* 1992; 72:865–874.

30. Akeson W, Amiel D, Woo S. Immobility effects on synovial joints. The pathmechanics of joint contracture. *Biorheology* 1980;17:95.

31. Frank C, Akeson W, Woo S. Physiology and therapeutic value of passive joint motion. *Clin Orthop.* 1984;184:113.

32. Williams P, Watt P, Bicik V, Goldspink G. Effect of stretch combined with electrical stimulation on the type of sarcomeres produced at the ends of muscle fibers. *Exp Neurol.* 1986;93(3):500–509.

33. Goldspink DF, Easton J, Winterburn SK, Williams PE, Goldspink GE. The role of passive stretch and repetitive electrical stimulation in preventing skeletal muscle atrophy while reprogramming gene expression to improve fatigue resistance. *J Card Surg.* 1991;6(1Suppl):218–224.

34. Moseley A, Herbert R, Sherrington C, Maher C. Evidence for physiotherapy practice: A survey of the Physiotherapy Evidence Database (PEDro). *Aust J Physiotherapy.* 2002;48:43–49.

35. Bandy WD, Irion JM, Briggler M. The effect of static stretch and dynamic range of motion training on the flexibility of the hamstring muscles. *J Orthop Sports Phys Ther.* 1998;27(4):295–300.

36. Bandy WD, Irion JM, Briggler M. The effect of time and frequency of static stretching on flexibility of the hamstring muscles. *Phys Ther.* 1997; 77(10):1090–1096.

37. Bandy WD, Irion JM. The effect of time on static stretch on the flexibility of the hamstring muscles. *Phys Ther.* 1994;74(9):845–850.

38. Bohannon RW. Effect of repeated eight-minute muscle loading on the angle of straight-leg raising. *Phys Ther.* 1984;64(4):491–497.

39. Godges J, Mattson-Bell M, Thorpe D, Shah D. The immediate effects of soft tissue mobilization with proprioceptive neuromuscular facilitation on glenohumeral external rotation and overhead reach. *J Orthop Sports Phys Ther.* 2003;33:713–718.

40. Halbertsma JP, Goeken LN. Stretching exercises: effect on passive extensibility and stiffness in short hamstrings of healthy subjects. *Arch Phys Med Rehabil.* 1994;75(9):976–981.

41. Leivseth G, Torstensson J, Reikeras O. Effect of passive muscle stretching in osteoarthritis of the hip. *Clin Sci (Lond).* 1989;76(1):113–117.

42. Magunsson S, Simonsen E, Aagaard P, Kjaer M. Biomechanical responses to repeated stretches in human hamstring muscle in vivo. *Am J Sports Med.* 1996;24:622–628.

43. McCarthy P, Olsen J, Smeby I. Effects of contract-relax stretching procedures on active range of mo-

44. Pollard H, Ward G. A study of two stretching techniques for improving hip flexion range of motion. *J Manipulative Physiol Ther.* 1997;20(7):443–447.

45. Reid DA, McNair PJ. Passive force, angle, and stiffness changes after stretching of hamstring muscles. *Med Sci Sports Exerc* 2004;36(11):1944–1948.

46. Roberts J, Wilson K. Effect of stretching duration on active and passive range of motion in the lower extremity. *Br J Sports Med.* 1999;33:259–263.

47. Starring DT, Gossman MR, Nicholson GG Jr, Lemons J. Comparison of cyclic and sustained passive stretching using a mechanical device to increase resting length of hamstring muscles. *Phys Ther.* 1988;68(3):314–320.

48. Steffen TM, Mollinger LA. Low-load, prolonged stretch in the treatment of knee flexion contractures in nursing home residents. *Phys Ther.* 1995;75(10): 886–895.

49. Tanigawa M. Comparison of the hold-relax procedure and passive mobilization on increasing muscle length. *Physiol Ther.* 1972;52:725–735.

50. Voss D, Ionta M, Myers B. *Proprioceptive neuromuscular facilitation, patterns and techniques.* 3rd ed. Philadelphia; Harper Row Publishers: 1985.

51. Etnyre BR, Abraham LD. Gains in range of ankle dorsiflexion using three popular stretching techniques. *Am J Phys Med.* 1986;65(4):189–196.

52. Goodridge J. Muscle energy technique: Definition, explanation, methods of procedure. *J Am Osteopathic Assoc.* 1981;81:249–254.

53. Ballantyne F, Fryer G, McLaughlin P. The effect of muscle energy technique on hamstring extensibility: the mechanism of altered flexibility. *J Osteopath Med.* 2003;6:59–63.

54. Ferber R, Osternig L, Gravelle D. Effect of PNF stretch techniques on knee flexor muscle EMG activity in older adults. *J Electromyography Kinesiology.* 2002;12:391–397.

55. Lenehan K, Fryer G, McLaughlin P. The effect of muscle energy technique on gross trunk range of motion. *J Osteopathy Med.* 2003;6:13–18.

56. Schenk R, MacDiarmid A, Rousselle J. The effects of muscle energy technique on lumbar range of motion. *J Manual Manipulative Ther.* 1997;5:179–183.

57. Schenk R, Adelman K, Rousselle J. The effects of muscle energy technique on cervical range of motion. *J Manual Manipulative Ther.* 1994;2: 149–155.

58. Winters M, Blake C, Trost S, Marcello-Brinker T, Lowe L, Garber M, Wainner R. Passive versus active stretching of hip flexor muscles in subjects with limited hip extension: a randomized trial. *Phys Ther.* 2004;84:800–807.

tion of the cervical spine in the transverse plane. *Clin Biomech.* 1997;12:136–138.

59. Grieve G. *Common vertebral joint problems.* 2nd ed. Edinburgh; Churchill Livingstone: 1988
60. Shekelle PG. Spinal manipulation. *Spine.* 1994;19: 858–861.
61. Whittingham W, Nilsson N. Active range of motion in the cervical spine increases after spinal manipulation. *J Manipulative Physiol Ther.* 2001;24:552–555.
62. Andersen S, Fryer G, McLaughlin P. The effect of talocrural joint manipulation on range of motion at the ankle joint in subjects with a history of ankle injury. *Australas Chiropract Osteopathy.* 2003;11:57–62.
63. Brantingham J, Williams A, Parkin-Smith G, Weston P, Wood T. A controlled, prospective pilot study of the possible effects of chiropractic manipulation in the treatment of osteoarthritis of the hip. *Eur J Chiropract.* 2003;53:149–166.
64. Cassidy JD, Lopes AA, Yong-Hing K. The immediate effect of manipulation versus mobilization on pain and range of motion in the cervical spine: a randomized controlled trial. *J Manipulative Physiol Ther.* 1992;15(9):570–575.
65. Fryer G, Mudge J, McLaughlin P. The effect of talocrural joint manipulation on range of motion at the ankle. *J Manipulative Physiol Ther.* 2002;25: 384–390.
66. Pollard H, Ward G. The effect of upper cervical or sacroiliac manipulation on hip flexion range of motion. *J Manipulative Physiol Ther.* 1998;21:611–616.
67. Wood T, Collaca C, Matthews R. A pilot randomized clinical trial on the relative effect of instrumental (MFMA) versus manual (HVLA) manipulation in the treatment of cervical spine dysfunction. *J Manipulative Physiol Ther.* 2001;24:260–271.
68. Angstrom L, Lindstrom B. (abstract). Treatment effects of traction and mobilization of the hip joint in patients with inflammatory rheumatological diseases and hip osteoarthritis. *Nordisk Fysoterapi.* 2003;7:17–27.
69. Collins N, Teys P, Vicenzino B. The initial effects of a Mulligan's mobilization with movement technique on dorsiflexion and pain in subacute ankle sprains. *Man Ther.* 2004;9:77–82.
70. Conroy D, Hayes K. The effect of joint mobilization as a component of comprehensive treatment for primary shoulder impingement syndrome. *J Orthop Phys Ther.* 1998;28:3–14.
71. Gibson H, Ross J, Allen J, Latimer J, Maher C. The effect of mobilization on forward bending range. *J Man Manipulative Ther.* 1993;1:142–147.
72. Ginn K, Cohen M. Conservative treatment for shoulder pain: Prognostic indicators of outcome. *Arch Phys Med Rehabil.* 2004;85:1231–1235.
73. Green T, Refshauge K, Crosbie J, Adams R. A randomized controlled trial of a passive accessory joint mobilization on acute ankle inversion sprains. *Phys Ther.* 2001;81:984–994.
74. Hjelm R, Draper C, Spencer S. Anterior-inferior capsular length insufficiency in the painful shoulder. *J Orthop Sports Phys Ther.* 1996;23:216–222.
75. Hoeksma H, Dekker J, Ronday K, Heering A, van der Lubbe N, Vel C, Breedveld F, van den Ende C. Comparison of manual therapy and exercise therapy in osteoarthritis of the hip: a randomized clinical trial. *Arthritis Rheumatism.* 2004;51:722–729.
76. Randall T, Portney L, Harris B. Effects of joint mobilization on joint stiffness and active motion of the metacarpal-phalangeal joint. *J Orthop Sports Phys Ther.* 1992;16:30–36.
77. Shamus J, Shamus E, Gugel R, Brucker B, Skaruppa C. The effect of sesamoid mobilization, flexor hallucis strengthening, and gait training on reducing pain and restoring function in individuals with hallux limitus: a clinical trial. *J Orthop Sports Phys Ther.* 2004;34:368–376.
78. Haldeman S. The clinical basis for discussion of mechanisms of manipulative therapy. In: Korr I. (ed). *The neurobiologic mechanisms in manipulative therapy.* New York; Plenum: 1978.
79. Raftis K, Warfield C. Spinal manipulation for back pain. *Hosp Pract.* 1989;15:89–90.
80. Glover J, Morris J, Khosla T. Back pain: a randomized clinical trial of rotational manipulation of the trunk. *Br J Physiol.* 1947;150:18–22.
81. Denslow JS. Analyzing the osteopathic lesion. 1940. *J Am Osteopath Assoc.* 2001;101(2):99–100.
82. Farfan H. The scientific basis of manipulation procedures. In: Buchanan W, Kahn M, Rodnan G, Scott J, Zvailfler N, Grahame R (eds). *Clinics in rheumatic diseases.* London; WB Saunders: 1980.
83. Giles L. *Anatomical basis of low back pain.* Baltimore; Williams and Wilkens: 1989.
84. Terrett AC, Vernon H. Manipulation and pain tolerance. A controlled study of the effect of spinal manipulation on paraspinal cutaneous pain tolerance levels. *Am J Phys Med.* 1984;63(5):217–225.
85. Vernon H, Dhami M, Howley T, Annett R. Spinal manipulation and beta-endorphin: a controlled study of the effect of a spinal manipulation on plasma beta-endorphin levels in normal males. *J Manipulative Physiol Ther.* 1986;9:115–123.
86. Petersen N, Vicenzino B, Wright A. The effects of a cervical mobilization technique on sympathetic outflow to the upper limb in normal subjects. *Physiotherapy Theory Practice.* 1993;9:149–156.
87. Vicenzino B, Collins D, Wright A. Sudomotor changes induced by neural mobilization techniques in asymptomatic subjects. *J Manual Manip Ther.* 1994;2:66–74.
88. Chiu T, Wright A. TO compare the effects of different rates of application of a cervical mobilization technique on sympathetic outflow to the

upper limb in normal subjects. *Man Ther.* 1996;1:198–203.

89. Wyke B: Articular neurology: a review. *Physiotherapy* 1972;58(3):94–99.

90. Wyke BD. The neurology of low back pain. In Jayson MIV, ed. *The lumbar spine and back pain.* 3rd ed. Edinburgh, UK; Churchill-Livingstone: 1987.

91. Wyke B. The neurology of joints. *Ann R Coll Surg Engl.* 1967l;41(1):25–50.

92. McLain R, Pickar J. Mechanoreceptor ending in human thoracic and lumbar facet joints. *Spine.* 1998;23:168–173.

93. Sakamoto N, Yamashita T, Takebayashi T, Sekine M, Ishii S. An electrophysiologic study of mechanoreceptors in the sacroiliac joint and adjacent tissues. *Spine.* 2001;26:468–471.

94. Korr IM. Proprioceptors and somatic dysfunction. *J Amer Osteopath Assoc.* 1975;74:638–650.

95. Zusman M. Spinal manipulative therapy: review of some proposed mechanisms and a hew hypothesis. *Australian J Physio* 1986;32:89–99.

96. Sung P, Kang YM, Pickar J. Effect of spinal manipulation duration on low threshold mechanoreceptors in lumbar paraspinal muscles. *Spine.* 2004;30:115–122.

97. Dishman J, Bulbulian R. Spinal reflex attenuation associated with spinal manipulation. *Spine.* 2000;25:2519–2525.

98. Murphy B Dawson N, Slack J. Sacroiliac joint manipulation decreases the H-reflex. *Electromyog Clin Neurophysiol.* 1995;35:87–94.

99. Besson JM, Chaouch A. Peripheral and spinal mechanisms of nociception. *Physiol Rev.* 1987;67(1):67–186.

100. Wright A. Hypoalgesia post-manipulative therapy: a review of a potential neurophysiologic mechanism. *Man Ther.* 1995;1:1–16.

101. Lovick TA, Li P. Integrated function of neurones in the rostral ventrolateral medulla. *Prog Brain Res.* 1989;81:223–232.

102. Lovick T. Interactions between descending pathways from the dorsal and ventrolateral periaqueductal gray matter in the rat. In: Depaulis A, Bandler R. (eds) *The midbrain periaqueductal gray matter.* New York; Plenum Press: 1991.

103. Cannon JT, Prieto GJ, Lee A, Liebeskind JC. Evidence for opioid and non-opioid forms of stimulation-produced analgesia in the rat. *Brain Res.* 1982;243(2):315–321.

104. Zusman M. Mechanisms of musculoskeletal physiotherapy. *Physical Therapy Reviews.* 2004;9:39–49.

105. Sterling M, Jull G, Wright A. Cervical mobilization: concurrent effects on pain, sympathetic nervous system activity and motor activity. *Man Ther.* 2001;6:72–81.

106. Vicenzino B, Paungmali A, Buratowski S, Wright A. Specific manipulative therapy treatment for chronic lateral epicondylalgia produces uniquely characteristic hypoalgesia. *Man Ther.* 2001;6:205–212.

107. Picker J. Neurophysiologic effects of spinal manipulation. *Spine J.* 2002;2:357–371.

108. Sizer PS, Matthijs O, Phelps V. Influence of age on the development of pathology. *Curr Rev Pain* 2000; 4:362–373.

109. Wright A, Thurnwald P, Smith J. An evaluation of mechanical and thermal hyperalgesia in patients with lateral epicondylalgia. *Pain Clin.* 1992;5:199–282.

110. Wright A, Thurbwald P, O'Callaghan J. Hyperalgesia in tennis elbow patients. *J Musculoskel Pain.* 1994;2:83–89.

111. Simon R, Vicenzino B, Wright A. The influence of an anteroposterior accessory glide of the glenohumeral joint on measures of peripheral sympathetic nervous system function in the upper limb. *Man Ther.* 1997;2(1):18–23.

112. Melzack R, Wall P. Pain mechanisms: a new theory. *Science.* 1965;150:971–979.

113. Pickar J, Wheeler J. Response of muscle proprioceptors to spinal manipulative-like loads in the anesthetized cat. *J Manipulative Physiol Ther.* 2001; 24:2–11.

114. Lederman E. Overview and clinical application. In *Fundamentals of manual therapy.* London: Churchill Livingstone, 1997;213–220.

115. Placebo effect accounts for fifty percent of improvement in depressed patients taking antidepressants. Accessed January 26, 2005, at: *http://www.apa.org/releases/placebo.html.*

116. Dodes, J. (1997) The mysterious placebo effect. Accessed January 26, 2005, at: *http://www.csicop.org/si/9701/placebo.html.*

117. Breen A, Breen R. Back pain and satisfaction with chiropractic treatment: what role does the physical outcome play? *Clin J Pain.* 2003;19(4):263–268.

118. Curtis P, Carey TS, Evans P, Rowane MP, Jackman A, Garrett J. Training in back care to improve outcome and patient satisfaction. Teaching old docs new tricks. *J Fam Pract.* 2000;49(9):786–792.

119. Licciardone J, Stoll S, Fulda K, Russo D, Siu J, Winn W, Swift J. Osteopathic manipulative treatment for chronic low back pain: a randomized controlled trial. *Spine.* 2003;28:1355–1362.

120. Cherkin D, Deyo R, Battie M, Street J, Barlow W. A comparison of physical therapy, chiropractic manipulation, and provision of an educational booklet for the treatment of patients with low back pain. *N Engl J Med.* 1998;339(15):1021–1029.

121. Williams S, Weinman J, Dale J, Newman S. Patient expectations: what do primary care patients want from the GP and how far does meeting expectations affect patient satisfaction? *Fam Pract.* 1995; 12(2):193–201.

122. Goldstein M. *Alternative health care: medicine, miracle, or mirage?* Philadelphia; Temple University Press: 1999.

123. Oths K. Communication in a chiropractic clinic: how a D.C. treats his patients. *Cult Med Psychiatry.* 1994;18(1):83–113.

124. Main CJ, Watson PJ. Psychological aspects of pain. *Man Ther.* 1999;4(4):203–215.

125. Axen I, Rosenbaum A, Robech R, Wren T, Leboeuf-Yde C. Can patient reactions to the first chiropractic treatment predict early favorable treatment outcome in persistent low back pain? *J Manipulative Physiol Ther.* 2002;25(7):450–454.

126. Melzack R, Casey K. Sensory, motivational and central control determinants of pain. In: Kenbshalo D (ed). *The skin senses.* Springfield, MA; Charles Thomas Publishing: 1968.

127. Epping-Jordan JE, Wahlgren DR, Williams RA, Pruitt SD, Slater MA, Patterson TL, Grant I, Webster JS, Atkinson JH. Transition to chronic pain in men with low back pain: predictive relationships among pain intensity, disability, and depressive symptoms. *Health Psychol.* 1998;17(5):421–427.

128. Haldeman S. Neck and back pain. In Evans R. *Diagnostic testing in neurology.* Philadelphia; Saunders Group: 1999.

129. Peters M, Vlaeyen J, Weber W. The joint contribution of physical pathology, pain-related fear and catastrophizing to chronic back pain disability. *Pain.* 2005;115:45–50.

130. de Jong J, Valeyen J, Onghena P, Goosens M, Geilen Mulder M. Fear of movement/(re)injury in chronic low back pain: Education or exposure in vivo as mediator to fear reduction? *Clin J Pain.* 2005;21:9–17.

131. Bruehl S, Chung O, Burns J, Biridepalli S. The association between anger expression and chronic pain intensity: evidence for partial mediation by endogenous opiod dysfunction. *Pain.* 2003;106:317–324.

132. DeGood D, Shutty M, Turk D, Melzack R. *Handbook of pain assessment.* New York; Guilford Press: 1992.

133. Schultz I, Crook J, Berkowitz S, Meloche W, Milner R, Zubervier O, Meloche G. Biopsychosocial multivariate predictive model of occupational low back disability. *Spine.* 2002;27(23):2720–2725.

134. Jordan A, Bendix T, Nielsen H, Hansen FR, Host D, Winkel A. Intensive training, physiotherapy or manipulation for patients with chronic neck pain: a prospective, single-blinded, randomized clinical trial. *Spine.* 1998;1:23(3):311–318.

135. Alaranta H, Rytokoski U, Rissanen A, Talo S, Rommemaa T, Puukka P, Karppi S, Videman T, Kallio V, Slatis P. Intensive physical and psychosocial training program for patients with chronic low back pain. A controlled clinical trial. *Spine.* 1994;19(12):1339–1349.

136. van Tulder MW, Koes BW, Bouter LM. Conservative treatment of acute and chronic nonspecific low back pain: A systematic review of randomized controlled trials of the most common interventions. *Spine.* 1997;22:2128–2156.

# 2

# Orthopedic Manual Therapy Assessment

## Objectives

- Outline and review selected manual therapy backgrounds.
- Compare and contrast selected manual therapy backgrounds and their assessment philosophies.
- Determine if any of the philosophical elements of manual therapy are best supported by scientific evidence.

- Describe the three elements of assessment.
- Describe the purposes, types, and necessities of a manual therapy diagnosis.
- Describe the combined pathological- and impairment-based assessment model.

## ASSESSMENT MODELS

### Manual Therapy Backgrounds

Farrell and Jensen[1] define a **manual therapy philosophical approach** as a set of general beliefs, concepts, and attitudes. They suggested that the philosophical approach dictates how a clinician performs the specific mechanics of the patient assessment process. Although most manual therapy philosophies demonstrate similarities in the examination process, variations of the role of applied anatomy, biomechanics, and the origin of structures often dictate the perspective of a particular model. Because physical therapy educators have different philosophical backgrounds, variation in the education of manual therapy in physical therapy schools is widespread.

In 1988, the most prevalent manual therapy assessment models taught in prelicensure settings were Kaltenborn and Maitland, followed by Paris and Cyriax.[3] A more recent investigation (1997) found that the Maitland approach was emphasized the most (22%), followed by McKenzie (17%), with Paris and Osteopathic tied for third (14% each).[3] A 2004 survey by Cook and Showalter[4], which asked practicing clinicians to identify the background they have adopted for their manual therapy assessment approach, found that the McKenzie approach was the most common assessment model with 34.7%, followed by Maitland (20.9%) and eclectic (10.6%). A follow-up study that

was comprised of APTA, board-certified orthopedic specialists (OCS), and/or Fellows of the *American Academy of Orthopedic Manual Therapists* (AAOMPT) also provided a report of manual therapy background.[5] The most common reported backgrounds included Maitland (24.1%), Osteopathic (19.4%), McKenzie (14.7%), Paris (12.3%), and Kaltenborn (8.2%). Because 99% of physical therapy schools teach manual therapy within the curriculum[3], there is a significant chance that exposure to one specific philosophy occurs prior to actual clinical practice.

Studies involving clinicians in other countries have also demonstrated background preferences. The four most popular postgraduate courses attended by respondents to a survey in Northern Ireland were Maitland peripheral short courses (48.0%), Maitland spinal short courses (42.1%), McKenzie A (76.3%), and McKenzie B (65.8%).[6] Respondents indicated that 71.4% of patients with low back pain were treated with McKenzie techniques, 43.8% were treated with Maitland mobilization, and 5.9% were treated with Cyriax techniques.[6] Foster et al.[7] surveyed physiotherapists in Great Britain and Ireland managing nonspecific low back pain, and found that 53.9% attended postgraduate Maitland vertebral mobilization classes and 53.2% attended McKenzie Part A courses. For spinal treatment, Maitland mobilizations were used by 58.9% of therapists and McKenzie techniques were used by 46.6% of therapists.[7] A survey of Canadian physiotherapists found that 67% of respondents reported using Maitland techniques and 41% reported using Cyriax techniques for cervical spine treatments.[8]

## Philosophical Differences

In 1979, Cookson[9] and Cookson and Kent[10] published comparative data among four popular manual therapy philosophies for treatment of the spine and extremities, respectively. Discussion of the principle philosophies for the extremity and spinal treatment philosophies included the Cyriax, Kaltenborn, Maitland, and Mennell approaches. There were notable differences regarding the method in which each philosophy converted examination findings to treatment methods. In an overview of assessment of extremities, Cookson noted that Cyriax and Kaltenborn based examination results on the presence of capsular patterns and the results of resisted testing. Both backgrounds used Cyriax's etiological philosophy for identification of guilty lesions. Cyriax's selection of treatment depended greatly on the examination findings and the classification of the impairments. For example, the selection of a physiological movement, accessory movement, or other form of treatment was dependent on the pain level, end feel, capsular pattern, and presence of a contractile or noncontractile lesion.

For selection of specific treatment techniques, Kaltenborn extrapolated the findings of the examination toward the theoretical relationship of arthrokinematic movements. These arthrokinematic movements were based on the convex/concave rules originally developed from the work of MacConail.[11] Kaltenborn's philosophy was to divide joints into hyper- or hypomobilities and to restore movement or stabilize as needed. The philosophy for treatment of hypomobility includes mobilization methods such as traction and accessory glides, often incorporating procedures at the end ranges to target selective stiffness.

Mennell uses a concept of joint dysfunction, which was based on onset, presence of trauma, and subjective findings. For treatment of joint dysfunction, the Mennell approach used quick thrusts designed to increase range of motion upon findings of joint limitation.[12] Often, active movements followed mobilization to encourage "muscular reeducation." One notable belief was the exclusion of therapeutic movements in the presence of inflammation.

The Maitland approach targeted treatments that affected the comparable sign of the patient. The comparable sign was defined as the motion or combination of motions that reproduces the pain or stiffness of the patient. Maitland divided the oscillatory-based application into four primary grades.[10] These grades differed in force, amplitude, and objective and were ascertained during patient assessment. Maitland's treatment approach was independent of capsular patterns, arthrokinematic patterns, or other biomechanical regulations.

There were similar differences found in the philosophical treatment of the spine.[9] Of the four approaches outlined for treatment of the spine, the Maitland and Mennell approach advocated the affiliation of examination and treatment techniques. Maitland focused more on oscillatory movements for joints that were considered either hypo- or hypermobile, while Mennell used a series of traction and positioning techniques for pain relief. Like the peripheral analysis, the Kaltenborn approach was based on biomechanical classification. Three treatment methods are used, depending on the examination findings, which range from mobilization to treatment procedures. Cyriax used a priori clustering of selected pathologies, but essentially maintained that the disk was the primary pathology of most spine ailments. Treatment generally consisted of generalized mobilization techniques or reduction traction methods if radiculopathy was perceptible.[9]

A similar analysis of manual therapy philosophies was performed in 1992 by Farrell and Jensen[1] with the addition of two approaches: Osteopathic and McKenzie. Like the Cookson series[9,10], Farrell and Jensen[1] reported numerous differences among the representative philosophies. For example, Cyriax's assessment system was dedicated toward his interpretation of applied anatomy and use of capsular patterns. Mennell's philosophy was oriented toward joint dysfunction-based techniques. Although Maitland, McKenzie, and Kaltenborn have many examination elements that were similar to Cyriax, Maitland assigns less credence to diagnostic or pathological labels and supports the use of reexamination to verify treatment effectiveness. McKenzie uses a series of repeated movements and postural (positioning assessment) to determine patient response during clinical examination. Often, McKenzie assigns a classification of the spinal impairment into one of three groups: postural, derangement, or dysfunction. The Osteopathic method emphasized the interpretation of three potential findings: a positional fault, restriction fault, and/or segmental or multisegmental impairment. Table 2.1 summarizes the findings of the three articles and outlines the similarities and differences of these approaches.

## Summary

- Numerous manual therapy assessment models have been taught in educational settings. The most commonly reported models are those of Maitland, McKenzie, Kaltenborn, Osteopathic, and eclectic.
- The most common continuing education courses, both nationally and internationally, are those provided by Maitland, McKenzie, Osteopathic, Kaltenborn, and Paris.
- The most commonly recognized manual therapy assessment approaches have notable similarities and differences. Past studies have outlined those comparisons and contrasts.

**TABLE 2.1    A Summary of the Philosophical Properties of Each Manual Therapy Theory**

| | Cyriax | Kaltenborn | Maitland | McKenzie | Mennell | Osteopathic |
|---|---|---|---|---|---|---|
| Philosophy adopts selected biomechanical and arthrological constructs | Yes | Yes | No | Yes and no | Mixed | Mixed |
| Approach places an emphasis on patient education | Yes | Yes | Yes | Yes | Yes | Yes |
| Evaluative criteria | Isolation of anatomical guilty structure | Biomechanical analysis of joint and soft tissue pathology | Identify relevant patient signs and symptoms | Interpretation of whether impairment is a dysfunction, derangement, or postural syndrome | Assessment of joint dysfunction | Identification of positional fault, restriction fault, or single vs. multisegmental findings |
| Key concepts | Diagnosis of soft tissue lesions and isolate of contractile vs. noncontractile components | Assessment of somatic involvement and application of biomechanical-based treatment systems | Examination and treatment methods are highly interrelated | Examination and treatment methods are highly related; selected positions may encourage certain disorders | Joint play assessment is critical | Assessment of somatic involvement; assessment focuses on the presence of asymmetry, restriction of movement, and palpations of soft tissue |

## Philosophical Analysis

It is apparent that numerous manual therapy philosophies exist. Upon face analysis, there appears to be three discrete assessment philosophical approaches or bases among the multiple manual therapy backgrounds. The first assessment format focuses on arthrokinematic and biomechanical principles. This **biomechanical–pathological assessment method** utilizes priori selected biomechanical theories for assessment of abnormalities in movement and positioning then targets treatments using similar arthrokinematic principles. Treatment techniques are based on theoretical relationships between anatomical contributions and pathological presentations. Often, these relationships are extrapolated into determination of a specific pathology or diagnosis. Some approaches rely on a given pathology or diagnostic label prior to administration of treatment. For example, the presence of a movement restriction based on the presence of Cyriax's

capsular pattern is often labeled adhesive capsulitis of the glenohumeral joint.[13] Assessment formats that use this process of assessment and treatment would then extrapolate the arthrological findings to related arthrological theories, most notably the convex–concave rule. Since external rotation is typically the range of motion that has the highest ratio of loss, and since the humerus is a convex structure moving on a concave glenoid fossa, a posterior-to-anterior glide mobilization would be considered the appropriate mobilization direction.[14]

The second method, the **patient response model**, addresses pain reproduction (using pain provocation and reduction methods) with various movements and does not rely on specific biomechanical models for diagnostic assessment. The patient response model assesses the response of singular or repeated movements and/or positions on the patient's comparable complaint of pain or abnormality of movement. Treatment techniques are often similar to the direction and form of assessment method. The particular treatment technique is based on the movement method that reproduces the patient's pain in a way designed to yield a result that either reduces pain or increases range of motion. The direction, amplitude, force, and speed of the treatment would depend on the patient response during and after the application. For example, using the same example of adhesive capsulitis; a provocation assessment would target the movement that most reproduced the patient's symptoms in a desirable fashion. The clinician may have found that during the application of an anterior-to-posterior (AP) glide, the result was an improvement in external rotation and a reduction in pain, therefore validating the selection of that method.

The third model uses a mixture of both methods. Both anatomical and biomechanical theories are used to initiate treatment, and variations that occur during treatment outside the rigid boundaries of biomechanical theory are often warranted. There are three potential forms of a **mixed model.** First, a model may follow a patient response-based assessment, and adopt biomechanical-based treatment parameters. Second, the assessment may be biomechanical-based, but the clinician adopts a patient response-based treatment. Third, the clinician may adopt a variety of both biomechanical-based and patient response-based parameters during examination and treatment, and truly uses an eclectic model.

---

## Summary

- There appear to be three primary assessment approaches in manual therapy.
- The first approach consists of biomechanical analysis, consisting of assessments using capsular patterns, coupling motions of the spine, biomechanical movement theory, and treatment methods using convex–concave rules.
- The second approach is a patient response approach, which consists of movements and treatments based on patient reports of symptoms provocation and resolution.
- The third approach consists of parameters of both assessment models. This combined approach may rely more heavily on biomechanical assessment and patient response treatment, vice versa, or will use an eclectic model used ad hoc.

---

## What Is the Best Approach?

Unfortunately, there is no direct evidence to determine which assessment philosophy reigns superiorly over another. Therefore, it is inappropriate to make conclusive judgments regarding the different approaches since no direct comparisons involving patient outcome assessment

are known to exist. At present, only indirect suppositions are plausible. Nevertheless, there is evidence that some methods of manual therapy assessment have performed less successfully during methodological scrutiny and could result in inappropriate, inaccurate, or invalid assessment.

### The Convex–Concave Rule

The **convex–concave rule** is a standard of biomechanical-based assessment methods that is not universally applicable to all regions. The convex–concave theory of arthrokinematic motion was first described by MacConail.[11] This theory asserts that the joint surface geometry dictates the accessory movement pattern during physiological movement.[15] The convex–concave rule states that when a concave surface rotates about a convex surface that rolling and gliding will occur in the same direction.[16] Conversely, if a convex surface rotates on a concave surface, rolling and gliding occur in opposite directions.[16] This pattern is purported to be irrespective of muscle movement or passive contributions of surrounding structures, pathology, and is purely a product of articular geometry.[17] To some extent, there is reasonable data to support that this process is predictive in the knee and ankle.[18,19] Indeed this model is often used to describe spinal-related movements, especially during end-range physiological activities.[20] Nonetheless, there is sizeable evidence that the shoulder fails to conform to the convex–concave guidelines. Numerous studies indicate that the glenohumeral joint does not always move as a ball and socket joint, but occasionally displays translatory-only movements during pathology.[15,21,22] Because of this, it appears that the selection of a technique that focuses on a specific direction based solely on the convex–concave rule may not yield values any better than the antagonistic direction at the shoulder.[22–24]

An additional problem is that some joints demonstrate irregularities of anatomy. The joint surfaces of C1 on C2 have been described as both convex on concave and convex on convex.[25] Often, the acromioclavicular joint demonstrates irregularity as well.[26] Because variations are so minute, it is difficult for a clinician to alter their biomechanical examination and treatment paradigm based on palpatory or observation-based findings. These irregularities may lead to variations in treatment and in theory such as the inappropriate direction during treatment application.

Although this evidence is condemning for use at the shoulder joint and in a situation where anatomical variation is present, one additional bit of information may be just as troublesome. The assertion that a manual therapist is able to apply a selected accessory-based movement that is biomechanically designed to replicate the active physiological movement of the patient is unsupported.[27] There is no evidence that lends credibility to the doctrinaire assertion that selected accessory techniques must be applied at specific angles or planes.

## Isometric Tension Testing

Cyriax had three principles for examination by **selective tissue tension.** The first involves isometric contraction of contractile tissue to determine if pain or weakness were present during loading. Cyriax proposed that contractile tissues (muscle, tendon, and bony insertion) are painful during an applied isometric contraction and inert structures (capsule, ligaments, bursae) are painful during passive movement. He furthered this definition by providing subdefinitions to the findings or the provocation tests. Franklin et al.[28] found some consistencies and inconsistencies with Cyriax's theory. First, as Cyriax noted, patients with minor contractile tissue lesions did display initially unchanged passive range of motion and pain with increased resistive activity.[29] However, in contrast to Cyriax's parameters, active range did worsen over time, as did strength. This questions the parameter "strong and painful," and supports the existence of another category, weak and painful. Table 2.2 outlines Cyriax's selective tension testing.

## Cyriax's Capsular Pattern

The second component of Cyriax's selective tissue tension concept is the capsular pattern. Several studies have demonstrated mixed value regarding Cyriax's definition of **capsular pattern theory.**[13,30–32] Klassbo and Harms-Ringdahl[29] and Bijl et al.[32] found a poor relationship between hip range-of-motion losses secondary to osteoarthritis and evidence of a capsular pattern. Klassbo and Harms-Ringdahl[31] also investigated the modified definition of the hip capsular patterns suggested by Kaltenborn[33] that also failed to demonstrate association. The findings in the knee are mixed. Hayes et al.[30] used a strict interpretation of the ratio of flexion to extension loss of the knee in their investigation of a capsular pattern. Using a strict definition, they found poor validity among their population of knee patients. Mitsch et al.[13] discovered variability in the capsular pattern in patients diag-

nosed with adhesive capsulitis of the shoulder. Bijl et al.[32] also did not find consistency. In contrast, Fritz et al.[34] found that the capsular pattern to be useful and consistent. The reason why each group found differences may lie in the interpretation and patient selection. It appears that Fritz et al.[34], Hayes et al.[30], and Mitsch et al.[13] placed some consideration on physician diagnosis, while Bijl et al.[32] used Altmann's clinical classification criteria for arthritis. Subsequently, some conflict exists regarding a stable capsular pattern at the hip and shoulder and possibly at the knee. If selecting the proper individual to meet Cyriax's criteria is essential for the use of this assessment method, then the benefit of the assessment model may be substantially reduced.

## Cyriax's End Feel Classification

The last aspect of Cyriax's selective tissue tension concept is the classification of the end feel. One study questions the validity of reliability in identification of discrete **end feel** categorization.[30,35] Cyriax[29] describes an end feel as "the extreme of each passive movement of the joint (that) transmits a specific sensation to the examiner's hands." He identified five specific end feels, which are outlined in Table 2.3. End feel tends to suffer from poor interrater reliability but seems to exhibit better reliability when the presence of pain is assessed during detection of abnormal end feel[36] or when an additional educational tool is used concurrently.[37]

## Directional Coupling of the Cervical Spine

Assessment of upper cervical **directional spine coupling** may also suffer a lack of validity. Many disciplines still report the use of two-dimensional theories[38], most notably the so-called *Laws of Physiologic Spinal Motion* outlined by Fryette.[39] In 1954, Fryette's findings were published and were largely based on the findings of Lovett.[40] Fryette's perception of coupling of the cervical region was that "sidebending is accompanied by rotation of the bodies of

**TABLE 2.2** Potential Findings During Resisted Movement Testing (Cyriax & Cyriax, 1993)

| Classification | Description |
|---|---|
| Strong and Painless | This finding suggests that the contractile tissue is not involved. |
| Strong and Painful | This finding suggests that there is a minor lesion of the contractile tissue. |
| Weak and Painless | This finding suggests there may be signs of a complete rupture of the contractile tissue or it may be a disorder of the nervous system. |
| Weak and Painful | This finding suggests a major lesion has occurred. |
| All Painful | Once all sinister pathologies are ruled out, the therapist should consider that the affective component may be the chief generator of pain. Additionally, this could be a gross lesion lying proximally; usually capsular and produced with joint movement is not fully restrained. |
| Painful on Repetition | If the movement is strong and painless but hurts after several repetitions, the examiner should suspect intermittent claudication. |

**TABLE 2.3**   End Feel Classification (Cyriax & Cyriax, 1993)

| End Feel Classification | Description |
| --- | --- |
| Bone to bone | The end feel of the joint is hard as when a bone engages another bone. |
| A spring block | This may suggest internal derangement but may also represent a capsular or ligamentous end feel. |
| An abrupt check | An unexpected restriction imposed by a muscular spasm. |
| Soft-tissue approximation | A normal end feel where the joint can be pushed no further secondary to engagement to another body part. |
| Empty end feel | No end feel is felt since the movement is too painful and the examiner is unable to push the joint to its end range. |

the vertebrae to the concavity of the lateral curve, as in the lumbar [spine]."[39] Recent three-dimensional analyses have confirmed that Fryette was correct on his assumption of cervical coupling direction from the cervical levels of C2-3 to C7-1, but was incorrect at the levels of C0-1 through C1-2. Recent three-dimensional analyses of the cervical spine have demonstrated that variations in the upper cervical spine are present, thus exhibiting coupling patterns that are inconsistent.[41–45] Dogmatic use of Fryette's law during assessment of the upper cervical spine should be questioned.

### Directional Coupling of the Lumbar Spine

Several authors have suggested that lumbar coupling biomechanics and Fryette's first and second *Laws of Physiological Spinal Motion* are poorly reliable and lack validity.[38,40,46] Recently, Cook[40] outlined the disparity between lumbar coupling directional movements, specifically at lumbar segments L1–2, L4–5, and L5–S1. There seems to be little evidence to support that knowledge of lumbar spine coupling characteristics are important in understanding and treating patients with low back pain.[47] Many manual therapy techniques use coupling-based mobilizations and the validity of this approach is questionable. Several authors have suggested that the use of symptom reproduction to identify the level of pathology is the only accurate assessment method.[48–54] Because no pathological coupling pattern has shown to be consistent, an assessment method in absence of pain provocation or reduction methods may yield inaccurate results. Therefore, upper cervical and lumbar biomechanical coupling theory may only be useful if assessed with pain provocation or reduction within a clinical examination.[40,55]

### Postural Asymmetry and the Relationship to Impairment

A potential misjudgment is the emphasis placed on observational asymmetries found during assessment of spinal abnormalities. McKenzie[56] writes, "there is a mistaken belief among some physical therapists that articular asymmetry is a contributing factor to the onset of backache." In fact, there are no studies that have calculated any predictive observational relationship with any form of progression or predisposition to spinal impairment. Commonly identified maladies such as pelvic obliquity are as recognizable in patients with pain as those without pain.[57] Postural asymmetry in the absence of a well-defined anatomical anomaly has no correlation with back pain and other forms of pelvic asymmetry are even less conclusive.[58] Additionally, it has been reported that asymmetries associated with the pelvis are too small to detect by manual examination, thus abnormalities have a high potential of being speculative assumption only.[59–61]

### Assessment of Passive Accessory Spinal Movement

Passive spinal assessment methods such as **passive accessory intervertebral movements** (PAIVMs) are widely used in joint mobilization.[62–64] One particular method the posterior–anterior (PA) mobilization applied specifically to the spinous process is purported to be a fundamental technique in clinical judgment.[62,65–67] Use of PA mobilization has been found to have a reasonable intertherapist reliability in the detection of the symptomatic lumbar segment level when accompanied with the verbal response of the subject.[68–70] Nonetheless, studies that have measured interrater reliability of forces without verbal response of the subject have reported a high degree of variability.[71–76] Additionally, studies that have focused on the presence of R1, defined as the point where stiffness is first perceived where the "feel" of the motion presents resistance to the therapist[1,70,71,77–79], have demonstrated poor reliability.[1,80] There are many theories for the poor reliability, some of which include inconsistencies within the clinician education process[77,81–85], differences in postgraduate training[1,27,84,86], years of experience[1,27,84], conflicting therapists' concept of stiffness[70,85,87,88], the angle of mobilization force[89], position of the patient during mobilization[90,91], and teaching method.[64] Most notably, it appears that assessment of finite motions in the absence of patients' verbal feedback may lead to questionable findings.

The finite movement associated with a PAIVM involves displacements that are more complicated than a straight translation. In an *in-vivo* analysis, Keller et al.[92] reported peak shear movements of 0.3 mm, axial movements of 1 millimeter, and sagittal rotation of 1 degree during manipulation forces. Mean movements of around half a millimeter for medial to lateral, anterior to posterior, and axial displacement were recorded and represent true spinal displacement.[92] Although evidence does exist that movements of this magnitude are therapeutic, there is conflicting evidence to support that a clinician can "feel" such diminutive displacement, let alone discriminate between axial rotation and translation.

### Biomechanic Theory of Disc Displacement with Repeated Movements

Well-substantiated evidence to support the use of repeated end-range movements for patients with a suspected herniated disc exists.[93] In studies where patients have performed movements of this nature and have exhibited **centralization** of symptoms, outcomes have been favorable.[93] However, there is limited evidence to support that remodeling of the disc is the reason behind the benefit. Variations have been reported in studies that have examined the movement of intradiscal matter during repeated flexion and extension movements.[94,95] In some individuals and/or specimens, the discal matter moved anterior, posterior, or in both directions.

In place of remodeling of the disc there are other theories that may have merit. There is some evidence to support that benefit to repeated movements may be associated with a change in the tension placed upon a nerve root during repeated loadings. In a cadaveric study, Schnebel et al.[96] reported that repeated extension decreased the tension and compression on the L5 nerve root. Repeated movements that reduce the tension and/or compression of a chemically sensitized disc would demonstrate the same patient-reported benefit as an alteration of a disc bulge.

### An Overreliance on the Diagnostic Value of Special Testing

There appears to be questionable validity associated with approaches that focus excessively on the use of "special" clinical tests to identify pathology or provide a diagnostic label prior to treatment. When examining reports on the diagnostic accuracy of a special test, a cohort of patients is subjected to at least two types of mutually exclusive testing: an index test (the special test) and the reference test, the latter usually being the best method available to detect the target condition. The accuracy of the index test is expressed in terms of sensitivity, specificity, or likelihood ratios.[97] These terms are discussed in detail in Chapter 3. Many commonly used special tests are subject to likelihood values that offer little conclusive diagnostic use to the clinician. The sacroiliac joint has a wealth of tests that have performed poorly in diagnostic studies[98], as does other anatomical regions of the body such as the shoulder and knee. An overreliance on special tests may also reduce the pertinent information necessary during treatment selection.

### Is Anything Substantiated?

Although many of the traditional principles developed by the pioneers of manual therapy have suffered attack, there are some theories that have weathered well under scrutiny. The patient response method, a philosophy that fits agreeably within the guidelines of the *Guide to Physical Therapist Practice*[99], does appear to yield useful and valid findings.

## *Summary*

- There is strong evidence to support that the convex–concave rule does not apply to the glenohumeral joint. There is some evidence that the rule is effective for the ankle and knee.
- There is fair evidence that the Cyriax theory of selective tension is not applicable to all conditions.
- There is conflicting evidence that the Cyriax capsular pattern theory lacks complete validity and depends substantially on how patients are selected for assessment.
- There is some evidence that questions the reliability of Cyriax's end feel classification.
- There is strong evidence to support that upper cervical spine coupling direction is unpredictable, thus Fryette's laws of physiological motions are invalid.
- There is substantial evidence to support that there is not predictable coupling pattern for the lumbar spine, thus Fryette's laws at the lumbar spine are invalid.
- There is moderate evidence to support that postural asymmetry is not directly correlated to a specific impairment.
- There is moderate evidence that supports that the disc does not move in a specific direction or behave in a specific manner with repeated movements or specific postural positioning.
- There is strong evidence that suggests that manual therapy approaches that overutilize special tests will harbor inappropriate diagnoses and findings.
- There is fair evidence to support the use of a patient response-based system for assessment.

The patient response model is designed to determine selected impairments and does not focus on the isolation of a dedicated pathology. For example, the use of repeated end-range movements or postural positioning designed to determine if a patient exhibits centralization behavior has been shown to exhibit validity and is a patient response-based assessment and treatment. A patient who demonstrates centralizing symptoms has been associated with better outcomes than comparative patients who failed to centralize, regardless of the identified pathology. The use of a patient response model relies less on theory and more on the immediate response of the patient. Using the previous example, determining whether disc-related changes occur is insignificant and is considered secondary information when compared to assessment of patient response.

# The Three Elements of Assessment

Despite the inherent differences among the selected models there are notable commonalities that do exist. First, the majority of methods focus on a patient-centered approach to examination. The majority identify potential impairments based on the interplay between subjective and objective findings. Second, all models harbor selected theoretical reasoning behind each manual therapy procedure, although in many cases, this clinical reasoning differs among pioneers. Third, and perhaps most impor-

tantly, all orthopedic manual therapy models use a systematic process of assessment. This process consists of (1) clinical examination, (2) treatment, and (3) reexamination (Figure 2.1). Farrell and Jensen[1] stated that this implicit dimension suggests that the values and behaviors that are central to the work of a manual therapist may be the most important contribution to manual therapy.

The clinical examination is the systematic process of identifying the dysfunction, recognizing potential pathobiological mechanisms, isolating the source of the symptoms or dysfunction, recognizing contributing factors, and managing the condition.[100] This process is performed during the history and subjective and the physical examination. Treatment is the application of a skilled hand movement intended to improve tissue extensibility, increase range of motion, reduce pain, or improve overall function. Reexamination is the systematic process of reevaluating the effect of each treatment technique to determine its specific effectiveness. Chapter 4 discusses treatment and reexamination.

## Summary

- All manual therapy models use an element of assessment that consists of examination, treatment, and reexamination.
- All models contain some form of clinical reasoning that guides practice patterns.

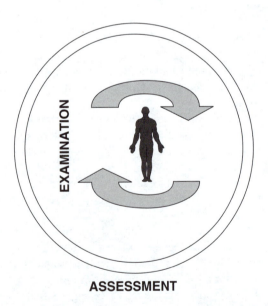

**Figure 2.1**  The three components of effective assessment consist of the examination, the treatment, and the reexamination. This figure represents the nonlinear and direct relationship of treatment and reexamination. Examination occurs within the first session but from then on reexamination is the process associated with treatment.

## Creating a Diagnosis

The *Guide to Physical Therapist Practice* outlines that a **diagnostic label** is assigned as a result of a systematic process of integrating and evaluating the data obtained during assessment. Delitto and Snyder-Mackler[101] argued that most clinicians create a workable diagnosis based on signs and symptoms, and clinical classification of recognizable clusters of information. This identification of the impact of the dysfunction is obtained through the history, signs, symptoms, examination, and tests that are performed by the clinician.[102] In essence, all clinicians create a diagnosis during treatment, with an understanding that many of the symptoms may vary within a single diagnostic label.

A logical and appropriate clinical examination is the cognitive foundation of the clinical assessment process and is required prior to assigning a diagnostic label. Two forms of diagnostic examination exist: a pathology-based and impairment-based.

### *Pathology-Based Assessment*

In traditional medical diagnosis, clinicians use **pathology-based assessment models** to classify clinical phenomena into diagnostic labels, accordingly assigning a diagnostic label to a specific pathology.[103–106] Selected clinical tests and measures are used to strengthen the likelihood that the clinician isolates the pathology and appropriately assigns the diagnostic label. Although this method is frequently used and substantially investigated, there are some limitations. Unfortunately, no diagnostic laboratory or clinical test for pathology is completely specific.[97,107,108] Many diagnostic testing methods yield results that are unrelated to the impairment at hand.[109] Tests that have a high sensitivity and are indicative of the presence of a disease typically have low specificity, indicating the negative presence of the disease.[97,107] Clusters of tests improve the diagnostic value but research is incomplete regarding which tests are appropriate for clustering within a given region. Given these challenges, it is apparent that the use of a pathology-based examination may yield inaccuracies and, potentially, the selection of inappropriate treatment.

Within medicine, many diagnostic titles are inadequate to explain a patient's condition and may be merely linked to patterns of symptoms or suppositions.[110,111] Commonly, patients present with problems that aren't easily transposed into pathological patterns and/or diagnostic labels. The usefulness of diagnostic labels seldom guide clinical decisions related to the prognosis or treatment of patients.[27] Furthermore, diagnostic labels provide little insight on the severity, irritability, nature, and stage of the disorder.[112]

There is often poor agreement among medical clinicians regarding appropriate diagnostic test results, which tests to use, and the outcome of those tests.[113] X-rays, MRIs, CT-scans, and other forms of static diagnostic equipment are not designed to measure movement-related disorders.[114] Traditional diagnostic tests seldom offer sufficient information on the source of the disorder and/or the mechanisms of symptoms. These methods may convey misleading information, such as abnormal changes unrelated to the present disorder.[115] Additionally, most patients exhibit concurrent psychosocial problems that complicate their interpretation and reaction from their problem.[100] Despite overwhelming evidence suggesting the use of an alternative paradigm, there is continued adherence to an anatomically based, nociceptive-centered pathology-based assessment model.[116]

## Impairment-Based Assessment

An alternative to the pathology-based assessment model is the use of an **impairment-based assessment model** referenced by clinical subjective and objective findings[117] and patient response.[56] The impairment-based examination model advocates the use of independent examination findings to drive the selection of various treatments. The underlying philosophy suggests that the relationship between the impairment and each sign and symptom is of greater importance than the label of a diagnosis.[118] The

*Guide to Physical Therapist Practice*[99] recognizes that in some cases the physical therapist may administer interventions even when the diagnostic process does not yield an identifiable cluster of information for categorization into a diagnostic label. They do so by administering interventions based on alleviation of symptoms or remediation of impairments, guided primarily by patient response during reexamination.

## Combining Pathology- and Impairment-Based Diagnosis

Often, clusters of symptoms provide useful information for diagnostic labeling, and offers even greater benefit for selection of treatment. Although this situation may focus more heavily on an impairment-based examination, the clusters of information allow the clinician to address both forms of examination. Several authors have provided models designed to address both issues and improve the clinical reasoning capabilities during examination. Jones[119] and others[100,120] have proposed the application of hypotheses categories that consist of discrete clusters of related concepts. These clusters represent key treatment cues for an orthopedic manual therapist for appropriate selection of treatment application. These categories consist of:

1. Functional Limitations and Disability
2. Pathobiological Mechanisms
3. Source of Symptoms
4. Contributing Factors
5. Precautions and Contraindications
6. Prognosis
7. Management

These hypotheses categories may yield greater information than a stand alone diagnostic label, or identification of impairment. Additionally, this method may improve the process in which manual therapists extract useful information from an examination for later use. Others have explored the use of this method during clinical reasoning among manual clinicians and these hypotheses appear accurate in representing the treatment decision-making model of experienced clinicians.[121] The model allows flexibility among clinicians and emphasizes the one-on-one interaction between the clinician and the patient. By using the selected categories, the clinician is able to examine multiple components of disability, including features potentially outside the boundaries of care. Applying hypotheses categories is useful in reducing errors associated with sinister pathological conditions and determining if a patient is appropriate for the clinician's domain of expertise.

## Summary

- All clinicians create a workable diagnosis during the manual therapy assessment process.
- A pathology-based diagnosis may yield less useful information, is wrought by poor reliability, and provides the manual therapy clinician with limited treatment options.
- An impairment-based diagnosis often yields useful treatment-based information and relies heavily on the signs and symptoms of a patient's condition.

# THE PATIENT RESPONSE-BASED MODEL

Within this textbook, the "flavor" of the assessment most resembles a patient response-based model. First, it is imperative to recognize that the adoption of this particular model does not suggest that other forms (i.e., biomechanical, mixed) of models are not effective and/or beneficial methods for manual therapists. As stated previously, there is no direct evidence to determine which assessment philosophy reigns over another. It is quite apparent that manual therapy pioneers such as James Cyriax, Freddy Kaltenborn, Andrew Still, selected pioneering chiropractors, and others who have advocated a biomechanical or mixed model have provided an invaluable framework for manual therapists. Their contribution has been substantial and it would be inappropriate to assume anything otherwise.

Nonetheless, the investigation of the literature does suggest that a patient response-based model, although not perfect, provides the greatest validity for evidence-based assessment in manual therapy. Additionally, this model, when performed in a sequential and specific manner, provides a rigorous system of what amounts to data collection and processing that is used to guide the clinician through a logical treatment format.[122] In a situation in which the patient and the clinician work together, the consequence of the assessment is irrefutable. Primarily, the pioneers of this particular approach include G.D. Maitland, Robin McKenzie, numerous Australian-based researchers and physiotherapists, Brian Mulligan, Gregory Grieve, and selected osteopathic approaches that have analyzed patient symptoms primarily with less emphasis on observation-based, visual abnormalities. It is the approach of these pioneers that is reflected within this textbook, and to these clinical vanguards we are eternally grateful.

## *Advantages of the Patient Response-Based Approach*

There are several advantages to a patient response-based approach. These advantages are outlined as follows:

1. Adaptability to each patient and variability of symptoms.
2. Treatment is specific since it is driven by a positive response from the patient.
3. The model is not based on biomechanical principles and since some biomechanical principles lack validity, have questionable validity, or are only valid in selected situations, the chance of error is substantially reduced.
4. The approach is similar to the philosophical guidelines of the *Guide to Physical Therapist Practice*, which dictate an impairment-based approach that respects and selects a diagnosis, but bases much of the treatment decision making on impairment-based findings.
5. The model does not rely on the hypothetical presentation or protocol-based algorithm from a diagnostic label.
6. The treatment selection changes as the patient's symptoms change.
7. Several well-documented manual therapy models use a similar philosophy.
8. The model is intuitive and is relatively easy to learn.

## *Disadvantages of the Patient Response-Based Approach*

Gregory Grieve[118] once wrote, "no test is perfect." Correspondingly, no clinical assessment method is perfect either. The patient response-based method does have notable flaws, which are listed below.

1. The patient-response model is more time-intensive because patient examination and treatment is not easily compartmentalized into common criteria.
2. The model ignores many traditionalistic assessment methods commonly used in manual therapy. As such,

## Summary

- This textbook has adopted a patient-response approach.
- The patient-response approach is similar to those pioneered by G.D. Maitland, Robin McKenzie, numerous Australian researchers and physiotherapists, Brian Mulligan, and selected osteopaths who are not overly committed to purportedly visual biomechanical constructs.
- Both strengths and weaknesses of the patient response-based system are apparent. No assessment approach is perfect, yet the patient response-based system provides a fair amount of validity when both clinician and patient are committed to an effective outcome.

it is often identified as an outsider or is considered maverick.

3. The model requires dedicated communication between the clinician and the patient and will fail without concerted effort from both. In some situations where there lacks a patient's commitment, the result may yield poor outcomes. Nonetheless, this is evident with any approach.

4. Because diagnostic labeling is considered inconsequential to the outcome of the patient, comparative research analysis with other disorders is less conclusive. In some cases (not all) the clinician may treat without a specific diagnosis since this rarely impacts the outcome or selection of treatment techniques.

5. Although no single model has been comparatively measured against another in a randomized clinical trial, the ability to indicate that the patient-response model is better than another form of assessment model does not exist.

## Chapter Questions

1. Describe the three manual therapy philosophical approaches. Compare and contrast assessment methods.
2. Outline the weaknesses of the discussed manual therapy areas and how they could alter assessment.
3. Outline the strengths of selected manual therapy areas and discuss how they lead to pertinent assessment.
4. Define the three elements of assessment and identify how each element is related both directly and circuitously.
5. Describe how the pathological- and impairment-based assessment models can fit together. Define the role of the diagnostic label in manual therapy.

## References

1. Farrell J, Jensen G. Manual therapy: a critical assessment of role in the professional of physical therapy. *Phys Ther.* 1992;72:843–852.
2. Ben-Sorek S, Davis CM. Joint mobilization education and clinical use in the United States. *Phys Ther.* 1988;68:1000–1004.
3. Bryan JM, McClune LD, Rominto S, Stetts DM, Finstuen K. Spinal mobilization curricula in professional physical therapy education programs. *J Physical Ther Education.* 1997;11:11–15.
4. Cook C, Showalter C. A survey on the importance of lumbar coupling biomechanics in physiotherapy practice. *Man Ther.* 2004;9:164–172.
5. Cook C. Subjective and objectives identifiers of clinical lumbar spine instability: A delphi study. *Man Ther.* 2006;11:11–21.
6. Gracey J, Suzanne M, Baxter D. Physiotherapy management of low back pain: A survey of current practice in Northern Ireland. *Spine.* 2002;27(4):406–411.
7. Foster N, Thompson K, Baxter D, Allen J. Management of nonspecific low back pain by physiotherapists in Britain and Ireland. *Spine.* 1999;24:1332–1342.
8. Hurley L, Yardley K, Gross A, Hendry L, McLaughlin L. A survey to examine attitudes and patterns of practice of physiotherapists who perform cervical spine manipulation. *Man Ther.* 2002;7(1):10–18.
9. Cookson J. Orthopedic manual therapy—an overview. Part II: The spine. *Phys Ther.* 1979;59:259–267.
10. Cookson J, Kent B. Orthopedic manual therapy—an overview. Part I: The extremities. *Phys Ther.* 1979;59:136–146.
11. MacConail M. Joint movement. *Physiotherapy.* 1964;50:363–365.
12. Mennell J. Back pain: *Diagnosis and treatment using manipulative techniques.* Boston, MA; Little, Brown and Co.: 1960.
13. Mitsch J, Casey J, McKinnis R, Kegerreis S, Stikeleather J. Investigation of a consistent pattern of motion restriction in patients with adhesive capsulitis. *J Manual Manipulative Ther.* 2004;12:153–159.
14. Wadsworth C. *Manual examination and treatment of the spine and extremities.* Baltimore, MD; Williams and Wilkins: 1988.
15. McClure P, Flowers K. Treatment of limited should motion: a case study based on biomechanical considerations. *Phys Ther.* 1992;72:929–936.
16. Kaltenborn FM. *Manual mobilization of the extremity joints* (4th ed.). Minneapolis: OPTP; 1989.
17. MacConaill M, Basmajian J. Muscles and movement: A basis for human kinesiology. Baltimore, MD: Williams & Wilkins; 1969.
18. Frankel V, Burstein A, Brooks D. Biomechanics of internal derangement of the knee; Pathomechanics as determined by analysis of the instant centers of motion. *J Bone Joint Surg (Am).* 1971;53:945–962.
19. Sammarco G, Burstein A, Frankel V. Biomechanics of the ankle: a kinematic study. *Orthop Clin North Am.* 1973;4:75–96.

20. Mercer S, Bogduk N. Intra-articular inclusions of the cervical synovial joints. *British Journal of Rheumatology.* 1993;32:705–710

21. Baeyens J, Van Roy P, De Schepper A, Declercq G, Clarijs J. Glenohumeral joint kinematics related to minor anterior instability of the shoulder at the end of the later preparatory phase of throwing. *Clin Biomech.* 2001;16:752–757.

22. Baeyens J, Van Roy P, Clarjjs J. Intra-articular kinematics of the normal glenohumeral joint in the late preparatory phase of throwing: Kaltenborn's rule revisited. *Ergonomics.* 2000;10:1726–1737.

23. Hsu A, Ho L, Hedman T. Joint position during anterior-posterior glide mobilization: its effect on glenohumeral abduction range of motion. *Arch Phys Med Rehabil.* 2000;81:210–214.

24. Harryman et al. (1990). Translation of the humeral head on the glenoid with passive glenohumeral motion. *J Bone Jnt Surg.* 1990;79A(9):1334–1343.

25. White A, Panjabi M. *Clinical biomechanics of the spine.* Philadelphia: J.B. Lippincott Co, 1990; p. 94.

26. Harryman D, Lazarus M. The stiff shoulder. In: Rockwood C, Matsen F, Wirth M, Lippitt S. *The shoulder.* Vol 2. 3rd edition. Philadelphia; W.B. Saunders: 2004.

27. Riddle D. Measurement of accessory motion: critical issues and related concepts. *Phys Ther.* 1992;72:865–874.

28. Franklin M, Conner-Kerr T, Chamness M, Chenier T, Kelly R, Hodge T. Assessment of exercise-induced minor muscle lesions: the accuracy of Cyriax's diagnosis by selective tension paradigm. *J Ortho Sports Phys Ther.* 1996;24:122–129.

29. Cyriax J, Cyriax P. *Cyriax's illustrated manual of orthopaedic medicine.* Oxford; Boston; Butterworth-Heinemann: 1993.

30. Hayes K, Peterson C, Falconer J. An examination of Cyriax's passive motion tests with patients having osteoarthritis of the knee. *Phys Ther.* 1994;74:697–707.

31. Klassbo M, Larsson G. Examination of passive ROM and capsular patterns of the hip. *Physiotherapy Res International.* 2003;8:1–12.

32. Bijl D, Dekker J, van Baar M, Oostendorp R, Lemmens A, Bijlsma J, Voorn T. Validity of Cyriax's concept capsular pattern for the diagnosis of osteoarthritis of hip and/or knee. *Scand J Rheumatol.* 1998;27:347–351.

33. Kaltenborn F. *Manual mobilization of the joints. The Kaltenborn method of joint mobilization and treatment.* 5th edition. Oslo; Olaf Norlis Bokhandel: 1999.

34. Fritz J, Delitto A, Erhard R, Roman M. An examination of the selective tissue tension scheme, with evidence for the concept of a capsular pattern of the knee. *Phys Ther.* 1998;78:1046–1056.

35. Hayes K, Peterson C. Reliability of assessing end-feel and pain and resistance sequence in subjects with painful shoulders and knees. *J Orthop Phys Ther.* 2001;31:432–445.

36. Peterson C, Hayes K. Construct validity of Cyriax's selective tension examination: association of end-feels with pain at the knee and shoulder. *J Orthop Sports Phys Ther.* 2000;30:512–521.

37. Chesworth B, MacDermid J, Roth J, Patterson S. Movement diagram and "end-feel" reliability when measuring passive lateral rotation of the shoulder in patients with shoulder pathology. *Phys Ther.* 1998;78:593–601.

38. Gibbons P, Tehan P. Patient positioning and spinal locking for lumbar spine rotation manipulation. *Man Ther.* 2001;6(3):130–138.

39. Fryette H. *The principles of osteopathic technique.* Carmel, CA; Academy of Applied Osteopathy: 1954; p. 21.

40. Cook C. Lumbar Coupling biomechanics—A literature review. *J Manual Manipulative Ther.* 2003;11(3):137–145.

41. Panjabi M, Oda T, Crisco J, Dvorak J, Grob D. Posture affects motion coupling patterns of the upper cervical spine. *J Orthop Research.* 1993;11:525–536.

42. Mimura M, Hideshige M, Watanbe T, Takahashi K, Yamagata M, Tamaki T. Three-dimensional motion analysis of the cervical spine with special reference to axial rotation. *Spine.* 1989;14:1135–1139.

43. Penning L. Normal movements of the cervical spine. *Am J Roentgenology.* 1978;130:317–326.

44. Iai H, Hideshige M, Goto S, Takahashi K, Yamagata M, Tamaki T. Three-dimensional motion analysis of the upper cervical spine during axial rotation. *Spine.* 1993;18:2388–2392.

45. Oda T, Panjabi M, Crisco J. Three-dimensional translation movements of the upper cervical spine. *J Spinal Disorders.* 1991;4:411–419.

46. Harrison D, Harrison D, Troyanovich S. Three-dimensional spinal coupling mechanics: Part one. *J Manipulative Physiol Ther* 1998;21(2):101–113.

47. Panjabi M, Oxland T, Yamamoto I, Crisco J. Mechanical behavior of the human lumbar and lumbosacral spine as shown by three-dimensional load-displacement curves. *Am J Bone Jnt Surg.* 1994; 76:413–424.

48. Keating J, Bergman T, Jacobs G, Finer B, Larson K. The objectivity of a multi-dimensional index of lumbar segmental abnormality. *J Manipulative Physiol Ther.* 1990;13:463–471.

49. Hardy G, Napier J. Inter- and intra-therapist reliability of passive accessory movement technique. *New Zealand J Physio.* 1991;22–24.

50. Vilkari-Juntura E. Inter-examiner reliability of observations in physical examinations of the neck. *Phys Ther.* 1987;67(10):1526–1532.

51. Lee M, Latimer J, Maher C. Manipulation: Investigation of a proposed mechanism. *Clin Biomech.* 1993; 8:302–306.

52. Maher C, Adams R. Reliability of pain and stiffness assessments in clinical manual lumbar spine examinations. *Phys Ther.* 1994;74(9):801–811.

53. Maher C, Latimer J. Pain or resistance: The manual therapists' dilemma. *Aust J Physiother.* 1992;38(4):257–260.

54. Boline P, Haas M, Meyer J, Kassak K, Nelson C, Keating J. Interexaminer reliability of eight evaluative dimensions of lumbar segmental abnormality: Part II. *J Manipulative Physiol Ther.* 1992;16(6):363–373.

55. Li Y, He X. Finite element analysis of spine biomechanics. *J Biomech Engineering.* 2001;18(2)288–289, 319.

56. McKenzie R. Mechanical diagnosis and therapy for disorders of the low back. In: Twomey L, & Taylor J. *Physical therapy of the low back.* 3rd ed. New York; Churchill Livingstone: 2000.

57. Fann A. The prevalence of postural asymmetry in people with and without chronic low back pain. *Arch Phys Med Rehabil.* 2002;83:1736–1738.

58. Levangie PK. The association between static pelvic asymmetry and low back pain. *Spine.* 1999;15;24(12):1234–1242.

59. Dreyfuss P, Michaelsen M, Pauza K, McLarty J, Bogduk N. The value of medical history and physical examination in diagnosing sacroiliac joint pain. *Spine.* 1996;21:2594–2602.

60. Freburger J, Riddle D. Using published evidence to guide the examination of the sacroiliac joint region. *Phys Ther.* 2001;81:1135–1143.

61. Sturesson B, Uden A, Vleeming A. A radiosterometric analysis of movements of the sacroiliac joints during the standing hip flexion test. *Spine.* 2000;25:354–368.

62. Battie M, Cherkin D, Dunn R, Ciol M, Wheeler K. Managing low back pain: Attitudes and treatment preferences of physical therapist. *Phys Ther.* 1994;4(3):219–226.

63. Fitzgerald G, McClure P, Beattie P, Riddle D. Issues in determining treatment effectiveness of manual therapy. *Phys Ther.* 1994;74(3):227–233.

64. Petty N, Bach T, Cheek L. Accuracy of feedback during training of passive accessory intervertebral movements. *J Manual Manipulative Ther.* 2001;9(2):99–108.

65. Di Fabio R. Efficacy of manual therapy. *Phys Ther* 1992;72(12):853–864.

66. Harms M, Milton A, Cusick G, Bader D. Instrumentation of a mobilization couch for dynamic load measurements. *J Med Engineering Tech.* 1995;9(4):119–122.

67. Goodsell M, Lee M, Latimer J. Short-Term effects of lumbar posteroanterior mobilization in individuals with low-back pain *J Manipulative Physiol Ther.* 2000;23(5):332–342.

68. Jull G, Bogduk N, Marsland A. The accuracy of a manual diagnosis for cervical zygapophysial joint pain syndromes. *Med J Australia.* 1998;148:233–236.

69. Behrsin J, Andrews F. Lumbar segmental instability: Manual assessment findings supported by radiological measurement. *Aust J Physiotherapy.* 1991;37:171–173.

70. Bjornsdottir S, Kumar S. Posteroanterior spinal mobilization: State of the art review and discussion. *Disability Rehabil.* 1997;19(2):39–46.

71. Matyas T, Bach T. The reliability of selected techniques in clinical arthrometrics. *Aust J Physiotherapy.* 1985;31:175–199.

72. Carty G. A comparison of the reliability of manual tests of compliance using accessory movements in peripheral and spinal joints. Abstract. *Aust J Physiotherapy.* 1986;32:1,68.

73. Gibson H, Ross J, Alien J, Latimer J, Maher C. The effect of mobilization on forward bending range. *J Manual Manipulative Ther.* 1993;1:142–147.

74. McCollam R, Benson C. Effects of poster-anterior mobilization on lumbar extension and flexion. *J Manual Manipulative Ther.* 1993;1:134–141.

75. Simmonds M, Kumar S, Lechelt E. Use of spinal model to quantify the forces and motion that occur during therapists' tests of spinal motion. *Phys Ther.* 1995;75:212–222.

76. Binkley J, Stratford P, Gill C. 1992 Intertherapist reliability of lumbar accessory motion mobility testing. In: Proceedings of the International Federation of Orthopaedic Manipulative Therapists 5th International Conference, Vail Colorado. 150–151.

77. Lee M, Mosely A, Refshauge K. Effects of feedback on learning a vertebral joint mobilizations skill. *Phys Ther.* 1990;10:97–102.

78. Harms M, Cusick G, Bader D. Measurement of spinal mobilisation forces. *Physiotherapy.* 1995;81(10):559–604.

79. Maitland GD. *Maitland's vertebral manipulation.* 6th ed. London; Butterworth-Heinemann: 2001.

80. Viner A, Lee M. Direction of manual force applied during assessment of stiffness in the lumbosacral spine. *J Manipulative Physiol Ther.* 1997;18(7):441–447.

81. Maitland G, Hickling J. Abnormalities in passive movement: Diagrammative representation. *Physiotherapy.* 1970;56:105–114.

82. Latimer J, Lee M, Adams R. The effect of training with feedback on physiotherapy students' ability to judge lumbar stiffness. *Man Ther.* 1996;1(5):26–70.

83. Latimer J, Adams R, Lee R. Training with feedback improves judgments of non-biological linear stiffness. *Man Ther.* 1998;3(2):85–89.

84. Chiradenjnant A, Latimer J, Maher C. Forces applied during manual therapy to patients with low

back pain. *J Manipulative Physiol Ther.* 2002;25(6): 362–369.

85. Maher C, Simmonds M, Adams R. Therapists' conceptualization and characterization of the clinical concept of spinal stiffness. *Phys Ther.* 1998;78: 289–300.

86. Cook C, Turney L, Ramirez L, Miles A, Haas S, Karakostas T. Predictive factors in poor inter-rater reliability among physical therapists. *J Manual Manipulative Ther.* 2002;10(4):200–205.

87. Yahia L, Audet J, Drouin G. Rheological properties of the human lumbar spine ligaments. *J Biomed Eng.* 1991;13:399–406.

88. Shirley D, Ellis E, Lee M. The response of posteroanterior lumbar stiffness to repeated loading. *Man Ther.* 2002;7:19–25.

89. Caling B, Lee M. Effect of direction of applied mobilization force on the posteroanterior response in the lumbar spine. *J Manipulative Physiol Ther.* 2001; 24:71–78.

90. Edmondston S, Allison G, Gregg S, Purden G, Svansson G, Watson A. Effect of position on the posteroanterior stiffness of the lumbar spine. *Man Ther.* 1998;3(1):21–26.

91. Lee R, Evans J. An *in-vivo* study of the intervertebral movements produced by posteroanterior mobilization. *Clin Biomech.* 1997;12:400–408.

92. Keller TS, Colloca CJ, Gunzburg R. Neuromechanical characterization of in vivo lumbar spinal manipulation. Part I. Vertebral motion. *J Manipulative Physiol Ther.* 2003;26(9):567–578.

93. Wetzel FT, Donelson R. The role of repeated end-range/pain response assessment in the management of symptomatic lumbar discs. *Spine J.* 2003;3(2): 146–154.

94. Seroussi RE, Krag MH, Muller DL, Pope MH. Internal deformations of intact and denucleated human lumbar discs subjected to compression, flexion, and extension loads. *J Orthop Res.* 1989;7(1): 122–131.

95. Edmondston SJ, Allison GT, Gregg CD, Purden SM, Svansson GR, Watson AE. Effect of position on the posteroanterior stiffness of the lumbar spine. *Man Ther.* 1998;3(1):21–26.

96. Schnebel BE, Watkins RG, Dillin W. The role of spinal flexion and extension in changing nerve root compression in disc herniations. *Spine.* 1989;14(8): 835–837.

97. Mol BW, Lijmer JG, Evers JL, Bossuyt PM. Characteristics of good diagnostic studies. *Semin Reprod Med.* 2003;21(1):17–25.

98. Laslett M, Young S, Aprill C, McDonald B. Diagnosing painful sacroiliac joints: a validity study of a McKenzie evaluation and sacroiliac provocation tests. *Aust J Physiotherapy.* 2003;49:89–97.

99. Guide to Physical Therapist Practice. 2nd ed. *Phys Ther.* 2001;81:9–744.

100. Gifford LS, Butler DS. The integration of pain sciences into clinical practice. *J Hand Ther.* 1997; 10(2):86–95.

101. Delitto A, Snyder-Mackler L. The diagnostic process: examples in orthopedic physical therapy. *Phys Ther.* 1995;75:203–211.

102. Sahrmann SA. Diagnosis by the physical therapist—a prerequisite for treatment. A special communication. *Phys Ther.* 1988;68(11):1703–1706.

103. Deyo RA, Phillips WR. Low back pain. A primary care challenge. *Spine.* 1996;21(24):2826–2832.

104. Deyo RA. Fads in the treatment of low back pain. *N Engl J Med.* 1991;325(14):1039–1040.

105. Hart LG, Deyo RA, Cherkin DC. Physician office visits for low back pain. Frequency, clinical evaluation, and treatment patterns from a U.S. national survey. *Spine.* 1995;20(1):11–19.

106. Hollander J. Painful joints: clues to early diagnosis. *Postgrad Med.* 1978;64:50–56,60.

107. Glas AS, Lijmer JG, Prins MH, Bonsel GJ, Bossuyt PM. The diagnostic odds ratio: a single indicator of test performance. *J Clin Epidemiol.* 2003;56(11): 1129–1135.

108. Wainner RS, Fritz JM, Irrgang JJ, Boninger ML, Delitto A, Allison S. Reliability and diagnostic accuracy of the clinical examination and patient self-report measures for cervical radiculopathy. *Spine.* 2003; 28(1):52–62.

109. Fritz JM, Wainner RS. Examining diagnostic tests: an evidence-based perspective. *Phys Ther.* 2001;81 (9):1546–1564.

110. Boden SD. The use of radiographic imaging studies in the evaluation of patients who have degenerative disorders of the lumbar spine. *J Bone Joint Surg Am.* 1996;78(1):114–124.

111. Maitland GD. *Peripheral manipulation.* 3rd ed. London; Butterworth-Heinemann: 1986.

112. Sprague R. Differential assessment and mobilization of the cervical and upper thoracic spine. In: Donatelli R, Wooden M. *Orthopaedic physical therapy.* Philadelphia; Churchill Livingston: 2001.

113. Tomberline J, Saunders D. *Evaluation treatment and prevention of musculoskeletal disorder.* Vol. 2. Chaska, MN; The Saunders Group: 2004

114. Harrison D, Harrison D, Troyanovich S, Hansen D. The anterior–posterior full-spine view: The worst radiographic view for determination of mechanics of the spine. *Chiropractic Technique.* 1996;8:163–170.

115. McCowin PR, Borenstein D, Wiesel SW. The current approach to the medical diagnosis of low back pain. *Orthop Clin North Am.* 1991;22(2):315–325.

116. Twomey L, Taylor J. *Physical therapy of the low back.* 3rd ed. New York; Churchill Livingstone: 2000.

117. Spitzer W, LeBlanc F, Dupuis M. Scientific approach to the assessment and management of activity-related spinal disorders. A monograph for clinicians. Report of the Quebec Task Force on spinal disorders. *Spine*. 1987;12:S1–59.
118. Grieve G. *Common vertebral joint problems*. 2nd ed. Edinburgh; Churchill Livingstone: 1988.
119. Jones M. Clinical reasoning in manual therapy. *Phys Ther*. 1992;72:875–884.
120. Gifford L. Pain, In: *Rehabilitation of movement: theoretical basis of clinical practice*. London; Saunders Publishing: 1997.
121. Rivett D, Higgs J. Hypothesis generation in the clinical reasoning behavior of manual therapists. *Phys Ther Educ*. 1997;11:40–45.
122. Twomey L. Introduction. *Aust J Physiotherapy*. 1986; 31:174.

# 3

# Orthopedic Manual Therapy Clinical Examination

## Objectives

- Define the purpose of the clinical examination.
- Outline the essential elements of the clinical examination.
- Review the two components of observation.
- Analyze the essential aspects of the subjective/history.
- Analyze the essential aspects of the objective/physical history.
- Review the purpose of a clinical test.
- Associate the findings of the examination and the clinical reasoning hypotheses.

## THE CLINICAL EXAMINATION PROCESS

The purpose of a clinical examination is to outline the movements, positions, or activities that produce, reduce, or selectively modify a patient's "familiar sign and symptoms," (**concordant sign**). Only during a systematic examination can a clinician outline the behavior of a patient's symptoms. This scheme is described as the *patient-response method*, a method that relies less on theory and more on immediate patient response. The patient-response model is designed to determine selected impairments and does not focus on the isolation of a dedicated pathology.

Gregory Grieve[1] wrote, "the meaning of each sign and symptom in itself has much greater importance for treatment indications than for diagnosis. It is not especially difficult to decide 'this is a degenerative joint condition'. We have to note how, and in what kind of patient . . . (examples of multiple variables associated with patient type) . . . and has a bearing on how we proceed, as does coexistent disease and past history."

Three different examination domains—observation, subjective (historical), and objective (physical)—impart essential information for treatment planning and endorse hypotheses of the type of physical impairment and related functional, physical, psychological, and social problems. These examination domains are outlined in detail in the following section of this chapter. Throughout the text-book, each region-specific section will follow the format outlined below.

1. Observation
2. Subjective (Patient History)
3. Objective Clinical Examination
   a. Structural Differentiation Tests
   b. Active Physiological Movements
   c. Passive Physiological Movements
   d. Passive Accessory Movements
   e. Clinical Special Tests

Structural differentiation tests are not always performed and may consist of highly sensitive clinical special tests or active movements with overpressure to "clear" a region. Although structural differentiation tests are generally performed earlier in the examination than clinical special tests, these tests are discussed further in the clinical special tests section of this chapter.

## OBSERVATION

**Observation** is informally divided into two categories: general inspection and introspection. The process of general inspection includes the examination of outwardly apparent factors that may or may not associate to the patient's impairment. Introspection includes the aggregation of outwardly apparent information with selected psychological and social factors potentially related to the patient's condition.

### General Inspection

The purpose of the **general inspection** is to examine visible static and movement-related defects for analysis during the subjective (history) and objective (physical) examination. Commonly, the static general inspection consists of skin (integument) inspection, posture, and body symmetry. Skin inspection may yield valuable information on past injuries (scars), inflammatory processes (redness, swelling), and sympathetic contributions to pain. Although posture and body symmetry alone do not dictate the presence of impairment, it is feasible to assume that these conditions may contribute to underlying pathologies. At present, there are no studies that have calculated any direct-predictive observational relationship with any form of progression or predisposition to spinal impairment.[2] Postural asymmetry has no correlation with back pain, and other forms of pelvic asymmetry are even less conclusive.[3] Nonetheless, dramatic postural faults are worth further investigation and can be the basis for future exploration in many anatomical regions, especially when examined in conjunction with other assessment concepts.[4–6] Although the observations may not be exclusively predictive, they can provide clinically useful information that improves the expansion of the treatment hypothesis.

### Introspection

**Introspection** allows the clinician to step back and analyze the relationship of nonphysical findings with physical findings. Examples include patient attitude, facial expressions during movement, expressions of pain, gender and the potential association to selected impairments, and believability. Patients may express a decreased willingness to move a finding that has been related to poor treatment outcomes.[7,8] Avoidance of certain movements because of fear of reinjury or increased pain is common in patients with chronic low back impairment.[8] This reluctance to move may lead to a cascade of further problems associated with disuse.

## Summary

- Observation involves the careful identification of potential contributors to the patient's impairments.
- The presence of a postural fault or body asymmetry does not dictate a pathology or impairment.
- Introspection involves the careful examination of both physical and non-physical contributors to the impairment.

# THE SUBJECTIVE/PATIENT HISTORY EXAMINATION

The *Guide to Physical Therapist Practice*[9] defines the history as the "systematic gathering of data, from both the past and the present." The history is a useful guide in outlining the ease in which symptoms are aggravated, the activities that contribute to the concordant sign, and the relationship to the physical measures assessed.[10] Generally, there are three major goals of a subjective examination. The first goal is to characterize the problem and to establish potential causes. The second goal is to determine the effect of the problem on patient lifestyle, and the third, to monitor the response to treatment for examination of effectiveness.[11]

Although history taking is often considered the most important aspect of a clinical evaluation, few studies have evaluated how subjective findings contribute to problem solving for treatment application.[11] Nonetheless, those that have investigated history taking are also stratified into diagnostic- and impairment-based methods. For clinicians who use a diagnostic-based examination method, history taking appears to play a favorable part, providing significant value in the diagnostic process.[12]

For clinicians who have adopted the impairment-based examination method, history and subjective findings have also demonstrated usefulness when combined with a purposeful physical examination. In studies that examined the history-taking strategies of clinical experts, engagement with the family and patient was more extensive, often prompting questions regarding the nature of the disorder versus questions that attempt to isolate a specific pathology.[10] Those who used the impairment-based model focused more on how the symptoms were related to movements and activities and less on how the symptoms were related to a diagnosis.[10]

The subjective consultation involves both clinician and patient expectations. Patients aspire to fully characterize their current symptoms and the impact of the disorder in both physical and psychological terms. Often, clinicians are interested in clustering selected signs and symptoms for the appropriate selection of a treatment intervention[11,13] or interpreting the nature and severity of the condition at hand.[10] In many cases, the desires of the two are not the same or may address different purposes.

Some evidence exists that supports that effective history taking is related to a desired outcome. Walker et al.[14] identified that subjective history, specifically report of activity requirements, was associated with future outcome and performance. By means of systematically obtaining information, a clinician can obtain information to the origin, contribution, and potential prognosis of a condition. Table 3.1 outlines the appropriate components of an effective subjective/history examination.

**TABLE 3.1**    The Systematic Process of the Subjective/History Examination

| Category | Primary Purpose |
|---|---|
| Mechanism and description of problem | To determine the cause of the injury and to elicit a careful explanation of the symptoms. |
| Concordant sign | To determine the movement associated with the pain of the individual. |
| Nature of the condition | To determine the severity, irritability, kind, and stage of the impairment. |
| Behavior of the symptoms | To understand how the symptoms change with time, movement, and activities. |
| Pertinent past and present medical history | To determine if potential related medical components are associated to this disorder, or may lead to retardation of healing. |
| Patient goals | To understand the patient's goal behind organized care. |
| The baseline (function or pain) | To elicit a baseline measure to reevaluate over time. |

## Mechanism and Description of Injury

The mechanism of the injury is the detailed recital of what the patient was doing when he or she injured him- or herself. In some circumstances, the mechanisms can provide useful information to the identification of the potential tissue. More importantly, the description of the injury provides a documentation of the "essence" of the problem. This involves two forms: (1) explanation and description of the injury-related pain; and (2) the timing of when the event occurred. The identification of the pain from the injury is further expounded during the discussion of the concordant sign and nature of the problem whereas the timing of the event is closely associated with the stage of the disorder. Both components enable the patient to meet their expectations of discussing the condition at hand.

## Concordant Sign

The concordant pain response is an activity or movement that provokes the patient's "familiar sign."[15] Laslett et al.[15] define the concordant "familiar sign" as the pain or other symptoms identified on a pain drawing and verified by the patient as being the complaint that has prompted one to seek diagnosis and treatment. Maitland[16] describes a similar focal point identified as the **comparable sign.** A comparable joint or neural sign refers to any combination of pain, stiffness, and spasm that the examiner finds upon examination and considers comparable with the patient's symptoms. This text uses the two terms synonymously and recognizes that Maitland's contribution to this concept has been more significant to orthopedic manual therapists.

Laslett et al.[15] suggests that one should focus on a patient's concordant (comparable) sign, and should distinguish this finding from other symptoms produced during physical assessment. They identify a finding that may be painful or abnormal, but not related to the concordant sign as the "discordant pain response." Essentially, a discordant pain response is the provocation of a pain that is unlike the pain for which the patient sought treatment.

Maitland[16] identifies a similar term, called the "joint sign." Like a **discordant sign,** the joint sign may appear to implicate a guilty structure but may not be associated with the pathology whatsoever. Maitland[16] suggests avoidance of the tendency to focus on joint signs, which he defines as any aspect of a movement that is "abnormal." Because the term "joint sign" is somewhat confusing and infers that the pain or abnormality of the region is solely associated with a joint, the term "discordant sign" is used within this textbook.

Although the concordant sign is queried during the patient history, this phenomenon is also a physical response determined during the objective exam, requires inspection during the physical assessment, and requires further examination throughout the length of the intervention. The concordant sign is often used as a litmus test to determine both mechanical and pain-related changes over time.

## The Nature of the Condition

The nature of the condition is a reflection of the internalization of a patient's condition. The nature of the condition may alter how the examination and treatment is performed and may influence the aggressiveness of the clinician. Although many manual therapy models use variations of "nature," there are typically three representative aspects explored by each: (1) severity, (2) irritability, and (3) stage.

### Severity of the Disorder

Severity is the subjective identification of how significantly this impairment has affected the patient. Typically, a severe problem will result in a reduction in activity of daily living functions, work-related problems, social disruption, and leisure activities. Severity may be associated with unwanted alterations or changes in lifestyle. The clinician should endeavor to determine where the patient's impairment lies on a continuum of nuisance or disability. Many functional outcomes scales are designed to measure the severity of the impairment and are effective in collecting aggregate data.

### Irritability

**Irritability,** or "reactivity," is a term used to define the stability of a present condition. In essence, irritability denotes how quickly a stable condition degenerates in the presence of pain-causing inputs. Irritable patients may often be leery of aggressive treatment because they will typically worsen with selected activities.[16-19] Patients who exhibit irritable symptoms may respond poorly to an aggressive examination and treatment approaches. Irritability is operationally defined using three criteria: (1) what does the patient have to do to set this condition off?, (2) once set off, how long do the symptoms last and how severe are the symptoms?, and (3) what does the patient have to do to calm the symptoms down? The irritability of the patient will guide the aggressiveness of the treatment and will dictate the selection of treatment procedures. Fundamentally, irritability dictates the aggressiveness of the treatment application.

One common pitfall is the assumption that acute disorders are always irritable. Although irritability is seen more commonly in acute disorders, chronic disorders may also demonstrate irritability. Subjective clues to the likely presence of irritability are: interrupted sleep, heavy doses of medications, limited levels of activity or activity avoidance, and/or a diagnosis suggesting serious pathology. Patients presenting with recent trauma, arachnoiditis, fractures, and acute arthritis are prone to being irritable. However, patients with chronic arthritis, especially osteoarthritis related to stiffness, are usually not irritable and may respond well to vigorous treatment.

Another pitfall is the supposition that irritability is synonymous with the "*super-pain*" patient. This thinking ignores that patients without pain, or without significant pain, can be irritable. Patients with serious pathology may not always present with significant pain. Patients with noteworthy neurological changes are often irritable and may demonstrate little or no pain. Overlooking the presence of irritability can cause serious consequences.[20]

Figure 3.1 illustrates the collective aspects of irritability. Because the three domains of irritability are dichotomous, the likelihood of all three being present synonymously is not 100%. Although irritability is often considered a single dimensional concept, in reality it is multidimensional, difficult to isolate using a binary definition, and may require the clinical judgment of the manual therapist.

### Stage

Most impairments change over time. A skilled manual clinician is able to understand the path or progression of the disorder, a concept identified as the "stage."[16] The stage of an injury or impairment involves a snapshot of how the patient identifies their current level of dysfunction as compared to a given point in the past. This allows examination of whether the condition has stabilized, stagnated, or progressed. Consequently, there are only three potential reports for the stage of a disorder: worse, better, or the same.

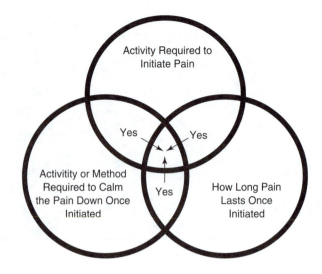

**Figure 3.1**    The Three Dichotomous Stages of Irritability

The stage of a disorder identifies the "snapshot" of that patient's condition in a cycle of natural progression. The cycle of an injury is very complicated and involves numerous steps. The onset of an injury often leads to an inflammatory process and a consequential cascade of comorbidities. First, muscle inhibition is common and can lead to decreased active stability at the sight of an injury. Decreased stability can lead to increased capsuloligamentous laxity and hypermobility.[21] As demand is placed upon the joint segment, reflexogenic spasm attempts to stabilize the region.[22-25] Unfortunately, this mechanism often contributes to muscular pain, ineffective stabilization, and supplementary weakness.[26,27] The joint no longer tracks or responds efficiently to required demands. Because the joint is unable to stabilize effectively against outside forces, continued trauma leads to degeneration of the segments. Throughout the process of degeneration, reflexive spasms continue in a subconscious attempt to stabilize the segment.[28] This degeneration culminates into boney, cartilage, and ligamentous changes that modify the arthrokinematics of the segment.[29] These changes are the hallmark components associated with losses in range of motion.[30] Figure 3.2 outlines the lifespan of an unopposed injury and suggests the potential stages along the cycle.

### Behavior of Symptoms

There are three aspects of the "behavior" of the pain: (1) time, (2) response to movements, and (3) area. First, it is critical to determine how the pain changes over a 24-hour period. Conditions associated with inflammation may worsen during rest or aggressive movements.[16] Noninflammatory conditions may worsen during very aggressive, unguarded movements. Sinister problems (nonmechanical disorders that are potentially life threatening) often yield worsening symptoms at night. Second, the behavior of the symptoms is necessary to determine whether a specific

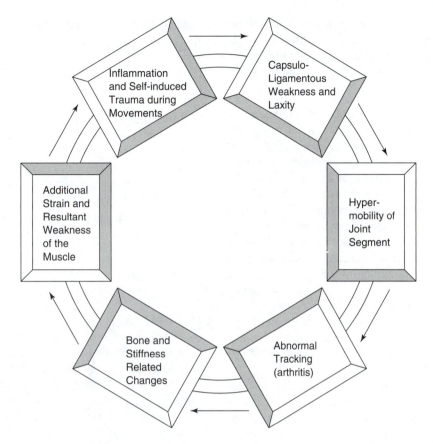

**Figure 3.2**    The Lifespan of an Unopposed Injury

movement pattern exists. Some conditions are worse in various postures or positions whereas others demonstrate improvement or deterioration during repeated movements. Third, isolation of the area of the symptoms is necessary to determine potentially contributing structures. In some conditions, there may be more than one site of pain.[31] Regardless of the tissue diagnosis, the patient should be questioned regarding neighboring tissues. Failure to ascertain the total area of symptoms may lead to inappropriate or incomplete administration of treatment.

## Pertinent Past and Present History

The pertinent past and present history assist in identifying contributing components that may affect the presence of the impairment. An investigation of similar past conditions, related disorders, and general health considerations yields valuable information. One may ask relevant medical questions as well within this domain, including information to distill potential red flags to recovery (Chapter Five). Lastly, associative medications, surgeries, and comparable past and present treatment may generate ideas for effective care.

The *Guide to Physical Therapist Practice*[9] suggests the administration of a systems review when assessing pertinent medical history. The systems review is a brief or limited examination of the anatomical and physiological status of the cardiopulmonary, integumentary, and neuromuscular systems as well as the affect, cognitive status, and learning style of the patient. Exploring the potential contributions of these components to a musculoskeletal-based problem assists the clinician in identifying possible problems that require outside consultation to a more appropriate provider.[9]

## Patient Goals

The patient's goals will drive what the patient hopes to get out of the rehabilitation experience. The goals should also influence the treatment plan since these will be the milestones for the patient. Although there is little research in this area, there does appear to be a relationship between the selected goals and the patient and the likelihood of accomplishing the outcome. In a recent study that investigated return-to-work, the patient's return-to-work date (goal) was the single best predictor of return to work outcome. In contrast, increased number of premorbid jobs, compensation status, and the patient's race and sex were not predictive. This suggests that the assessment of an individual's motivation (by using goal-setting) may be a key factor in predicting a favorable outcome.[32]

Another benefit of obtaining a list of patients' goals is the ability to assess their perception or expectations of their outcome. It is probable that that patient who does not expect an efficacious treatment outcome will not recover as quickly as one who expects an efficacious outcome. Additionally, the patient goal is a reflection of his or her perceived assessment of the nature of the problem.

### The Baseline

The **baseline** is the base performance or pain indicator prior to the treatment intervention. For a quick reference, one can use an iteration of a visual analog scale (a 0–10 pain scale)[32,33], appropriate range-of-motion measurements, or some other easily repeatable value. Since the baseline is measured during each assessment position, each treatment, and during the beginning and end of each session, this simple comparative value should lack complexity but represent an overall picture of the condition at hand. Additionally, a baseline measure of function provides comparable and essential information for future measurement. Numerous functional outcome measurement scales exist that measure general or region-specific constructs. Functional outcome measurement scales allow quantification of the impact of the impairment on the performance of common activities of daily living, psychological impact, and socially related changes.[34,35,36]

Two forms of measurement scales—generic- and region-specific—exist, each with professed benefits. Region-specific scales are thought to exhibit greater sensitivity to change and display greater content validity[37], while generic-specific questionnaires are considered more psychometrically sound and may have the capability of measuring health status across multiple bodily dimensions.[37]

Functional outcome scales are characterized by their properties of reliability, validity, and responsiveness to clinical changes. These properties ensure that data are collected and interpreted in a systematic and reproducible way, allowing comparison between different patient populations.[37]

Reliability is a property that measures consistency and reproducibility. Two forms of reliability—internal consistency and temporal stability—are required. Internal consistency indicates whether the items constituting a scale are highly intercorrelated, measuring the same concept or construct.[37] Temporal stability is the ability of the instrument to provide repeatable information over a given period of time.

Validity indicates that the measure criteria within the outcome scale principally measures the construct it is intended to measure rather than some other related construct.[37] Four types of validity are commonly reported: face, content, criterion-related, and construct validity.

Responsiveness is the ability of an instrument to detect small but important clinical changes.[37] The minimal clinically important difference (MCID) is the pre-to-post change in instrument value that is determined to be significantly improved or worsened. A highly responsive instrument is capable of detecting a "clinically important change," as a result of the treatment or patient perception.

### Putting the Subjective/History Examination Findings Together

By the end of the subjective/history, the clinician should have the following criteria:

1. Post-subjective set of competing hypotheses (an educated guess of the primary structures involved and the potential pain generators). The post-subjective hypotheses may allow the clinician to isolate certain components of the objective examination for more specific findings.

2. An understanding of the patient's applicability for manual therapy. Some clues within the subjective ex-

## Summary

- The history is a useful guide in outlining the ease in which symptoms are aggravated, the activities that contribute to the concordant sign, and the relationship to the physical measures assessed.
- The history is often considered the most important aspect of the examination.
- There are seven primary components of the subjective history: the mechanism and description of injury, the concordant sign, the nature of the problem, the behavior of the symptoms, the pertinent past and present medical history, the patient's goals, and the baseline. Each has a specific purpose.
- The purpose of the mechanism and description of the injury is to determine the cause of the injury and to elicit a careful explanation of the symptoms.
- The purpose of determining the concordant sign is to determine the movement associated with the pain of the individual.
- The purpose determining the nature of the problem is to determine the severity, irritability, kind, and stage of the impairment.
- The purpose of determining the behavior of the symptoms is to understand how the symptoms change with time, movement, and activities.
- The purpose of determining the pertinent past and present medical history is to determine if potential related medical components are associated to this disorder, or may lead to retardation of healing.
- The purpose in determining the patient's goals is to understand the patient's goal behind organized care.
- The purpose behind eliciting a baseline measure is to reevaluate over time.

amination (such as report of stiffness) may drive the selection of manual therapy methods of examination and treatment.

3. The nature of the problem. The nature of the problem is characterized by the severity, irritability, and stage of the condition. These three areas provide information that can modify the vigor of the examination and treatment.

4. The patient's expectations and prediction of the outcome (through goals). Often, the patients' goals and expectations will drive their participation within the program. Additionally, this provides communication between the patient and clinician for use later during the intent of the treatment.

5. The concordant sign of the patient and a hypothesis of what physical activities may be associated with it. The concordant sign will drive the examination and the treatment. The concordant sign, although also a manifestation of the physical examination, is the most important aspect of the manual therapists' examination.

# THE OBJECTIVE/PHYSICAL EXAMINATION

The objective/physical examination's principal aim is to establish the effect of movement on the patient's concordant symptoms that were described during the subjective/history.[9,31] By assessing movement, the clinician is more likely to determine the contributory muscles, joint, or ligaments involved in the patient's condition that are responsible for the concordant signs and symptoms. Most importantly, the use of movement to alter symptoms enables determination of an appropriate treatment method and how that method would positively or negatively contribute to the patient's condition. This irrefutable evidence is specific for that single patient and improves the likelihood of a positive outcome during treatment.

Orthopedic manual therapy treatment areas encompass innumerable methods of classification. In essence, most techniques will take the form of three particular categories, each based on the method of application and participation by the patient. For clarification, these skilled methods are outlined in the following three categories:

1. *Active movements* (including active physiological techniques performed exclusively by the patient).

2. *Passive movements* (including passive physiological, passive accessory, and combined passive movements performed exclusively by the clinician).

3. *Clinical special testing* (includes palpation, muscle provocation testing, upper and lower motor screening, differentiation tests, neurological testing, and any specific clinical tests designed to implicate a lesion).

## Active Movements

**Active movements** are any form of physiological movements performed exclusively by the patient (Figure 3.3). In a clinical examination, the purpose of an active movement is to identify and examine the effect of selected active movements on the concordant sign. By determining the behavior of the concordant sign to selected movements, the clinician can effectively identify potential active physiological treatment approaches.

It has been suggested that the pattern associated with active movements may be beneficial in identifying selected impairments. McKenzie has developed a classification scheme for the lower back using this philosophy.[38] Using McKenzie's approach the patient's response to postural and repeated movements is recorded and classified for potential treatment application. Active movement patterns have also been suggested as helpful in implicating contractile versus noncontractile components; when scrutinized, this method of assessment is not precise and has not held up irrefutably.[39,40] Additionally, selected active movements are often assigned as home exercise programs and adjuncts to passive treatments.

The recommended procedure within this textbook for exploring the benefit of active movement assessment involves three stages of movements and an examination of the patient response during these stages. The initial movement involves a single active movement to the initiation of pain, if pain occurs prior to the limit or end range. The movement is held in this position and the patient's pain is assessed for change. This procedure is followed by movement past the pain to the limit (if the patient is able to move to this point). Again, the patient is asked to hold this position to determine the behavior of the pain. Lastly, the patient is asked to repeat the movement at end range to further assess the response of the patient.

1. The patient moves to the first point of pain (response is assessed).

2. The patient then moves beyond the pain and holds (response is assessed).

3. The patient then repeats the movement to determine if pain or range changes (response is assessed).

In the absence of pain, an **overpressure** is applied. The use of overpressure is designed to "rule out" potential joints, which do not contribute to the patient's impairment and may be useful in isolating various impairments.[41,42] Overpressure is less effective when one attempts to dictate the presence of a specific pathology based on "feel" of the end range. An overpressure should be limited to differentiation between the concordant signs versus discordant signs and symptoms, or to identify when no symptoms are present.

There are several conjectures to examine when evaluating the effect of active movement on impairment. First, positive patient responses include an increase of range of

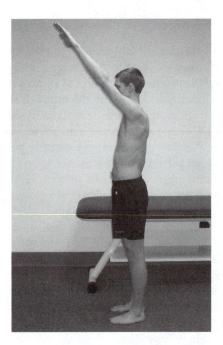

**Figure 3.3**    Active Movement (Shoulder Flexion)

motion, a reduction of pain, or both. The procedure (i.e., movement into flexion, abduction, internal rotation, etc.) that was responsible for the greatest abolition of pain or increase in range is considered the best potential selection for treatment. Second, if symptoms were produced, how did the symptoms respond to single or repeated movements? Often, repeated movements will abolish symptoms, especially during mechanical dysfunction.[43] Third, where within the range did the symptoms worsen? End-range pain is typically associated with a mechanical impairment while mid- or through-range pain may be indicative of an inflammatory impairment or instability.[16,44] Fourth, it is imperative to investigate how the patient yields to a particular movement. Since the intent to treat may require repeated movements into a movement that is initially painful, it is important to consider how faithful the patient would commit to adoption of this potential strategy. Lastly, are there other factors that could potentially contribute to this problem? Is the movement sequential? Does there appear to be a range restriction or hypermobility? Is weakness a consideration?

## Passive Movements

**Passive movements** are any planar or physiological motions that are performed exclusively by the clinician. The purpose of a passive movement is to identify and examine the effect of selected passive movements (repeated or static) on the concordant sign. Passive movements include (1) passive physiological motions, (2) passive accessory movements, and (3) combined passive movements.

### Passive physiological movements

Maitland[31] describes passive physiological movement (Figure 3.4) as "movement which is actively used in the

many functions of the musculoskeletal system." Passive physiological movements are commonly defined in kinesiological literature as osteokinematic motions and generally are categorized using planer-based descriptors such as flexion, extension, adduction, abduction, and medial or lateral rotation. Passive physiological movements occur simultaneously with accessory motions; the degree of freedom and the availability of motion is a product of that accessory mobility.

Assessment of passive physiological movement is useful to differentiate total range of motion at a particular joint segment. Cyriax[40] claimed that passive physiological movements were necessary to assess the contribution of ligaments, capsule, and other inert structures to the cause of the impairment. In occasions where patients are unable or are fearful to move the joint to the end range, the apparent range may be mistakenly assessed as limited. To determine the true range of motion, a passive physiological movement is required.

The examination procedure for passive physiological movements is similar to the active physiological process. First, the patient is moved passively to the first point of pain identified by the patient. At that point, the amount and intensity of the pain is recorded by the clinician. Next, the patient is moved beyond the first point of pain and held in that position. Again, the patient is examined for response. Lastly, the patient is moved repeatedly near the limit of motion and changes in range or pain are recorded.

*Procedure for Examination of Passive Physiological Range*

1. The patient's selected body part is moved to the first point of reported pain (response is assessed).
2. The patient is then moved beyond the pain and held (response is assessed).
3. The clinician then repeats the movement to determine if pain or range changes (response is assessed).

This within-session process of examining symptoms has been shown to correctly identify the patients who are most likely to demonstrate between-session changes.[45] Al-

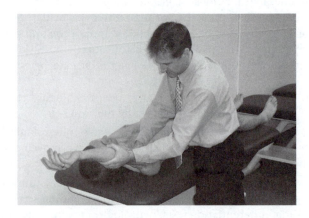

**Figure 3.4**    Passive Physiological Movement (Shoulder Flexion)

though laborious, this process provides the most specific marriage between the examination and potential treatment options.

### Passive Accessory Movements

Grieve[1] indicates that a passive accessory movement (Figure 3.5) is "any movement mechanically or manually applied to a body with no voluntary muscular activity by the patient." Passive accessory mobilizations are best divided into two forms: regional and local mobilizations. Regional mobilizations involve directed, passive movement to more than one given area, segment, or physiological component, while local mobilization is specific and directed to one segmental and/or joint region.[1] Within the spine, the majority of mobilization procedures advocated within this textbook involve regional mobilizations. Posterior–anterior (PA) mobilizations involve three-point movements of the primary targeted and neighboring segments.[46,47] To date, the specific selection of the mobilization technique used on the spine is less essential as the ability to correctly identify the appropriate targeted segments.[48]

Techniques that qualify as local mobilization require a locking of the adjacent joint segments to foster greater movement at the targeted level. Generally, locking occurs through a procedure called apposition, which occurs when joint surfaces are most congruent and when ligamentous structures are maximally taut.[49] When treating the spine, targeting the appropriate level leads to better outcomes than when a randomly selected joint is treated.[50] Whether or not the specific locking of a joint is required to achieve this benefit is still unknown.

Some authors have suggested that passive accessory movements are effective for passively engaging selected components of the capsule and ligament. For optimum assessment, passive assessment should occur at multiple ranges throughout the physiological availability to determine range–pain behavior. Additionally, passive movements throughout the range of motion will provide range–pain behavior. Some authors identify the range differences as "open-packed" and "closed-packed" positions. Closed-packed positions are those that theoretically tighten the ligaments and capsule maximally and create maximal congruency of a joint. Open-packed positions are those positions that do not place maximal tension on the capsule, and have been described by Cyriax[40] and Kaltenborn.[51] Mobilization at end range or the closed-packed position may be useful if stiffness is the primary concern. A particular close-packed position could vary from one individual to another or may be associated with the pathological condition of the individual. Despite the widespread use of paradigms such as capsular patterns and theoretical closed-packed positions, this method of categorizing inert tissue has not stood up well to scrutiny and may be inappropriate for selected tissues.[52–55]

During the examination procedure for passive accessory movements, the articular movements are evaluated for reproduction of the concordant sign. Using either a translatory or rolling motion, the patient's segment is moved passively to the first point of pain identified by the patient; the intensity of the pain is then recorded by the clinician using some mechanism of scale. Next, the clinician applied a force that moves the segment beyond the first point of pain. The joint is held in that position and the response of the patient is re-elicited. Lastly, the clinician uses repeated movements near the limit of motion to determine if changes in range or pain have occurred.

1. The patient's selected body part is moved to the first point of reported pain (response is assessed).
2. The patient is then moved beyond the pain and held (response is assessed).
3. The clinician then repeats or sustains the movement to determine if pain or range changes (response is assessed).

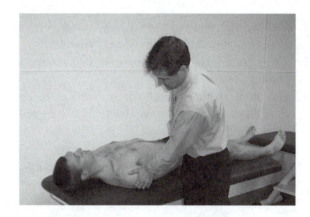

**Figure 3.5**   Passive Accessory Movement (Shoulder Flexion)

### Combined Movements

Brian Edwards[9] purported that **combined movements** (Figure 3.6) are habitual movements of the spine, and that "movements of the vertebral column occur in combination across planes rather than as pure movements in one plane." Movements of the periphery are also adopted in this definition. Therefore, a physical examination should be expanded to include combined movements since the standard movements of lateral flexion, extension and flexion, and occasionally rotation are single-plane movements.

Combined movements are frequently used during manipulative procedures. Often, coupling movements are termed in osteopathic literature as a "locked" position.[49] Grieve[1] states that "the appreciation of the difference between the feel of a 'locked' joint and one that has not achieved a 'crisp or locked' end-feel is vital in determining the appropriate combined movement."[56] Cyriax[40] has proposed a measurement system to describe end feels among various joints. Although the end feel characterization is not combined-movement specific, the reliability of end feel assessment based on Cyriax's theories is mixed.[52,57] Those studies that examined the presence of pain and abnormal end feel concurrently[58] or provided further education constructs associated with end feel[59] demonstrated the best interrater reliability. The reliability of ligamentous detection methods that do not use a categorical system such as Cyriax has fared much worse.[60,61]

In the periphery, combined movements are often necessary to place tension on selected ligamentous and capsular structures. For example, in the shoulder, maximal tension for the posteroinferior glenohumeral ligament occurs during internal rotation and elevation whereas maximal tension of the posterosuperior capsule occurs during internal rotation at lower shoulder elevations.[62] Subsequently, to engage the numerous capsular and ligamentous components, one would be required to move the shoulder into combined, multiphysiological positions.

The same process as active and passive movement examination is relevant for combined movements.

1. The patient's selected body part is moved to the first point of reported pain (response is assessed).
2. The patient is then moved beyond the pain and held (response is assessed).
3. The clinician then repeats the movement to determine if pain or range changes (response is assessed).

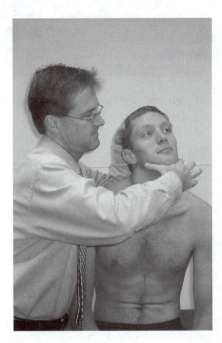

**Figure 3.6**    Combined Movement of the Upper Cervical Spine

Combined movements may have many flavors. For example, two active movements can be combined, as can two physiological or accessory motions. Additionally, the combination of an active physiological with a passive physiological, active physiological with a passive accessory, or a passive accessory with a passive physiological can increase the number of potential movements dramatically.

### Fine-Tuning Mechanisms

Like active movement assessment, there are several conjectural considerations to examine when evaluating the effect of passive movement on impairment. For the most part, they are the same as those found during active movements. If the patient reports decreased pain, increased range, or both during the movement, the action that was responsible for the greatest abolition of pain or increase in range is considered the best potential selection for a treatment. The movements should be assessed for best response, whether it is single or repeated. If the pain is at end range, repeated movements should abolish the symptoms versus mid-range movements for patients with pain dominance. Often, an assessment is made whether a patient is applicable for manipulation during both passive physiological and passive accessory movements.[63]

Since assessment of passive accessory movement mandates an analysis of concordant pain behavior through various means, one should optimize the use of differentiation of targeted pain generators (i.e., one spine level versus another; the origin of pain from the shoulder versus the cervical spine). Many forms of impairment have associated aches and pains, yet the concordant sign is the passive movement that most appropriately isolates the true impairment.[15]

Lee et al.[64] outline variables that may alter both assessment findings and treatment outcome during application of accessory movements. Although the authors presented these variables with respect to application during spinal examination and treatment, there is overlay to peripheral tissues. Because each variable may be altered by the manual therapy clinician, we will discuss these in the context of examination in this chapter, and in the context of treatment in Chapter 4.

### Magnitude of Force

The magnitude of the force will clearly affect the amount of joint displacement.[64] In studies that have investigated the spine, a reasonable pattern has emerged. Increases in applied force will result in corresponding increases in linear displacement.[65] Most studies have suggested that a critical threshold exists before linear movement occurs. Prior to reaching the threshold, low load forces will most likely move soft tissues and will not result in linear movements. Lee et al.[64] claim that the range for linear assessment appears to exist in the order of 30–100 Newtons. Edwards[66] suggests that although the force for initial assessment is typically taken to the first point of pain, in some cases, it is necessary to push beyond to acquire reasonable joint behavioral characteristics. Often (i.e., with inflammatory conditions, the first point of pain occurs early within the assessment and may not engage the 30–100 threshold. Failure to meet each joint's specific threshold most likely represents failure to comprehensively analyze the movement of that given segment.

## Rate of Increase of Force

Fung[67] suggests that increases in the frequency of mobilization will result in an increase in resistance to deformation. Thus, it is expected that during a manual assessment, an increase in frequency during linear assessment of a given segment may appear stiffer. Consequently, frequency of the accessory motion during the assessment will alter the clinician's identification of stiffness and this creates another intrinsic variable that alters interrater reliability.

## Duration of Loading

There is some controversy regarding the effects of tissue mobility during the application of load over a given time. Lee et al.[64] reports that prolonged load results in an increase in deformation. Shirley et al.[68] reported an increase in stiffness and displacement. Subsequently, repeated loads over time will lead to greater stiffness assessment at end range, although linear movements prior to end range should increase.

## Targeted Tissue to Which the Force Is Applied

In the spine, the segment is a significant predictor of the detection of stiffness. Contributions from the pelvis, other segments, and from the respiratory system[68] can alter the assessment of stiffness per segment. Morphological characteristics may alter findings as well, since soft tissue is both a supportive mechanism during application in force and is generally the first tissue displaced during assessment.

## Location of Manual Force in Relation to Center of the Targeted Structure

Maitland suggests that for optimum reliability across assessments, the starting point of assessment should be near the center of the targeted structures.[16] Lee[69] confirmed that a substantial effect does exist depending on where the force is applied on the targeted segment.

## Direction of Force

The direction of mobilization forces can alter the amount of stiffness measured by machines and perceived by therapists. Caling and Lee[70] determined that stiffness measured at plus or minus 10° from a perpendicular base direction (defined as the mean direction of force applied by experienced therapists), was from 7 to 10% less than the stiffness measured in the perpendicular direction. Minor variations in joint assessment position can theoretically alter the response of the patient. However, Chiradejnant et al.[48] reported that the direction of the technique made little difference in the outcome of the patient. Randomly selected spine mobilization techniques performed at the targeted level demonstrated no difference when compared to therapist-selected techniques.

## Contact Area over Which the Force Is Applied

Lee et al.[64] state, "Although for many purposes, a manual force can be considered to be applied at one point, in reality there is a distribution of force over a finite area of skin surface." Consequently, differences of interpretation of joint mobility may occur based on the method used for skin contact. Several common assessment methods are currently used, including the thumbs, pisiform, and other contact points of the hand.

# Clinical Special Testing

There are three purposes of a **clinical special test.** First, a series of clinical special tests are often used to provide the examiner with additional information regarding the nature of the condition. For example, palpation and manual provocation tests lend support to the findings of certain impairments but yield little information in the absence of the movement examination. The second purpose is to provide diagnostic value to a set of findings. Third, clinical special tests may be useful in ruling out (structural differentiation) a particular region if the tests demonstrate a high degree of sensitivity. We will initially discuss the first proposed set of benefits of a clinical special test.

## The Use of Clinical Special Tests as Supportive Information

### Palpation

Cyriax writes, "Palpation used by itself regularly deceives."[40] Palpation may be useful when performed near the end of treatment once the clinician has identified the series of concordant movements by the patient. Yet when used early or without clarification of a movement-based assessment, palpation may be of limited value. Palpation demonstrates poor reliability when tested during motion detection of the spine, but does yield useful information during analysis of the rotator cuff, temporomandibular joint, and tendonitis.[71–73] Additionally, palpation is useful to implicate a pain generator when referred pain of the patient's concordant sign occurs during palpation of a particular structure.[40]

### Muscle Provocation Testing

The purpose of **muscle provocation testing** is to determine the "guilt" of contractile versus noncontractile tissue. A method described as "selective tension testing" was first acknowledged by Cyriax.[40] He proposed that contractile tissues (muscle, tendon, and bony insertion) are painful during an applied isometric contraction and inert structures (capsule, ligaments, bursae) are painful during passive movement. He furthered this definition by providing subdefinitions to the findings of the provocation tests. He suggested that a finding of *strong* and *painless* suggests that contractile tissue is not involved. *Strong* and *painful* indicates there is a minor lesion of the contractile tissue. *Weak* and *painless* may be a sign of complete rupture of the contractile tissue or it may be a disorder of the nervous system. *Weak* and *painful* indicates a major lesion. If all movements are painful one should consider that affective component or a sinister pathology may be the chief generator of pain. Lastly, if the tested muscle group is strong and painless but hurts after several repetitions the examiner should suspect intermittent claudication.

As discussed in Chapter 2, the scientific evidence to support this elaborate set of findings is mixed. Pellecchia et al.[74] and Fritz et al.[75] found acceptable reliability and clinical usefulness with this tool. Others[39,52] have reported that the model lacks validity and reliability.

Finally, the traditional **manual muscle test** is also used as a clinical special test to implicate weakness at selected muscles. The studies are also mixed[76–78] but a growing amount of evidence supports the use of this testing method when a handheld device is used for a more specific detection[79–82] and when the plus and minus categories are discarded.[78] Standardized criteria are outlined in Table 3.2.

## The Use of Clinical Special Tests for Diagnostic Value

The second purpose of a clinical special test is to provide **diagnostic value.** Diagnostic value may take two forms: (1) to evaluate and form a hypothesis for labeling a specific pathology or (2) to classify a cluster of symptoms for selection of an intervention. Essentially, high-quality clinical special tests are designed to discriminate a subgroup of homogeneous characteristics from a heterogeneous pool of patients with dysfunction[83] or to confirm a tentative diagnosis to make a differential diagnosis to differentiate between structures or to unravel difficult signs and symptoms.[84]

There are four characteristics to a well-performed analysis of a clinical special test. First, the clinical special test must be compared to a reference standard that best defines the condition of interest.[85,86] In most cases, the best reference standard is surgical intervention. Unfortunately, the majority of studies have used more readily available methods such as traditional diagnostic tests.

Given the relative diagnostic values of many traditional diagnostic tests such as the MRI, CT-scan, and others, many clinical special tests have inherent flaws. Additionally, the reference point should be independent of the test itself. One challenge in using patient report of symptoms or clinician interpretation is the risk of bias. Independent methods reduce the risk since they do not coincide with the application of the clinical special test.

Second, the study should be free from spectrum bias.[86] Spectrum bias is present when study subjects are not representative of the population in which the test is generally applied, or may occur when the only population that is tested is highly impaired and has a greater than average likelihood of having the impairment. Often, spectrum bias will overtly improve the sensitivity of a test and bias the diagnostic value. Unfortunately, the very tool that increases the validity of a clinical special test, the reference standard, can also increase the spectrum bias of a study. For example, if the clinical special test was performed only on patients who were to receive a selected form of surgical intervention, the likelihood of obtaining a sensitive response is high, thus biasing the sensitivity of the test.

Third, the clinical special test should lack variance in application, should dictate specific procedural processes that all study members follow, and should have appropriate blinding by examiners. Many clinical special tests lack uniformity, thus reduce the ability for cross-comparison of different studies. In some studies, the procedure is either poorly described or lacks any technical description for reproduction. Since many clinical studies lack blinding by the examiners these studies may be subject to selection bias. Some clinicians may have a predisposition to select a positive or negative consequence based on past experience or personal preference.

Lastly, the clinical special test should contain the appropriate threshold or cut-off score. Altering the cut-off point that determines whether a test is positive or negative can significantly affect the sensitivity and specificity of a test. In some cases the results of a clinical special test are inconclusive and do not yield findings that are above or below the threshold. Bossuyt et al.[87] recommend the use

**TABLE 3.2**    The Five Categories of a Graded Traditional Manual Muscle Test

| Grade | Description |
| --- | --- |
| V | Patient holds the position against maximum resistance throughout the complete range of motion. |
| IV | Patient holds the position against strong to moderate resistance and demonstrates full range of motion. |
| III | Patient tolerates no resistance but performs the movement through the full range of motion. |
| II | Patient demonstrates movement all or partial range of motion in the gravity-eliminated position. |
| I | The muscle/muscles are palpable while the patient is performing the action in the gravity-eliminated position. |
| 0 | No contractile activity is felt in the gravity-eliminated position. |

of a third category to define tests that are indeterminate. Because the failure to find a positive or negative could significantly affect the diagnostic usefulness of a test, this consequence should be identified in clinical special test studies.

Along with methodological strength during testing, a discriminatory clinical special test should be reliable, sensitive, and/or specific. Reliability is the estimate to which a test score is free from error and if erroneous the degree in which the value varies from a true score.[88] The sensitivity of a test is the ability of the test to identify a positive finding when the targeted diagnosis is actually present while few who have the disorder are mistakenly missed.[89] Specificity is the discriminatory ability of a test to identify if the disease or condition is absent when in actuality it truly is absent.[89] The sensitivity and specificity values are then used to calculate positive and negative likelihood ratios and a diagnostic odds ratio. A positive likelihood ratio (+LR) identifies the strength of a test in determining the presence of a finding. A value of 1 indicates an equivocal strength of diagnostic power; values that are higher suggest greater strength. The likelihood ratio for a negative result (−LR) identifies how much the odds of the disease decrease when a test is negative. The lower the value the better the ability of the test to determine the chance the disease is actually present in the event the finding is negative. A number closer to one indicates that a negative test is equally likely to occur in individuals with or without the disease.

Consider the following example involving a study of the straight leg raise (SLR) and the likelihood of ruling in or out the presence of a herniated disc. In our hypothetical example, the reference standard with surgery and the population of individuals included patients with and without disc herniation. The administrators were blinded to the subject's classification and all the preceding methodological suggestions were followed. One hundred sixty seven individuals were included in the study and 29 were found by the reference standard to exhibit a positive disc herniation. Of the 29, nine exhibited a positive SLR (true positive) and 20 did not (false negative). Of the 138 asymptomatic patients included in the study, 16 presented with a positive test (false positive), and 122 did not (true negative). Upon post-test analysis, the sensitivity of the SLR for reproduction of radicular pain was 31% (9/29). The specificity of the SLR was 88.4% (122/138). The +LR ratio for the SLR was 2.68 (.31/(1 − .884)) a likelihood measurement indicating those who demonstrate a positive test are over two and a half times as likely to rule in the presence of low back pain pathology. The −LR was 0.79 ((1 − .31)/.884), a number representing greater odds in ruling out pathology. Because a higher number for a negative likelihood ratio represents a poorer discriminatory value (number closer to zero is better at ruling out a disorder), this finding suggests weak inequitable selection power.[89]

It is essential to recognize that only when a clinical special test demonstrates good reliability and diagnostic value may it effectively contribute to appropriate differential diagnosis and/or treatment decision making. An astounding number of clinical special clinical tests demonstrate poor diagnostic value, are overused or used out of context, and often lend very little to a clinician's examination process.[90] Table 3.3 provides a guideline for acceptable diagnostic values of a clinical special test.

**TABLE 3.3    Diagnostic Value Guidelines (Revised from Jaeschke et al.[112])**

| +LR | Interpretation |
|---|---|
| > 10 | Large and often conclusive increase in the likelihood of disease |
| 5–10 | Moderate increase in the likelihood of disease |
| 2–5 | Small increase in the likelihood of disease |
| 1–2 | Minimal increase in the likelihood of disease |
| 1 | No change in the likelihood of disease |

| −LR | Interpretation |
|---|---|
| 1 | No change in the likelihood of disease |
| 0.5–1.0 | Minimal decrease in the likelihood of disease |
| 0.2–0.5 | Small decrease in the likelihood of disease |
| 0.1–0.2 | Moderate decrease in the likelihood of disease |
| < 0.1 | Large and often conclusive decrease in the likelihood of disease |

+LR = Positive likelihood ratio
−LR = Negative likelihood ratio

## *The Use of Clinical Special Tests as Structural Differentiation Tests*

The third benefit of clinical special tests is for use during region and structure differentiation. Structural identification allows the clinician to target movement assessment at the appropriate bodily regions. Cues collected from the subjective examination outline which area the clinician should focus the tests and measures. Generally, the clinician performs one to several structural differentiation tests to confirm the correct origin of the dysfunction. This is necessary when a patient is unable to provide a definitive region or when the symptoms suggest overlap or confusion between different bodily regions; the clinician should differentiate each region using quick structural differentiation tests. Quality differentiation tests demonstrate a high degree of sensitivity and are easily provoked when impairment is present. Since the clinician is interested in differentiating structures, a negative test (for a test and measure with high sensitivity) is telling and suggests that symptoms are not present in that region. Selected clinical special tests with high sensitivity such as the hip scour and cervical and lumbar quadrant may be useful at ruling out regions. Otherwise, the use of overpressures after active movements help rule out a particular region as well.

## Summary

- The purpose of the objective/physical examination's principal aim is to establish the effect of movement on the patient's symptoms that were described during the subjective/history.
- There are three primary areas of the objective/physical examination: (1) active movements, (2) passive movements, and (3) clinical special tests.
- Active movements include all motions performed exclusively by the patient.
- Passive movements include all motions performed by the clinician and may be physiological, accessory, or combined.
- Clinical special tests include clinical special tests, palpation, and manual muscle testing.

## Putting the Objective/Physical Examination Findings Together

By the end of the objective/physical examination the clinician should have the following criteria:

1. A strong understanding of the causal pain-generating region.
2. An understanding of which active movements increase or decrease the pain associated with the concordant sign.
3. An understanding of which active movements increase, decrease, or normalize range of motion.
4. An understanding of which passive movements increase or decrease the pain associated with the concordant sign.
5. An understanding of which passive movements increase, decrease, or normalize range of motion.
6. An understanding of the potential pain generator based on movement, positional, and palpatory findings.
7. An understanding of a potential diagnosis based on the examination and clinical test findings.
8. A strong association between the subjective and objective findings (a marriage of the information).

## Summary

- By the end of the objective/physical examination the clinician should have an understanding of which movements alter the concordant sign, which movements alter the range of motion, and which potential treatment methods could be associated with the examination results.

# POST-EXAMINATION CLINICAL REASONING

Upon completion of the examination, the data presented by the patient should allow two primary theoretical conclusions. First, the clinician should have a strong understanding of the movements that negatively or positively affect the concordant sign of the patient. Second, the clinician should have a moderate understanding of where the patient presents regarding **stiffness** (mechanical) and pain (inflammatory) dominance. This is accomplished by analyzing the motion-induced pain during both active and passive movement examinations. Pain during the initiation and/or midrange of movement is typically caused by inflammatory changes whereas pain near end range is mechanical or stiffness by nature.[91]

Within the primary stiffness and pain characterization, there are four highly variable, potential patient presentations. These include: (1) corresponding pain-dominance and hypomobility; (2) corresponding pain-dominance with hypermobility; (3) corresponding hypomobility and limited or no pain; and (4) corresponding limited or no report of pain with hypermobility. Within the four variables, different presentations are possible and one area may be emphasized over another. Of the four extreme selections, the fourth choice, limited or no pain but hypermobility, is less frequently treated by manual therapists because the patient will often demonstrate no functional impairment.

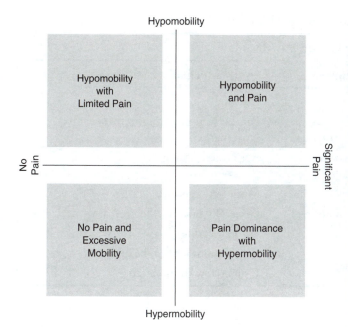

**Figure 3.7**   The Pain/Stiffness Grid

Figure 3.7 outlines the pain and stiffness grid and is adapted from the conceptualizations of others.[31,92,93] The grids represent potential characteristics based on the two potential linear presentations of pain and stiffness. The quadrangle not only allows variations of pain and stiffness but variations within a specific quadrant. For example, a patient may present with significant stiffness but only moderate to severe pain. Although the patient would present in the quadrant "hypomobility and pain," the primary emphasis could be directed toward the Y-axis, representing a more substantial stiffness presentation than pain.

For orthopedic manual therapists, the presentation most commonly encountered is **hypomobility** with some iteration of pain. Several conditions are causal to this presentation including reflexogenic spasm, capsuloligamentous stiffness, and age-related arthritic changes. **Pain-dominant problems** are generally associated with inflammation and pain-mediated responses.

To demonstrate adequate validity, the manual therapist should be able to pull reliable evidence from the examination that would specifically target an effective treatment technique. Unfortunately, many of the historic methods designed to isolate pathological patterns of abnormal movements (coupling, capsular patterns, and end feels) have demonstrated questionable validity.[94–97] Additionally, the reliability of many of the pathological movement-based evaluation methods is poor, suggesting the potential of disparate findings among practitioners. Multiple studies have shown that the manual evaluation of factors such as bony anomalies, tissue texture, muscle tension, joint com-

pliance, and range of motion are variable when performed by physical therapists, chiropractors, and physicians whereas tests that rely on patient response are more reliable.[94] This substantially challenges our ability to dictate whether a patient is truly a hypo- or hypermobility based on objective examination alone.

One proposed solution to the problem of accurately assessing stiffness is to omit this information from the examination process.[98] Examination and treatment would rely solely on the response of the patient to the treatment applied and would require direct application to the patient's concordant sign using pain provocation–based maneuvers. Using pain provocation–based maneuvers, the clinician would apply specific techniques until a positive change is elicited from the patient. Truly, this characteristic is an underlying theme in some patient response-based approaches. Often, repeated movements or manual therapy procedures are applied during the examination and the same movements are continued to determine patient response. Maher and Latimer[98] suggest this approach may sound extreme, yet to date there are no studies that have proven an alternative strategy is actually better. Nonetheless, most manual therapists (and certainly this author) would argue that detection of stiffness still has a reasonable place in examination.

Several authors have suggested that the use of symptom reproduction to identify the level of pathology is the only accurate evaluative method[99–104] and have promoted this approach concurrently with movement assessment.[103–107] To some extent, this assists in substantiating the detection of stiffness during the objective exam, but only during concurrent assessment of pain. This process has been defined as a form of diagnostic differential assessment. Differential assessment is largely hypothesis testing, which takes place before, during, and after all phases of the patient's visit. Mark Jones[108] terms physical differentiation as a method of evaluation that "involves altering the pain provoking position or movement in such a way that one structure is implicated as a source, while another is eliminated from contention." Adopting this philosophy dictates that the purpose of physical differentiation is to stress only one area, ensuring that the symptoms are produced from that area alone; thus, the other area(s) are ruled out as a source of the disorder. A key to differential assessment is to determine the source of the symptoms manually rather than labeling the disorder as a syndrome based on a collection of symptoms.

Some may argue that the failure to produce a workable diagnosis may lead to an inappropriate treatment selection. Yet most likely, skilled clinicians are used to working in the absence of complete information, and have mastered the capacity to appropriately treat when the underlying diagnosis remains uncertain. Jensen et al.[109] identified that expert orthopedic clinicians were comfortable with ambiguity and had the capacity to self-monitor their data collection and thinking patterns. They are able to do this by combining

**TABLE 3.4**    Pain- and Stiffness-Related Subjective Symptoms (Adapted from Showalter and Sprague[113])

| Subjective Examination Variables | | |
|---|---|---|
| **Variables** | **Pain Reduction** | **Mechanical Stiffness** |
| Mechanism | Acute | Chronic |
| Concordant complaint | Painful throughout the range of selected movements | Painful near end range with selective movements |
| Effects of repeated concordant activity | Aggravated by mild activity | Aggravated by vigorous activity |
| Severity | Often disabling | More of a nuisance |
| Irritability | Typically irritable (not always) | Generally not irritable (not always) |
| Stage | Unpredictable | Unpredictable |
| Frequency | Constant/variable | Intermittent (driven by activity) |
| Pain report | Usually high >5 | Usually low to moderate <5 |

clusters of information together into workable sets, based on past experience and cooperative decision making.[110] The *Guide to Physical Therapist Practice*[9] outlines that in situations where determination of a specific pathology is evasive, interventions for the alleviation of symptoms and remediation of impairments are still useful and appropriate. The clinician is then guided by the responses to those interventions and can proceed accordingly.[9]

Some have proposed that certain elements of the examination lend credence to the ability to associate a particular patient's condition to stiffness- versus pain-dominance (Table 3.4). Although this material has not been rigorously evaluated, it provides the examining clinician with guidelines on how to appropriately manage the treatment approach. This method requires a coordinated effort of patient verbal feedback and elicitation of nonverbal responses detected by skilled clinicians.[99]

At the end of the clinical examination, the clinician should have a strong understanding of the patient's concordant sign and which activities negatively or positively affect the sign. Failure to identify a concordant sign during examination will either yield three different consequences. First, since no mechanical pattern of symptoms was isolated, the patient could potentially receive a treatment approach that may or may not be associated with their impairment. Second, if the clinician is unable to isolate symptoms using appropriate clinical examination methods, it is possible that the patient exhibits a nonmechanical disorder and may be outside the scope of an orthopedic manual therapist's care. If manual therapy clinical examination methods that are mechanical in nature do not positively or negatively affect the patient's concordant sign, the patient may not benefit from manual therapy. The patient may be best served by referring to a more appropriate medical provider. Third, some patients require preloading or cumulative loading of tissues to reproduce the concordant pain. This consequence occurs in many sports or occupation-related injuries that require repetition before onset of symptoms.

Since the purpose of the clinical examination was to analyze the response of the concordant sign to multiple movements, the clinician should have a strong understanding of which techniques improve or aggravate the patient's condition. Treatment selection should be based on these findings, and less on theoretical analysis or conjecture. The individual patient findings are absolute, irrefutable evidence. Since these methods are provided in a controlled setting, with controlled application totals and frequencies, a strong understanding of the patient response is likely.

In Chapter 2, we discussed the application of hypotheses categories into discrete clusters of related concepts. These clusters could represent key treatment cues for an orthopedic manual therapist for appropriate selection of treatment application. This concept, promoted by Jones[108] and others[111], hypothesizes a theoretical framework for examination modeling. Along with the systematic collection of data, this philosophy ensures consistency and thoroughness of the examination and provides a framework for reexamination.

## *Summary*

- Most methods that involve movement detection of finite quantities have demonstrated poor reliability and validity.
- Most methods that utilize patient report of symptoms during clinician-driven provocation procedures have demonstrated good reliability and validity.
- Clinical reasoning that focuses on pain provocation and alteration of techniques to patient response is the focus of this textbook.

# Chapter Questions

1. Describe the benefits and pitfalls of using observation-based methods during examination.
2. Define the concordant and discordant sign. How can an overemphasis on the discordant sign lead to false findings during an examination?
3. Define the irritability of a patient. Describe how irritability is a multidimensional concept.
4. Identify measures that are appropriate for a patient baseline. Please describe how these methods are used during treatment and reexamination.
5. Describe the appropriate procedural process of an active movement examination.
6. Describe the factors (methods) within a passive movement examination.
7. Describe the appropriate procedural process of a passive movement examination.
8. Outline the qualities of clinical special tests and the necessary elements required for validity.
9. Describe how the patient response-based method provides usable information for a potential treatment program. Why is this method effective?

# References

1. Grieve G. *Common vertebral joint problems.* 2nd ed. Edinburgh; Churchill Livingstone: 1988
2. Fann A. The prevalence of postural asymmetry in people with and without chronic low back pain. *Arch Phys Med Rehabil.* 2002;83:1736–1738.
3. Levangie PK. The association between static pelvic asymmetry and low back pain. *Spine.* 1999;15;24(12):1234–1242.
4. Pearsall A, Speer K. Frozen shoulder syndrome: diagnostic and treatment strategies in the primary care setting. *Med Sci Sports Ex.* 1998;30:33–39.
5. Astrom M, Arvidson T. Alignment and joint motion of the foot. *J Orthop Sports Phys Ther* 1995;22:216–222.
6. Harris G, Wertsch J. Procedures for gait analysis. *Arch Phys Med Rehabil.* 1994;75:216–225.
7. Fritz J, George S. Identifying psychosocial variables in patients with acute work-related low back pain: The importance of fear-avoidance beliefs. *Phys Ther.* 2002;82:973–983.
8. Kilpikoski S, Airaksinen O, Kankaanpaa M, Leminen P, Videman T, Alen M. Interexaminer reliability of low back pain assessment using the McKenzie method. *Spine.* 2002;27(8):E207–214.
9. Guide to Physical Therapist Practice. 2nd edition. *Phys Ther.* 2001;81:9–744.
10. Edwards B. *Manual of combined movements.* Oxford; Butterworth-Heinemann: 1999
11. Woolf AD. How to assess musculoskeletal conditions. History and physical examination. *Best Pract Res Clin Rheumatol.* 2003;17(3):381–402.
12. McGregor AH, Dore CJ, McCarthy ID, Hughes SP. Are subjective clinical findings and objective clinical tests related to the motion characteristics of low back pain subjects? *J Orthop Sports Phys Ther.* 1998;28(6):370–377.
13. Luime J, Verhagen A, Miedema H, Kupier J, Burdorf A, Verhaar J, Koes B. Does this patient have an instability of the shoulder or a labrum lesion? *JAMA.* 2004;292:1989–1999.
14. Walker W, Cifu D, Gardner M, Keyser-Marcus L. Functional assessment in patients with chronic pain: Can physicians predict performance? *Spine.* 2001;80:162–168.
15. Laslett M, Young S, Aprill C, McDonald B. Diagnosing painful sacroiliac joints: a validity study of a McKenzie evaluation and sacroiliac provocation tests. *Aust J Physiotherapy.* 2003;49:89–97.
16. Maitland GD. *Maitland's Vertebral Manipulation.* 6th ed. London; Butterworth-Heinemann: 2001.
17. Zusman M. Irritability. *Man Ther.* 1998;3(4):195–202.
18. Koury M, Scarpelli E. A Manual therapy approach to evaluation and treatment of a patient with a chronic lumbar nerve root irritation. *Phys Ther.* 1994;74(6):548–559.
19. Tovin B. *Evaluation and treatment of the shoulder: an integration of the guide to physical therapist practice.* Philadelphia; F.A. Davis Company: 2001.
20. Sprague R. Differential assessment and mobilization of the cervical and upper thoracic spine. In: Donatelli R, Wooden M. *Orthopaedic physical therapy.* Philadelphia; Churchill Livingston: 2001.
21. Jonsson H, Riklund-Ahlstrom K, Lind J. Positive pivot shift after ACL reconstruction predicts later osteoarthrosis: 63 patients followed 5–9 years after surgery. *Acta Orthop Scand.* 2004;75(5):594–599.
22. McLain RF. Mechanoreceptor endings in human cervical facet joints. *Spine.* 1994;19(5):495–501.
23. Fryer G, Morris T, Gibbons P. Paraspinal muscles and intervertebral dysfunction: part one. *J Manipulative Physiol Ther.* 2004;27(4):267–274.
24. McQuillen MP, Tucker K, Pellegrino ED. Syndrome of subacute generalized muscular stiffness and spasm. *Arch Neurol.* 1967;16(2):165–174.
25. Kang YM, Choi WS, Pickar JG. Electrophysiologic evidence for an intersegmental reflex pathway

between lumbar paraspinal tissues. *Spine.* 2002;27 (3):E56–63.

26. Fitzgerald GK, Piva SR, Irrgang JJ. Reports of joint instability in knee osteoarthritis: its prevalence and relationship to physical function. *Arthritis Rheum.* 2004;51(6):941–946.

27. Svanborg A. Practical and functional consequences of aging. *Gerontology.* 1988;34 Suppl 1:11–5.

28. Williams M, Solomonow M, Zhou BH, Baratta RV, Harris M. Multifidi spasms elicited by prolonged lumbar flexion. *Spine.* 2000;25(22):2916–2924.

29. Borenstein D. Does osteoarthritis of the lumbar spine cause chronic low back pain? *Curr Pain Headache Rep.* 2004;8(6):512–517.

30. Mariani PP, Santori N, Rovere P, Della Rocca C, Adriani E. Histological and structural study of the adhesive tissue in knee fibroarthrosis: a clinical-pathological correlation. *Arthroscopy.* 1997;13(3): 313–318.

31. Maitland GD. *Peripheral manipulation.* 3rd ed. London; Butterworth-Heinemann: 1986.

32. Tan V, Cheatle M, Mackin S, Moberg P, Esterhai J. Goal setting as a predictor of return to work in a population of chronic musculoskeletal pain patients. *Int J Neurosci.* 1997;92:161–170.

33. Davies A. Rating systems for total knee replacement. *Knee.* 2002;9:261–266.

34. Flaherty S. Pain measurement tools for clinical practice and research. *AANA J.* 1996;64:133–140.

35. Patrick D, Deyo R. Generic and disease-specific measures in assessing health status and quality of life. *Med Care.* 1989;27:S217–S232.

36. Westaway M, Stratford P, Brinkley J. The patient-specific functional scale: validation of its use in persons with neck dysfunction. *J Orthop Sports Phys Ther.* 1998;27:331–338.

37. Pietrobon R, Coeytaux R, Carey T, Richardson W, DeVellis R. Standard scales for measurement of functional outcome for cervical pain or dysfunction. *Spine.* 2002;27:515–522.

38. Donelson R. The McKenzie approach to evaluating and treating low back pain. *Orthopedic Review.* 1990;8:681–686.

39. Franklin M, Conner-Kerr T, Chamness M, Chenier T, Kelly R, Hodge T. Assessment of exercise-induced minor muscle lesions: the accuracy of Cyriax's diagnosis by selective tension paradigm. *J Ortho Sports Phys Ther.* 1996;24:122–129.

40. Cyriax J, Cyriax P. *Cyriax's illustrated manual of orthopaedic medicine.* Oxford; Butterworth-Heinemann: 1993.

41. Niere KR, Torney SK. Clinicians' perceptions of minor cervical instability. *Man Ther.* 2004;9(3): 144–150.

42. Yelland M. Back, chest and abdominal pain. How good are spinal signs at identifying musculoskeletal causes of back, chest or abdominal pain? *Aust Fam Physician.* 2001;30:980–912.

43. Wetzel FT, Donelson R. The role of repeated end-range/pain response assessment in the management of symptomatic lumbar discs. *Spine J.* 2003;3(2): 146–154.

44. O'Sullivan PB. Lumbar segmental 'instability': clinical presentation and specific stabilizing exercise management. *Man Ther.* 2000;5(1):2–12.

45. Hahne A, Keating J, Wilson S. Do within-session changes in pain intensity and range of motion predict between-session changes in patients with low back pain? *Aust J Physiotherapy.* 2004;50:17–23.

46. Lee R, Evans J. An in vivo study of the intervertebral movements produced by posteroanterior mobilization. *Clin Biomech.* 1997;12:400–408.

47. Lee R, Tsung BY, Tong P, Evans J. Bending stiffness of the lumbar spine subjected to posteroanterior manipulative force. *J Rehabil Res Dev.* 2005;42(2): 167–174.

48. Chiradejnant A, Maher C, Latimer J, Stepkovitch N. Efficacy of therapist selected versus randomly selected mobilization techniques for the treatment of low back pain: A randomized controlled trial. *Aust J Physiotherapy.* 2003;49:233–241.

49. Hartman L. *Handbook of Osteopathic Technique.* 3rd ed. San Diego, CA; Singular Pub Group: 1997.

50. Chiradejnant A, Latimer J, Maher C, Stepkovitch N. Does the choice of spinal level treated during posteroanterior (PA) mobilization affect treatment outcome? *Physiotherapy Theory Practice.* 2002;18:165–174.

51. Kaltenborn F. Manual mobilization of the joints. *The Kaltenborn method of joint mobilization and treatment.* 5th ed. Oslo; Olaf Norlis Bokhandel: 1999.

52. Hayes K, Peterson C, Falconer J. An examination of Cyriax's passive motion tests with patients having osteoarthritis of the knee. *Phys Ther.* 1994;74:697–707.

53. Klassbo M, Larsson G. Examination of passive ROM and capsular patterns of the hip. *Physiotherapy Res International.* 2003;8:1–12.

54. Mitsch J, Casey J, McKinnis R, Kegerreis S, Stikeleather J. Investigation of a consistent pattern of motion restriction in patients with adhesive capsulitis. *J Manual Manipulative Ther.* 2004;12:153–159.

55. Bijl D, Dekker J, van Baar M, Oostendorp R, Lemmens A, Bijlsma J, Voorn T. Validity of Cyriax's concept capsular pattern for the diagnosis of osteoarthritis of hip and/or knee. *Scand J Rheumatol.* 1998;27:347–351.

56. Grieve G. *Mobilisation of the spine: A primary handbook of clinical method.* 5th ed. New York; Churchill Livingstone: 1991.

57. Hayes K, Peterson C. Reliability of assessing end-feel and pain and resistance sequence in subjects with painful shoulders and knees. *J Orthop Sports Phys Ther.* 2001;31:432–445.

58. Peterson C, Hayes K. Construct validity of Cyriax's selective tension examination: association of end-feels with pain at the knee and shoulder. *J Orthop Sports Phys Ther.* 2000;30:512–521.

59. Chesworth B, MacDermid J, Roth J, Patterson S. Movement diagram and "end-feel" reliability when measuring passive lateral rotation of the shoulder in patients with shoulder pathology. *Phys Ther.* 1998;78:593–601.

60. Cooperman J, Riddle D, Rothstein J. Reliability and validity of judgments of the integrity of the anterior cruciate ligament of the knee using the Lachman's test. *Phys Ther.* 1990;70:225–233.

61. McClure P, Flowers K. Treatment of limited should motion: a case study based on biomechanical considerations. *Phys Ther.* 1992;72:929–936.

62. Harryman D, Lazarus M. The stiff shoulder. In: Rockwood C, Matsen F, Wirth M, Lippitt S. *The shoulder.* Vol 2. 3rd ed. Philadelphia: W.B. Saunders. 2004.

63. Haldeman S. Spinal manipulative therapy. A status report. *Clin Orthop.* 1983;(179):62–70.

64. Lee M, Steven J, Crosbie R, Higgs J. Towards a theory of lumbar mobilization-the relationship between applied manual force and movements of the spine. *Man Ther.* 1996;2:67–75.

65. Lee M, Svensson NL. Effect of loading frequency on response of the spine to lumbar posteroanterior forces. *J Manipulative Physiol Ther.* 1993;16(7):439–446.

66. Edwards B. Examination. In: Maitland GD. *Maitland's vertebral manipulation.* 6th ed. London; Butterworth-Heinemann: 2001.

67. Fung Y. Biomechanics. *Mechanical properties of living tissues.* 2nd ed. New York; Springer-Verlag: 1993.

68. Shirley D, Ellis E, Lee M. The response of posteroanterior lumbar stiffness to repeated loading. *Man Ther.* 2002;7:19–25.

69. Lee M. Mechanics of spinal joint manipulation in the thoracic and lumbar spine: A theoretical study of posteroanterior force techniques. *Clin Biomech.* 1989;4:249–251.

70. Caling B, Lee M. Effect of direction of applied mobilization force on the posteroanterior response in the lumbar spine. *J Manipulative Physiol Ther.* 2001;24:71–78.

71. Wolf EM, Agrawal V. Transdeltoid palpation (the rent test) in the diagnosis of rotator cuff tears. *J Shoulder Elbow Surg.* 2001;10(5):470–473.

72. Manfredini D, Tognini F, Zampa V, Bosco M. Predictive value of clinical findings for temporomandibular joint effusion. *Oral Surg Oral Med Oral Pathol Oral Radiol Endod.* 2003;96(5):521–526.

73. Cook JL, Khan KM, Kiss ZS, Purdam CR, Griffiths L. Reproducibility and clinical utility of tendon palpation to detect patellar tendinopathy in young basketball players. Victorian Institute of Sport tendon study group. *Br J Sports Med.* 2001;35(1):65–69.

74. Pellecchia GL, Paolino J, Connell J. Intertester reliability of the Cyriax evaluation in the assessing patients with shoulder pain. *J Orthop Sports Phys Ther.* 1996;23:34–38.

75. Fritz J, Delitto A, Erhard R, Roman M. An examination of the selective tissue tension scheme, with evidence for the concept of a capsular pattern of the knee. *Phys Ther.* 1998;78:1046–1056.

76. Jepsen J, Laursen L, Larsen A, Hagert C. Manual strength testing in 14 upper limb muscles: a study of inter-rater reliability. *Acta Orthop Scand.* 2004;75:442–448.

77. Perry J, Weiss W, Burnfield J, Gronley J. The supine hip extensor manual muscle test: a reliability and validity study. *Arch Phys Med Rehabil.* 2004;85:1345–1350.

78. Frese E, Brown M, Norton B. Clinical reliability of manual muscle testing. Middle trapezius and gluteus maximus muscles. *Phys Ther.* 1987;67:1072–1076.

79. Ottenbacher K, Branch L, Ray L, Gonzales V, Peek M, Hinman M. The reliability of upper- and lower-extremity strength testing in a community survey of older adults. *Arch Phys Med Rehabil.* 2002;83:1423–1427.

80. Kelly B, Kadrmas W, Speer K. The manual muscle examination for rotator cuff strength. An electromyographic investigation. *Am J Sports Med.* 1996;24:581–588.

81. Hsieh C, Phillips R. Reliability of manual muscle testing with a computerized dynamometer. *J Manipulative Physiol Ther.* 1990;13:72–82.

82. Wadsworth C, Krishnan R, Sear M, Harrold J, Nielson D. Intrarater reliability of manual muscle testing and hand held dynametric muscle testing. *Phys Ther.* 1987;67:1342–1347.

83. Hicks G, Fritz J, Delitto A, Mishock J. Interrater reliability of clinical examination measures for identification of lumbar segmental instability. *Arch Phys Med Rehabil.* 2003;84(12):1858–1864.

84. Ombregt L, Bisschop P, ter Veer H, Van de Velde T. *A system of orthopedic medicine.* London; W.B. Saunders Co: 1995.

85. Jaeschke R, Meade M, Guyatt G, Keenan SP, Cook DJ. How to use diagnostic test articles in the intensive care unit: diagnosing weananability using f/vt. *Crit Care Med.* 1997;25:1514–1521.

86. Fritz JM, Wainner RS. Examining diagnostic tests: an evidence-based perspective. *Phys Ther.* 2001;81(9):1546–1564.

87. Bossuyt P, Reitsma J, Bruns D, Catsonis C, Glasziou P, Irwig L, Lijmer J, Moher D, Rennie D, de Vet H. Towards complete and accurate reporting of studies of diagnostic accuracy: the STARD initiative. *Family Practice.* 2004;21:4–10.

88. Portney L, Watkins M. *Foundations of clinical research: Applications to practice.* 2nd ed. Upper River Saddle, NJ; Prentice Hall Health: 2000.

89. Glas AS, Lijmer JG, Prins MH, Bonsel GJ, Bossuyt PM. The diagnostic odds ratio: a single indicator of test performance. *J Clin Epidemiol.* 2003;56(11):1129–1135.

90. Deyo RA, Rainville J, Kent DL. What can the history and physical examination tell us about low back pain? *JAMA* 1992;268(6):760–765.

91. Dvorak J. Epidemiology, physical examination, and neurodiagnostics. *Spine* 1998;23:2663–2672.

92. Sprague R. The acute cervical joint lock. *Phys Ther.* 1983;63(9):1439–1144.

93. Matyas TA, Bach TM. The reliability of selected techniques in clinical arthrometrics. *Aust J Physiotherapy.* 1985;31:175–197.

94. Cook C. Lumbar Coupling biomechanics—A literature review. *J Manual Manipulative Ther.* 2003;11(3):137–145.

95. Cook C Showalter C. A survey on the importance of lumbar coupling biomechanics in physiotherapy practice. *Man Ther.* 2004; 9:164–172.

96. Gibbons P, Tehan P. Patient positioning and spinal locking for lumbar spine rotation manipulation. *Man Ther.* 2001;6(3):130–138.

97. Hsu AT, Hedman T, Chang JH, Vo C, Ho L, Ho S, Chang GL. Changes in abduction and rotation range of motion in response to simulated dorsal and ventral translational mobilization of the glenohumeral joint. *Phys Ther.* 2002;82(6):544–556.

98. Maher C, Latimer J. Pain or resistance-the therapists' dilemma. *Aust J Physiotherapy.* 1993;38:257–260.

99. Phillips DR, Twomey LT. A comparison of manual diagnosis with a diagnosis established by a uni-level lumbar spinal block procedure. *Man Ther.* 2000;1(2):82–87.

100. Petty N, Bach T, Cheek L. Accuracy of feedback during training of passive accessory intervertebral movements. *J Manual Manipulative Ther.* 2001;9(2):99–108.

101. Di Fabio R. Efficacy of manual therapy. *Phys Ther.* 1992;72(12): 853–864.

102. Harms M, Milton A, Cusick G, Bader D. Instrumentation of a mobilization couch for dynamic load measurements. *Journal of Medical Engineering Technology.* 1995;19(4):119–122.

103. Goodsell M, Lee M, Latimer J. Short-Term effects of lumbar posteroanterior mobilization in individuals with low-back pain. *J Manipulative Physiol Ther.* 2000;23(5):332–342.

104. Fitzgerald G, McClure P, Beattie P, Riddle D. Issues in determining treatment effectiveness of manual therapy. *Phys Ther.* 1994;74(3):227–233.

105. Jull G, Bogduk N, Marsland A. The accuracy of manual diagnosis for cervical zygopophyseal joint pain syndromes. *Med J Aust.* 1988;148(5):233–236.

106. Boline PD, Haas M, Meyer JJ, Kassak K, Neslon C, Keating JC. Inter-examiner reliability of eight evaluative dimensions of lumbar segmental abnormality: Part II. *J Manipulative Physiol Ther.* 1992;16:363–373.

107. Sandmark H, Nisell R. Validity of five common manual neck pain provoking tests. *Scand J Rehabil Med.* 1995;27(3):131–136.

108. Jones M. Clinical reasoning in manual therapy. *Phys Ther.* 1992;72:875.

109. Jensen G, Gwyer J, Shepard K, Hack L. Expert practice in physical therapy. *Phys Ther.* 2000;80:28–43.

110. Jensen G, Shepard K, Hack L. The novice versus the experienced clinician: insights into the work of the physical therapist. *Phys Ther.* 1990;70:314–323.

111. Gifford LS, Butler DS. The integration of pain sciences into clinical practice. *J Hand Ther.* 1997;10(2):86–95.

112. Jaeschke R, Guyatt G, Sackett D. Users' guides to the medical literature: III. How to use an article about a diagnostic test: B. What are the results and will they help me in caring for my patients? *JAMA.* 1994;271:703–707.

113. Sprague R, Showalter C. MT-2. Intermediate spine. Maitland Australian Physiotherapy Seminars. Cutchogue, NY; MAPS: 2002.

# 4

# Treatment and Reexamination

## Objectives

- Define the patient response treatment philosophy.
- Outline the method suggested to describe grades of mobilization.
- Define how the different determinants of treatment alter the outcome of the treatment.

- Describe the various treatment techniques used by orthopedic manual clinicians.
- Describe the patient's role in "intention to treat" and how this role may alter the outcome of the treatment.

## TREATMENT

### Treatment Philosophy

The purpose of treatment, the second element of assessment, is to apply purposeful techniques that reduce, centralize, or abolish the patient's signs and symptoms. The selection of a set of treatment techniques follows the same philosophy as the examination. As discussed in Chapter 3, a clinician's examination is determined by performing movements that alter the patient's report of signs and symptoms[1], a procedure defined as the patient-response method. The patient-response method requires a diligent effort of the patient and the clinician to determine the behavior of the patient's pain and/or impairment by analyzing concordant movements and the response of the patient's pain to repeated or applied movements. The repeated or sustained movements that positively or negatively alter the signs and symptoms of the patient deserve the highest priority for treatment selection[2,3] and should be similar in construct to the concordant examination movements. Examination methods that fail to elicit the patient response may offer nominal or imprecise value as do methods that focus solely on treatment decision making based on a single diagnostic label.[4]

Although some may argue that the failure to produce a definitive diagnosis may lead to an inappropriate treatment selection, in reality, few situations allow clinicians to have

100% certainty of a diagnosis. A definitive diagnosis that provides a pathological label is not always possible in a clinical setting.[4] Even when data-collecting capabilities are comprehensive, clinicians demonstrate poor interrater reliability during identification of diagnostic labels of selected anatomical regions[5] and are biased toward selected forms of pathologies.[6] A diagnostic label is generally inadequate to explain the patient's condition and is often created based on a contrived pattern of patient symptoms or clinicians' suppositions.[2,7] And when created, the diagnostic label generally offers little insight on the severity, irritability, nature, and stage of the disorder.[8]

## Summary

- Treatment is based on the patient response method and should accurately reflect the findings during the examination.
- Examination methods that fail to elicit the patient response may offer nominal or imprecise value.
- A definitive diagnosis that provides a pathological label is not always possible in a clinical setting.
- A diagnostic label generally offers little insight regarding the severity, irritability, nature, and stage of the disorder specifically in association with treatment.

## The Intention of Treatment

Christensen et al.[9] state, "A patient's full understanding of and participation in the management of his or her problem, resulting in an increase in understanding and, in turn, self-efficacy, is thought to have a significant positive impact on treatment outcomes." The idea of involving the patient in their own care is not new and is purported to lead to beneficial outcomes.[10] By empowering the patient to participate in the treatment, the patient improves their ability to adjust to symptomatic changes.

To accomplish this concept, the patient must be made aware of the intention of treatment. The intention of treatment is the cooperative understanding of the goals of the treatment, developed in a format in which the patient can understand. Although there are several goals to a manual therapist's intervention, there are essentially three potential treatment objectives: (1) pain reduction, (2) alteration of stiffness (either more or less), and (3) education of the patient to allow self-treatment. By involving the patient in the intention of the treatment, they are more likely to understand how each selected intervention applies toward on of the three objectives. For example, if the objective of the treatment is to alter stiffness, specifically when the goal is to increase range of motion, then the patient must be made aware that some treatment mechanisms may result in stretching, mobilization of stiff tissues, and some pain.

There are few instances when the intention to treat is limited only to reduction of pain. Nonetheless, in cases where a patient exhibits symptoms associated with inflammation, reduction of pain should be at least one of the objectives. Inflammatory conditions are generally described using pain-related verbiage and frequently patients with this primary disorder are considered "pain dominant."[11,12] It has been suggested that inflammatory-based pain demonstrates characteristics that are different from stiffness-related pain such as resting pain or pain that is described as "through range." Since pain-dominant characteristics are associated with many factors in addition to inflammation, a comprehensive assessment of movement-related dysfunctions is critical.

With the pain-dominant patient, pain reduction is the intent of the treatment. The objective of pain reduction can assume many forms. There is no specific prescription for a manual therapy procedure to reduce pain; truly, this varies from one patient to another. Some patients respond well to lighter grades of motion whereas others function better with heavier grades. The ability to predict this prior to examination is abstruse. Pain reduction techniques are typically borne out of the examination and are fine-tuned as the patient's symptoms and presentation change.

Alteration of stiffness may be the most challenging component of the three objectives since detection of stiffness lacks validity in absence of concurrent patient report of symptoms. Stiffness may take many different physiological forms, including reflexogenic spasm and/or degenerative capsuloligamentous tightness.[13] Furthermore, the term "stiffness" may encompass differences in theoretical constructs among physical therapist.[14] It is highly likely that one clinician's assessment of stiffness will differ from the assessment of others. Since so many different variables can modify the detection of stiffness, the ability to reliably assess the exact quantity of resistance during an examination may be beyond the skills of a manual therapist.

Maher and Latimer[11] suggested that the treatment focus should remain on the concordant sign and modifications based on the response of the patient should dictate the progression of the treatment plan. Treatment is directed to the source of the problem and may result in a temporary increase in the patient's resting symptoms. This concept is very different from competing philosophies, which prescribe guilt to neighboring segments that may or may not be associated to the cause, and/or observable asymmetries, stiffness variability, and biomechanical findings. Subsequently, direct application of treatment to the concordant sign may produce a more compelling reproduction or reduction of symptoms than treating adjunct regions. Because the technique's objective is to reproduce or reduce the patient's pain during the treatment process, the patient must be made well aware of the intent and the prospected outcome.

The patient response to the movements within the examination and treatment will guide the treatment techniques selected by the clinician. There is little question that this assessment approach presents with as much face validity as other competing approaches. Nonetheless, it is helpful to

## *Summary*

- A patient's full understanding and participation in the management of his or her problem should have a significant positive impact on treatment outcome.
- There are essentially three treatment objectives during orthopedic manual therapy: (1) pain reduction, (2) alteration of stiffness, and (3) education of the patient to allow self-treatment.
- Inflammatory conditions are generally described using pain-related verbiage, and frequently patients with this primary disorder are considered "pain dominant."
- Although the assessment of stiffness is questionably valid, certain clues regarding a stiffness-dominant patient improve the understanding of a mechanically-based dysfunction that responds well to aggressive movements.

**TABLE 4.1    Pain versus Stiffness Guidelines (Adapted from Showalter and Sprague[75])**

| Subjective Examination Variables | | |
|---|---|---|
| **Variables** | **Pain Reduction** | **Mechanical Stiffness** |
| Mechanism | Acute | Chronic |
| Concordant complaint | Painful throughout the range of selected movements | Painful near end range with selective movements |
| Effects of repeated concordant activity | Aggravated by mild activity | Aggravated by vigorous activity |
| Severity | Often disabling | More of a nuisance |
| Irritability | Typically irritable (not always) | Generally not irritable (not always) |
| Stage | Unpredictable | Unpredictable |
| Frequency | Constant/variable | Intermittent (driven by activity) |
| Pain report | Usually high >5 | Usually low to moderate <5 |
| **Objective/Physical Examination Variables** | | |
| **Variables** | **Pain Reduction** | **Mechanical Stiffness** |
| Active movements | Often afraid to move | Limited by range and less by fear |
| Repeated movements | If vigorous, may worsen condition | May to vigor to improve the condition |
| Postural positioning | Usually have little effect | May or may not be beneficial |
| Passive physiological movements | Usually demonstrates through-range pain | Usually demonstrates end-range pain |
| Passive accessory movements | P1 occurs before R1 | R1 occurs prior to P1 |
| Special testing | Tests are generally overly sensitive | Tests are generally less sensitive |
| **Intention to Treat** | | |
| **Variables** | **Pain Reduction** | **Mechanical Stiffness** |
| Intent of exam | Reduce pain | Increase range |
| Barriers | At pain | At stiffness |
| Dominance | Pain | Stiffness |
| Focus of assessment | Pain behavior | Range, function |
| Preferred treatment movement | Freest | Most restricted |
| Suggested origin | Inflammation | Mechanical |

use guidelines during treatment application that may make the clinician more efficient. For example, during treatment of stiffness versus pain, selected grades and intensities of mobilization may demonstrate greater effectiveness. Because the intent to treatment for stiffness-dominant patients requires a mechanism to improve range of motion, patients with this impairment respond better to higher, more aggressive grades, performed at end ranges. Conversely, since pain reduction is the goal of a pain-dominant patient, and the likelihood of an inflammatory process contributing to the presence of pain is high, individuals with this impair-

ment tend to respond better to lower grades performed at midranges in loosely packed positions. The following guidelines are untested, but are suggestive of a patient representation of pain or mechanical stiffness-related conditions (Table 4.1). Essentially, this process is based on the philosophy of G.D. Maitland and Gregory Grieve.

## *The Goal of the Treatment*

The purpose of physical differentiation tests during the examination is to so stress one area that the symptoms are produced from that area alone, thus the other area(s) are

**TABLE 4.2**    Goals of Manual Therapy Treatment

| Objectives | Description |
|---|---|
| **Objective One—Reduction of pain** | 1. Relief of pain and reduction of muscle spasm. |
| | 2. Relief from chronic postural or occupational stress. |
| **Objective Two—Alteration of stiffness** | 1. Restoration of normal tissue pliability and extensibility. |
| | 2. Correction of muscle weakness or imbalance. |
| | 3. The stabilization of unstable segments. |
| | 4. Restoration of adequate control of movement. |
| **Objective Three—Patient education** | 1. Prevention of reoccurrence. |
| | 2. Restoration of psychological well-being and confidence. |

ruled out as a source of the disorder. This method assists in targeting appropriate choices involved in selection of treatment techniques, dosage, and progression.[9] It emphasizes the suggestion that techniques by themselves offer little in isolation and should always represent a means to an end.[2] The selection of a technique is based on the presentation of the particular patient, indicating that the technique selection will most likely be different from patient to patient and will often change throughout the course of the patient's progression. The determination of method, dosage, and progression is dependent on the direct response of the patient and will differ over time.

Gregory Grieve[15] outlined common treatment-related goals in his 1988 textbook. If analyzed, Grieve's eight goals reflect the three principle objectives of treatment that include reduction of pain, alteration of stiffness, and patient education for self-treatment. The eight goals are listed in Table 4.2, broken down into the three objectives with some degree of overlap.

dic manual therapy techniques encompass five major categories: (1) repeated active movements, (2) positioning methods, (3) mobilization, (4) manipulation, and (5) combined techniques.

## Repeated Active Movements

**Repeated active movements** (Figure 4.1) are active physiological techniques performed exclusively by the patient. Generally, active movements are regionally applied, meaning that the methods of treatment are poorly localized. For use during treatment, the preferred direction of movement for the delivery of repeated movements and the need for progression of the loading forces, repetitions, or positional aspects are all determined by patient response during the initial and subsequent assessments.

---

### *Summary*

- In short, the purpose of physical differentiation procedures used during the examination is to so stress one area that the symptoms are produced from that area alone, thus the other area(s) are ruled out as a source of the disorder.
- Identifying the concordant pain generator allows the clinician to target the lesion specifically.
- By targeting the lesion the clinician may accomplish the three principle objectives of: (1) alteration of pain, (2) reduction of stiffness, and (3) patient education.

## Manual Therapy Techniques

Most manual therapy techniques are highly specified and require a formal education and skill levels beyond an entry-level practitioner.[16] The preponderance of orthope-

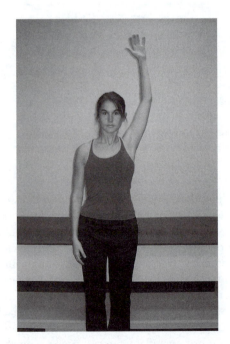

**Figure 4.1**    Repeated Active Movement of Shoulder Flexion

## Summary

- Repeated active movements are active physiological techniques performed exclusively by the patient.
- Active movements are regional applications indicating that the methods of treatment are poorly localized.

## Sustained Holds or Positioning Methods

**Sustained holds or positioning methods** (Figure 4.2) are desired or targeted postural positions, near end or selected ranges, designed to cause pain, abolish pain, or move the pain to a desired location.[17] In essence, positional techniques are most likely either static stretching methods or techniques that target neurophysiological changes by reducing irritation on selected mechanoreceptors. Frequently, positioning techniques are used in the treatment of cervical or lumbar patients. Nonetheless, there is little evidence to suggest that positioning methods alter disc biomechanics since the movement of the nucleus in an intervertebral disc is generally unpredictable.[3,18]

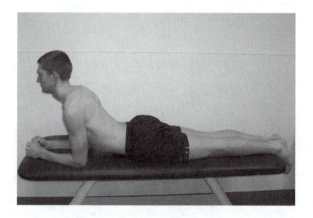

**Figure 4.2**   Sustained Hold or Postural Positioning Method

## Summary

- Positioning methods are desired or targeted postural positions, near end or selected ranges, designed to provoke, abolish, or move the pain to a desired location.
- Positional techniques function primarily to target neurophysiologic changes by reducing irritation on selected mechanoreceptors and may provide little alteration to tissue restructuring.

## Mobilization

Mobilizations typically fall within the treatment domain of passive movements.[16] Mobilization methods may involve segmental/joint or soft-tissue mobilization. There are two forms of segmental/joint mobilizations: regional and local. **Regional mobilizations** involve directed passive movement to more than one given area, segment, or physiological component, while **local mobilization** is specific and directed to one segmental and/or joint region.[14]

### Segmental/Joint Mobilization

Segmental/joint mobilization techniques are designed to restore a full painless joint function by rhythmic, repetitive passive movements to the patients' tolerance, in voluntary and/or accessory range and graded according to examination findings.[14] Generally, segmental/joint techniques involve static and/or oscillatory movements. Static techniques (prolonged stretch into restricted tissue) are sustained forces applied manually or mechanically to one aspect of a body part, to distract the attachments or shortened soft tissue. Oscillatory techniques (small or large passive movements) are applied movements to a segment/joint anywhere in a range, while the joints are held or compressed.[2] Both techniques appear to exhibit similar mechanical characteristics.

Motion at a joint is the result of movement of one joint surface in relation to the other.[19] Mobilization movements of a segmental region may include any biomechanical form of accessory motion including distraction, compression, sliding, spinning, and rolling.

Techniques that encourage distraction (joint surface separation without injury or dislocation of the parts) are sustained or rhythmic in nature, manual or mechanical, and are applied in a longitudinal manner that results in the distancing of two joint surfaces (Figure 4.3). Mennell[20] and Cyriax[21] frequently described distraction mobilization as useful treatment methods.

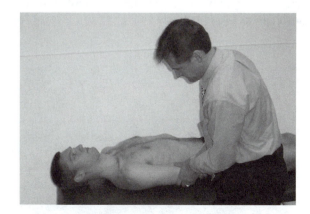

**Figure 4.3**   Mobilization Procedure of Distraction of the Shoulder

Techniques that encourage compression result in joint surfaces that are compressed together, allowing shorter distances between articular structures. Several authors have suggested the benefit of compression mobilization, although in most cases, the compressions were actually combined with other accessory movements such as gliding or rolling.

Techniques that encourage sliding (Figure 4.4) refer to the gliding of one articular component over another. The majority of simple planer mobilizations are sliding techniques. The convex–concave rule particularly emphasizes the proposed benefit to following appropriate sliding rules during mobilization application.[22]

### Soft-Tissue Mobilization

Soft-tissue mobilization techniques (Figure 4.6) are typically defined as massage or myofascial release. Soft tissue mobilization is the intentional and systematic manipulation of the soft tissues of the body to enhance health and healing.[23] Multiple forms of soft-tissue techniques exist, and may include gliding, sliding, percussion, compression, kneading, friction, vibrating, stretching, and holding.[23] This textbook does not describe soft-tissue mobilization in detail.

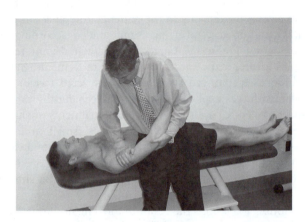

**Figure 4.4**    Mobilization Techniques that Encourage Sliding of the Shoulder

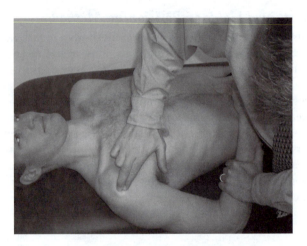

**Figure 4.6**    Friction Massage Technique Applied to the Shoulder

Techniques that encourage rolling (Figure 4.5) refer to the rolling of one body surface over another. For example, when a convex surface moves osteokinematically on a fixed concave surface, the majority of the hypothetical movement should include rolling. Nonetheless, this pattern has been justifiably questioned by recent studies specifically at the glenohumeral joint. Whether or not rolling and the convex–concave rule are transferable to all synovial joints is questionable.

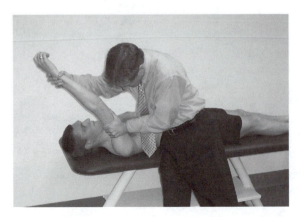

**Figure 4.5**    Mobilization Techniques that Encourage Rolling of the Shoulder

## Summary

- Regional mobilizations involve directed passive movement to more than one given area, segment, or physiological component, while a local mobilization is specific and directed to one segmental and/or joint region.
- Segmental/joint mobilization techniques are designed to restore a full painless joint function by rhythmic, repetitive passive movements to the patient's tolerance, in voluntary and/or accessory range and graded according to examination findings.
- Segmental/joint techniques involve static (prolonged stretch) and/or oscillatory (repeated passive motion) movements.
- Mobilization movements of a segmental region may include any biomechanical form of accessory motion including distraction, compression, sliding, spinning, and rolling.
- Soft-tissue mobilization is the intentional and systematic manipulation of the soft tissues of the body to enhance health and healing.

## Manipulation

Manipulations are used in both passive and assisted movements.[16] Grieve[15] defines a manipulation as an accurately localized, single, quick, and decisive movement of small amplitude, following careful positioning of the patient. Typically manipulation techniques are classified as localized or general.

### Localized Manipulation

**Localized manipulative** techniques involve the intent of applying a passive or assisted movement toward one specific functional region (i.e., spinal unit or single joint).[24] These techniques are occasionally termed "short-lever" manipulative procedures (Figure 4.7). During a localized manipulative technique the application of a high-velocity, low-amplitude thrust occurs at the end of range of movement for the joint. Generally, the joint is appropriately prepositioned in such a manner that allows an end-range feel to be produced in a combination of midrange positions.[25] Thus the high-velocity, low-amplitude thrust is applied in a position where the joint was placed in a clinician-determined end range of movement, in a particular combination of plane movements to allow application isolated to that segment.[26] Manipulation is distinguished from mobilization by the prepositioning, the administration of the high velocity, low amplitude thrust, and that the clinician manages the direction force and application beyond the patient's control.

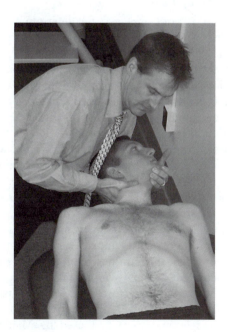

**Figure 4.7**    Localized Manipulation of the Cervical Spine

### Generalized Manipulation

**Generalized manipulative** techniques (Figure 4.8) involve less defined prepositioning methods and are designed in such a manner as to isolate the thrust to a dedicated region. These techniques are frequently de-

scribed as "long-lever" manipulative techniques. Force is directed through a long lever arm, which is distant from the specific contact.[27] Generalized manipulative techniques allow the thrust to transcend throughout the regional anatomical site dispensing the force through multiple segmental levels or peripheral joints. Muscle energy techniques used for manipulation purposes are examples of a generalized manipulation technique.

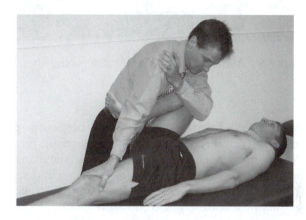

**Figure 4.8**    Generalized Manipulation of the SI Joint

### Summary

- Manipulation involves a clinician-driven method that is accurately localized, singularly performed, and involves a quick and decisive small amplitude movement.
- Localized manipulative techniques involve the intent of applying a passive or assisted movement toward one specific functional region.
- Generalized manipulative techniques involve less defined prepositioning methods and are designed in such a manner as to isolate the thrust to a dedicated region.

## Combined Techniques

Any method that combines any of the previously described techniques is considered a combined method. Selected combined techniques include (1) manually assisted movements (Figure 4.9) and (2) **muscle energy techniques.**

One popular form of manually assisted movement is "mobilization with movement," a term coined by Brian Mulligan. Mobilization with movement is defined as the application of an accessory glide during the patient-driven active physiological movement.[28–30] The underlying principle recommends accessory application along biomechanical joint orientations.[31] This concept may involve the application of sustained, through-range, manually derived forces that guide the joint in such a manner that

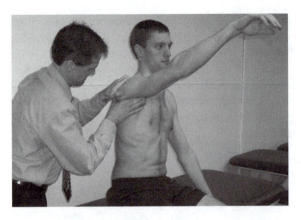

**Figure 4.9**    Manually Assisted Movement of the Shoulder

superimposed active movement, which previously produced pain, can then occur painlessly. Essentially, the nature of these techniques involves the simultaneous combination of passive accessory mobilization and active patient-originated movement.[32] Mobilization with movement has its foundation based on Kaltenborn's principles of restoring the accessory component of active and passive physiological joint movement.[31]

Muscle energy techniques (METs) are a technique in manual therapy where the patient actively uses their muscles, on request, while maintaining a targeted preposition, against a distinctly executed counterforce.[33] METs may be classified as isotonic or isometric contractions, each with opposite desired outcomes. In an isometric contraction, the overall muscle length (of the activated muscle) shortens, while during an isotonic contraction the muscle can shorten (concentric) or lengthen (eccentric).[34] For example, a muscle energy technique involves an active movement (by the patient) and a localized stabilization force (by the therapist). The result is a localized active movement, mobilization, or manipulation method that may consist of distraction, compression, gliding, or rolling of the segmental/joint surface. Goodridge[33] suggests that localization of force by appropriate patient positioning is essential to the benefit of MET, and is more important than force intensity.

A well-established method used in the application of a muscle energy technique is proprioceptive neuromuscular facilitation (PNF). PNF techniques make use of proprioceptive stimulus for strengthening or inhibition, of selected and targeted muscle groups.[35] Some of the application methods include hold–relax and contract–relax stretching applied by targeting the agonist or antagonist of the desired movement. Wilson[36] suggests that manually assisted techniques such as those associated with mobilization with movement or PNF methods are helpful by combining neuromuscular contraction and articular input concurrently to stimulate or inhibit a specific muscle group. It is suggested that methods such as PNF may re-

duce the reflexive components of muscle contraction, promoting muscle relaxation and subsequently increasing joint range of motion.[37]

## Summary

- Any method that combines active and/or passive movements is considered a combined method.
- The most common methods of combined movements involve mobilization with movement, muscle energy techniques, and proprioceptive neuromuscular facilitation.

## Fine-Tuning the Techniques

There is little evidence that suggests that there is one "right" way to do a specific technique. In fact, there is more evidence to the opposite: the non-specific nature of selected applications (various techniques) yield similar consequences.[38,39] Fundamentally, there are many different ways to apply techniques and many methods to alter the selected technique once chosen. The fine-tuning mechanisms suggested by Lee et al.[40] outline variations of both examination and treatment that could yield different outcomes of the concordant sign.

### *Magnitude of Force*

There is not a "gold standard" for determining the ideal magnitude of force applied during applied segmental movements.[41–46] In theory, the "ideal" force should vary from subject to subject and will directly rely on the type and location of the signs and symptoms of the patient. For example, if a patient exhibits inflammatory-based pain, light movements designed to alter the affected substance composition may encourage normalization of the tissue chemical environment.[47] Symptoms associated with segmental restrictions may require treatment techniques that lengthen the tissue and provide a mechanical change. Mechanical symptoms associated with muscle reflexive spasm may require forces that result in a reduction in protective spasm, thus allowing osteokinematic movements.

In recognition of this dilemma, G. D. Maitland[48] fashioned a movement diagram designed to explore the relationship of patient sign and symptom presentation and the theoretically appropriate force for optimal treatment. Movement diagrams generally function as prospective learning models, and were first used by Maitland as a teaching aid and means of communication. Maitland[2] detailed, "the movement diagram is a dynamic map representing the quality and quantity of passive movement perceived by the manipulative physiotherapist during the examination of any passive movement direction." Spatial and temporal learning consists of a pattern of active movements defined in terms of space and time, anticipated through visual information.[49–50] The concept has merit since visual modeling has been shown to improve motor learning, specifically in situations that involve exposure to stimuli that require new learning.[51–52]

The visual information provided in a movement diagram defines objective constructs associated for the appropriate amount of graded mobilization forces.[13,52–55] The selection of the proper grade is theoretically dependent upon the tissue relationship and the pathology. The key concept within this relationship is the concept of R1. R1 is the location where stiffness is first perceived by the clinician. This stiffness is perceived as the first point in which the "feel" of the joint assessment presents an objectively identifiable resistance to the clinician. R1 has also been reported by Kaltenborn who identified this concept as the "first stop."[42] Theoretically, the determination of R1 is a prerequisite to selecting grades of manual therapy mobilization.[24]

An example of a stiffness-dominant movement diagram is provided in Figure 4.10. The X-axis (line A-B) is used to indicate the onset of pain or resistance, whichever is depicted first. The Y-axis defines the force associated with the mobilization movement. The first point of pain is identified by P1; the first point of resistance, R1; maximum pain, P2; and maximum resistance, R2. Typically, lines are drawn by the therapist upon evaluation of the detected resistance of the joint. If one adopts this concept, each grade of motion should vary from subject to subject. The selection of the grade should depend on the presence of the first point of resistance felt within the tissue and the pain of the patient.[56] Based on the Maitland model, oscillatory forces for Grades I and II should be below R1, whereas forces applied for Grades III and IV should exceed R1 with some degree of overlap.[57] In the presence of these subjective guidelines, it may be reasonable and pertinent to quantify the applied magnitude, amplitude, and frequency of oscillations in order to appropriately select the correct therapeutic force.[42,54]

Since manual therapy clinicians are taught to identify the difference between normal joint resistance and abnormal joint resistance[41,53], this method of theorizing applied force has conceptual merit. Movement diagrams have been shown to be effective teaching methods for recording the stiffness–force relationship in manual therapy mobilization of the shoulder[46,58], but have demonstrated poor outcomes during assessment of the lumbar spine.[59] Assessment of R1 has generally demonstrated poor interclinician reliability, even when visually demonstrated using a movement diagram.[41] This may be one reason why clinicians demonstrate poor interrater reliability during application of selective grades of mobilization.[54,59] Another weakness of the movement diagram is its primary association with mobilization and manipulation techniques. Nonetheless, the concept can be extrapolated to static stretching.

Although there is a theoretical concept associated with the ideal force during treatment, there are few examples within the literature of measured forces during mobilization and manipulation among various professions. While the reliability and consistency of force during application is somewhat suspect, the forces can be generalized based on several studies. Measurement devices have ranged from subjective scales, force platforms, pinch grips, and a mechanical spinal mobilization device. The difficulty in standardizing a measurement point may be one of the reasons for the sparseness within the literature. Many studies have utilized a posterior–anterior (PA) force to the spine as their measurement point within studies.

In a study performed to measure the educational effects of using the force plate, Lee, Moseley, and Refshauge[55] found that most physical therapy students applied consistent mobilization forces that ranged from 20–45 Newtons. Latimer, Lee, and Adams[60] determined the range of applied force of manual therapists varied from 30–200 Newtons. The authors suggested that most clinicians routinely applied forces of 30–429 Newtons during mobilization. Others have reported[61] average mobilization forces ranging from 50.1 Newtons to 194.8 Newtons during actual patient care intervention of the lumbar spine. The lower numbers reflected lower grades and correspondingly, the upper numbers reflected upper grades.

Herzog et al.[62] reported consistent use of 500–600 Newtons of force during the fourth thoracic vertebral (T4) manipulation techniques from chiropractors. Additionally, most chiropractic techniques require a preload of forces that are often higher than a mobilization-based force. Cervical and sacroiliac techniques were observed with smaller torque values, 100 Newtons and 300-plus Newtons, respectively. These forces occurred with a population of symptomatic patients without incident or plastic failure.

Based on the literature it is reasonable to assume normal treatment ranges for both mobilization and manipulation from 30–500 Newtons of force. This force application must be selective toward the proper target

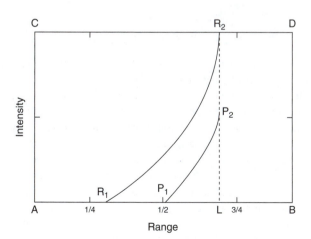

**Figure 4.10** An Example of a Movement Diagram— Stiffness Dominance

tissue. For instance, the connective tissue of the lower back, including the shear forces absorbed by the disc and surrounding tissues, may tolerate more force than the connective tissue of the anterior talofibular ligament.

### Rate of Increase of Force

It has been suggested that the rate of increase in force application can alter the perception of stiffness.[40] A similar suggestion from Maitland[2] hypothesizes that differences in frequency are necessary depending on the response of the patient to various mobilization movements. Variations include faster frequencies during the application "on" and slower frequency for load "off" or a steady pace when patients exhibit fair to strong symptoms.

### Duration of Loading

Maitland[57] also suggests that a sustained load in the presence of a muscle spasm may yield positive responses and a reduction in muscle spasm. Nonetheless, there is little information to support the suggestion that duration significantly alters the treatment outcome. Essentially, modification of the duration of the load is purely patient response based and may yield different results with each patient.

### Targeted Tissue to Which the Force Is Applied

New information has suggested that a technique applied any direction within the region of the spine is as beneficial as a therapist-selected force to the pathological segment.[38,39] This concept is a paradigm shift from most philosophies and further studies are suggested. Furthermore, evidence exists that manual therapy to the thoracic spine is helpful for patients complaining of a cervical spine disorder.[39] This suggests a link between various aspects of the cervical and thoracic spine pain generators.

### Location of Manual Force in Relation to Center of the Targeted Structure

Maitland[57] recognizes that mobilization methods performed at various locations on the targeted structure (i.e., interspinous space, laminar trough, transverse process, and zygopophyseal joint) will yield different results. Since the application of a technique that identifies the patient's most concordant reproduction is the goal of the treatment, movements outside the "center" of the targeted structure are warranted. The manner in which the symptoms are reproduced demonstrate equal importance to the diagnosis of the patient.[57]

### Direction of Force

Selected authors have suggested that patient position and direction (angle) of force may lead to differences in stiffness detection.[53,63] Increased stiffness, or resistance, begins as soon as force is applied to a spinous process during a posterior–anterior mobilization and is increased or decreased by changing the position of the spine.[53] Edmondston et al.[53] found that prepositions of flexion or extension by the patient during prone lying significantly in-

creased the stiffness coefficient of the lumbar spine. To maintain continuity between raters, the patient is required to assume the exact position he or she assumed from the previous rater. This difficulty in maintaining a standard position for assessment, combined with the small overall joint movement expected during a movement assessment, will reduce the possibility of obtaining reliable results.[64,65]

The direction of mobilization forces can alter the amount of stiffness measured by machines and perceived by therapists. Caling and Lee[65] determined that stiffness measured at plus or minus 10° from a perpendicular base direction (defined as the mean direction of force applied by experienced therapists) was from 7 to 10% less than the stiffness measured in the perpendicular direction.

### Contact Area over Which the Force Is Applied

Several common treatment methods currently use different contact aspects of a clinician's hands. For example, the use of the thumbs, pisiform, and/or other contact points of the hand could alter the pain reproduction associated with the treatment approach. It is common to produce "false pain" during a treatment that is purely associated with a painful contact versus the movement reproduction of the pain.

> ## Summary
>
> - Fundamentally, there are many different ways to apply techniques and many methods to alter the selected technique once chosen.
> - Methods to alter the treatment include changes in force magnitude and direction, contact area, duration of loading, rate of increased force, and alterations in the tissue in which the force is applied.

# REEXAMINATION

## The Purpose of Reexamination

The careful marriage of examination and treatment results in reduction of pain or normalization of range of motion. These impairment-based changes should result in an improvement in dysfunction or reduction in disability. In essence, a patient's condition is capricious and requires an ever-changing clinician's response. Analysis of the patient's change is the purpose behind careful reexamination. Additionally, the reexamination determines when and how the treatment would benefit from modification based on new findings.

Sizer et al.[66] reported that adaptation to patient response was one of the most imperative aspects of orthopedic manual therapy treatment. Included within these skill descriptors were force management, technique modifications, and velocity management methods. Ladyshewsky and Gotjamanos[67] suggested that adaptation is only possible during affective verbal and nonverbal communication between the patient and the clinician. Others have identified this form of communication as an essential trait of orthopedic clinical experts.[68]

In Chapter 2, we discussed the treatment–reexamination cycle and emphasized how each depends on the outcome of the other. The first initiation of the treatment is predicated on the outcome of the examination and from then on is based on the findings of the reexamination. All three of these components are encompassed in the global concept of "assessment."

There are two primary considerations during reexamination of a patient. First, since effective examination and treatment should lead to noticeable changes in the patient's concordant sign, a reexamination of each patient's concordant sign is necessary at each intervention. An outcome based on the concordant sign defines whether the "familiar" signs and symptoms of the patient have changed. Reexamining the concordant sign assumes that every individual is different and that the consequence of the pathology is specific to that one person and is generally well received by the patient. By focusing on the concordant sign the clinician is able to disseminate findings from changes that may not be related to a positive outcome of the patient (discordant signs). By focusing treatment on a discordant sign or some form of theoretical construct, the clinician may waste considerable time and effort toward a method that may demonstrate only moderate effectiveness.

It is expected that techniques will be modified during alterations in the patient's condition, tissue resistance, and force management.[66] Others have reported that changes in the patient's concordant signs and symptoms require modification of the treatment method, specifically velocity and force production of the procedure to ensure positive outcomes.[69]

Second, changes in the patient's report of function provide the clinician with additional data for analytical assessment. Multiple functional scales exist, each measuring different constructs, having different levels of responsiveness, and having variable floor and ceiling effects. **Generic-specific scales** that measure activities of daily living, function, and general well-being are considered more psychometrically sound and may have the capability of measuring health status across multiple bodily dimensions.[70] **Region-specific scales** are thought to exhibit greater sensitivity to change and display greater content validity.[70] Additionally, most region-specific scales have physiometric measures designed to demonstrate physical, social, and mental changes. Both are standardized measures that provide valuable insight to recovery that go beyond assessment of the concordant sign.

By using both methods during assessment, the accurate ability to quantify changes in a patient's conditions signifi-

cantly improves. Bias associated with discordant measures or by analyzing methods that are steeped in clinician perception is reduced dramatically. Perhaps most importantly, since the model is patient response based, alterations in the treatment are applied automatically, and are based on the results of a patient's concordant and functional changes.

## Summary

- Reexamination involves the analysis of the change associated with the targeted intervention.
- There are two primary considerations during reexamination of a patient: changes in the patient's concordant sign and alterations in the baseline function of the patient.

## *Troubleshooting*

Despite best efforts by manual therapists some patients do not respond positively to treatment. There are two possible reasons for a poor outcome. First, the patient may have a sinister disorder that requires medical care beyond the capacity of a manual therapist. Second, the manual therapist may have made errors in his or her assessment of the patient. Commonly, errors occur in the areas of (1) inappropriate examination, (2) inappropriate treatment, and (3) failure to assess and guide the patient in his or her role during treatment.

### *Inappropriate Examination*

Christensen et al.[9] identify three reasons that the clinical examination may demonstrate undesirable results. First, the clinician may place an overemphasis on biomedical or perceived clinical knowledge. Second, the clinician may make assumptions during the patient response-based assessment without clarifying the outcomes. Third, the clinician may have adopted a dogmatic assessment method that fails to enclose the signs and symptoms presented by the patient at hand. Additionally, if the patient is not committed to the process of the examination, the clinician runs the risk of obtaining less than beneficial data.

### *Inappropriate Treatment*

Inappropriate treatment may represent many forms. First, many appropriate techniques are performed using incorrect amounts of force. If the clinician provides too little force the outcome will be less than substantial. Too much force may worsen the condition. Force directed in the wrong direction may also worsen the condition. Movements as little as 10 degrees[63] can alter the perception of stiffness and may modify the clinician's perception of the condition. Essentially, force production problems are mostly associated with a failure to adapt the forces provided to the response of the patient. A hallmark of the patient-response method is modifying the treatment force to the patient's outcome.

Another treatment failure is associated with application strategy. Clinicians who blindly follow treatment recipes or protocols are more likely to miss the key aspects associated with progressive care.[9] Selecting treatments based on fad versus clinical reasoning is another common mistake made. Many clinicians attend "techniques" courses only to fail to discern when to use the specific techniques. Furthermore, attending only to those features that support a favorable hypothesis and either neglecting or not testing alternative hypotheses may lead to poor treatment outcomes.[9] By practicing lateral thinking, the clinician is more apt to keep an open mind when treating unfamiliar conditions.

### Failure to Appropriately Engage the Patient

Another common error is the failure to accurately assess and discuss the patient's role in his or her rehabilitation. In cases where a patient is familiar with a passive approach to his or her recovery, active methods may seem foreign and unnecessary. In some cases where a patient is asked to endure some discomfort during the procedure, especially when the patient has not "bought in" to the treatment method, the patient may not demonstrate commitment to the approach. Outside variables such as social, demographic, and emotional variables have a significant influence on the outcome of a patient and should also be considered as covariates to recovery.

---

## Summary

- Essentially, there are three possible reasons for failure to improve during reexamination: (1) inappropriate examination, (2) inappropriate treatment, and (3) failure to adequately engage the patient.

---

## Key Considerations for Orthopedic Manual Therapy

### Communication

Communication between clinician and patient is essential. During the examination, the communication between the clinician and patient is what determines the concordant sign, the irritability, the understanding of the area, and behavior of the symptoms and the assessment of the outcome of the treatment. Orthopedic manual therapists use verbal and nonverbal feedback to make a diagnosis.[71]

### Pain or Stiffness

Often, a patient is classified into a pain-dominant or stiffness-dominant condition.[11] These terms are synonymous with mechanical and inflammatory conditions. By understanding where a patient's symptoms most appropriately fit, the clinician may select the appropriate treatment technique.

### Selecting the Appropriate Grade

In orthopaedic manual therapy, a common assumption is that the movement of a joint determined during manual assessment will dictate the grade of application selected.[71] Those dominated by pain during movement may not tolerate aggressive, end-range movements. It has been suggested that through-range pain is best treated with lower grades.

#### Understanding Abnormal Tissue

It has been suggested that orthopedic manual therapists are taught to identify the difference between normal joint resistance and abnormal joint resistance (stiffness) through various training regimens.[55,72] Abnormal stiffness is the detection of motion availability within the examined joint and has been reliably detected in pathological individuals.[73,74] When assessment of abnormal stiffness is combined with detection of the concordant sign, the information provided is specific for that condition.

---

# Chapter Questions

1. Why is a careful analysis of the patient's response a necessity in determining the appropriate treatment technique selection?
2. Outline the various passive treatment techniques. Compare and contrast the methods.
3. Describe the philosophy of and a favorable response to an approach for a "pain-dominant" individual.
4. Describe the philosophy of and a favorable response to an approach for a "stiffness-dominant" individual.
5. What impact does the patient have on their outcome?

---

# References

1. Edwards B. *Manual of combined movements.* Oxford; Butterworth-Heinemann: 1999.
2. Maitland GD. *Peripheral manipulation.* 3rd ed. London; Butterworth-Heinemann: 1986.
3. Edmondston SJ, Allison GT, Gregg CD, Purden SM, Svansson GR, Watson AE. Effect of position on the posteroanterior stiffness of the lumbar spine. *Man Ther.* 1998;3(1):21–26.

4. Trott P. Management of selected cervical syndromes. In: Grant R. *Physical therapy of the cervical and thoracic spine.* 3rd ed. New York; Churchill Livingstone: 2002.

5. Deyo RA, Rainville J, Kent DL. What can the history and physical examination tell us about low back pain? *JAMA.* 1992;268(6):760–765.

6. Riddle D. Measurement of accessory motion: critical issues and related concepts. *Phys Ther.* 1992;72:865–874.

7. Boden SD, Riew KD, Yamaguchi K, Branch TP, Schellinger D, Wiesel SW. Orientation of the lumbar facet joints: association with degenerative disc disease. *J Bone Joint Surg Am.* 1996;78(3):403–411.

8. Sprague R. Differential assessment and mobilization of the cervical and upper thoracic spine. In: Donatelli R, Wooden M. *Orthopaedic physical therapy.* Philadelphia; Churchill Livingston: 2001.

9. Christensen N, Jones M, Carr J. Clinical reasoning in orthopedic manual therapy. In: Grant R. *Physical therapy of the cervical and thoracic spine.* 3rd ed. New York; Churchill Livingstone: 2002.

10. Gifford L. Pain, the tissues and the nervous system: a conceptual model. *Physiotherapy.* 1998;84:27.

11. Maher C, Latimer J. Pain or resistance-the therapists' dilemma. *Aust J Physiotherapy.* 1993;38:257–260.

12. Jones M. Clinical reasoning in manual therapy. *Phys Ther.* 1992;72:875–884.

13. Vicenzino B, Collins D, Wright A. Sudomotor changes induced by neural mobilization techniques in asymptomatic subjects. *J Manual Manipulative Ther.* 1994;2:66–74.

14. Maher C, Adams R. Reliability of pain and stiffness assessments in clinical manual lumbar spine examination. *Phys Ther.* 1994;74:10–18.

15. Grieve G. *Common vertebral joint problems.* 2nd ed. Edinburgh; Churchill Livingstone: 1988.

16. Guide to Physical Therapist Practice. 2nd ed. *Phys Ther.* 2001;81:9–744.

17. McKenzie R. Mechanical diagnosis and therapy for disorders of the low back. In: Twomey L, Taylor J. *Physical therapy of the low back.* 3rd ed. New York; Churchill Livingstone: 2000.

18. Seroussi RE, Krag MH, Muller DL, Pope MH. Internal deformations of intact and denucleated human lumbar discs subjected to compression, flexion, and extension loads. *J Orthop Res.* 1989;7(1): 122–131.

19. Norkin C, Levangie P. Joint Structure and Function: *A comprehensive analysis.* 2nd ed. Philadelphia; F. A. Davis Company: 1992.

20. Mennell J. Back pain: *Diagnosis and treatment using manipulative techniques.* Boston; Little, Brown and Co.: 1960.

21. Kaltenborn F. Manual mobilization of the joints. *The Kaltenborn method of joint mobilization and treatment.* 5th ed. Oslo; Olaf Norlis Bokhandel: 1999.

22. Cyriax J, Cyriax P. *Cyriax's illustrated manual of orthopaedic medicine.* Oxford; Butterworth-Heineman: 1993.

23. Benjamin P, Tappan F. *Tappan's handbook of healing massage techniques.* 4th ed. Upper Saddle River, NJ; Prentice Hall: 2004.

24. Herzog W. *Clinical biomechanics of spinal manipulation.* London; Churchill Livingstone: 2000.

25. McCarthy CJ. Spinal manipulative thrust technique using combined movement theory. *Man Ther.* 2001; 6:197–204.

26. Nyberg R. Manipulation: definition, types, application. In: Basmajian J, Nyberg R. (eds). *Rational manual therapies.* Baltimore; Williams and Wilkens: 1993.

27. Grice A, Vernon H. Basic principles in the performance of chiropractic adjusting: historical review, classification and objectives. In: Haldeman S, ed. *Principles and practice of chiropractic,* 2nd ed. Norwalk; Appleton & Lange: 1992;443–458.

28. Mulligan B. Mobilisations with movement (MVM's). *J Manual Manipulative Ther.* 1993;1:154–156.

29. Mulligan B. *Manual therapy "NAGS", "SNAGS", "MWM's" etc.* 4th ed. Wellington; Plane View Services Ltd.: 1999.

30. Mulligan BR. Spinal mobilisation with leg movement (further mobilisation with movement). *J Manual Manipulative Ther.* 1995;3(1):25–27.

31. Exelby L. The Mulligan concept: its application in the management of spinal conditions. *Man Ther.* 2002;7(2):64–70.

32. Konstantinou K, Foster N, Rushton A, Baxter D. The use and reported effects of mobilization with movement techniques in low back pain management; a cross-sectional descriptive survey of physiotherapists in Britain. *Man Ther.* 2002;7(4):206–214.

33. Goodridge JP. Muscle energy technique: definition, explanation, methods of procedure. *J Am Osteopath Assoc.* 1981;81(4):249–254.

34. Hubbard A. Homokinetics. Muscular function in human movement. In: Johnson W, Buskirk R. *Science and medicine of exercise and sport.* New York; Harper and Row: 1974.

35. Ferber R, Osternig L, Gravelle D. Effect of PNF stretch techniques on knee flexor muscle EMG activity in older adults. *J Electomyography Kinesiology.* 2002; 12:391–397.

36. Wilson E. Central facilitation and remote effects: treating both ends of the system. *Man Ther.* 1997; 2(3):165–168.

37. Prentice W. A comparison of static stretching and PNF stretching for improving hip joint flexibility. *Athletic Training.* 1983;18:56–59.

38. Childs J. Risk associated with the failure to offer manipulation for patients with low back pain. Platform Presentation. American Academy of Orthopaedic

Manual Physical Therapists Conference. Louisville, KY. 2004.

39. Cleland J, Childs J, McRae M, Palmer J. Immediate effects of thoracic spine manipulation in patients with neck pain: a randomized clinical trial. Platform Presentation. American Academy of Orthopaedic Manual Physical Therapists Conference. Louisville, KY. 2004.

40. Lee M, Steven J, Crosbie R, Higgs J. Towards a theory of lumbar mobilization-the relationship between applied manual force and movements of the spine. *Man Ther*. 1996;2:67–75.

41. Anson E, Cook C, Comacho C, Gwillian B, Karakostas K. The use of education in the improvement in finding R1 in the lumbar spine. *J Manual Manipulative Ther*. 2003;11(4):204–212.

42. Bjornsdottir SV, Kumar S. Posteroanterior spinal mobilization: State of the art review and discussion. *Disabil Rehabil*. 1997;19:39–46.

43. Yahia L, Audet J, Drouin G. Rheological properties of the human lumbar spine ligaments. *J Biomed Eng*. 1991;13:399–406.

44. DiFabio R. Efficacy of manual therapy. *Phys Ther*. 1992;72(12):853–864.

45. Petty N, Messenger N. Can the force platform be used to measure the forces applied during a PA mobilization of the lumbar spine? *J Manual Manipulative Ther*. 1996;4(2):70–76.

46. Chesworth B, MacDermid J, Roth J, Patterson S. Movement diagram and "end-feel" reliability when measuring passive lateral rotation of the shoulder in patients with shoulder pathology. *Phys Ther*. 1998; 78:593–601.

47. Holm S, Nachemson A. Variations in the nutrition of the canine intervertebral disc induced by motion. *Spine*. 1983;8:866–873.

48. Maitland G, Hickling J. Abnormalities in passive movement: Diagrammative representation. *Physiother*. 1970;56:105–114.

49. Carroll W, Bandura A. The role of visual monitoring in observational learning of action patterns: Making the unobservable observable. *J Motor Behavior*. 1982; 14:153–167.

50. Carroll W, Bandura A. Representational guidance of action production in observational learning: A causal analysis. *J Motor Behavior*. 1990;22:85–97.

51. Yahia L, Audet J, Drouin G. Rheological properties of the human lumbar spine ligaments. *J Biomed Eng*. 1991;13:399–406.

52. Lee R, Latimer J, Maher C. Manipulation: Investigation of a proposed mechanism. *Clin Biomech*. 1994; 8:302–306.

53. Edmondston S, Allison G, Gregg S, Purden G, Svansson G, Watson A. Effect of position on the posteroanterior stiffness of the lumbar spine. *Man Ther*. 1998;3(1):21–26.

54. Hardy GL, Napier JK. Inter and intra-therapist reliability of passive accessory movement technique. *NZ J of Physiotherapy*. 1991;22–24.

55. Lee M, Mosely A, Refshauge K. Effects of feedback on learning a vertebral joint mobilizations skill. *Phys Ther*. 1990;10:97–102.

56. Cook C. The effect of a pre-perceptual educational instrument on inter-rater reliability in physical therapists. *Internet Journal of Allied Health and Sciences*. 2003;1,2.

57. Maitland GD. *Maitland's vertebral manipulation*. 6th ed. London; Butterworth-Heinemann: 2001.

58. MacDermid JC, Chesworth BM, Patterson S, Roth JH. Validity of pain and motion indicators recorded on a movement diagram of shoulder lateral rotation. *Aust J Physiother*. 1999;45(4):269–277.

59. Cook C, Turney L, Miles A, Ramirez L, Karakostas T. Predictive factors in poor inter-rater reliability among physical therapists. *J Manual Manipulative Ther*. 2002;10(4):200–205.

60. Latimer J, Lee M, Adams RD. The effects of high and low loading forces on measured values of lumbar stiffness. *J Manipulative Physiol Ther*. 1998;21: 157–163.

61. Chiradejnant A, Latimer J, Maher CG. Forces applied during manual therapy to patients with low back pain. *J Manipulative Physiol Ther*. 2002;25(6):362–369.

62. Herzog W, Conway PJ, Kawchuk GN, Zhang Y, Hasler EM. Forces exerted during spinal manipulative therapy. *Spine* 1993;18(9):1206–1212.

63. Caling B, Lee M. Effect of direction of applied mobilization force on the posteroanterior response in the lumbar spine. *J Manipulative Physiol Ther*. 2001; 24:71–78.

64. Lee R, Evans J. An *in-vivo* study of the intervertebral movements produced by posteroanterior mobilization. *Clin Biomech*. 1997;12:400–408

65. Frank C, Akeson WH, Woo SLY, Amiel D, Coutts RD. Physiology and therapeutic value of passive joint of motion. *Clin Ortho*. 1984;185:113–124.

66. Sizer P. Manual therapy skills: results of the Delphi study. Breakout Presentation. American Academy of Orthopaedic Manual Physical Therapists Conference. Reno, NV. 2003.

67. Ladyshewsky R, Gotjamanos E. Communication skill development in health professional education: the use of standardised patients in combination with a peer assessment strategy. *J Allied Health*. 1997;26(4): 177–186.

68. Jensen G, Shepard K, Hack L. The novice versus the experienced clinician: insights into the work of the physical therapist. *Phys Ther*.1990;70:314–323.

69. Chiu T, Wright A. To compare the effects of different rates of application of a cervical mobilization technique on sympathetic outflow to the upper limb in normal subjects. *Man Ther*. 1996;198–203.

70. Pietrobon R, Coeytaux R, Carey T, Richardson W, DeVellis R. Standard scales for measurement of functional outcome for cervical pain or dysfunction. *Spine*. 2002;27:515–522.
71. Phillips DR, Twomey LT. A comparison of manual diagnosis with a diagnosis established by a uni-level lumbar spinal block procedure. *Man Ther*. 2000;1(2):82–87.
72. Threlkeld AJ. The effects of manual therapy on connective tissue. *Phys Ther*. 1992;72(12):893–902.
73. Jull G, Treleaven J, Versace G. Manual examination of spinal joints. Is pain provocation a major diagnostic clue for dysfunction? *Aust J Physiotherapy*. 1997:43:125.
74. Jull G, Bogduk N, Marsland A. The accuracy of manual diagnosis for cervical zygapophysial joint pain syndromes. *Med J Aust*. 1988;148(5):233–236.
75. Showalter C, Sprague, R. MT-2. Basic Spinal. Maitland Australian Physiotherapy Seminars. Cutchogue, NY; MAPS. 2002.

# 5

# Medical Screening

## Objectives

- Define the purpose of the medical screen.
- Recognize the presence of "red flags" during a screen and understand the appropriate mechanism and outside referral (if necessary).
- Define the key aspects of the upper and lower quarter screen.

- Demonstrate the ability to differentiate between somatic and visceral referred pain, radiculopathy, and myelopathy.
- Outline the contraindications of selected methods of manual therapy.

## THE MEDICAL SCREEN

The *Guide to Physical Therapist Practice*[1] recognizes **medical screening** as an essential element of an initial evaluation. Key constituents of the *Guide* include cardiovascular/pulmonary, skin integumentary, neuromuscular, communication, and musculoskeletal assessment.[1] Medical screening is an essential aspect of a manual therapist's evaluation because it promotes awareness of comorbidities that may contribute or potentially harm a patient's recovery and/or function. Common comorbidities such as high blood pressure, arthritis, depression, and others are probable in physical therapy practice.[2,3] Other disorders such as a neurological illness, fracture, or neoplasm represent comorbidities that are potentially threatening to the patient.

A medical screen is a constituent of the history taking, database analysis, physical examination, and monitoring of the patient's condition.[4] Discerning findings in each of these categories may warrant the use of a lower or upper quarter testing designed specifically to determine if the patient would benefit from additional medical consultation. These discerning findings are identified as "red flags."

**Red flags** are signs and symptoms that may tie a disorder to a serious pathology.[4] When combinations or singular representations of selected red flag features are encountered during an examination, a clinician may im-

prove their ability to assess the risk of a serious underlying pathology.[5] Red flag features are stratified into three primary categories: (1) patient history and situational prevalence, (2) present complaint characteristics, and (3) physical examination and laboratory findings.[5]

### Patient History and Situational Prevalence

Swenson[5] outlines several patient history or situational components considered as red flags. A history of cancer, history of a disorder with predilection for infection or hemorrhage, long-term corticosteroid use, a history of a metabolic bone disorder, a recent history of unexplained weight loss, and an age greater than 50 years may contribute negatively toward treatment. Triggers associated with situational prevalence increase the likelihood of the presence of selected conditions based on underlying characteristics and have been recognized to increase the potential of sinister phenomenon such as cancer, spinal osteomyelitis, or fracture.[6] Furthermore, the presences of some of these phenomena are contraindications to selected manual therapy procedures.

### Present Compliant Characteristics

Present compliant characteristics include physical system changes, poor response to conservative care, and conditional aspects. Physical system changes include pathological changes in bowel and bladder, patterns of symptoms not compatible with mechanical pain, blood in sputum, an impairment precipitated by recent trauma, bilateral or unilateral radiculopathy or parathesia, numbness or parathesia in the perianal region, writhing pain, nonhealing sores or wounds, unexplained significant lower or upper limb weakness, and a progressive neurological deficit. Components demonstrating poor response to conservative care include lack of pain relief with prescribed bed rest, pain that is worse during rest than activity, pain worsened at night or not relieved by any position, and poor success with comparable treatments. Conditional characteristics such as litigation for the current impairment, long-term worker's compensation, and poor relationship with the employment supervisor[7] have been linked to poor recovery for orthopedic conditions.

## Physical Examination and Laboratory Findings

Numerous physical examination and laboratory findings exist that deserve recognition. These include but are not limited to pulsatile abdominal masses, fever, neurological deficit not explained by monoradiculopathy, clonus, gait defects, abnormal reflexes, and an elevated sedimentation rate. Physical examination findings are often examined using special tests with high levels of sensitivity or specificity. High levels of sensitivity indicate that a negative test has the capacity to rule out a particular disorder. High levels of specificity indicate a positive test has the capacity to rule in a disorder.

The presence of some red flags suggests a serious pathology outside the realm of care of manual therapists. Some "red flag" findings such as radiculopathy are common and simply require further differentiation. Table 5.1 delineates which red flag findings warrant immediate medical attention and which require further investigation.

How an orthopedic manual therapist responds to each of the three categories of red flags depends on the intent of treatment. Many of the history and situational prevalence components are absolute or relative contraindications for treatment. Information obtained from present complaints may range from solicitation of appropriate medical consultation to the use of a multidisciplinary treatment plan. Any of the physical examination and labo-

**TABLE 5.1    Categorical Classification of "Red Flag" Findings during Medical Screening**

| | |
|---|---|
| Category 1: Factor that requires immediate medical attention | • Pathological changes in bowel and bladder<br>• Patterns of symptoms not compatible with mechanical pain (after physical exam)<br>• Blood in sputum<br>• Numbness or parathesia in the perianal region<br>• Progressive neurological deficit<br>• Pulsatile abdominal masses<br>• Neurological deficit not explained by monoradiculopathy<br>• Elevated sedimentation rate |
| Category 2: Factors that require subjective questioning or contraindications to selected manual therapy techniques | • Impairment precipitated by recent trauma<br>• Writhing pain<br>• Nonhealing sores or wounds<br>• Fever<br>• Clonus (could be related to past CNS disorder)<br>• Gait defects<br>• History of cancer<br>• History of a disorder with predilection for infection or hemorrhage<br>• Long-term corticosteroid use<br>• History of a metabolic bone disorder<br>• Recent history of unexplained weight loss<br>• Age > than 50<br>• Litigation for the current impairment<br>• Long-term worker's compensation<br>• Poor relationship with the employment supervisor |
| Category 3: Factors that require further physical testing and differentiation analysis | • Bilateral or unilateral radiculopathy or parathesia<br>• Unexplained significant lower or upper limb weakness<br>• Abnormal reflexes |

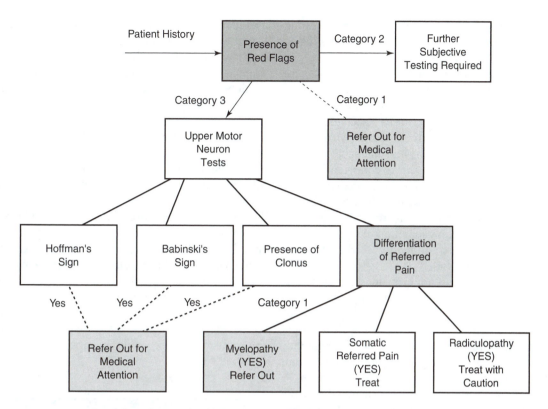

**Figure 5.1**    Guideline for Medical Screening of "Red Flags"

ratory findings may function as a trigger to perform either neurological testing or upper and lower quarter screening, or both. Figure 5.1 outlines the screening process when red flags are encountered during the clinical examination.

## Summary

- Red flag features are signs and symptoms that may tie a disorder to a serious pathology.
- During a regional examination, red flag features are distilled during investigation of three primary areas: (1) patient history and situational prevalence), (2) present compliant characteristics, and (3) physical examination and laboratory findings.
- The existence of selected red flags warrants outside medical attention; others are contraindications to selected manual therapy approaches.

# UPPER AND LOWER QUARTER SCREENING

An orthopedic manual therapist may elect to perform an upper or lower quarter screen upon identification of red flags during the clinical examination. The purpose of the **upper quarter screen** and **lower quarter screen** is to further distill the origin of the signs and symptoms and determine the patient's applicability for care. One sign and symptom that is considered a trigger for further assessment beyond the traditional examination is referred pain into the extremities. Upper and lower quarter screening is designed to identify the behavior of the referred pain and further delineate its characteristic.

Upper and lower quarter screen involves four components: (1) **sensation testing** (dermatomes); (2) regional muscle strength testing **(myotome)**; (3) **reflex testing;** and (4) **differentiation of referred pain.** The assessment of these four methods is commonly used in impairments associated with cervical and lumbar radiculopathy, although limitations do exist.

It is quite common for upper and lower quarter screening to lead to variable findings. Many of the conditions that are associated with referred pain such as a herniated or bulging disc demonstrate inconsistent presentations and may or may not yield sensation, strength, or reflex changes. This variable impairment characteristic (VIC) behavior is suggestive of the unpredictability of the disorder, and less so the weakness of the testing methods.

## Sensation Testing

Sensation testing consists of light touch, pain, vibration, and thermo-testing (temperature). Sensation testing has been described in many ways and consists of a wide variety of application methods. In most cases, sensation testing involves comparative analysis between extremities using any of the aforementioned sensations.

It has been suggested that clinical application of these methods are not reliable because they require consistent reproducible application and assessment among multiple examiners.[8] This finding is most likely associated with a failure to standardize the application method. Most errors occur when the clinician fails to blind the subject to the area tested or when the clinician fails to consistently apply a side-to-side examination within a short time span. The best way to apply sensory testing is to provide comparative applications bilaterally for each dermatome, during blinding, using a battery of different sensation methods. Asking the properties of "sameness" and whether they feel the sensation or not are both advised.

When carefully evaluated, abnormalities found during current perception threshold testing do implicate a dysfunction of peripheral nerve fibers.[9–11] Therefore, one can ascertain a dysfunction of some form causing either compression or traction, resulting in a pathological phenomenon. Unfortunately, the testing does not implicate the cause of the dysfunction nor is the test designed to have specificity to do so. Because the causes of peripheral referred pain often exhibit variable impairment characteristics, in many cases, the impairments do not exhibit sensation changes.

A clinician may find improved use of sensation testing upon understanding of the prevalence of variable impairment characteristics. Aronson and Dunsmore[12] indicated that sensory deficits to pin prick involving L3-L4 were noted in 39% of patients with L2-L3 disc herniation, and in 30% of patients with problems at L3-L4, verified intraoperatively. Others[13] found 60% had sensory impairments at L3-L4, 52% at L4-L5. Jonsson et al.[14] reported that dermatome sensory disturbance was present in 60% of patients with sciatica. Blower[15] found 62% of patients with sensory disturbances and Jensen[16] reported that just 56% of patients with sciatica of a L4-5 distribution demonstrated neighboring sensory disturbance and L5-S1 distributions. Lauder et al.[17] found a sensitivity of 55% in a population of patients with lumbar radiculopathy and abnormal electrodiagnostic test values. Specificity scores were slightly higher (77%), yielding a +LR of 3.91.

The diagnostic strength of cervical sensory testing is unclear. Several authors have reported high levels of sensitivity[18–21] verified during surgical identification of a herniated disc and/or spondylopathy. Others have reported low sensitivity levels[22–24] using both surgically documented analysis and needle EMG diagnosis of cervical radiculopathy. In what appears to be the most comprehensive sensory assessment, Wainner et al.[25] reported poor diagnostic values for all cervical levels except C5. In fact, dermatome testing of the levels C6 through T1 demonstrated positive likelihood values below one suggesting no value to the diagnostic process. Furthermore, other studies have reported that various forms of sensation testing lack the ability to detect the level of the lesion. Nygaard and Mellgren[26] suggested that thermo and vibratory tests are not suitable for predicting the level of lesion, because there is no significant difference between an ipsilateral nerve root sensation change and the compressed nerve root. Others have reported that patients with sciatica may complain of altered heat, cold, and mechanical thresholds as compared with nonsymptomatic extremities.[27–29]

Standalone sensation testing may or may not yield useful information, but is certainly an important characteristic of a screen when used in concert with other findings. The presence of sensation change does provide very useful information and may be indicative of pathology when combined with other measures. The absence of a sensation change does not rule out the presence of a disc pathology or sinister phenomenon and has been commonly reported within the literature.

Figure 5.2 identifies common sensory dermatomes within the body. Figures 5.3 through 5.6 outline the appropriate forms of sensibility testing.

## Summary

- Sensation testing consists of light touch, pain, vibration, and temperature assessments.
- Standalone sensation testing may or may not yield useful information, but is certainly an important characteristic of a screen.
- Several studies have suggested that sensation testing is not discriminatory enough to determine the level of a specific pathology, or determine the presence of a particular disorder.
- Sensation is best performed during blinding of the patient and bilateral performance of the sensation stimuli.

## Regional Muscle Strength Testing

Myotome testing, or "muscle strength testing," is a method designed to identify if abnormalities in muscle strength are present during a one-repetition manual muscle test. Like sensation testing, myotome testing may yield variable findings that are characteristic of the unpredictable findings of the impairment (VIC). Additionally, two factors, the level of the actual lesion (spine level) and the multiplicity of levels that innervate selected muscle groups, can lead to inconclusive findings. Hakelius and Hindmarsh[30] reported that quadriceps weakness was present in only 1% of the population operated for disc herniation, including any level. Aronson and Dunsmore[12] found much higher values, 30% of individuals with L2-L3 disc

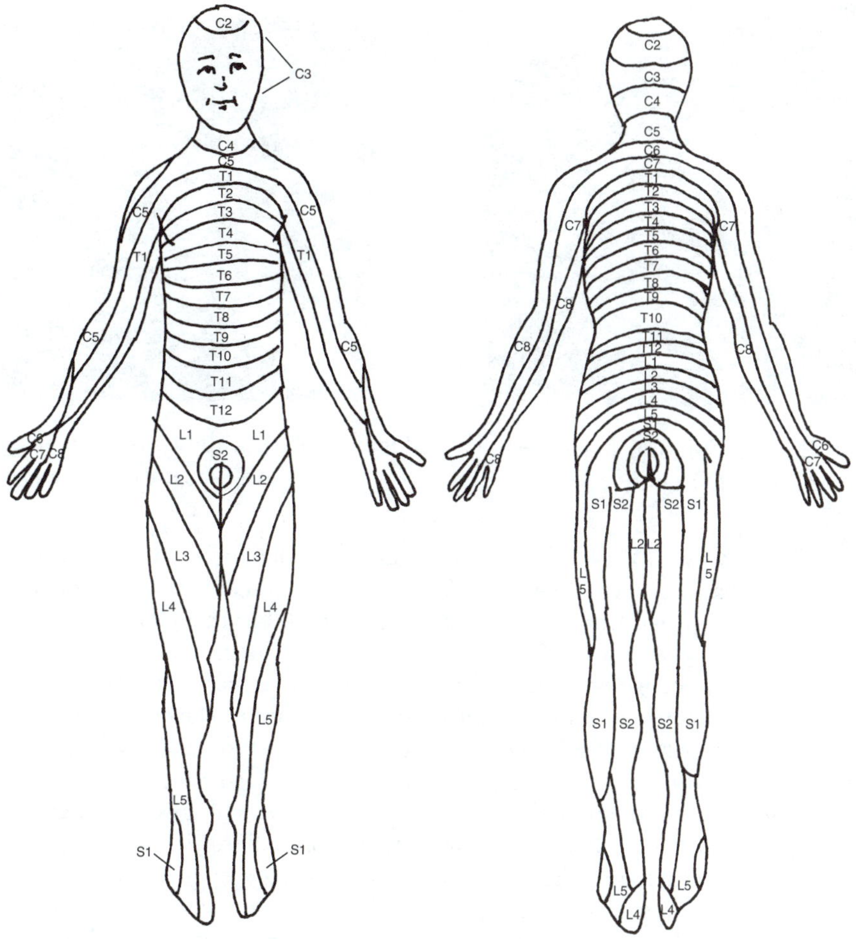

**Figure 5.2**    Sensory Dermatomes

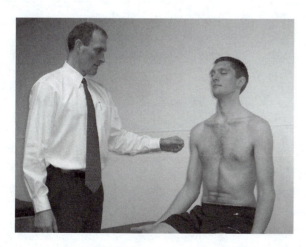

**Figure 5.3**    Sensibility Testing: Soft Touch Sensory Assessment

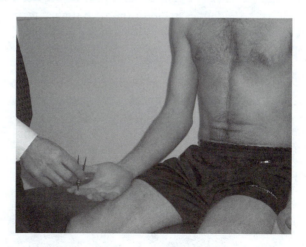

**Figure 5.4**    Sensibility Testing: Sharp/Dull Sensory Assessment

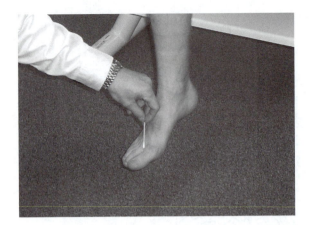

**Figure 5.5**    Sensibility Testing: Soft Touch Sensory Assessment Lower Extremity

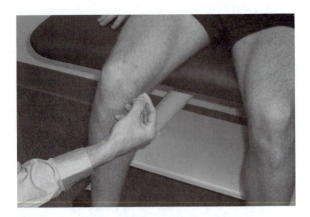

**Figure 5.6**    Sensibility Testing: Sharp/Dull Sensory Assessment Lower Extremity

herniation and 37% of individuals with L3-L4 disc herniation. Rainville et al.[13] found quadriceps weakness in 70% of patients at L3-L4 and 56% of patients at L4-L5. The authors found ankle DF weakness (30%) at L4-5 and just 9% with extensor hallicus longus weakness at the same level. Lauder et al.[17] evaluated any form of lower extremity weakness and recorded a sensitivity of 69%, specificity of 61%, and a +LR of 3.44.

The method of testing quadriceps strength varies among investigators and clinicians.[13] Methods have ranged from asking the patient to straighten the leg then offering resistance[31,32] to asking the individual to push against his or her resistance while the knee remains flexed.[33,34] The use of body weight to evaluate potential strength loss indicating the validity of the test most likely represents muscular strength has been previously suggested.[34] McCombe et al.[35] reports that reliability between therapists for knee flexion and knee extension testing is good, but reliability among physicians and physical therapists is poor.

Rainville et al.[13] reported that of four methods of quadriceps testing (knee extension, step-up test, knee-flexed test, and the sit to stand tests), the most reliable method for patients with L2-L3 impairment is the sit to stand test. The sit to stand test requires the patient to rise upon a single extremity using his or her own body weight as the resistance. This suggests that myotome testing should be performed with both vigor and temporal qualities (hold the force up to 3 seconds) to lessen the risk of falsely identifying muscle strength as "normal." This concept, known as the overload principle, suggests that forces placed upon the muscle should be higher than those that normally occur.[13]

**TABLE 5.2**    The Five Categories of a Graded Traditional Manual Muscle Test

| Grade | Description |
|---|---|
| V | Patient can hold the position against maximum resistance and through complete range of motion. |
| IV | Patient can hold the position against strong to moderate resistance, has full range of motion. |
| III | Patient can tolerate no resistance but can perform the movement through the full range of motion. |
| II | Patient has all or partial range of motion in the gravity-eliminated position. |
| I | The muscle/muscles can be palpated while the patient is performing the action in the gravity-eliminated position. |
| 0 | No contractile activity can be felt in the gravity-eliminated position. |

**TABLE 5.3**    Myotome Levels for Muscle Testing

| Spinal Level | Muscle Testing Action |
|---|---|
| C-1 | Resisted Cervical Rotation |
| C2,3,4 | Resisted Shoulder Shrug |
| C-5 | Resisted Shoulder Abduction |
| C-6 | Resisted Elbow Flexion |
| C-7 | Resisted Wrist Flexion |
| C-8 | Resisted Thumb Extension |
| T-1 | Resisted Finger Abduction |
| L1-2 | Resisted Hip Flexion (sitting) |
| L3-4 | Resisted Knee Extension |
| L4-5 | Heel Walking |
| L5 | Resisted Great Toe Extension |
| L5-S1 | Single Leg Stance (Hip Abduction Sign) |
| S1 | Toe Walking |

Muscle testing for the cervical spine myotomes has yielded conflicting results. Wainner et al.[25] reported that muscle testing of the biceps, triceps, and deltoid provided beneficial diagnostic value during a study. Nonetheless, testing of the extensor carpi radialis brevis/ longus, flexor carpi radialis, first dorsal interosseus, and abductor pollicus brevis yielded +LR values near or below 1.0, providing very little or no diagnostic benefit in detecting cervical radiculopathy.

Davidson et al.[36] found high sensitivity for loss of muscle strength (91% of the sample) as did Yoss et al.[22] (75%). Lauder et al.[23] reported moderate diagnostic value of muscle strength testing (+LR 4.56) on patients positively diagnosed with cervical or upper extremity pain confirmed during electrodiagnosis. Conversely, others[24,37] reported low sensitivity.

The following photos (Figures 5.7–5.19) outline the procedure used for upper and lower quarter regional

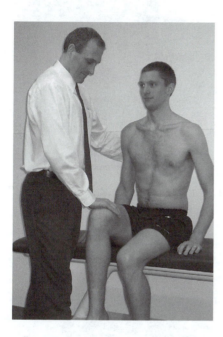

**Figure 5.7**   Lower Quarter Regional Muscle Strength Testing: Resisted Hip Flexion (L1-2)

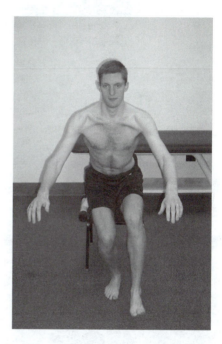

**Figure 5.8**   Lower Quarter Regional Muscle Strength Testing: Resisted Knee Extension-Unilateral Sit to Stand (L3-4)

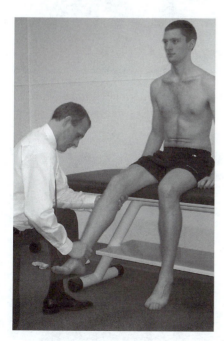

**Figure 5.9**   Lower Quarter Regional Muscle Strength Testing: Alternative, Resisted Knee Extension (L3-4)

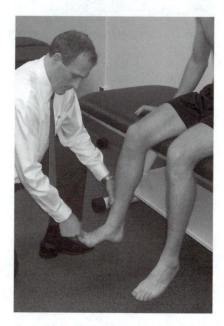

**Figure 5.10**   Lower Quarter Regional Muscle Strength Testing: Resisted Great Toe Extension (L5)

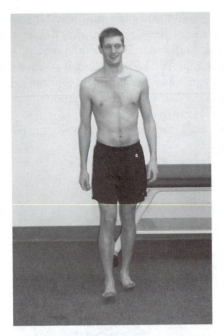

**Figure 5.11**    Lower Quarter Regional Muscle Strength Testing: Heel Walking (L4-5)

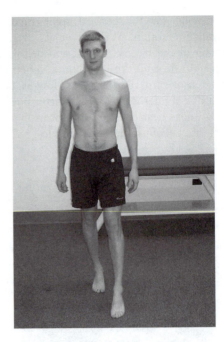

**Figure 5.12**    Lower Quarter Regional Muscle Strength Testing: Toe Walking (S1)

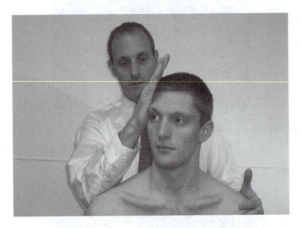

**Figure 5.13**    Upper Quarter Regional Muscle Strength Testing: Resisted Cervical Rotation (C1)

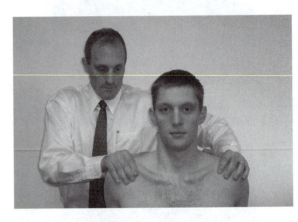

**Figure 5.14**    Upper Quarter Regional Muscle Strength Testing: Resisted Shoulder Shrug (C2,3,4)

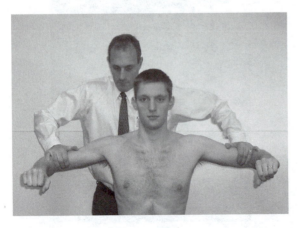

**Figure 5.15**    Upper Quarter Regional Muscle Strength Testing: Resisted Shoulder Abduction (C5)

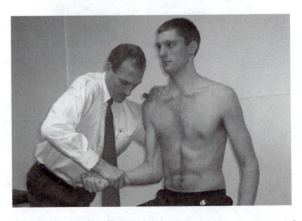

**Figure 5.16**    Upper Quarter Regional Muscle Strength Testing: Resisted Elbow Flexion (C6)

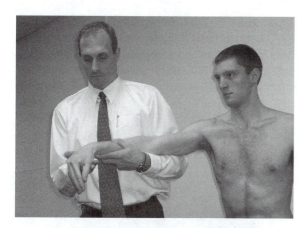

**Figure 5.17**    Upper Quarter Regional Muscle Strength Testing: Resisted Wrist Flexion (C7)

## Summary

- Myotome testing, or "muscle strength testing," is a method designed to identify if abnormalities in muscle strength are present during a one-repetition manual muscle test.
- Several studies have suggested that myotome testing may yield variable findings in the presence of radiculopathy.
- Variations in the method applied for muscle testing may lack the discrimination for isolating selected levels of impairment.

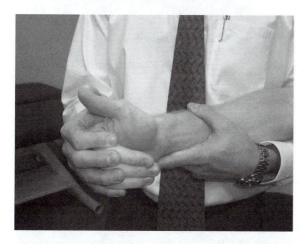

**Figure 5.18**    Upper Quarter Regional Muscle Strength Testing: Resisted Thumb Extension (C8)

muscle strength testing. Tables 5.2 and 5.3 outline muscle grading and myotome levels for testing.

## Deep Tendon Reflex Testing

Muscle stretch reflex testing (termed "deep tendon reflex testing," or DTR) is assessed by tapping over a selected muscle tendon with an appropriate testing device. The clinical utility of the test is based on the quality and magnitude of the response for normalcy. Like sensation and myotome testing, reflex testing is often hampered by variable impairment characteristics.

Spangfort[38] reported that unilateral impaired patella reflexes were evident in 35% of patients who required surgery for L2-3, 48% for L3-4, 6% for L4-5 and L5-S1 combined. Patella reflex abnormalities were noted by others[13] in 60% of patients with impaired L3, 65% in patients with impaired L4. In their study, many of the subjects with normal clinical reflex tests concurrently demonstrated impaired quadriceps strength. Lauder et al.[17] reported that the clinical utility of the patella reflex resulted in higher diagnostic values than the Achilles reflex test (+LR = 3.27 versus +LR = 2.09). The patient population in the study included individuals with lumbar radiculopathy, verified through electrodiagnostic testing.

Historically, findings of reflex alterations in patients diagnosed with a cervical herniated disc and/or cervical spondylopathy are inconclusive. Although many older studies demonstrated moderate sensitivity[19,20,22], recent studies have found much lower values.[21,23,24,36] These findings appear to be independent in the method used to diagnose the cervical disorder. In a recent study that examined cervical radiculopathy, only the biceps reflex test demonstrated good diagnostic value.[17]

It does appear that the clinical utility of reflex testing may suffer during traditional testing. Selected authors[39,40] have reported that reflex testing demonstrated abnormal Hoffman reflexes in 100% of patients with radiculopathy; however, they were able only to establish this by use of electrodiagnostic means. Since most clinicians do not have electrodiagnostic means for assessment, the clinical

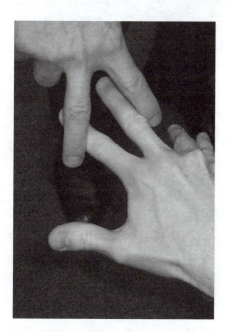

**Figure 5.19**    Upper Quarter Regional Muscle Strength Testing: Resisted Finger Abduction (T1)

**TABLE 5.4** Normative Values for Reflex Testing

| Grade | Evaluation | Response Characteristics |
|-------|-----------|--------------------------|
| 0+ | Absent | No visible or palpable muscle contraction with reinforcement |
| 1+ | Tone Change | Slight, transitory impulse, with no movement of the extremities |
| 2+ | Normal | Visible, brief movement of the extremity |
| 3+ | Exaggerated | Full movement of the extremities |
| 4+ | Abnormal | Compulsory and sustained movement, lasting for more than 30 seconds |

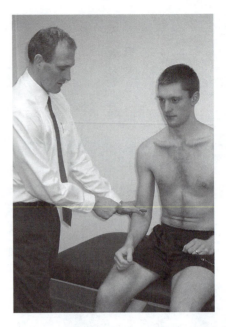

**Figure 5.20** Deep Tendon Reflex Testing; (C5,6) Biceps

threshold of a reflex test is what must be assessed. The clinical threshold in the absence of electrodiagnostic means often provides poor sensitivity.[41] One possible explanation for the variability in findings is that 25–30% of patients with abnormal reflexes demonstrate abnormalities in afferent and efferent pathways that are different from those tested by a clinical deep tendon reflex test.[39]

These findings suggest that electrodiagnostic findings may not always extrapolate into clinical findings. One method designed to improve the outcome of the reflex test is the Jendrassik maneuver. The Jendrassik maneuver is performed when the patient hooks together the fingers of the hands and attempts to pull them apart during the clinical reflex testing procedure.[42] When effective, the maneuver produces a more pronounced elicitation of the reflex for comparative analysis. Tables 5.4 and 5.5 outline the normative values for reflex testing and difficulty in performing the manuevers. Figures 5.20–5.25 demonstrate appropriate deep tendon reflex testing.

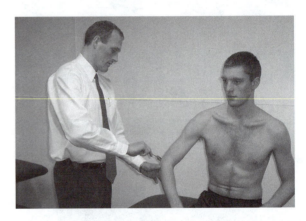

**Figure 5.21** Deep Tendon Reflex Testing; (C7,8) Triceps

**TABLE 5.5** Deep Tendon Reflexes and Appropriate Spinal Root Levels

| DTR | Difficulty to Elicit | Spinal Root Level |
|-----|---------------------|-------------------|
| Biceps Reflex[79,80] | Easy | C5,C6 |
| Brachioradialis[79,80] | Difficult | C5,C6 |
| Triceps[81] | Moderate | C7,C8 |
| Patellar Reflex[79,80] | Easy | L3 |
| Achilles Reflex[79,80] | Easy | S1 |

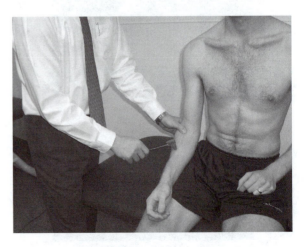

**Figure 5.22** Deep Tendon Reflex Testing; (C6) Brachioradialis

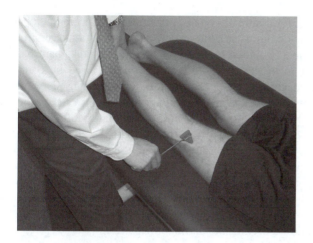

**Figure 5.23**    Deep Tendon Reflex Testing; (L5,S1,S2) Hamstrings

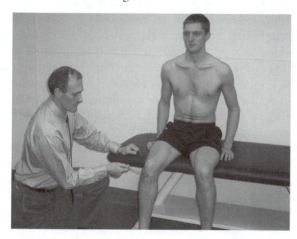

**Figure 5.24**    Deep Tendon Reflex Testing; (L2,L3,L4) Patellar

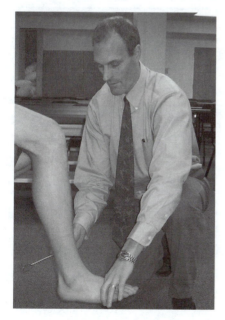

**Figure 5.25**    Deep Tendon Reflex Testing; (S1,S2) Ankle Achilles

## Summary

- Muscle stretch reflex testing is assessed by tapping over selected muscle tendons with an appropriate testing device.
- The clinical method of reflex testing may lack the discriminatory capabilities of electrodiagnostic methods.
- In recent studies, clinical reflex testing yielded mixed results.

## Differentiation of Referred Pain

Referred pain is defined as "pain perceived as arising or occurring in a region of the body innervated by nerves or branches of nerves other than those that innervate the actual source of pain."[43] The pain perceived by the patient is felt in an area other than where the pain generator originates. This process of pain referral associated with a nerve root is not completely understood[26] and may take many forms, including pain, parathesia, sensory deficits, and motor weakness.[26]

Historically, referred pain was commonly associated with nerve root compression; however, mechanical nerve root compression does not explain all forms of upper and lower limb radiculopathy. Several authors have outlined the biochemical interaction between intervertebral disc injury and nerve roots, which can result in referred pain.[44,45] Olmarker and Rydevik[46] found that changes in the nucleus pulposis altered nerve root velocities in the absence of nerve root compression. Chemical components of the disc have been shown to penetrate nerve roots to sensitize the nerve root fibers.

Referred pain is not always associated with an intervertebral disc.[35,47,48] Bogduk[48] stated, "Virtually any source of local lumbar or lumbosacral pain is capable of producing somatic referred pain." These structures can include ligaments, vertebrae musculature zygopophyseal joints, and the outer border of the annulus.[49] Often, the referral distribution patterns overlap. This suggests that the presence of referred pain in a specific location is not predictive of the origin of the referred pain.

Referred pain is present in four forms: visceral, somatic, nerve root, and the spinal cord. Generally, these referred pain components are defined somatic referred (visceral and somatic), radiculopathy, and myelopathy, respectively. **Somatic referred pain** from ligaments, capsule, and the annulus is often treated through various manual therapy means. These referred symptoms can be reproduced during provocation of these selected somatic elements. Typically, somatic referred pain does not follow a dermatome pattern as does radiculopathy.

**Radiculopathy** is a chemical or nerve root compression that causes referred pain. Radiculopathy is commonly caused by a herniation of a cervical or lumbar disc and results in nerve inflammation, impingement, or both.[25] Other factors such as degenerative changes, stenosis, and soft tissue growths may also be associated with radiculopathy.[50]

**Myelopathy** is common during upper motor neuron lesion or central nervous system dysfunction and may be outside the scope of manual therapy treatment. Myelopathy is characterized by the clinical finding that the lower extremities are affected first, with subsequent spasticity and paresis. The patient often complains of a gait disturbance due to abnormalities in the corticospinal tracts and spinocerebellar tracts. Later the upper extremities become involved with loss of strength and difficulty in fine finger movements.[51]

**Visceral referred pain** is pain generated from an organ such as the prostate, heart, or bladder. Visceral pain is a poorly defined, midline sensation but after minutes or hours becomes "referred" to a somatic region when it becomes sharper and better localized. Typically, visceral pain (1) arises from visceral tissues and is initially often poorly localized and diffuse, (2) is often referred to more superficial structures, (3) is the site of referred pain from the viscera and may also show hyperalgesia, and (4) occurs in disease states, where the afflicted viscera may also become hyperalgesic.[49] Generally, visceral pain is not within the scope of a manual therapist and warrants the outside intervention of appropriate medical practitioners.

There is another reason in addition to identifying whether the patient is appropriate for manual therapy that the orthopedic manual therapist should identify the structure that causes the referred pain. The outcome of treatment is often dependent on the recognition of the pain generator and the appropriate application of the desired treatment. Within this textbook, the use of the patient response method often requires the recreation of the patient's signs and symptoms, which is examined during repeated movements at various ranges. A condition such as lumbar or cervical radiculopathy typically responds poorly to provocative movements, often yielding a worsening of symptoms. On the other hand, a patient with somatic referred pain typically responds well to repeated movements. A patient who is stiffness-dominant often benefits from techniques intended to stretch or squeeze tissue for range-of-motion improvement.[52] Often, a patient who exhibits stiffness-dominant characteristics also demonstrates somatic referred pain. Somatic referred pain is less predictable and often will exhibit acharacteristic patterns among symptomatic individuals. Referred pain may manifest either with or without hyperalgesia. Hyperalgesia is more common and can be demonstrated by changes in pain threshold.[53]

Pain dominant–related structures such as radiculopathy may be best treated in loosely packed positions using techniques designed for pain reduction. Radicular pain has its origin in the nerve root and is often caused by complex mechanisms. Radicular pain is typically caused by compression and/or mechanical stimulation of a nerve root[49]; however, the nerve root must exhibit preexisting damage.[54] In essence, for radiculopathy to occur the environment for the nerve root must be chemically sensitized.[55] Inflammatory causes generally include the disc; studies have shown that inflammation without compression can cause paresthesia, numbness, and motor loss.[56] Mixed evidence suggests that upper and lower extremity radiculopathies will follow a predictable dermatome pattern.[49]

There are several methods to differentiate referred pain. The first is recognition of the "red flags" associated with myelopathy. Signs and symptoms of myelopathy are generally associated with an insidious onset of neck stiffness; unilateral or bilateral deep, aching neck, arm, and shoulder pain; and possibly stiffness or clumsiness while walking.[57] Neurological testing investigates the presence of an **upper motor neuron lesion.** The presence of an upper motor neuron lesion may indicate that a central cord or central nervous system impairment is present.[58] Central cord compression may place pressure on the spinal cord, which results in spinal nerve tissue lesions. These forms of lesions can lead to demyelinization of the descending and ascending pathways[49] and subsequent dysfunction. Upper motor neuron dysfunction may take on many different symptoms (see Table 5.6).

**TABLE 5.6   Signs and Symptoms of Neurological Dysfunction**

| | |
|---|---|
| Observable patient symptoms | • Widely diffuse pain<br>• Atrophy in the small hands[82,83]<br>• Gait abnormalities |
| Symptoms identified during special testing | • Pathologically increased reflexes<br>• Positive Babinski's sign<br>• Absent abdominal reflexes<br>• Decreased vibratory sense in lower extremities<br>• Hyperactive scapulohumeral reflex[84]<br>• Hoffmann's reflex (sign) |
| Symptoms discernible during testing and observation | • Electric pain down the spine (Lhermitte's sign)<br>• Tetraspasticity[85]<br>• Clonus |

Because the existence of an upper motor neuron prompts the necessity of medical intervention, it is important that tests designed to rule in the presence of the disorder are sensitive. Several studies have shown that a positive Hoffmann's reflex is 94% likely to rule in a cervical upper motor neuron lesion.[60–62] A positive **Hoffman's sign** (Figure 5.27) appears to be isolated to an upper motor neuron lesion in the cervical spine versus thoracic and lumbar[63], although other components (abdominal reflexes, lower limb deep tendon reflexes, and **Babinski's sign** (Figure 5.26)) of upper neuron dysfunction do not differentiate between upper or lower motor neuron problems.[64] Handle et al.[65] reported that the presence of a positive Hoffmann's reflex and hyperreflexia were the most sensitive tests and had the highest accuracy for diagnosis of cervical myelopathy. In their study, patients with a positive Hoffmann's sign also exhibited a positive **clonus** (Figure 5.28) and Babinski when a patient exhibits evidence of neural compression.

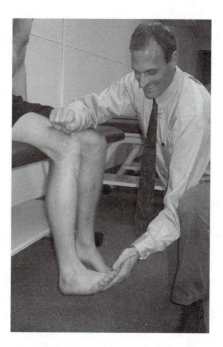

**Figure 5.28**    Clonus

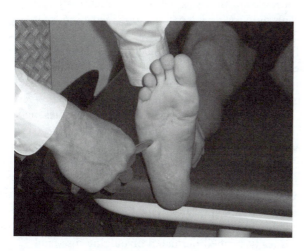

**Figure 5.26**    Babinski's Sign

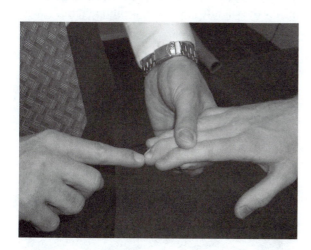

**Figure 5.27**    Hoffmann's Sign

## *Summary*

- Referred pain is defined as "pain perceived as arising or occurring in a region of the body innervated by nerves or branches of nerves other than those that innervate the actual source of pain."
- Referred pain may be visceral, somatic, radiculopathy, or myelopathy.
- The presence of myelopathy is associated with an upper motor neuron lesion.
- The clinical tests of Hoffmann's sign, Babinski's sign, and clonus are useful in detecting an upper motor neuron lesion.

## *Clinical Tests for Characterization of Referred Pain in the Upper Extremity*

In conjunction with prudent use of the Hoffmann's test, other clinical tests that are designed to characterize the form of referred pain are valuable resources. As discussed, the identification of myelopathy is essential because the patient may require pertinent medical attention. Radicular pain differs from somatic and visceral referred pain through the mechanism of the pain generator. While visceral referred pain is beyond the scope of a manual therapist, both somatic and radicular pain are commonly treated using manual approaches.

Two tests are purported to aid in differentiation of radicular symptoms. In 2003, Wainner et al.[25] reported on the reliability and diagnostic value of the **upper limb tension test** (ULTT) in detecting cervical radiculopathy. The ULTT

(Figure 5.29) is highly sensitive, thus a negative finding is a good predictor of absence of cervical radiculopathy. However, the +LR of a variation of the ULTT, commonly described as the median nerve tension test, was only 1.3. The upper limb tension test was hampered from the low specificity of the test and correspondingly low negative likelihood ratio. Subsequently, diagnosing a condition based on the ULTT median nerve tension test is not advised.

Another test developed by Spurling is the **Spurling's compression test** (Figure 5.30).[66] In the original design of this test, passive side flexion is performed to the patient's symptomatic side and an overpressure is added. Tong et al.[66] reported strong specificity scores (93%) and low sensitivity values (30%) with the Spurling's test, resulting in a positive likelihood ratio of 4.5. Wainner et al.[25] reported a similar value of 3.5, further supporting the use of this test. Of the two methods of radiculopathy differentiation, the Spurling's test demonstrates the highest diagnostic value while the ULTT is best at ruling out the presence of cervical radiculopathy.

## Summary

- There are two purported methods to differentiate cervical referred pain (somatic referred vs. radiculopathy): the upper limb tension test and Spurling's sign.
- Of the two forms of differentiation, only Spurling's sign demonstrates strong diagnostic value.

## *Clinical Tests for Characterization of Referred Pain in the Lower Extremity*

The **straight leg raise** (SLR) (Figure 5.31) and the **slump sit test** (SS) (Figure 5.32) are purported measures of neural tension, and in past studies have demonstrated similar diagnostic values. Several authors[67–71] found very high sensitivity (89–97%) and low specificity (10–17%) values in their surgically confirmed populations of patients with herniated nucleus pulposis. Lauder et al.[17] obtained a sensitivity score of 21% and a specificity of 87%. Most likely the variances in findings are reflective of the dissimilarities in population selection. The Lauder et al.[17] study was the only investigation that limited spectrum bias and included all patients consecutively referred within multiple general practices. The studies that exhibited higher sensitivity values included samples of patients with a high degree of severity (surgical candidates). Deyo et al.[72] suggest that in studies that generate high specificity values, the presence of a positive finding is more valuable than the presence of a negative finding.

Only one study has measured the diagnostic value of the SS. Stankovic et al.[73] reported a sensitivity of 82.6% and a specificity of 54.7% in their population of patients with diagnostically verified herniated or bulging disc, and 12 patients with no positive findings on the diagnostic imaging. Like many of the previously discussed SLR studies, spectrum bias was evident in this study, which most likely accounts for the slightly improved likelihood ratio.

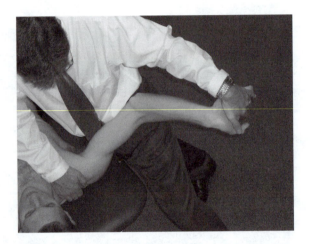

**Figure 5.29**    Upper Limb Tension Test A. The Median Nerve Tension Test

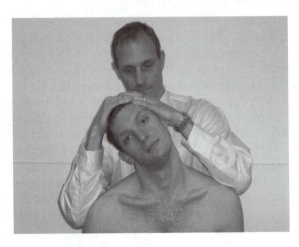

**Figure 5.30**    Spurling's Test

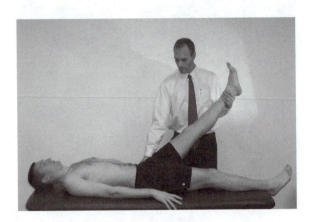

**Figure 5.31**    The Straight Leg Raise

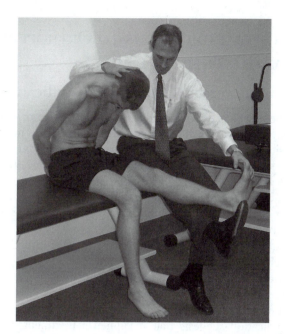

**Figure 5.32**    The Slump Sit Test

Another clinical test that has yet to be examined is the so-called **Kemp test**[74] (Figure 5.33) for the lumbar spine. The test is procedurally similar to Maitland's lumbar quadrant test.[75] During the maneuver, the patient side flexes, rotates, and extends to the concordant side of pain. Reproduction of the radiculopathy is considered a positive test. Table 5.7 outlines the differentation of reffered pain.

## Summary

- There are three purported methods to differenti-ate lumbar referred pain (somatic referred vs. radiculopathy): the straight leg raise, the slump sit test, and the Kemp (lumbar quadrant) test.
- Both the straight leg raise and the slump test demonstrate comparable and fair diagnostic value.
- The Kemp test (and lumbar quadrant) has been untested. Thus diagnostic value is unknown.

**TABLE 5.7**    Differentiation of Referred Pain Characteristics

| Characteristic | Radiculopathy | Myelopathy | Somatic Referred Pain | Visceral Pain |
|---|---|---|---|---|
| Axial distribution | + | + | + | + |
| Upper extremity muscle weakness | + | + | − | − |
| Lower extremity muscle weakness | + | + | − | − |
| Upper extremity sensory disturbance | + | + | − | − |
| Lower extremity sensory disturbance | + | + | − | − |
| Clumsiness | − | + | − | − |
| Gait disturbance | + or − | + | − | − |
| Spurling's sign | + | − | + or − | − |
| Sensory deficit | + or − | + or − | − | − |
| Loss of vibratory sense | − | Yes (LE) | − | − |
| Tendon reflex changes | Diminished + or − | Increased | − | − |
| Muscle wasting | Unilateral + or − | Bilateral | − | − |
| Babinski's sign | − | + | − | − |
| Hoffman's sign | − | + | − | − |
| Muscle tone | Normal | Increased | Normal | Normal |
| Limb tension test | + | + or − | − | − |

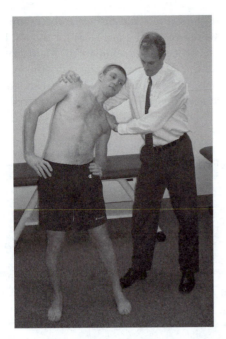

**Figure 5.33**    The so-called "Kemp test" or Lumbar Quadrant

# CONTRAINDICATIONS TO ORTHOPEDIC MANUAL THERAPY

## Absolute versus Relative Contraindications

Some red flags discovered during the subjective or objective examination will distill comorbidities that do not necessitate the referral to appropriate medical personnel but do require special consideration. In these cases, where risk may outweigh the benefit of a specific procedure, contraindications for selected manual therapy procedures exist. Two forms of contraindications are evident: absolute and relative.

An **absolute contraindication** involves any situation in which the movement, stress, or compression placed on a particular body part involves high risk of a deleterious consequence. A **relative contraindication** involves a situation that requires special care.[76] The presence of a relative contraindication suggests that if applied a treatment runs a high risk of injury and should involve considerable reflection prior to use. Because selected treatments have dissimi-

**TABLE 5.8**    Absolute and Relative Contraindications of Active Movement

| Absolute contraindications | Malignancy of the targeted physiological region |
|---|---|
| | Cauda equina lesions producing disturbance of bowel or bladder |
| | Red flags including signs of neoplasm, facture, or systemic disturbance |
| | Rheumatoid collagen necrosis |
| | Vertebral basilar insufficiency (unless active movements involve stabilization procedures) |
| | • Drop attacks, blackouts, loss of consciousness |
| | • Nausea, vomiting, and general lack of wellness |
| | • Dizziness or vertigo |
| | • Disturbance of vision including diplopia |
| | • Unsteadiness of gait and general feelings of weakness (intermittent) |
| | • Tingling or numbness (especially dysaethesia, hemianaesthesia, or facial sensation) |
| | • Dysarthria or swallowing difficulty |
| | • Hearing disturbances |
| | • Headaches |
| | Unstable upper cervical spine (unless active movements involve stabilization procedures) |
| Relative contraindications | Active, acute inflammatory conditions |
| | Significant segmental stiffness |
| | Systematic disease |
| | Neurological deterioration |
| | Irritable patient |
| | Osteoporosis (depending on the intent and direction of movement) |
| | Condition is worsening with present treatment |
| | Hamstring and upper limb stretching on acute nerve root irritations |

lar elements of risk, the contraindications are divided into treatment categories versus a single list of factors.

## Active Movements

There are a variety of techniques utilized within physical medicine for the treatment of associated range-of-motion losses, most notably, static stretching, mobilization, and manipulation. Nonetheless, active range is a method that is used occasionally for increase in elected movement and may be beneficial for use in a home exercise program (Table 5.8).

## Passive Movements

### Static Stretching, Mobilization, and Manually Assisted Movements

In theory, static stretching, mobilization, and manually assisted movements demonstrate comparable force magnitudes, directions, and principles of application. Because of this, the three methods have been consolidated. Few studies have reported dire complications associated with the application of these techniques; nonetheless, a prudent

**TABLE 5.9**    Absolute and Relative Contraindications to Passive Movements (i.e., mobilization, stretching, and manually assisted movements)

| | |
|---|---|
| **Absolute contraindications** | a. Malignancy of the targeted physiological region |
| | b. Cauda equina lesions producing disturbance of bowel or bladder |
| | c. Red flags including signs of neoplasm, fracture, or systemic disturbance |
| | d. Rheumatoid collagen necrosis |
| | e. Unstable upper cervical spine (unless active movements involve stabilization procedures) |
| | f. Vertebral basilar insufficiency |
| | • Drop attacks, blackouts, loss of consciousness |
| | • Nausea, vomiting, and general unwellness |
| | • Dizziness or vertigo |
| | • Disturbance of vision including diplopia |
| | • Unsteadiness of gait and general feelings of weakness (intermittent) |
| | • Dysarthria or swallowing difficulty |
| | • Hearing disturbances |
| | • Headaches (unless headache lessons with continued application) |
| | • Tingling or numbness (especially dysaethesia, hemianaesthesia, or facial sensation) |
| **Relative contraindications** | a. Previously defined relative contraindications |
| | • Active, acute inflammatory conditions |
| | • Significant segmental stiffness |
| | • Systematic disease |
| | • Neurological deterioration |
| | • Irritable patient |
| | • Osteoporosis (depending on the intent and direction of movement) |
| | • Condition is worsening with present treatment |
| | b. Acute nerve root irritation (radiculopathy) |
| | • When subjective and objective symptoms don't add up |
| | • Any patient condition (handled well) that is worsening |
| | • Use of oral contraceptives (if cervical spine) |
| | • Long-term oral corticosteroid use (if cervical spine) |
| | c. Immediately postpartum (if noncervical spine) |
| | d. Blood clotting disorder |

manual therapist must be well aware of the associative contraindications (Table 5.9).

### Manipulation

In general, the question of safety risks associated with manipulation (and mobilization) is relatively answered. Recently, Hurwitz et al.[77] performed a large-scale randomized trial that consisted of manipulation- and mobilization-based treatments. The authors reported that complications associated with manipulation- and mobilization-based treatments were minimal with respect to the total procedures performed. A majority of complications are associated with treatment of the cervical spine and occurred during treatment, which negatively affected the vertebral basilar artery insufficiency. Although some patients reported the occurrence of some symptoms associated with vertebral basilar artery insufficiency testing, those individuals who recorded negative consequences had premeditating components associated with potential stroke such as smoking, hypertension, or arteriosclerosis. These considerations should be apparent during the patient history far prior to the application of mobilization or manipulation (Table 5.10).

**TABLE 5.10    Absolute and Relative Contraindications to Manipulation**

| | |
|---|---|
| **Absolute contraindications** | a. Previously defined absolute contraindications<br>• Malignancy of the targeted physiological region<br>• Cauda equina lesions producing disturbance of bowel or bladder<br>• Red flags including signs of neoplasm, facture, or systemic disturbance<br>• Rheumatoid collagen necrosis<br>• Vertebral basilar insufficiency<br>• Unstable upper cervical spine (unless active movements involve stabilization procedures)<br>b. Practitioner lack of ability<br>c. Spondylolithesis<br>d. Gross foraminal encroachment<br>e. Children/teenagers<br>f. Pregnancy<br>g. Fusions<br>h. Psychogenic disorders<br>i. Immediately postpartum |
| **Relative contraindications** | a. Previously defined relative contraindications<br>b. Active, acute inflammatory conditions<br>c. Significant segmental stiffness<br>d. Systematic disease<br>e. Neurological deterioration<br>f. Irritable patient<br>g. Osteoporosis (depending on the intent and direction of movement)<br>h. Condition is worsening with present treatment<br>i. Acute nerve root irritation (radiculopathy)<br>j. When subjective and objective symptoms don't add up<br>k. Any patient condition (handled well) that is worsening<br>l. Use of oral contraceptives (if cervical spine)<br>m. Long-term oral corticosteroid use (if cervical spine)<br>n. Immediately postpartum (if noncervical spine)<br>o. Blood clotting disorder |

In a comprehensive literature review, Di Fabio[78] suggested that mobilization and manipulation may be effective for the treatment of cervical conditions, but use does involve a risk of injury involving lesions of the brain stem, most specifically with disruption of the vertebral artery during cervical manipulation. Physical therapists were less involved than other practitioners in injury totals, which accounted for less than 2%.[78] Physical therapists tend to be less involved in potential incidents, with less than one event for every 1,573 manipulations, while chiropractors were involved in one for every 476 cervical manipulations.

## Summary

- Contraindications to manual therapy exist in two forms: relative and absolute.
- A relative contraindication involves a situation that requires special care, but does not negate the use of the technique.
- An absolute contraindication involves any situation in which the movement, stress, or compression placed on a particular body part involves a high risk of a deleterious consequence.
- Of the litany of manual therapy techniques, manipulation displays the highest quantity of contraindications.
- Of the areas of the body that demonstrate the highest risk for manual therapy, the upper cervical spine has been linked to the most complications.

# Chapter Questions

1. Describe key components of a medical screen and the criteria each is designed to identify.
2. Compare and contrast the different forms of "red flags" and outline why some are definitive causes for referral to appropriate medical personnel and others require additional screening.
3. Briefly provide an explanation of the diagnostic value of sensation, myotome, and reflex testing for identifying a specific level of lesion, identifying the presence of an upper motor neuron lesion, and differentiating somatic referred and radicular symptoms.
4. Describe the tests designed to differentiate somatic referred and radicular symptoms that display the highest diagnostic value.
5. List the contraindications to the selected treatment components of manual therapy.

# References

1. Guide to Physical Therapist Practice. 2nd ed. *Phys Ther.* 2001;81:9–744.
2. Boissonnault WG, Koopmeiners MB. Medical history profile: orthopaedic physical therapy outpatients. *J Orthop Sports Phys Ther.* 1994;20(1):2–10.
3. Boissonnault WG. Prevalence of comorbid conditions, surgeries, and medication use in a physical therapy outpatient population: a multicentered study. *J Orthop Sports Phys Ther.* 1999;29(9):506–19; discussion 520–525.
4. Sobri M, Lamont A, Alias N, Win M. Red flags in patients presenting with headache: clinical indications for neuroimaging. *Br J Radiology.* 2003;76:532–535.
5. Swenson R. Differential diagnosis. *Neurologic Clinics of North America.* 1999;17:43–63.
6. Haldeman S. Neck and back pain. In: Evans R. *Diagnostic testing in neurology.* Philadelphia; Saunders: 1999.
7. Schultz I. Crook J, Berkowitz J, Meloche G, Milner R, Zuberbier O, Meloche W. Biopsychosocial multivariate predictive model of occupational low back disability. *Spine.* 2002;27(23):2720–2725.
8. Yamashita T, Kanaya K, Sekine M, Takebayashi T, Kawaguchi S, Katahira G. A quantitative analysis of sensory function in lumbar radiculopathy using current perception threshold testing. *Spine.* 2002;27: 1567–1570.
9. Chado H. The current perception threshold evaluation of sensory nerve function in pain management. *Pain Digest.* 1995;5:127–134.
10. Consensus report. Quantitative sensory testing: A consensus report from the peripheral neuropathy association. *Neurology.* 1993;43:1050–1052.
11. Liu S, Kopacz D, Carpentart R. Quantitative assessment of differential sensory nerve block after lodocaine spinal anesthesia. *Anesthesiology.* 1995;1:60–63.

12. Aronson H, Dunsmore R. Herniated upper lumbar discs. *J Bone Joint Surg Am.* 1963;45:311–317.

13. Rainville J, Jouve C, Finno M, Limke J. Comparison of four tests of quadriceps strength in L3 or L4 radiculopathies. *Spine.* 2003; 28:2466–2471.

14. Jonsson B, Stromquist B. Symptoms and signs in degeneration of the lumbar spine. *J Bone Joint Surg Br.* 1993;75:381–385.

15. Blower P. Neurologic patterns in unilateral sciatica: A prospective study of 100 new cases. *Spine.* 1982;6: 175–179.

16. Jensen O. The level-diagnosis of a lower lumbar disc herniation: the value of sensibility and motor testing. *Clin Rheumatol.* 1987;6:564–569.

17. Lauder T, Dillingham T, Andary M, Kumar S, Pezzin L, Stephens R, Shannon S. Effect of history and exam in predicting electrodiagnostic outcome among patients with suspected lumbosacral radiculopathy. *Arch Phys Med Rehabil.* 2000;79:60–68.

18. Semmes R, Murphy F. The syndrome of unilateral rupture of the sixth cervical intervertebral. *JAMA.* 1943;121:1209–1214.

19. Michelsen J, Mixter W. Pain and disability of shoulder and pain due to herniation of the nucleus pulposis of cervical intervertebral disks. *N Engl J Med.* 1944; 231:279–287.

20. Spurling R, Scoville W. Lateral rupture of the cervical intervertebral discs. *Surg Gyencol Obstet.* 1944;78: 350–358.

21. Waylonis G. Electromyographic findings in chronic cervical radicular syndromes. *Arch Phys Med Rehabil.* 1968;49:407–412.

22. Yoss R, Corbin K, MacCarty C, Love J. Significance of symptoms and signs in localization of involved root in cervical disc protrusion. *Neurology.* 1957;7(10): 673–683.

23. Lauder T, Dillingham T, Andary M, Kumar S, Pezzin L, Stephens R. Predicting electrodiagnostic outcome in patients with upper limb symptoms: are the history and physical examination helpful? *Arch Phys Med Rehabil.* 2000;81:436–441.

24. Hong C, Lee S, Lum P. Cervical radiculopathy: clinical, radiographic and EMG findings. *Orthop Rev.* 1986;15:433–439.

25. Wainner R, Fritz J, Irrgang J, Boninger M, Delitto A, Allison S. Reliability and diagnostic accuracy of the clinical examination and patient self-report measures for cervical radiculopathy. *Spine.* 2003;28:52–62.

26. Nygaard O, Mellgren S. The function of sensory nerve fibers in lumbar radiculopathy: Use of quantitative sensory testing gin the exploration of different populations of nerve fibers and dermatomes. *Spine.* 1998;23:348–352.

27. Zwart J, Sand T, Unsgaard G. Warm and cold thresholds in patients with unilateral sciatica: C-fibers are more severely affected than A-delta fibers. *Acta Neurol Scand.* 1998;97:41–45.

28. Mosek A, Yarnitsky D, Korczyn A, Niv D. The assessment of radiating low back pain by thermal sensory testing. *Eur J Pain.* 2001;5:347–351.

29. Schiff E, Eisenberg E. Can quantitative sensory testing predict the outcome of epidural steroid injections in sciatica? A preliminary study. *Anesth Analg.* 2003: 97:828–832.

30. Hakelius A, Hindmarsh J. The significance of neurological signs and myelographic findings in the diagnosis of lumbar root compression. *Acta Orthop Scand.* 1972;43:239–246.

31. Bates B, Bickley L, Hockelman R. *A guide to physical examination and history taking.* 6th ed. Philadelphia; J.B. Lippincott: 1995.

32. Swartz M. Physical diagnosis: *History and examination.* 3rd ed. Philadeliphia; WB Saunders: 1998.

33. Kendall F, McCreary E. *Muscle testing and function.* 3rd ed. Baltimore; Williams and Wilkins: 1983.

34. Katz L. Quadriceps femoris strength following patellectomy. *Phys Ther. Rev* 1952;32(8):401–414.

35. McCombe PF, Fairbank JCT, Cockersole BC, et al. Reproducibility of physical signs in low-back pain. *Spine.* 1989;14:908–917.

36. Davidson R, Dunn E, Metzmaker J. The shoulder abduction test in the diagnosis of radicular pain in cervical extradural compression monomradiculopathies. *Spine.* 1981;6:441–446.

37. Partanen J, Partanen K, Oikarinen H, Niemitukia L, Hernesniemi J. Preoperative electro-neuromyography and myelography in cervical root compression. *Electromyogr Clin Neurophysiol.* 1991;31:21–26.

38. Spangfort E. The lumbar disc herniations-a computer aided analysis of 2,504 operations. *Acta Orthop Scand.* 1972;(Suppl 142):1–93.

39. Miller T, Pardo R, Yaworski R. Clinical utility of reflex studies in assessing cervical radiculopathy. *Muscle Nerve.* 1999;22:1075–1079.

40. Sabbahi M, Khalil M. Segmental H-reflex studies in upper and lower limbs of patients with radiculopathy. *Arch Phys Med Rehabil.*1990;71:223–227.

41. Vroomen P, de Krom M, Wilmink J, Kester A, Knottnerus J. Diagnostic value of history and physical examination in patients suspected of lumbosacral nerve root compression. *J Neurol Neurosurg Psychiatry.* 2002; 72:630–634.

42. O'Sullivan S. Assessment of motor function. In: O'Sullivan S, Schmitz T. *Physical rehabilitation; assessment and treatment.* Philadelphia; F.A. Davis: 2001.

43. International Association for the study of Pain Task Force on Taxonomy Classification of chronic pain: description of chronic pain syndromes and definitions of pain terms. 2nd ed. Seattle; IASP Press: 1994.

44. McCarron R, Wimpee M, Hudkins P, Laros G. The inflammatory effect of nucleus pulposis: A possible element in the pathogenesis of low-back pain. *Spine.* 1987;12:760–764.

45. Saal J. The role of inflammation in lumbar pain. *Spine.* 1995;16:1821–1827.

46. Olmarker K, Rydevik B. (abstract). New information concerning pain caused by herniated disk and sciatica. Exposure to disk tissue sensitizes the nerve roots. *Lakartidningen.* 1998;95(49):5618–5622.

47. Charnley, J. Orthopaedic signs in the diagnosis of disc protrusion with special reference to the straight-leg-raising test. *Lancet.* 1951;1:186–192.

48. Bodguk N. *Clinical anatomy of the lumbar spine and sacrum.* 3rd ed. New York; Churchill Livingstone: 1997.

49. Robinson J. Lower extremity pain of lumbar spine origin: Differentiating somatic referred and radicular pain. *J Manual Manipulative Ther.* 2003;11:223–234.

50. Bigos S, Bowyer O, Braen T. Acute low back problems in adults 1994. AHRCPR publication 95-0642. Rockville, MD. Agency for Health Care Policy and Research, Public Health Service, U.S. Department of Health and Human Services.

51. Gorter K. Influence of laminectomy on the course of cervical myelopathy. *Acta Neurochirurgica.* 1976;33: 265–281.

52. Edwards B. Examination. In: Maitland GD. *Maitland's vertebral manipulation.* 6th ed. London; Butterworth-Heinemann: 2001.

53. Giamberardino MA, Vecchiet L. Visceral pain, referred hyperalgesia and outcome: new concepts. *Eur J Anaesthesiol Suppl.* 1995;10:61–66.

54. Kuslich S, Ulstrom C, Michael C. The tissue origin of low back pain and sciatica: A report of pain response to tissue stimulation during operations on the lumbar spine using local anesthesia. *Ortho Clin North Am.* 1991;22:181–187.

55. Takebayashi T, Cavanaugh J, Ozaktay C, Kallakuri S, Chen C. Effect of nucleus pulposis on the neural activity of dorsal root ganglion. *Spine.* 2001;26:940–945.

56. Ozaktay A, Kallakuri S, Cavanaugh J. Phospolipase A2 sensitivity of the dorsal root and dorsal root ganglion. *Spine.* 1998;23:1297–1306.

57. Adams RD, Victor M. Diseases of the spinal cord, peripheral nerve and muscle. In: Adams RD, Victor M, eds. *Principles of neurology.* 5th ed. New York; McGraw-Hill, Health Professions Division: 1993: 1100–1101.

58. York GK. Motor testing in neurology: an historical overview. *Semin Neurol.* 2002;22(4):367–374.

59. Dvorak J. Epidemiology, physical examination, and neurodiagnostics. *Spine.* 1998;23:2663–2672.

60. Fischground J, Herkowitz H. Cervical degenerative disease. In: Garfin S. Vaccaro A. (eds). *Orthopaedic knowledge update spine.* Rosemont; American Academy of Orthopedic Surgeons: 1997.

61. Healy J, Healy B, Wond W. Cervical and lumbar MRI and asymptomatic older male lifelong athletes: Frequency of degenerative findings. *J Comp Assist Tomogr.* 1996;20:107–112.

62. Lehto I, Tertti M, Komu M. Age-related MRI changes at 0.1 T in cervical disc in asymptomatic subjects. *Neurorad.* 1994;36:49–53.

63. Sung R, Wang J. Correlation between a positive Hoffmann's reflex and cervical pathology in asymptomatic individuals. *Spine.* 2001;26:67–70.

64. Doherty J, Burns A, O'Ferrall D, Ditunno J. Prevalence of upper motor neuron vs. lower motor neuron lesions in complete lower thoracic and lumbar spinal cord injuries. *J Spinal Cord Med.* 2002;25:289–292.

65. Handal JA, Hagopian J, Dellose S. The validity of clinical tests in the diagnosis of cervical myelopathy. Presented at the annual meeting of the North American Spine Society, San Francisco, California, October 30, 1998.

66. Tong H, Haig A, Yamakawa K. The Spurling test and cervical radiculopathy. *Spine.* 2002;27:156–159.

67. Hakelius A, Hindmarsh J. The comparative reliability of preoperative diagnostic methods in lumbar disc surgery. *Acta Orthop Scand.* 1972;43(4):234–238.

68. Hakelius A, Hindmarsh J. The significance of neurological signs and myelographic findings in the diagnosis of lumbar root compression. *Acta Orthop Scand.* 1972;43(4):239–246.

69. Kosteljanetz M, Bang F, Schmidt-Olsen S. The clinical significance of straight-leg raising in the diagnosis of prolapsed lumbar disc. Interobserver variation and correlation with surgical finding. *Spine.* 1988;13(4): 393–395.

70. Bolan RA, Adams RD. Effects of ankle dorsiflexion on range and reliability of straight leg raising. *Aust J Physiotherapy.* 2000;46:191–200.

71. Sizer PS, Phelps V, Dedrick, G, Matthijis, O. Differential diagnosis and management of spinal nerve root-related pain. *Pain Practice.* 2002;2(2):98–121.

72. Deyo RA, Rainville J, Kent DL. What can the history and physical examination tell us about low back pain? *JAMA.* 1992;268(6):760–765.

73. Stankovic R, Johnell O, Maly P, Willner S. Use of lumbar extension, slump test, physical and neurological examination in the evaluation of patients with suspected herniated nucleus pulposus. A prospective clinical study. *Man Ther.* 1999;4(1):25–32.

74. McGann WA. History and physical examination. In: Steinberg ME. The *hip and its disorders.* Philadelphia: W.B. Saunders Company: 1991.

75. Maitland GD. *Maitland's vertebral manipulation.* 6th ed. London; Butterworth-Heinemann: 2001.

76. Grieve G. *Common vertebral joint problems.* 2nd ed. Edinburgh; Churchill Livingstone: 1988.

77. Hurwitz EL, Morgenstern H, Harber P, Kominski GF, Belin TR, Yu F, Adams AH. A randomized trial of medical care with and without physical therapy and chiropractic care with and without physical modalities for patients with low back pain: 6-month follow-up outcomes from the UCLA low back pain study. *Spine.* 2002;27(20):2193–2204.

78. Di Fabio RP. Manipulation of the cervical spine: risks and benefits. *Phys Ther.* 1999;79(1):50–65.

79. Nolan M. *Introduction to the neurological examination.* Philadelphia; FA Davis: 1996.

80. Nick J. Deep tendon reflexes: the what, why, where, and how of tapping. *J Obstet Gynecol Neonatal Nurs.* 2003;32(3):297–306.

81. Seidel H, Ball J, Dains J, Benedict G. *Mosby's guide to physical assessment.* 4th ed. St. Louis; Mosby: 1999.

82. Ebara S, Yonenobu K, Fujinara K, Yamashita K, Ono K. Myelopathic hand characterized by muscle wast-ing. A different type of myelopathic hand in patients with cervical spondylosis. *Spine.* 1988;13:785–791.

83. Colebatch J, Gandevia S, The distribution of muscular weakness in upper motor neuron lesions affecting the arm. *Brain.* 1989;112:749–763.

84. Shimizu T, Shimada H, Shirakura K. Scapulohumeral reflex. *Spine.* 1993;18:2182–2190.

85. Mayer N. Clinicophysiological concepts of spasticity and motor dysfunction in adults with an upper motor neuron lesion. *Muscle Nerve.* 1997:S6:S1–S12.

# 6

# Manual Therapy of the Cervical Spine

## Objectives

- Outline the pertinent clinically relevant anatomy of the cervical spine.
- Outline the three-dimensional coupling patterns of the cervical spine.
- Outline and describe the anatomical considerations of the vertebral artery.
- Perform the clinical examination of the cervical spine.

- Outline an effective treatment program for various cervical spine impairments.
- Describe common cervical spine disorders treated by manual therapists: (1) cervical radiculopathy, (2) degenerative arthritis, (3) cervical instability, (4) whiplash, and (5) headaches.
- Identify the outcomes associated with manual therapy to the cervical spine.

## PREVALENCE

Cervical spine pain is a common musculoskeletal malady reportedly affecting 70% of individuals within their lifetime.[1] Many neck disorders can significantly affect physical and social function,[2,3] resulting in high levels of health-care use[4] and direct and indirect costs.[4] A large proportion of the direct health-care-related costs are attributed to visits to health-care providers such as physicians and physical therapists.[2,5]

Cervical disorders are almost as prevalent as low back pain[6] and, like low back pain, the actual origin of pain is often indefinable. Nonphysical issues are nearly as relevant to the outcome of cervical disorders as the measurable impairment.[7] Because of the high degree of prevalence and the variability associated with the physical and nonphysical impairments, cervical spine disorders are a troublesome and challenging disorder for orthopedic manual therapists.

## UPPER CERVICAL SPINE ANATOMY

The upper cervical segments (Figure 6.1) are formed by the articulation of the occiput on C1 (OA joint) and the articulation of C1 on C2 (AA joint) (Figure 6.2).[8] This region includes selective joints and ligaments but does not include an intervertebral disc.[9] Of the two aspects of the cervical spine, the upper cervical spine is the most complex and predisposed to injury by trauma.

Within the OA joint, the cup-like configuration provides anatomical structure and stability along with an extensive connective tissue arrangement. The occipital condyles and the superior articular facets of the atlas slope

## Summary

- Cervical disorders are nearly as common as low back impairments and are responsible for high levels of health-care use.
- Various physical, psychological, and social medical factors contribute to a patient's prognosis.

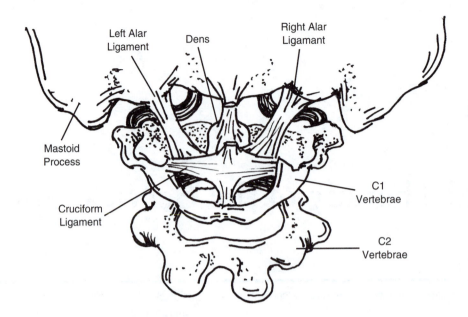

**Figure 6.1**    The Upper Cervical Spine Anatomy

downward and medially provide an orientation that promotes upper cervical extension.[10] The condylar arrangement leads to both an anterior and posterior atlanto-odontoid articulation within the OA joint.[10]

The atlas (C1) is peculiar when compared to other vertebral bones because it has no vertebral body. The atlas is essentially a ring-like hollow structure that is intimately attached to the axis. The atlas has no spinous process and consists of an anterior and a posterior arch and two lateral masses; the anterior arch forms about one-fifth of the ring. The atlas's anterior surface is convex, and presents at its center the anterior tubercle for the attachment of muscles.

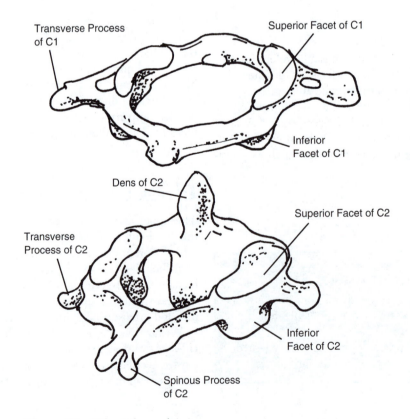

**Figure 6.2**    The Atlas and Axis

The axis (C2) is uniquely shaped as well and forms the pivot upon which the atlas rotates. The most distinctive characteristic of this structure is the strong odontoid process that rises perpendicularly from the upper surface of the body. The odontoid process of the axis is the attachment site of numerous ligaments and is considered an imperative structure of stability. The axis does have a bifid spinous process that is quite prominent and is the attachment site of numerous posteriorly oriented muscles.

An extensive connective tissue arrangement exists in the upper cervical region where the range of motion between vertebrae is greater than any other spine segmental region.[11] This complex arrangement is designed to control movement while providing stability through the interaction of various ligaments. The anterior longitudinal ligament, the anterior altanto-dental ligament, the tectorial membrane, the dentate ligaments, and the cruciform ligaments are recognized as crucial contributors to stability, while some of the connective tissue elements such as the ligamentum nuchae and the anterior longitudinal ligament are considered controversial.[12] The anterior longitudinal ligament, cruciform ligament, tectorial membrane, and nuchal ligament attach to the occiput, C1 and C2[10] and the anterior occipitoatloid membrane, atlanto-odontoid ligament, apical ligament of the dens, Alar ligaments, posterior occipitoatloid membrane, and the atlantoaxial membrane are limited in attachment to two of the three bones.[10]

White and Panjabi[12] state that the cruciform ligament is the most important ligament of the C0–C1–C2 complex. This ligament consists of both transverse and vertical portions, with the transverse portion providing the most important stabilizing function.[10] Fundamentally, the primary role of the cruciform ligament is to prevent the atlas from translating anterior on the axis during flexion. Uncontrolled translation would result in compromising the spinal cord, medulla, and potentially the vertebral arteries.

The dentate ligaments include the Alar and apical ligaments. The Alar ligaments are a pair of structures that attach to the dorsal-lateral surface of the dens and runs obliquely to the medial surfaces of the occipital condyles.[12] During side bending of the head on the neck, the occipital portion of the Alar ligament on the side that is side flexed toward is relaxed, while the Alar ligament on the side opposite of the relaxed band is tightened. During rotation, the Alar tightens on the side opposite the direction of rotation.[13] Subsequently, the left Alar ligament tightens and restricts rotation of the head and C1 to the right.[12]

The tectorial membrane is an extension of the posterior longitudinal ligament.[12] The tectorial membrane is located between the cruciform ligament and the atlas anteriorly and the anterior dura mater posteriorly and is thought to be a continuation of the anterior longitudinal ligament. It is proposed that this ligament may function to prevent traction-based movements.[12]

The muscles of the upper cervical spine are compartmentalized into three layers—the superficial, the middle, and the deep layer[14]—each layer providing different elements of mobility and stability to the upper cervical spine. Panjabi[15] described a form of dynamic stability responses, which is provided by muscular control during movements in mid- or early ranges. This concept is distinguished from passive stability, in which stabilization is obtained through passive structures such as ligaments, discs, bones, and joint capsules.

## Summary

- The upper cervical spine demonstrates unique bony and ligamentous stabilization systems.
- The complex arrangement of ligamentous structure in the upper cervical spine is responsible for movement control and stability.
- It is theorized that different muscles of the upper cervical spine are responsible for stabilization and movement initiation.

# LOWER CERVICAL SPINE ANATOMY

The lower cervical segments (Figure 6.3) include the segmental levels of C2-3 to C7-T1 and are noted more for their similarities than differences. All the segments exhibit intervertebral discs, uncinate processes, and spinous processes.[12] Additionally, passive spine integrity is imposed by a combined stabilization effort of the **zygopophyseal joints, uncinate processes,** intervertebral discs, and other passive structures. Although all vertebrae demonstrate significant similarities, Lysell[16] considered the C2 vertebral body unique as a transitional vertebra that divides the functions of the cervical spine.

There are five primary articulations between adjacent vertebrae. The first is the intervertebral disc, which cushions and controls movement between two vertebral bodies. Two uncinate processes articulate laterally and provide control of side flexion-based movements, and two zygopophyseal joints guide movements such as rotation. The intervertebral discs allow movement in all three planes, plus torsion. The zygopophyseal joints are considered translational joints and allow sliding motions that depend on the orientation of the joint plane. The uncinate processes allow sliding movements as well but are thought to be limited to those associated with convex and concave movements such as side flexion and sagittal movements.[12]

## *Cervical Intervertebral Disc*

Intervertebral discs (Figure 6.4) make up the fibrocartilagenous joints between adjacent cervical vertebral bodies and are present at the levels of C2-3 to C7-T1. The intervertebral discs share passive control of movement with the

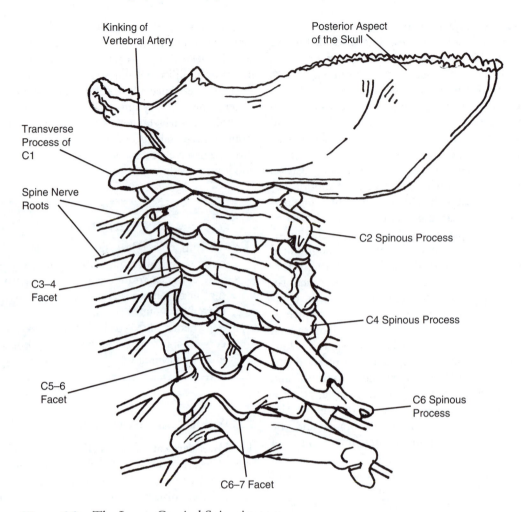

**Figure 6.3**  The Lower Cervical Spine Anatomy

uncinate processes and zygopophyseal joints and allow a specific range of motion throughout the cervical spine. Quality of range is dependent upon the thickness of the intervertebral discs relative to the horizontal dimensions of the vertebral bodies;[17] subsequently, younger individuals that display greater disc heights also demonstrate greater range of motion on average.

The cervical intervertebral disc has both similarities and dissimilarities to the lumbar disc. Like the lumbar disc, each intervertebral disc contains an **annulus fibrosis** and interiorly a gel-like **nucleus pulposis.** However, unlike the lumbar disc, an annulus is lacking posterior,[18] and the separate physical disc properties of a nucleus and annulus are reserved for younger populations. As one ages, the nucleus is replaced by fibrocartilage and other fiber components, typically occurring as early as the second decade of life.[19] An additional dissimilarity is the fiber direction of the annulus, which is not crossed concentrically as in the lumbar spine but arranged horizontally, converging upward toward the anterior aspect of the superior adjacent vertebral body.[18] Additionally, the annulus fibrosis does not encompass the entire perimeter of the disc,[18] potentially predisposing the disc to degenerative processes such as horizontal fibrillation. As Bogduk and Mercer[20] note, "The cervical annulus is well developed and thick anteriorly; but it tapes laterally and posteriorly towards the anterior edge of the uncinate process on each side."

Beyond the uncovertebral joint, the primary integrity of the posterior disc is enclosed by the posterior longitudinal ligament (PLL). The PLL is located on the posterior surface of the vertebral bodies within the spinal canal, and progresses from an attachment to the C2 vertebra to the dorsum of sacrum.[21] Essentially, the PLL is constructed in two layers: a thick anterior layer that is firmly attached to the posterior annulus and vertebral bodies, and a thin posterior layer loosely attached to the thick anterior layer, but completely unattached to the dura.[21] The PLL does contribute significantly to segmental stability specifically in patients with degenerative conditions[22], although its complete role during stabilization is controversial.

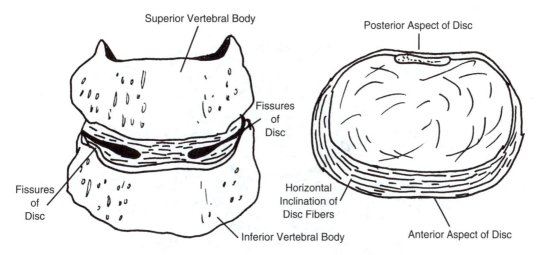

**Figure 6.4**    The Cervical Intervertebral Disc. Concept adapted from Mercer and Bogduk, 1999[18]

## The Cervical Facet (Zygopophyseal)

The cervical facet or zygopophyseal joints are progressively oblique from the cephalic segments to the caudal segments[23] and connect the lamina of each vertebral body. There are two facet joints between each pair of vertebrae, one left and one right. They are primarily designed to allow the vertebral bodies to rotate with respect to one another. The lower cervical segments are convex on concave and are nearly 45 degrees in inclination. There is some degree of angular change from cephalic to caudal in normal individuals, although this change is not constant or normative across subjects (Figure 6.5).[24]

In healthy individuals, the uneven surfaces within the zygopophyseal joints are filled by an invagination of the

posterior capsule called a **meniscoid**.[25] Meniscoids are fatty and highly innervated and frequently are involved in entrapment impairments on the cervical spine. Meniscoids function similarly to the meniscus of the knee in improving joint congruency. The posterior capsule is less thick than the anterior capsule, often integrates with a meniscoid and the multifidi musculature, and is vulnerable to injury.[17] During degenerative conditions, the posterior capsule becomes lax and allows possible displacement during neutral postures. Additionally, degenerative progression often causes the meniscoids to atrophy and virtually disappear, thus decreasing the integrity and stability of the zygopophyseal joints even further.[26] In normal subjects or those that experience early degenerative changes, articular facet impingements are common in large synovial folds while subluxation of the facet is more common when the meniscoids have degenerated or represent less space within the facet.[27] The anterior joints do not articulate with meniscoids and have capsules that are normally lax and permit large range of movements during neutral postures.[17]

## Uncinate Processes (The Joint of Luschka)

The uncinate processes are commonly identified as the joints of Luschka (Figure 6.6).[28] Uncinate processes are unique to the cervical spine and are found at levels C3 to C7. Essentially, these saddle-like formations increase the joint surface of the vertebral body of the above segment with the lower segment. Uncinate processes are developed during childhood and fully mature by the second decade.[28] Lateral fissures in the disc create a transformation that enlarges the lateral aspect of the annulus and encourages the articulation of the uncovertebral joints. By the second and third decade of life, the uncinate processes become fully articular with the development of

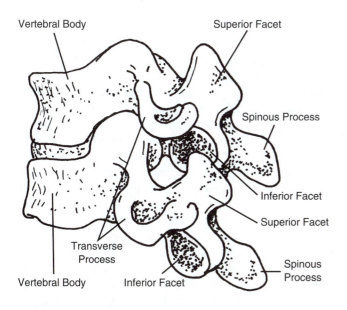

**Figure 6.5**    The Cervical Zygopophyseal Joints

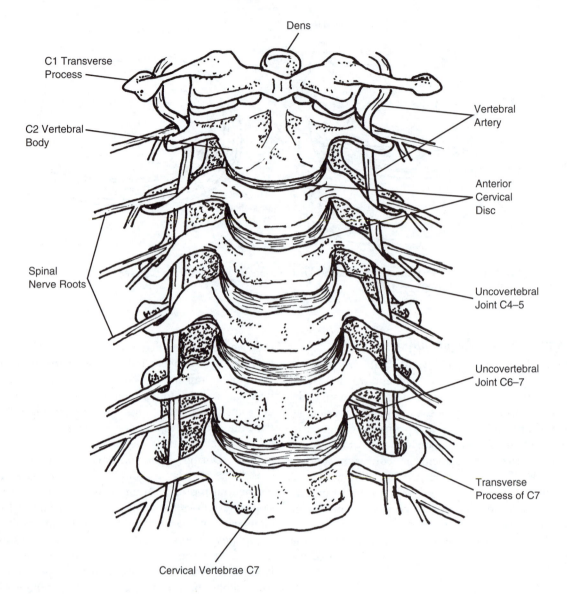

**Figure 6.6**    The Cervical Uncinate Processess

a pseudo-synovial joint.[28] The contact points are covered with articular cartilage and are considered true articulations but do exhibit a unique characteristic of both fibrocartilage and vascular contact points. The anterior part of the joint capsule of the uncovertebral joint blends with the annulus fibrosis of the disc.[26]

The uncinate processes contribute significantly to control of sagittal and coronal range of motion.[29] Degeneration of the uncinate processes is one of the chief reasons behind cervical spondylogenic changes and cervical radiculopathy.[26] These degenerative processes appear to coincide with intervertebral disc alterations of proteoglycan content.[28]

### Selected Muscular Anatomy

Bergmark[30] suggests that muscles within the trunk are best divided into **local muscle** and **global muscle** groups. The local muscles are deep and the global muscles are

generally superficial. The deep portions of some of the local muscles have their insertion and origin at the vertebrae in order to control the curvature of the spine and provide stiffness to maintain mechanical stability. Bergmark[30] also suggested that local muscles often attach directly to the joint capsules. Global muscles tend to be larger and are primarily responsible for transferring and balancing external loads during prime movements. Whereas global muscles undergo significant length change and function very little to control joint stability, local muscles undergo little length change. Most local muscles maintain an isometric contraction during their responsibility of stabilization, with specific focus of controlling shear forces at the insertion site. Subsequently, the role of the deep and local muscles is quite different from one another, a phenomenon that is very prevalent in patients with chronic neck pain.[31] Falla et al.[31] report that the deep cervical flexor muscles, longus capitis and colli, are related intimately with the cervical osseous and articular elements, and serve an important role in control of spinal elements, which cannot be replicated by the more superficial anterior muscles. Anatomically, sternocleidomastoid has no attachments to the cervical vertebrae and does not play a role in cervical stabilization. In some cases, cocontraction of the deep and superficial muscles is required for the muscles to stiffen or stabilize the segments, especially in functional midranges.[31] Protocols that have targeted local musculature have exhibited good outcomes for patients with chronic cervical pain and **cervicogenic headaches**.[32] Although less studied, the lateral and posterior muscles most likely contribute to postural dysfunctions and associative pain.

### The Vertebral Foramen and Nerve Roots

Each nerve root exits above the correspondingly numbered vertebral body from C2 to C7 in regions identified as intervertebral foramen. Nerve roots in the cervical spine are identified by the caudal segment of the intervertebral foramen. For example, the C3 nerve root exists above the C3 vertebral body, as does the C5 nerve root above the C5 body. This occurs because C1 exists between the occiput and atlas.[8]

The intervertebral canals are a special concern because these structures house the vertebral artery as it courses to the posterior aspect of the skull (Figure 6.7). The relatively large amount of rotation available at C1-2 allows a kinking to occur to the vertebral artery on the contralateral side in which the head is rotated[12], an action that is often the cause behind selected **vertebrobasilar insufficiency** responses in patients (Figure 6.8). White and Panjabi[12] suggested that 45 degrees of rotation is enough to kink the vertebral artery, thus potentially compromising blood flow.

The spinal column is surrounded by a variety of structures. The lateral aspect is covered posteriorly by the lateral aspects of a superior and inferior lamina. The ligamentum flavum provides the ventral cover and is attached to two-thirds of the undersurface of the superior lamina. Inferiorly the ligamentum flavum is attached to the superior edge of the lower lamina.[33] Posteriorly, from cephaled to caudal, the neural foramen's parameter is bound by 1–2 mm of the superior (descending) and inferior (ascending) facets. The superior and inferior boundaries of the neural foramen are formed by the superior and inferior vertebral pedicles.[33] Of all the vertebral spinal foramina, the largest diameter is at C2-C3, which progressively decreases in size to the C6-C7 level. In a nondamaged segment, the nerve root occupies between 25 and 33% of the foramina space.[8]

## Summary

- The lower cervical anatomy is dissimilar to the upper cervical anatomy.
- The cervical intervertebral discs exhibit dissimilar characteristics to those of the lumbar spine.
- The uncovertebral joint develops in the second decade of life and becomes more prominent with degenerative changes in the intervertebral disc.
- The intervertebral foramen and spinal column are predisposed to anatomical changes and may be the origins of cervical radiculopathy and myelopathy.

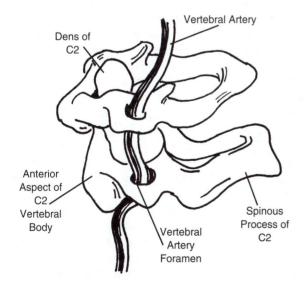

**Figure 6.7**    Normal Vertebral Artery Position during Neutral

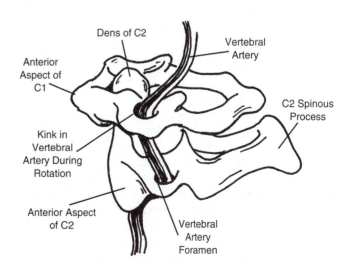

**Figure 6.8**    The Kinking of the Vertebral Artery during Rotation

# Biomechanics of the Cervical Spine

Fundamentally, there are two disparate regions to the cervical spine: the upper cervical spine and the lower cervical spine. Within this textbook, there are two points of consideration associated with biomechanics of the cervical spine: range of motion and **coupling behavior.** Range of motion is presented in two forms: gross cervical movement and individualized segmental movements. Using the 3 Space Isotrak measurement system, Trott et al.[34] outlined normative, average gross range-of-motion values for the age groups 20 through 59. They found the average flexion values were 45.1–57.5 degrees, average extension 60–76.1 degrees, average left rotation 63.4–71.7 degrees, average right rotation 70.4–78 degrees, average left lateral flexion, 32.4–45.5 degrees, and average right lateral flexion 35.4–47.6 degrees. The lower values represent the age group of 50–59, identifying a notable decline of range of motion with age.

Several methods of measurement for cervical range of motion are presented within the literature,[35,36] the more sophisticated and expensive the method, the more reliable the reported range-of-motion scores. Traditionally, most manual therapy clinicians measure three cardinal planes of motion (sagittal, coronal, and frontal) with a standard goniometer, a method that has exhibited fair reliability when specific guidelines are followed. Nilsson et al.[37] suggest that goniometric measurements exhibit good reliability when combined movements are measured (for instance, total range of motion of flexion and extension) versus selecting an arbitrary neutral or zero point as a starting reference. Others who have used the zero point method[37,38] have reported interclass coefficient values of 0.6–0.8, values that are moderately acceptable. For research purposes, a device that provides more accuracy in range of motion is beneficial, but for clinical purposes, the goniometric measure appears to be efficient and reliable.

## Upper Cervical Spine

### Range of Motion

The primary planar motion at C0-1 is flexion/extension, characterized by total segmental range-of-motion values of 25 degrees.[12] Unilateral lateral flexion is limited to 5 degrees, as is unilateral rotation.[12]

The axial-atlanto (AA) joint allows for 50% of all cervical rotation motion.[12] The occipital atlantal joint (OA) is responsible for 50% of flexion and extension of the complete cervical spine.[8] Unilateral side flexion accounts for 5 total degrees whereas flexion/extension measures 20 degrees during combined values.[12] It has been stated that the essential movement of the upper cervical spine occurs between the occiput and C2 and is regulated by the atlas.[9] In all motion initiations, whether proximal or distal to the upper cervical spine, C1 is mobile and the movement of the occiput and C2 predicates on the initiation of the movement.[9]

## Lower Cervical Spine

### Range of Motion

White and Panjabi[12] reported the mid-lower cervical range of motions values with a wide degree of variability. C2-3, C3-4, C6-7, and C7-T1 display the lowest segmental combined flexion/extension ranges whereas C4-5 and C5-6 exhibit the highest values. Unilateral side flexion progressively decline from cephaled to caudal, dropping from a peak of 10–11 degrees at C2-3, C3-4, and C4-5 to a low of 4 degrees at C7-T1. Unilateral rotation is greatest at C3-4 to C6-7, with nearly comparative values throughout. One exception is the lowest recorded value for unilateral rotation at C7-T1, with a reported range of 0–7 degrees.

## Coupling Biomechanics

Five studies qualified as three-dimensional analyses of coupling motion with side-bend initiation. Table 6.1 outlines those findings. Every study identified the simultaneous occurrence of the coupled movements of side flexion and rotation at all levels tested. Generally, there was remarkable agreement among all studies at the majority of segmental levels. All studies that tested C0-1, C2-3, C3-4, C4-5, C5-6, C6-7, and C7-1 found consistent side-bend and axial rotation to the same side. Two studies reported that side-bend and axial rotation occurred in opposition at C1-2 and two others found coupling movement to the same side.

Five studies measured rotation, two of which measured all levels (Table 6.2). Similar to side-bend initiation, axial rotation initiation demonstrated strong agreement among researchers. All studies that tested C0-1, C1-2, C3-4, C4-5, C5-6, C6-7, and C7-1 demonstrated absolute agreement. Levels C0-1 and C1-2 exhibited side-bend to the opposite direction as the initiated movement of axial rotation. The spinal levels C2-3, C3-4, C4-5, C5-6, C6-7, and C7-1 exhibit side-bend to the same direction as the initiated movement of axial rotation. Only two studies reported the movement values of C2-3 and C3-4 and found rotation and side flexion occurred to the same side.

White and Panjabi[12] stated that the coupling characteristics of the upper cervical spine were associated with some disagreement. At first analysis, coupling patterns may appear to differ across studies, but this is most likely a reflection of two methodological contributors that substantially alter the outcome of an analysis. First, failure to identify the motion that was used to initiate coupling could lead to inappropriate comparisons. It is notable that initiation of side-bend or rotation does appear to change the resultant directional coupling pattern of the upper cervical spine. This finding is similar to the report of Cook[45] regarding studies of lumbar spine coupling.

Second, the instrument used during the measurement process may also lead to variable results. Most studies that examined coupling using two-dimensional (2-D) analysis demonstrated conflicting findings in the upper cervical spine when compared at face value to three-dimensional

**TABLE 6.1   Coupled Cervical Motion with Side-Bend Initiation (Neutral Spine); 3-D Analyses**

| Side (Lateral)-Bend Initiation of Movement | | | | | | | | |
| --- | --- | --- | --- | --- | --- | --- | --- | --- |
| **Author** | **C0-1** | **C1-2** | **C2-3** | **C3-4** | **C4-5** | **C5-6** | **C6-7** | **C7-1** |
| Iai et al.[40] (in-vivo) | S | O | S | S | S | S | S | S |
| Panjabi et al.[43] (in-vitro) | NT | NT | S | S | S | S | S | S |
| Panjabi et al.[39] (in-vitro) | S | O | NT | NT | NT | NT | NT | NT |
| Panjabi et al.[44] (in vitro) | S | S | S | S | S | S | S | S |
| Penning et al.[9] (in-vivo) | S | S | S | S | S | S | S | S |

*S = Axial rotation coupling to the same side as side-bend. O = Axial rotation coupling to the opposite side of side-bend. NT = Not tested. V = Variable coupling pattern among specimens.*

(3-D) analysis. It has been identified that 2-D analysis of coupling motions fails to report accurate axial rotation and may be ineffective at measuring coupling direction and quantity.[20,46] 2-D imagery has been criticized because it may lead to magnification errors, projection of translations as rotations, and misleading results.[47,48] In order to represent the true accurate motion behavior of the spine, intervertebral coupling motion is best measured with 3-D instrumentation.[46,49] The 3-D instrumentation allows the measurement of finite movements in multiple planes.

It is worth noting that Fryette's laws of physiological motion[50] are not included in this chapter's discussion of coupling. In 1954, Fryette's findings were published and were largely based on the findings of Lovett.[45] Fryette's perception of coupling of the cervical region was that "sidebending is accompanied by rotation of the bodies of the vertebrae to the concavity of the lateral curve, as in the lumbar [spine]."[50] The findings of Fryette are not included because they did not include a systematic, investigatory method of evaluation and were 2-D at best.

Anatomical variation and structure may explain the variation found at C1-2. Earlier studies described the C1-2 motion as a convex-on-convex movement, based strictly on radiographic assessment,[12] although others have suggested that the structure may vary between convex or con-

cave because of variations in cartilage anatomy. Additionally, C0-1 demonstrates very little actual axial rotation, which limits accuracy in measurement.[9]

## Summary

- With reference to biomechanical movement, the upper cervical spine is mostly responsible for physiological rotation, flexion, and extension movements.
- Coupling patterns of the upper cervical spine at C1-2 are somewhat unpredictable during side flexion initiation but are predictable during rotation initiation.
- C1 is mobile during all forms of movement whether caudally or cephalically initiated.
- The lower cervical spine demonstrates equivocal percentages of biomechanical movements in all ranges of physiological motion.
- The lower cervical spine demonstrates a consistent and predictable coupling pattern regardless of the initiation of motion; side flexion and rotation occur to the same side.

**TABLE 6.2   Coupled Cervical Motion with Rotation Initiation (Neutral Spine); 3-D Analyses**

| (Axial) Rotation Initiation of Motion | | | | | | | | |
| --- | --- | --- | --- | --- | --- | --- | --- | --- |
| **Author** | **C0-1** | **C1-2** | **C2-3** | **C3-4** | **C4-5** | **C5-6** | **C6-7** | **C7-1** |
| Ishii et al.[42] (in-vivo) | O | O | NT | NT | NT | NT | NT | NT |
| Mimura et al.[41] (in-vivo)* | NT | NT | NR | NR | S | S | S | S |
| Panjabi et al.[39] (in vitro) | O | O | NT | NT | NT | NT | NT | NT |
| Panjabi et al.[44] (in-vitro) | O | O | S | S | S | S | S | S |
| Penning et al.[9] (in-vivo) | O | O | S | S | S | S | S | S |

*S = Axial rotation coupling to the same side as side-bend. O = Axial rotation coupling to the opposite side of side-bend. NT = Not tested. V = Variable coupling pattern among specimens. NR = Not reported.*
*\*Mimura et al. reported the movements of Occ.-C2, not C0-1 and C1-2 individually.*

# ASSESSMENT AND DIAGNOSIS

## Subjective Considerations

Gregory Grieve[51] suggested three mandatory questions for the cervical spine: (1) any dizziness (vertigo), blackouts, or "drop" attacks? (2) any history of rheumatoid arthritis or other inflammatory arthritis, or treatment by systemic steroid? and (3) any neurological symptoms in the legs? Often, dizziness, blackouts, and drop attacks are associated with vertebral basilar insufficiency (VBI), a disorder characterized by restriction of blood flow through the vertebral arteries, thus restricting the flow of blood to the rear portions of the brain, including the occipital lobe, cerebellum, and brainstem.[52] Further discussion of detection of VBI is provided in the pretesting section.

**Neurological symptoms** are frequent in patients with instability-based disorders. Rheumatoid arthritis (RA) is the most common inflammatory disorder to affect the cervical spine, with a predilection for the atlanto-axial joint complex.[53] RA is associated with instability and should always be determined prior to assessment. However, Cook et al.[54] outlined selected subjective symptoms associated with instability and neurological symptoms were not consensually identified as a factor associated with instability.

Neurological symptoms in the legs associated with cervical disorders or movements may be indicative of myelopathy. Myelopathy is characterized by the clinical finding that the lower extremities are affected first, with subsequent spasticity and paresis. The patient often complains of a gait disturbance due to abnormalities in the corticospinal tracts and spinocerebellar tracts. Later the upper extremities become involved with loss of strength and difficulty in fine finger movements. Chapter 5 detailed the symptoms and aetiology of myelopathy. Significant complaints associated with myelopathy are best served by referral to a medical physician trained in traditional diagnostic assessment.

Many patients' cervical signs and symptoms necessitate the use of a functional outcome questionnaire. These signs and symptoms may negatively influence functional activities in ways beyond the traditional investigation of physiological impairments. Functional outcome questionnaires comprise the ability to gauge the impact of the disease process on the performance of daily activities.[53] Region-specific functional outcome questionnaires concentrate on specific areas of the body and may measure dysfunction with greater responsiveness than a scale that measures overall health and wellness.[55]

Two region-specific questionnaires for the cervical spine are the **Neck Disability Index** (NDI)[56,57] and the **Neck Pain and Disability Scale** (NPAD).[58] The NDI is designed to measure activity limitations due to neck pain and disability,[56] whereas the NPAD purportedly measures report of problems with neck movements, neck pain intensity, effect of neck pain on emotion and cognition, and the level of interference during life activities.[58] Both scales have been regularly used in previous studies that have investigated functional status,[59–61] although the NDI has been used more frequently.[55]

## Summary

- Dizziness, blackouts, and drop attacks are associated with vertebral basilar insufficiency (VBI).
- VBI is a disorder characterized by restriction of blood flow through the vertebral arteries, thus restricting the flow of blood to the rear portions of the brain, including the occipital lobe, cerebellum, and brainstem
- Two region-specific questionnaires for the cervical spine are the Neck Disability Index (NDI) and the Neck Pain and Disability Scale (NPAD), both of which have been validated for use in various populations.

## Objective/Physical Examination

### Pretesting

The cervical spine is unique to other musculoskeletal regions because life-threatening consequences have been associated with a condition called **vertebral basilar insufficiency** (VBI). The most frequent "life-threatening" consequence is a cerebrovascular complication associated with spinal manipulative therapy.[62] Ernst[62] outlined several signs and symptoms associated with cerebrovascular complications taken from a review of multiple case reports. Table 6.3 outlines the complications and the associative technique involved prior to the complication.

Barker et al.[63] reported several important premanipulative testing procedures prior to selection of a manipulative maneuver. The cornerstones of their suggestions identify the risk factors associated with vertebral basilar insufficiency assessment using both subjective and objective criteria. They suggest that premanipulative tests such as VBI testing maneuvers should be performed upon patient consent prior to treatment intervention.

VBI is a localized or diffuse reduction in blood flow through the vertebrobasilar arterial system. This system supplies the posterior aspects of the brain and includes the brainstem, cerebellum, occipital lobe, medial temporal lobe, and thalamus. VBI-related problems associated with manipulation have been reported to range from one occurrence in 20,000 to five in 10 million cervical spine manipulations.[64] The most frequently reported form of injury is arterial dissection that results in a variety of outcomes, including death in 18% of cases.[52] Although the causes of arterial dissection associated with manipulation are not completely known, it is apparent that the most frequently

**TABLE 6.3**   Cerebrovascular Complications Associated with Cervical Manual Therapy (adapted from Ernst[62])

| Symptoms | Intervention | Outcome |
|---|---|---|
| Stroke | Cervical manipulation | Neurological deficit or death |
| Emboli released | Cervical manipulation | Visual field damage |
| Spinal epidural hematoma | Cervical manipulation | Full recovery |
| Cauda equina syndrome | Cervical manipulation | Good recovery, questionable relationship |
| Bilateral blindness | Cervical manipulation | Persistent visual disturbances |
| Vertebral arteriovenous fistula | Cervical manipulation | Recovery |
| Dural tear | Cervical manipulation | Unknown |
| Horner's syndrome | Cervical manipulation | Unknown |
| Subdural hematoma | Cervical manipulation | Full recovery after surgical intervention |
| Wallenberg syndrome | Cervical manipulation | Unknown |

injured site is at C1-C2. This is most likely because the artery experiences elongation and kinking during cervical rotation.[65] For example, during right rotation the left vertebral artery experiences elongation. Despite this relatively rare occurrence of arterial dissection, the devastating effects of these complications emphasize the importance of establishing a valid and sensitive test to identify those patients who may be at risk of developing VBI.

Two recent reviews by McKechnie[66,67] identified selected signs and symptoms associated with a positive VBI test. The most commonly cited VBI-related symptoms included dizziness and vertigo, nausea, vomiting, inability to stand, blurred vision, and loss of lower extremity control. Less common symptoms included loss of consciousness, facial numbness, and headaches. The most commonly cited pathological neurological signs included cerebellar symptoms such as ataxia, dyssynergia and dysmetria, rotatory nystagmus, facial nerve palsy, and parathesia. Lincoln[68] suggested that the prevalence of hypermobility in the upper cervical spine was more appropriately associated with potential VBI signs and symptoms. The significance and commonality of upper cervical instability was identified by Panjabi et al.[69] and includes the passive losses of stability from the ligaments and active losses of the muscles and neural control mechanisms. The long-term clinical observation that cervical range of motion declines with age is only partially correct. Dvorak et al.[70] found that gross lower cervical ranges do decrease with age, especially over 50 years of age, yet overall upper cervical range of motion does not decline with age. Nonetheless, recent evidence suggests that VBI complications linked to manipulation occur more often than previously reported in individuals less than 45 years of age.[71,72]

VBI tests are used with some degree of controversy. Johnson et al.[73] found unreliable evidence that upper cervical manipulation affects upper vertebral artery flow. However, participants for the study were a mean age of 33 and were asymptomatic with no VBI-related symptoms. In other experimental studies, tests have shown mixed overall results regarding the occlusion of blood flow to the brain with cervical motion. Some studies confirm that collateral circulation is present during the provocative movements whereas others have been inconclusive overall.[74–77]

Several testing methods have been defined within the literature. Maitland[78] suggests placing an individual in the premanipulative position prior to performing the procedure, in order to assess their tolerance to the position. Of all the tests identified, sustained end-of-range rotation of the cervical spine has long been suggested as the most effective method of VBI assessment of the upper cervical spine. This test was first described by Maitland in 1968,[79,80] and is currently recommended in the premanipulation guidelines for the cervical spine[63,79,81,82] that are used by physiotherapists and other manual therapists. The purpose of the test is to reproduce potential signs or symptoms of VBI in a safe, gradual progression of neck rotation. If central neurological signs or symptoms are reproduced, immediate referral to a physician for further testing is warranted.

It is the discretion of the clinician to perform a VBI test prior to treatment; however, screening for VBI should occur prior to every manipulative session.[63] Barker et al.[63] report that despite thorough screening, there is still an element of risk associated with spontaneous accident. Additionally, the subjective examination will often dictate who may have a positive VBI response prior to testing. Because there is some risk of causing a positive VBI using the testing method, it may be advisable to avoid the performance of the test or treatment in cases where subjective symptoms are commonly reported or past tests have demonstrated positive findings. In the event of a positive VBI during testing, the treatment should be stopped immediately and appropriate medical assistance should be sought.[63] Figure 6.9 outlines the algorithm for premanipulative testing.

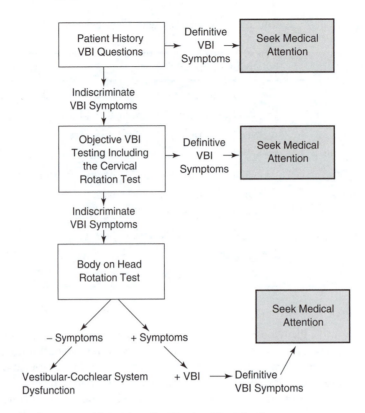

**Figure 6.9**    Algorithm for Testing Vertebral Basilar Insufficiency

---

## VBI Testing in Sitting

- Step One: The patient is interviewed to extract signs and symptoms of VBI (see Table 6.4). If remarkable, the patient is referred out for appropriate medical consult.
- Step Two: Prior to a comprehensive clinical examination, the clinician performs end-range cervical rotation tests on the patient in a sitting or supine position (Figures 6.10 and 6.11). The position is held for 10 seconds with observation for signs and symptoms of VBI.

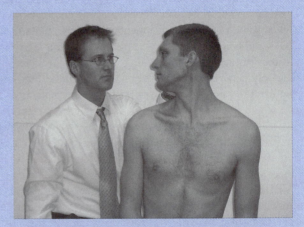

**Figure 6.10**    Cervical Rotation Test in Sitting

- Step Three: The head is returned to a neutral position and held for a minimum of 10 seconds.
- Step Four: Rotation is repeated to the opposite side (Figures 6.10 and 6.11) and the position is held for 10 seconds. The clinician observes for signs and symptoms of VBI. If remarkable, the patient is referred out for appropriate medical consult.

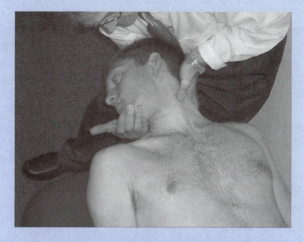

**Figure 6.11**   Cervical Rotation Test in Supine

- Step Five: If minor dizziness is present and the ability to differentiate if head movement and/or if the patient exhibits a history of vestibular symptoms associated with vestibulocochlear disorders, the clinician performs the body on head rotation test (see Figure 6.12). If this test is remarkable, the clinician should consider referring out for appropriate medical consult.
- Step Six: If dizziness abates during body on head rotation, the patient may exhibit a vestibulocochlear disorder and may benefit from vestibular rehabilitation. If symptoms are present during body on head but are "less" than the first assessments, the patient may exhibit cervical mechanoreceptor symptoms that mimic VBI. It is the discretion of the clinician at that point to evaluate the upper C-spine for signs of instability or stiffness as causal.

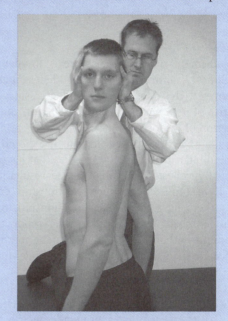

**Figure 6.12**   The Body on Head Rotation Test

- Step Seven: The last procedure performed is the premanipulative position test (see Figure 6.13) to determine the patient's tolerance to combined movements of the mid and lower cervical spine. The position is held for 10 seconds. If symptoms are remarkable, the patient is referred to appropriate medical personnel.

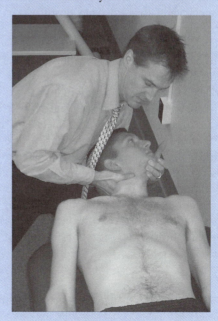

**Figure 6.13**   The Premanipulative Position

## Summary

- The cervical spine is unique to other musculoskeletal regions because of the consequences associated with vertebral basilar insufficiency. Consequently, premanipulative testing is required for safety considerations.
- Sustained end-of-range rotation of the cervical spine has long been suggested as the most effective method of VBI assessment of the upper cervical spine.
- Despite thorough VBI screening prior to the initiation of treatment, there is still an element of risk associated with spontaneous accident.

### Observation

Visual assessment of cervical posture is frequently used during clinical examination.[70,83] Nonetheless, Fedorak et al.[84] identified that the reliability of assessing postural asymmetry of the cervical spine was poor, specifically identification of lordosis.

It has long been postulated that posture directly affects craniomandibular pain (TMJ).[85] Studies that have investigated this hypothesis have found mixed results. Selected authors have reported no such relationship exists[85–88] whereas others have identified a relationship, most notably muscle imbalances.[89] Wright et al.[90] report that postural training with TMJ self-management methods was more effective than self-management methods alone. Further research is required for conclusion.

Selected authors[91,92] have reported a notable association between forward head posture and headaches. Watson and Trott[91] found that a preponderance of subjects examined with chronic headaches demonstrated abnormal posture, specifically forward head posture (Figure 6.14), whereas the control subjects did not.

A **"cock-robin" posture** (Figure 6.15) has been associated with atlanto-axial rotary subluxation.[12,93,94] This acute torticollis position, most typically found in children, is earmarked by side flexion, flexion, and rotation to one side. Individuals with connective tissue disorders may be predisposed to this condition and special care is warranted. Atlanto-axial subluxation requires differentiation from a similar postural abnormality associated with a herniated disc or cervical radiculopathy. Movements of side flexion, rotation, and extension to the same direction as a disc herniation or cervical spondylosis may provoke radiculopathic symptoms.[95] Consequently, the patient will often hold their head in a position of side flexion, rotation, and sagittal flexion.

### Introspection

A decreased willingness to move may be associated with spine instability or an upper cervical fracture. Because cer-

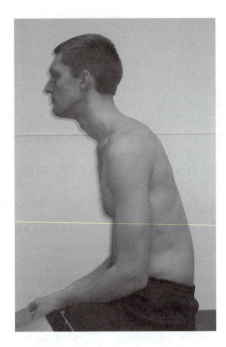

**Figure 6.14** Forward Head Posture

vical spine instability may only demonstrate subtle clinical examination features,[96,97] it is important to recognize certain attributes associated with this potentially serious complication. These attributes have been described as aberrant cervical movements,[98] referred shoulder pain,[32,98] radiculopathy and/or myelopathy,[99] paraspinal muscle spasms, decreased cervical lordosis,[98] tinnitus,[100]

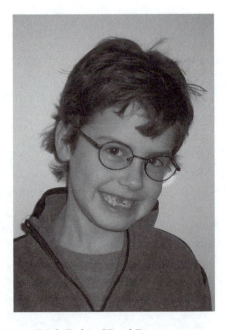

**Figure 6.15** Cock Robin Head Posture

pain during sustained postures,[98] and altered range of motion.[96,101–103] Because these symptoms are similar to other, less complicated disorders, it is essential to determine if a history of major trauma or repetitive microtrauma has predated the report of symptoms.[96]

In patients with cervical instability from a dens fracture, neurological symptoms associated with myelopathy may be present. Occasionally, these neurological symptoms are limited to one transitory episode of diffuse paresis following trauma, while in other patients, cervical myelopathy is notable and profuse. Progressive myelopathy causes weakness and ataxia, which predominates over sensory changes.[104] In severe cases a dens fracture may lead to neurovascular symptoms and vertebral artery compression. Subsequently, this compression may cause cervical and brainstem ischemia with signs and symptoms such as gait ataxia, syncope, vertigo, and visual disturbances. This serious phenomenon is beyond the scope of a manual therapist's treatment and should be discovered during the medical screening. Recent medical screening advances

have improved the likelihood of discovering cervical trauma and are worth noting.

Since less than 3% of trauma series have positive findings[105] and provided the very low yield of radiographic assessment, many authors consider universal C-spine radiography inefficient and costly.[106–109] Occasionally, to effectively clear the C-spine, repeated imaging attempts are required, a mechanism that adds to the total costs.[110] Subsequently, the **Canadian C-Spine rules** were devised to rule out those who may not need a radiograph after trauma. Bandiera et al.[111] have reported that the specificity of this instrument was higher than the clinical judgment of emergency room physicians demonstrating 100% specificity in a large population of patients with cervical spine trauma. Patients who are (1) cognitively intact and have no neurological symptoms, (2) are under the age of 65, (3) are not fearful of moving the head upon command, (4) who were not involved in a distraction-based injury, and (5) who demonstrate no midline pain are spared a radiograph.[111] Figure 6.16 outlines the Canadian C-Spine rules.

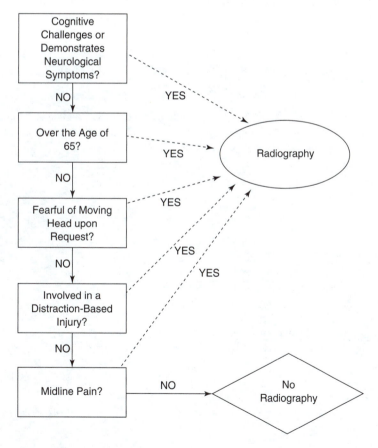

**Figure 6.16**    The Canadian C-Spine Rules for Determination of Necessity for a Radiograph (Modified from Bandiera et al. 2003[111])

## *Summary*

- Selected postures such as forward head and a "cock-robin" positions are commonly associated with cervical pain.
- There is mixed information regarding the postural contribution of the cervical spine to craniomandibular pain.
- After a traumatic incident, a decreased willingness to move could be a red flag associated with upper c-spine instability. The use of the Canadian C-Spine rules is beneficial in determining whether appropriate outside medical referral is beneficial.

# CLINICAL EXAMINATION

## Active Physiological Movements

Active movements are any form of physiological movements performed exclusively by the patient. In a clinical examination, the purpose of an active movement is to identify and examine the effect of selected active movements on the concordant sign. By determining the behavior of the concordant sign to selected movements, the clinician can effectively identify potential active physiological treatment approaches. Active physiological assessment of the cervical spine purportedly examines the contractile elements of the cervical spine.[26] Range of motion is an effective screening technique and is effective for assessment of age-related changes and degeneration. In many cases, degenerative changes of the cervical spine result in losses of range of motion in all movements except rotation.[26]

Sandmark and Nisell[112] deemed active assessment that consisted of visual observation of movement patterns insufficiently sensitive in detecting concordant patients' complaints. The authors used reproduction of pain as their sensitivity instrument during detection. Lee et al.[113] reported active range-of-motion differences between symptomatic and asymptomatic patients in a controlled comparison. Their findings indicate that when compared to normal subjects, symptomatic patients exhibited decreased lower cervical extension and left rotation but exhibited greater chin retraction. The work of Sterling et al.[114] indicates that the active range-of-motion values are consistent over time and do not reflect artifact from pain during the time of assessment. Subsequently, it appears that range-of-motion abnormalities, that also reproduce the patient's current complaint of pain, are helpful in identifying the impaired movement as compared to painful movements alone.

**Active Physiological Motion of the Upper Cervical Spine**
**Upper Cervical Flexion**

A systematic process is helpful in detecting the concordant sign of the patient and since multiple movements in several degrees of freedom are capable in the cervical spine, there are many movements to assess. The first motion of assessment is upper cervical spine flexion.

- Step One: The clinician positions the patient's head in a designated neutral position. Resting symptoms are assessed.
- Step Two: The clinician instructs the patient to retract his or her chin, "Make a double chin." The patient should be instructed to retract up to the first point of pain.
- Step Three: The clinician instructs the patient to retract beyond his or her first point of pain, or if no pain is present, go toward the end range.
- Step Four: The clinician then instructs the patient to gently nod his or her chin to detect provocation (repeated movements).

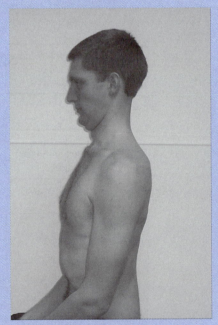

**Figure 6.17**  Upper C-spine Flexion

## Upper Cervical Extension

Upper cervical spine extension is a movement that is commonly associated with forward head postures. The following includes the steps associated with upper cervical spine extension.

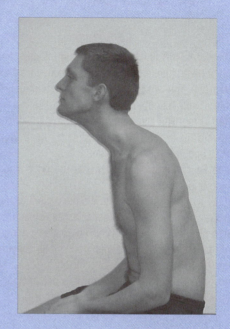

- Step One: The clinician positions the patient's head in a designated neutral position. Resting symptoms are assessed.
- Step Two: The clinician instructs the patient to protract his or her chin, "Stick your chin out." The patient should be instructed to protract up to the first point of pain.
- Step Three: The clinician instructs the patient to protract beyond his or her first point of pain, or if no pain is present, the patient is instructed to move toward the end range.
- Step Four: The clinician instructs the patient to gently nod his or her chin to detect provocation (repeated movements). The patient's signs and symptoms are readdressed.

**Figure 6.18**    Upper C-spine Extension

The use of overpressure may be useful in isolating various impairments and is designed to "rule out" potential joints that do not contribute to the patient's impairment.[96,115] Overpressure is less effective when one attempts to dictate the presence of the impairment based on "feel" of the end range. Assessment of end feel appears to be a valuable skill for manual therapists, although investigators have reported mixed outcomes regarding the reliability and clinical utility in several different joint systems.[116–119] Test effectiveness may vary according to other factors including the joint position, the tester's educational background,[120] and the presence of pain.[121]

## Active Physiological Motion of the Lower Cervical Spine
## Lower Cervical Flexion

The lower cervical spine harbors different movements and responsibilities when compared to the upper cervical spine. Subsequently, it is beneficial to disassociate the movement of the upper cervical spine motion. Because it is impossible to eliminate movement, the following provides a guideline that emphasizes the flexion-based motion to the lower cervical spine.

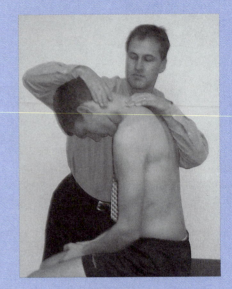

- Step One: The clinician positions the patient's head in a designated neutral position. Resting symptoms are assessed.
- Step Two: The clinician instructs the patient to retract his or her chin, "Make a double chin."
- Step Three: The clinician instructs the patient to bend the neck forward up to the first point of pain, "Keep your chin tucked, while bending your neck to your chest."
- Step Four: The clinician instructs the patient to move beyond the first point of pain.
- Step Five: The clinician instructs the patient to repeat gently the end range movement in order to assess change of condition.
- Step Six: (If no pain) The clinician applies a gentle overpressure into physiological flexion (pictured), while concurrently stabilizing the posterior neck. The clinician applies traction with the flexion-based overpressure and the patient's signs and symptoms are reassessed.

**Figure 6.19**   Lower Cervical Flexion with Overpressure

## Lower Cervical Extension

Forward head places the lower cervical spine into a position of flexion. Assessing extension is beneficial to determine if the postural problem is structural or positional. The following provides a guideline for examination of lower cervical spine extension.

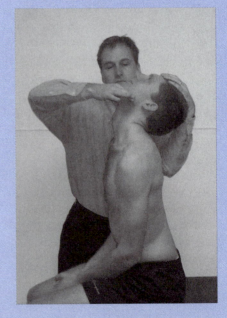

- Step One: The clinician positions the patient's head in a designated neutral position. Resting symptoms are assessed.
- Step Two: The clinician instructs the patient to retract his or her chin, "Make a double chin."
- Step Three: The clinician instructs the patient to bend the neck backward up to the first point of pain, "Keep your chin tucked in while bending your neck backward."
- Step Four: The clinician instructs the patient to move beyond the first point of pain to his or her end range.
- Step Five: The clinician instructs the patient to repeat gently the end range movement in order to assess change of condition.
- Step Six: (If no pain) The clinician applies a gentle overpressure into physiological extension using appropriate caution (pictured). The clinician should support the thoracic spine with his or her elbow and forearm while cupping the posterior aspect of the head for patient confidence. Upon completion, the patient's signs and symptoms are reassessed.

**Figure 6.20**   Lower Cervical Extension with Overpressure

## Physiological Side Flexion

Physiological side flexion is a movement that requires six degrees of accessory motion.[12] The following guidelines outline the examination process for side flexion.

- Step One: The clinician positions the patient's head in a designated neutral position. Resting symptoms are assessed.
- Step Two: The clinician instructs the patient to side flex the neck up to the first point of pain, "Touch your ear to your shoulder."
- Step Three: The clinician instructs the patient to move beyond the first point of pain to his or her end range.
- Step Four: The clinician instructs the patient to gently repeat the end range movement in order to assess change of condition.
- Step Five: (If no pain) The clinician gently applies overpressure into physiological side flexion (pictured). Typically, this is performed using the ulnar aspect of the hand for a "fulcrum" to the neck. The clinician should place his or her palm on the zygomatic arch of the patient while bifurcating the ear between the second and third fingers for maximum patient comfort. The patient's signs and symptoms should be reassessed.
- Step Six: Repeat on the opposite side.

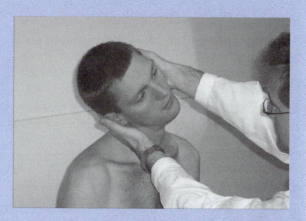

**Figure 6.21**    Side Flexion with Overpressure

## Physiological Rotation

Physiological rotation is guided primarily by zygopophyseal joint translation.[25] The following guidelines outline the examination process for side flexion.

- Step One: The clinician positions the patient's head in a designated neutral position. Resting symptoms are assessed.
- Step Two: The clinician instructs the patient to rotate the neck up to the first point of pain, "Turn to your right (or left) while keeping your eyes level."
- Step Three: The clinician instructs the patient to move beyond the first point of pain to his or her end range.
- Step Four: The clinician instructs the patient to gently repeat the end range movement in order to assess change of condition.
- Step Five: (If no pain) The clinician gently applies overpressure into physiological rotation (pictured). If right rotation, the right shoulder is stabilized with the clinician's left forearm (opposite for left rotation). The clinician places his or her palms on both zygomatic arches, while bifurcating the ears (as in side flexion). The forearm is used as a counterforce to prevent the body from turning. The patient's signs and symptoms are then assessed.
- Step Six: Repeat on the opposite side.

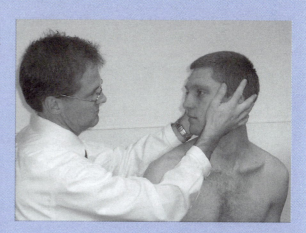

**Figure 6.22**    Rotations with Overpressure

### Combined Movements

Any method that combines the previously described techniques is considered a combined method. Selected combined movements may be beneficial to isolate the origin of the pain.[26]

## Active Cervical Flexion and Rotation

One well-documented movement is active cervical flexion combined with rotation. During flexion of the cervical spine, the segments below C2 are blocked.[26] Active physiological rotation in a position of physiological flexion analyzes movement at the AA joint whereas movement in extension focuses on the lower, middle, and upper cervical spine.[26] This method has shown validity in isolated cervicogenic headache pain generators, specifically those at C1-2.[122]

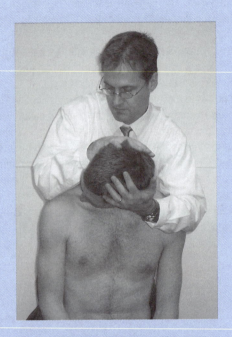

- Step One: The clinician positions the patient's head in a designated neutral position. Resting symptoms are assessed.
- Step Two: The clinician instructs the patient to forward flex the neck as far as possible forward (do not limit movement secondary to pain).
- Step Three: The clinician instructs the patient to rotate as far as possible to the right (or left). This movement assesses range-of-motion limitations as well as pain.
- Step Four: (If no pain) The clinician applies a gentle overpressure into physiological rotation. From behind the patient, the clinician places his or her palms on both zygomatic arches, while bifurcating the ears. Upon completion, the patient's condition is then reassessed.
- Step Five: Repeat on the opposite side.

**Figure 6.23**    Cervical Flexion and Rotation

Another well-described combined movement designed to narrow the anatomical space in the intervertebral foramen is the lower quadrant maneuver described by Maitland.[78] This test is similar to the Spurling's test and is consistently used during detection of cervical radiculopathy.[123] Maitland[78] reports that the quadrant test is effective in ruling out pain of cervical origin. A positive test could reflect nerve root compression of spondylogenic-based dysfunction on the side tested.

- Step One: The patient assumes a sitting position. The head is positioned in designated neutral position.
- Step Two: The clinician stands to the side of the patient on the tested side. The clinician then places their finger on the patient's scapular spinous process while the clinician stabilizes the patient's thorax with their forearm.
- Step Three: The clinician instructs the patient to look back to their finger (do not limit movement secondary to pain). The movement should consist of side flexion and rotation to the same side with extension. The patient should be instructed to stop at the first point of pain.
- Step Four: (If no pain) The clinician applies a gentle overpressure into the combined range of side flexion, rotation, and extension. The clinician then places the palm of their hand on the zygomatic arch and applies a very brief and quick force. Reassess pain.
- Step Five: Repeat on the opposite side.

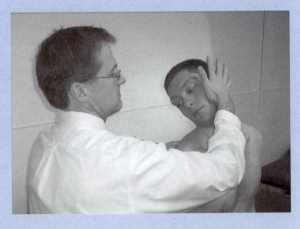

**Figure 6.24**    Lower Cervical Quadrant

## *Summary*

- Active physiological assessment of the cervical spine purportedly examines the contractile elements of the cervical spine, but also assesses the patient's tolerance to position.
- The use of overpressure may be useful in isolating various impairments and is designed to "rule out" joints that do not contribute to the patient's impairment.
- Selected combined movements may be beneficial to isolate the origin of the pain by increasing the tension or compression placed on articular and surrounding structures.
- Range-of-motion abnormalities that reproduce the patient's current complaint of pain are helpful in identifying the impaired movement as compared to strictly painful movements alone.

## Passive Movements

### *Passive Physiological Movements*

The movement planes applied during passive physiological examination are similar to those tested during active physiological movements, and are used to further confirm the concordant sign of the patient. In some cases, these movements are used only to determine abnormal mobility. Fjellner et al.[124] reported that passive physiological movements demonstrated acceptable interclinician reliability in six of the eight plane-based testing movements. Caution should be used when detecting abnormal movement in isolation from the concordant sign.

Passive physiological movements are commonly used to dictate the appropriate level for manipulation or mobilization of the cervical spine. In a recent study performed by Haas et al.,[125] manipulation based on clinical physiological end feel assessment was compared against a randomized selection of a targeted level. These findings were based on one day's worth of treatment and displayed no differences in pain or stiffness outcomes. This finding is analogous to the thoracic and lumbar spine that there is little information to support the need to identify a specific level for manipulative intervention.[126,127] Nonetheless, passive physiological movements have long been considered important for manual therapy assessment, thus it is intuitive to consider isolating the appropriate segment as crucial for appropriate care.

### Passive Physiological Flexion

The first passive physiological assessment method during examination is flexion. This procedure is not discriminatory in detecting concordant pain, but is helpful in detecting asymmetries in cervical flexion. The procedure is as follows:

- Step One: The patient assumes a supine position. The head should extend beyond the end of the plinth up to the T2 spinous process.
- Step Two: The head is stabilized using digits one and two to support the posterior articular pillars and the thumb anteriorly.
- Step Three: The clinician applies a gentle cephalic to caudal movement allowing passive flexion to occur in the spine, stopping at the first point of pain.
- Step Four: The clinician should feel for symmetry of motion and assess reproduction of pain while moving beyond the first point of pain and progressing to end range.
- Step Five: Repeated movements into flexion are then performed to assess the response of the patient.
- Step Six: If no pain is present the clinician may increase the sensitivity of the test by applying force through the top of the skull (using the abdomen to increase compression).

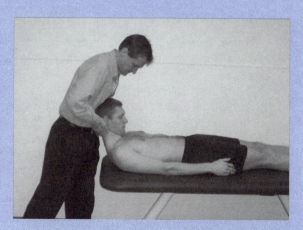

Figure 6.25    Passive Physiological Flexion

## Passive Physiological Extension

The second passive physiological assessment method during examination is extension. Because of the angle of the facets, this procedure provides fair discriminatory capabilities in detecting concordant pain, and is very helpful in detecting asymmetries in cervical extension. The procedure is as follows:

- Step One: The patient assumes a supine position. The head should extend beyond the end of the plinth up to the T2 spinous process.
- Step Two: The head is stabilized using digits one and two to support the posterior articular pillars and the thumb anteriorly.
- Step Three: The clinician applies a gentle cephalic to caudal movement allowing passive extension to occur in the spine. The head is extended to the T2 process but is stopped at the first reported presence of pain.
- Step Four: The clinician moves the patient's cervical spine into further extension beyond the first point of pain, while feeling for symmetry of motion and assessing reproduction of concordant pain.
- Step Five: The clinician applies repeated, extension-based movements near end range and reassesses the patient's response.
- Step Six: If no pain is present the clinician may increase the sensitivity of the test by applying force through the top of the skull (using the abdomen to increase compression).

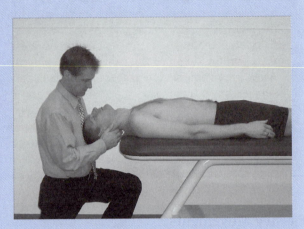

**Figure 6.26**    Passive Physiological Extension

## Chin Cradle Grip

The **chin-cradle grip** is an effective handling mechanism for assessment and treatment of the cervical spine.[78] The chin cradle grip permits one arm to perform the physiological movement activities while the other is free to apply force, palpate a segment, or stabilize a particular region.

- Step One: The patient assumes a supine position. The head should extend beyond the end of the plinth up to the T2 spinous process.
- Step Two: Using digits 4 and 5, the clinician "hooks" the chin of the patient and curls the forearm around and posterior to the ear in order to provide a stable "base" upon which the head can sit.
- Step Three: For rotations to the right, the right arm supplies the stabilization. For rotations to the left, the left arm supplies stabilization.
- Step Four: The clinician then places his or her shoulder gently on the patient's forehead and applies a gentle force to "lock" the head in the arm cradle.
- Step Five: For practice, the clinician may rotate the head "on a spit" using only the cradle arm and with posterior countersupport by the other hand.
- Step Six: Repeat on the opposite side to ensure bilateral mastery.

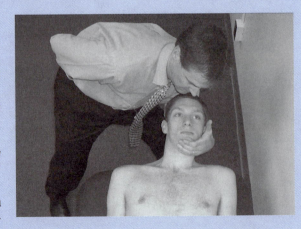

**Figure 6.27**    The Chin Cradle Grip

## Passive Physiological Side Flexion

The third passive physiological assessment method during examination is side flexion. This procedure assesses the collective mobility of all structures and may be helpful in assessing the uncovertebral joint. The procedure is as follows:

- Step One: The patient assumes a supine position. The head should extend beyond the end of the plinth up to the T2 spinous process.
- Step Two: The clinician uses the chin cradle grip to support the patient's cervical spine.
- Step Three: The clinician places his or her radial border of the first metatarsal joint against the posterior articular pillars of the desired cervical level and applies a fulcrum-like force with the metatarsal joint.
- Step Four: The clinician gently provides physiological side flexion toward the fulcrum force. The movement should "break" at the level of the ulnar border and should stop at the first reported pain response of the patient.
- Step Five: The patient is then moved beyond the first reported pain toward end range and the patient's response is again reassessed.
- Step Six: The clinician performs repeated movements at end range and reassesses the patient's response.
- Step Seven: To target different levels, the clinician may move the ulnar border up and down the posterior articular pillars to identify the "guilty" level.
- Step Eight: Repeat on the opposite side.

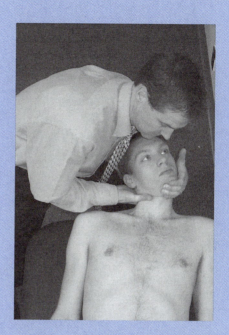

**Figure 6.28**    Side Flexion using Chin Cradle

## Passive Physiological Rotations

The fourth passive physiological assessment method during examination is rotation. This procedure assesses the collective mobility of all structures and may be helpful in assessing the zygopophyseal joints. The procedure is as follows:

- Step One: The patient assumes a supine position. The head should extend beyond the end of the plinth up to the T2 spinous process.
- Step Two: The clinician uses the chin cradle grip to support the patient's cervical spine.
- Step Three: The clinician then "grabs" the posterior tissue of the neck, "the scruff of the neck," to emphasize the rotation at that particular level, moving into rotation to the first point of the patient's pain. Assess concordant response.
- Step Four: The patient is then moved beyond the first reported pain toward end range and the patient's response is reassessed.
- Step Five: Repeated movements are performed at end range by the clinician while the patient's response is further assessed.

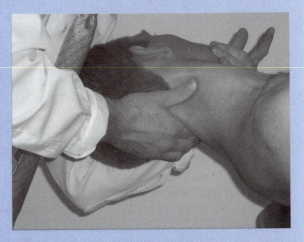

**Figure 6.29**    Posterior Hand Position for Rotation

- Step Six: The clinician may move the posterior grip up and down the cervical spine to isolate different cervical segments to identify the "guilty" level.
- Step Seven: Repeat on the opposite side.

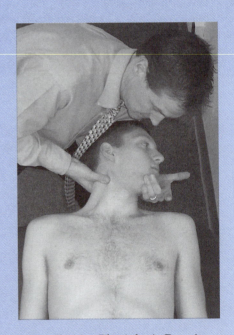

**Figure 6.30**    Passive Physiologic Rotation

### Combined Physiological Movements

Combined passive physiological movements are useful in detection of articular or capsular structures. Since there are several potential movements, it is helpful to divide the groups into supine and sitting assessment methods. The following three procedures are supine techniques.

## Premanipulative Position

Earlier, the premanipulative position was discussed as an assessment for VBI problems. This method is also a combined movement that increases the closing of vertebrae on the side that side flexion is initiated. Additionally, since many manipulations are based on apposition of the joints, this position is of importance. Apposition is a close packed, combined movement and is, in essence, the biomechanical opposite of a coupled movement. Apposition movements are frequently used during manipulative procedures and are termed in osteopathic literature as a "locked" position.[128] The procedure is as follows:

- Step One: The patient assumes a supine position. The patient's symptoms require a preassessment prior to the examination.
- Step Two: The patient's neck is side glided toward an end point.
- Step Three: Using the lateral aspect of the first metacarpalphalangeal joint, the clinician provides a fulcrum force to the neck. The contact point should consist of the articular pillars or the transverse processes.
- Step Four: The patient's neck is side flexed to the level of the contact point. Since combined movements are often used when single plane movements are less sensitive, pain should not be as critical a consideration.
- Step Five: The patient neck is rotated in the opposite direction as the side flexion, but not beyond.
- Step Six: The clinician should feel the neck "lock." The patient's condition should be reassessed, specifically for signs of VBI. Pain is respected and the same pattern of move to pain, move beyond pain, then repeating the movements should be implemented.

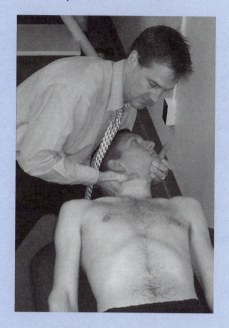

**Figure 6.31**    Premanipulative Position

## Extension and Rotation

The combined movement of extension and rotation can target different aspects of the articular regions beyond the assessment of a neutral position. The following describes the passive physiological combined movements of extension and rotation.

- Step One: The patient assumes a supine position. The head should extend beyond the table to approximately T2. The patient's symptoms require a preassessment prior to the examination.
- Step Two: Using the chin cradle grip, the clinician extends the cervical spine, carefully controlling the amount of upper cervical extension.
- Step Three: Upon completion of passive extension, the clinician then provides a rotational force toward the direction of the cradle arm (right hold, rotation right).
- Step Four: The clinician should feel the neck's range tighten up. The patient's condition should be reassessed for concordant pain but also for the possibility of VBI-related symptoms. Pain is respected and the same pattern of movement to pain, movement beyond pain, and repeated movement should be implemented.

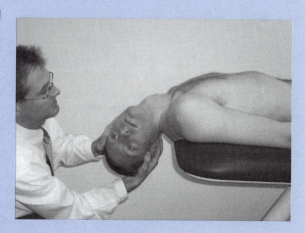

**Figure 6.32**    Combined Extension with Rotation

## Combined Flexion and Rotation

Following the combined movement of extension and rotation is the combined movement of flexion and rotation. This procedure primarily solicits movement from the upper cervical spine and may be useful in detecting cervicogenic headache complaints. The procedure is as follows:

- Step One: The patient assumes a supine position. The patient's symptoms require a preassessment prior to the examination.
- Step Two: Placing both hands behind the occiput, the clinician flexes the cervical spine, carefully controlling the amount of upper cervical extension.
- Step Three: Upon completion of passive flexion, the clinician then provides a rotational force until palpable end range.
- Step Four: The clinician should feel the neck's range tighten up. The patient's condition should be reassessed for concordant pain but also for the possibility of VBI-related symptoms. Pain is respected and the same pattern of movement to pain, movement beyond pain, and repeated movement should be implemented.

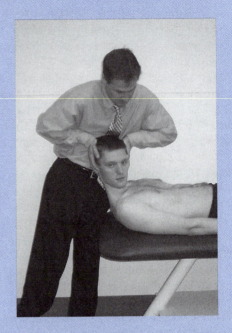

**Figure 6.33**    Combined Flexion with Rotations

## Cervical Distraction

Cervical distraction qualifies as a combined technique because it provides a general distraction to all segments. Cervical distraction is an assessment method that is very similar to the special test. As a treatment, distraction may be beneficial as a general relief maneuver. Typically, the movement is beneficial for pain relief.

- Step One: The patient assumes a supine position. The patient's symptoms require a preassessment prior to the examination.
- Step Two: The clinician drapes a towel posterior around the head of the patient, specifically targeting the occipital shelf of the neck.
- Step Three: The patient's head is secured by wrapping the towel around the ears and tension is placed longitudinally.
- Step Four: A traction force is applied and the patient's symptoms are reassessed. Pain is respected and the same pattern of movement to pain, movement beyond pain, and repeated movement should be implemented.

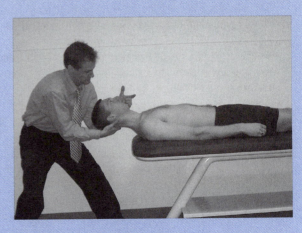

**Figure 6.34**    Cervical Distraction

# Upper Quadrant Examination

Combined movements are also performed in a sitting position. Maitland proposed that the upper cervical spine lock is useful in detecting difficult upper cervical lesions.[78] This method may be beneficial in ruling out upper cervical spine disorders. Since coupling of the upper cervical spine changes during motion initiation, it is prudent to adjust the procedure to the initiated motion. For example, Figure 6.35 outlines the upper c-spine quadrant during side-flexion initiation while Figure 6.36 displays the same procedure during rotation initiation. The coupling movements are in opposition because the initiation of the motion alters the locking position of the upper cervical spine. Because the movement is very provocative, it should only be used when the concordant sign is not found during normal assessment maneuvers. If pain occurs with any of the preceding examinations, the upper cervical quadrant is unnecessary. The following procedure outlines the upper quadrant during side flexion initiation.

- Step One: The head is positioned in designated neutral position.
- Step Two: The clinician stands to the side that he or she desires to assess.
- Step Three: The chin is protracted and a downward force is applied to the head.
- Step Four: The clinician then passively side glides the head away until a feeling of a tightening of the "slack" is interpreted.
- Step Five: The clinician then passively side-flexes the upper cervical spine (the spine should only move 5–10 degrees).
- Step Six: Passive rotation of the upper cervical spine by the clinician then follows (or to the same side as side flexion), with a concurrent gentle overpressure.
- Step Seven: Repeat on the opposite side.

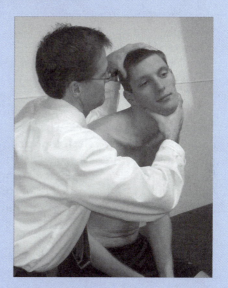

**Figure 6.35**  Upper Quadrant-Side Flexion Initiation-Upper C-spine Lock

Because the upper cervical spine changes its coupling pattern with a different initiation of movement, it is essential to discuss the upper cervical quadrant during rotation initiation. Like the other upper cervical spine quadrant test, it should only be used when the concordant sign is not found during normal assessment maneuvers.

- Step One: The head is positioned in designated neutral position.
- Step Two: The clinician stands to the side that they desire to assess.
- Step Three: The clinician protracts the chin and applies a downward force on the head.
- Step Four: The clinician passively side glides the head away until he or she feels a tightening of the "slack."
- Step Five: The clinician then passively rotates the upper cervical spine away (limit the movement to 5–10 degrees to ensure no recruitment from the lower cervical spine).
- Step Six: Passive side flexion of the neck toward the clinician then follows (the movement should be limited to 5–10 degrees) with a light application of an overpressure.
- Step Seven: Repeat on the opposite side.

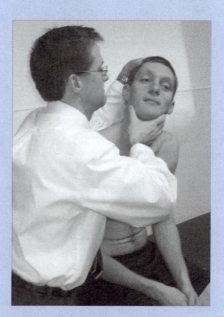

**Figure 6.36**  Upper Quadrant-Rotation Initiation-Upper C-Spine Lock

## Summary

- Passive physiological movement further localized cervical movements that contribute to concordant patient complaints.
- Passive physiological movements have demonstrated acceptable interclinician reliability.
- Passive physiological movements may be single plane or combined to engage the articular or surrounding structures.

### Passive Accessory Movements

Jull et al.[129] demonstrated 100% accuracy in isolating the appropriate level of pathology using passive accessory movements. They found that when used as a method to isolate the concordant sign the posterior anterior passive accessory movement is very useful. The authors used a combined assessment of stiffness detection and reproduction of the patient's concordant sign. The use of pain provocation during the examination is a concept supported by many authors.[129–131] A number of studies have shown the **intertester reliability** of examination methods that fail to concurrently elicit the joint movement and pain reproduction is abysmal.[124,130]

There may be several reasons for the poor reliability in these studies.[132] First, the majority of studies tested students versus experienced clinicians. Second, a preponderance of studies tested asymptomatic subjects. Third, the majority of the tests included stiffness detection in the absence of pain provocation. There is substantial evidence to support that this method of examination is unreliable secondary to the very small movements associated with passive neck glides.[132]

Nonetheless, some argue that a detection of stiffness is imperative to guide the clinician to appropriate treatment decision making. Jull et al.[129] write, "selection of a treatment technique . . . will differ if the tissue stiffness limiting movement is muscle spasm rather than capsular tightness." Subsequently, this textbook recognizes the importance of a stiffness assessment but also recognizes the weaknesses associated with stiffness assessment in absence of pain provocation. As discussed in Chapter Three, the passive accessory examination should be focused on the concordant movement or segment, allowing the clinician to further their analysis of the patient's response to movements and alterations in pain and stiffness.

### Central Posterior Anterior (CPA)

A central posterior anterior is often called a CPA. CPAs are used to detect concordant pain during a posterior-to-anterior glide. Maitland suggests that the CPA is beneficial for patients who demonstrate bilateral or midline pain.[78] The tests are commonly used in examination and are often used as treatment methods as well.[78]

- Step One: The patient may lie in prone or sidelying. The neck is positioned in neutral and resting symptoms are assessed.
- Step Two: The clinician palpates the C2 spinous process using the tips of the thumb. Using a thumb-to-thumb application, the clinician applies a gentle downward force up to the first point of the patient's complaint of pain and the pain response is assessed.
- Step Three: The clinician then pushes beyond the first point of pain, toward end range, and reassesses pain and quality of movement. Additionally, one should assess splinting or muscle spasm. Assess if pain is concordant.
- Step Four: The clinician repeats the movements toward end range while assessing pain. One should use caution if patient reports significant pain that is unrelenting.
- Step Five: The process is repeated on each spinous process to T4 to identify the concordant segment.

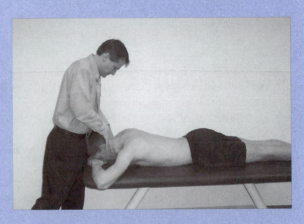

**Figure 6.37** CPA of the Cervical Spine

## Unilateral Posterior Anterior (UPA)

A unilateral posterior anterior is frequently called a UPA. The unilateral posterior anterior provides a combined extension-based movement with rotation to the same side the examination is applied. Maitland suggests that UPAs are useful in patients who demonstrate unilateral pain. UPAs are also commonly used as examination and treatment techniques and are useful in identifying the concordant sign of the patient.[129]

- Step One: The patient is positioned in prone or sidelying, and the neck is placed in neutral.
- Step Two: The clinician then pulls the paraspinals that lie just to the side of the spinous process medially. This will assist in exposing the articular pillars.
- Step Three: To isolate the articular pillar, the clinician finds the spinous process of C2, slides approximately a thumb width lateral, and moves his or her thumb in a caudal and cephalic direction. The raised area felt under the thumb is the articular pillar, the targeted region for the mobilization.
- Step Four: Using a thumb-to-thumb application, the clinician applies a gentle downward force up to the first point of the patient's complaint of pain. The pain is assessed for the concordant sign.
- Step Five: The clinician then pushes beyond the first point of pain toward end range, reassesses pain and quality of movement, and checks for splinting or muscle spasm. The pain is assessed for the concordant sign.
- Step Six: The clinician repeats the movements at end range while assessing pain, using caution if patient reports significant pain that is unrelenting.
- Step Seven: The clinician then repeats the process on each articular pillar to T4 attempting to identify the concordant segment.
- Step Eight: Repeat on the opposite side.

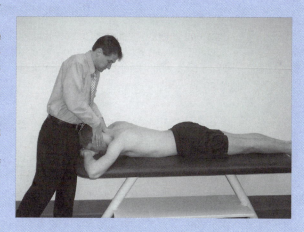

**Figure 6.38** UPA of the Cervical Spine

## Transverse Glides

Transverse glides are common methods that apply a lateral glide to the spinous processes of the spine. The technique is also commonly used in examination and treatment and has been well studied for its neurophysiologic effects.[134,135]

- Step One: The patient is positioned in prone or sidelying, and the neck is placed in neutral.
- Step Two: The clinician palpates the C2 spinous process using the tips of the thumb. Using one thumb pad, the clinician applies a very broad and deep contact to the side of the spinous process, applying more force on the base of the spinous than the posterior tip.
- Step Three: The clinician then aligns the forearm so that it is parallel to the force to the spinous process and pushes to the first point of reported pain. Concordant pain is assessed.
- Step Four: The clinician then pushes beyond the first point of pain toward end range, reassesses pain and quality of movement, and checks for splinting or muscle spasm. Concordant pain is assessed.
- Step Five: Passive repeated movements are performed at end range. Changes in pain level or determination if the pain is concordant are performed.
- Step Six: The process is repeated on each spinous process to T4 to identify the concordant segment.
- Step Seven: Repeat the process on the opposite side.

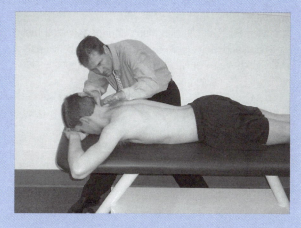

**Figure 6.39** Transverse Glide of the Cervical Spine

## Unilateral Anterior–Posterior (UAP)

Unilateral anterior–posteriors are often identified as a UAP. UAPs are also well studied[136] and are considered to have a very strong neurophysiologic effect on the spine and upper extremities. UAPs are often considered when referred pain to the upper extremity is reported during the history and subjective examination.

- Step One: The patient is positioned in prone or sidelying, and the neck is placed in neutral.
- Step Two: The patient is informed of the specifics of the technique. The patient should be informed that the hands of the clinician would be around the front of the throat.
- Step Three: Using a thumb, the clinician hooks the anterior cervical musculature (SCM specifically) and pulls the tissue medially. This will expose the anterior aspect of the transverse process.
- Step Four: The clinician then applies a broad and thick thumb contact (dummy thumb) to the anterior transverse processes while using the other thumb to apply a force downward on the "dummy" thumb. The clinician pushes to the first point of reported pain by the patient.

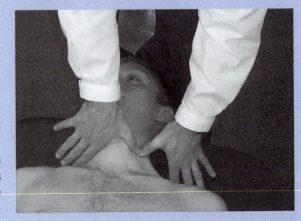

**Figure 6.40** Hand Placement for UAP

- Step Five: The clinician then pushes beyond the first point of pain, reassesses symptoms, and assesses if the pain is concordant.
- Step Six: The clinician then performs repeated movements toward end range while reassessing the patient's pain.
- Step Seven: Repeat the process on the opposite side.

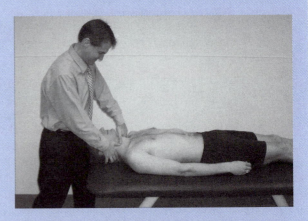

**Figure 6.41** UAP of the Cervical Spine

## CPA in Physiological Extension

Like passive physiological movements, passive accessory movements can be combined to increase the vigor of the movements. The combined movements may consist of active and passive physiological movements, or other passive accessory movements. The first movement, the CPA in physiological extension, may enhance the sensitivity of the technique.

- Step One: The patient is positioned in prone and the neck is placed in extension.
- Step Two: The clinician palpates the C2 spinous process using the tips of his or her thumb. Using a thumb-to-thumb application, the clinician applies a gentle downward force up to the first point of patient complaint of pain, assessing if the pain is concordant.
- Step Three: The clinician then pushes beyond the first point of pain toward end range, reassesses pain and quality of movement, and checks for splinting or muscle spasm.
- Step Four: The clinician performs repeated movements toward end range and reassesses pain.
- Step Five: The process is repeated on each spinous process to T4. Identify the concordant segment.

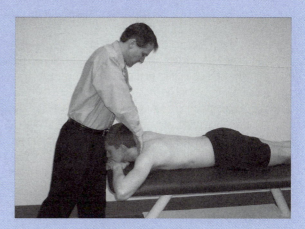

**Figure 6.42**    CPA in Extension

## UPA During Physiological Rotation

The UPA during physiological rotation enhances the movement that the UPA produces in isolation. Specifically, the procedure may increase the tension placed on the posterior capsule of the facet, an area thickened and altered during degenerative processes. Rotation increases the tension placed on this capsule.[12]

- Step One: The patient is positioned in prone and the neck is placed in rotation opposite of the direction of the targeted segment for the UPA.
- Step Two: The clinician pulls the paraspinals that lie just to the side of the spinous process medially, which exposes the articular pillars.
- Step Three: The clinician then finds the spinous process of C2, slides approximately a thumb width lateral, then moves their thumb in a caudal and cephalic direction to "feel" the articular pillar. The raised area felt under the thumb is the articular pillar.
- Step Four: Using a thumb-to-thumb application, the clinician applies a gentle downward force up to the first point of patient complaint of pain, assessing if the pain is concordant.
- Step Five: The clinician then pushes beyond the first point of pain toward end range, reassessing pain, quality of movement, and checking for splinting or muscle spasm.
- Step Six: The clinician the repeats the movements toward end range, reassessing pain and determining if the pain is concordant.
- Step Seven: This process is repeated on each articular pillar to T4. Identify the concordant segment.
- Step Eight: Repeat on the opposite side.

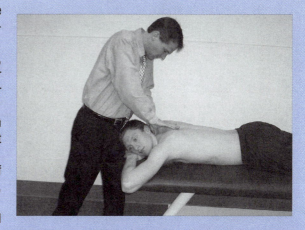

**Figure 6.43**    UPA in Physiological Rotation

## UPA During Physiological Side Flexion

The UPA during physiological side flexion may increase the tension placed on the anterior and posterior capsule of the facet and theoretically may be beneficial in individuals that have demonstrated degeneration associated with the uncovertebral joint.

- Step One: The patient is positioned in supine and the neck is positioned in side flexion toward the directed joint of interest.
- Step Two: The clinician pulls the paraspinals that lie just to the side of the spinous process medially, thus exposing the articular pillars.
- Step Three: The clinician palpates the spinous process of C2 and slides approximately a thumb width lateral; then moves their thumb in a caudal and cephalic direction. The raised area felt under the thumb is the articular pillar.
- Step Four: Using a thumb-to-thumb application, the clinician applies a gentle downward force up to the first point of patient complaint of pain, assessing if the pain is concordant.
- Step Five: The clinician then pushes beyond the first point of pain toward end range, reassessing the pain, quality of movement, and checking for splinting or muscle spasm.
- Step Six: The process is repeated toward end range, further assessing the pain.
- Step Seven: The clinician repeats the process on each articular pillar to T4 to identify the concordant segment.
- Step Eight: Repeat on the opposite side.

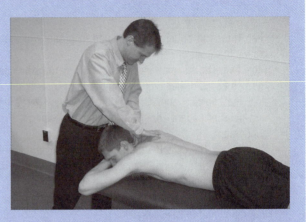

**Figure 6.44**   UPA in Physiological Side Flexion

## Combined UPA, UAP with Rotations

Perhaps the most difficult combined method to perform involves the combined movements of physiological rotation, a UAP, and a UPA. This procedure enhances the vigor of physiological rotation and concentrates the force of the examination on both sides of the joint segment.

- Step One: The patient is positioned in supine and the neck is placed in neutral.
- Step Two: The clinician holds the patient's head in a chin cradle grip.
- Step Three: Using the tips of digits 2 and 3, the clinician hooks the anterior aspect of the transverse processes on the same side of the neck in which rotation is initiated.
- Step Four: Using the thumb of the same hand, the clinician applies a direct force on the articular pillar of the same level as the anterior aspect of the transverse process hooked in Step Two.
- Step Five: In a combined sequence, the clinician provides a physiological rotation concurrently with the UAP and UPA motion. The process is performed up to the first point of pain, while assessing and targeting the pain that is concordant.
- Step Six: The clinician then takes the combined movement beyond the first reported point of pain and reassesses the patient, specifically the concordant sign.
- Step Seven: Furthermore, the clinician takes the combined movements to the end range, repeating the rotations while reassessing the patient.
- Step Eight: The clinician repeats this process at a different level, completely analyzing the cervical spine.
- Step Nine: Repeat on the opposite side.

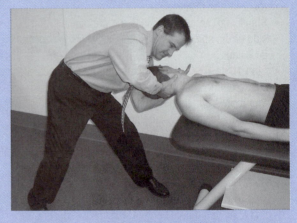

**Figure 6.45**   UPA and UAP during Physiological Rotation

## *Summary*

- Passive accessory movements, when combined with elicitation of the concordant sign of the patient, are reliable and useful assessment tools.
- Passive accessory movements used to isolate causal cervicogenic headache levels are useful and predictable among clinician assessors.
- Passive accessory movement in absence of elicitation of the concordant sign demonstrates little usefulness.

## Clinical Special Tests

There are two purposes of a clinical special test. First, a series of clinical special tests are often used to provide the examiner with additional information regarding the nature of the condition. The second purpose is to provide diagnostic value to a set of findings. Typically, palpation and muscle strength assessment provides additional data whereas clinical tests provide diagnostic information.

### *Palpation*

Several authors have purported the benefit of palpation during examination. Maigne suggests palpation is useful in identifying trigger points associated with cervical segments.[137] Others have reported that palpation is useful in detecting tenderness at C0 through C3 in patients with concurrent craniomandicular pain and cervical spine dysfunction.[138] Humphreys et al.[139] reported strong agreement among fourth-year chiropractic students during motion palpation in a sample of patients with a congenitally restricted cervical vertebra. Nonetheless, although palpation may demonstrate superficial tenderness in some structures, it does not implicate those structures as the concordant pain generator. Palpation should be used to confirm examination findings, yet when used in isolation is often deceiving and misleading.

### *Muscle Testing*

Typically, muscle strength tests are used to determine if weakness is present secondary to cervical radiculopathy. Chapter Five outlines the diagnostic benefit of muscle testing. Muscle testing for the cervical spine myotomes has yielded conflicting results. Wainner et al.[140] reported that muscle testing of the biceps (+LR 3.7), triceps, and deltoid yielded beneficial diagnostic values for patients with confirmed cervical radiculopathy. Davidson et al.[141] found high sensitivity (91% of the sample), as did Yoss et al.[142] (75%). Lauder[143] reported excellent diagnostic value of muscle strength testing (+LR 4.56) on patients positively diagnosed with cervical or upper extremity pain confirmed during electrodiagnosis. Conversely, others[144,145] reported low sensitivity.

Force measuring devices used to analyze cervical strength have been advocated as an alternative measure of strength and function of the cervical spine.[146] Authors have reported that patients with neck pain generally demonstrate weaker cervical muscles than normal controls, suggesting causation.[147] Strengthening of the cervical muscles has been linked to improvements in both pain and disability.[148]

### *Sensory Testing*

Chapter Five outlines the diagnostic benefit of sensory testing. Several authors have reported high levels of sensitivity[149–151] verified during surgical identification of a herniated disc and/or spondylopathy. Others have reported low sensitivity levels[152–155] using both surgically documented analysis and needle EMG diagnosis of cervical radiculopathy. In what appears to be the most comprehensive sensory assessment, Wainner et al[140] reported poor diagnostic values for all cervical levels expect C5. In fact, dermatome testing of the levels C6 through T1 demonstrated positive likelihood values below one suggesting no value to the assessment process. Furthermore, other studies have reported that various forms of sensation testing lack the ability to detect the level of the lesion. Nygaard and Mellgren[156] suggested that thermo and vibratory tests are not suitable for predicting the level of lesion, because there is no significant difference between an ipsilateral nerve root sensation change and the compressed nerve root. Others have reported increased heat, cold, and mechanical thresholds with sciatica as compared with nonsymptomatic extremities.[157–160] The dermatome levels are outlined in Chapter 5.

### *Reflex Testing*

Historically, findings of reflex alterations in patients diagnosed with a cervical herniated disc and/or cervical spondylopathy are inconclusive. Although many older studies demonstrated moderate sensitivity,[150,151,153] recent studies have found much lower values.[150,154,155] These findings appear to be independent in the method used to diagnose the cervical disorder. In a recent study that examined cervical radiculopathy, only the biceps reflex test demonstrated good diagnostic value.[140] Chapter Five outlines the clinical utility of reflex testing.

### *Clinical Special Tests*

Clinical special tests are designed to provide diagnostic value to a set of findings. This is accomplished by providing discriminatory power for ruling in and ruling out a disorder. There are several clinical special tests for the cervical spine, few of which have been exhaustively studied for diagnostic value. The following tests have been examined for diagnostic value.

## Spurling's Test

Spurling's test was first reported by Spurling and Scoville in 1944.[151] The test is designed to identify unilateral cervical radiculopathy through compression of the intervertebral foramen. Table 6.4 outlines the diagnostic value of the Spurling's test.

- Step One: The patient assumes a neutral cervical posture while sitting. Assess resting symptoms.
- Step Two: The patient is instructed to side flex their head to the side of their referred symptoms. Assess symptoms. If radicular pain is present, the test is positive.
- Step Three: (If no symptoms up to this point) The clinician then applies a combined compression and side flexion force in the direction of side flexion. Assess symptoms. If radicular pain is present, the test is positive.

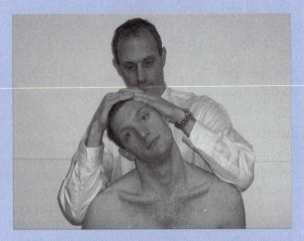

**Figure 6.46**   Spurling's Test

**TABLE 6.4**   Cervical Spine Clinical Special Tests: Diagnostic Values

| Study | Sensitivity | Specificity | +LR | −LR | Criterion Standard |
|---|---|---|---|---|---|
| **Spurling's Test** | | | | | |
| Spurling & Scoville[151] | NA | 100 | NA | NA | Disc herniation |
| Viikari-Juntura et al.[160] | 30.5 | 100 | NA | NA | Spondyl and disc herniation |
| Wainner et al.[140] | 50 | 86 | 3.5 | 0.58 | Cervical radiculopathy |
| **Upper Limb Tension Test (Median Nerve)** | | | | | |
| Wainner et al.[140] | 97 | 22 | 1.24 | .13 | Cervical radiculopathy |
| **Cervical Distraction Test** | | | | | |
| Viikari-Juntura et al.[160] | 21.5 | 100 | NA | NA | Spondyl and disc herniation |
| Wainner et al.[140] | 44 | 90 | 4.4 | 0.62 | Cervical radiculopathy |
| **Shoulder Abduction Test** | | | | | |
| Davidson et al.[141] | 68 | NA | NA | NA | Extradural defect |
| Viikari-Juntura et al.[160] | 36.5 | 100 | NA | NA | Spondyl and disc herniation |
| Wainner et al.[140] | 17 | 92 | 2.1 | 0.90 | Cervical radiculopathy |
| **Flexion-Rotation Test** | | | | | |
| Hall & Robinson[122] | 86 | 100 | NA | NA | Cervicogenic headache |

## The Upper Limb Tension Test (ULTT)

The upper limb tension test, commonly called the median nerve tension test, purportedly places selected tension on cervical nerve roots. Recently Kleinrensink et al.[161] identified of all the different movements of limb tension testing, the greatest amount of tension on the median nerve roots. Subsequently, it is proposed that the median nerve test should qualify for placing tension on all cervical nerve root branches. Butler[162] suggests the incidence of (1) reproduction of the concordant symptoms, (2) sensitizing of the pain with the movements of distal extremities, and (3) asymmetric symptoms are indications of a positive test. Table 6.4 outlines the diagnostic value of the ULTT for cervical radiculopathy.

- Step One: The patient assumes a supine position. The clinician assesses resting symptoms.
- Step Two: The clinician blocks the shoulder girdle to stabilize the scapulae. Symptoms are again assessed.
- Step Three: If no reproduction of symptoms has occurred, the glenohumeral joint is abducted to 110 degrees with slight coronal plane extension. Symptoms are again assessed.
- Step Four: If no reproduction of symptoms has occurred, the forearm is supinated completely and the wrist and fingers are extended. Ulnar deviation is implemented. Symptoms are again assessed.
- Step Five: If no reproduction of symptoms has occurred, elbow extension is applied. Symptoms are again assessed. One may measure the degree of elbow extension if range of motion is an objective.

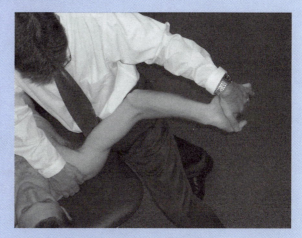

Figure 6.47   ULTT

## Cervical Distraction Test

The cervical distraction test is designed to measure the change in resting symptoms once distraction of the intervertebral foramen is implemented. The test may be beneficial in reducing the compression of a cervical nerve root, thus suggesting the incidence of nerve root compression. The test is classified as positive if the nerve root pain is relieved during the distraction maneuver.[163] Table 6.4 outlines the diagnostic value of the cervical distraction test for evidence of cervical radiculopathy.

- Step One: The patient assumes a sitting position. The clinician assesses resting symptoms. The test can be performed in supine as well.
- Step Two: The clinician provides a distraction force by cupping the chin and the occiput. Force is gradually applied and symptoms are assessed. If a reduction of symptoms has occurred, the test is considered negative. An alternative method of placing force on both mastoid processes is used when the patient exhibits TMJ symptoms or has dentures.

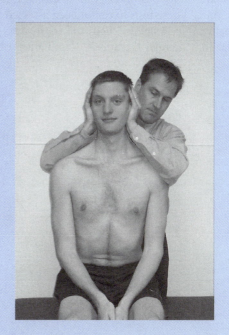

Figure 6.48   Cervical Distraction Test in Sitting

## Shoulder Abduction Test (Bakody's Sign)

The shoulder abduction test is designed to examine the presence of cervical radiculopathy on the lower cervical nerve roots. If the patient reports a relief of symptoms when the arm is placed on top of the head (while in sitting or supine) the test is considered positive. When the arm is placed on top of the head, the tension place on the nerve trunk is theoretically reduced.[141] Table 6.4 outlines the diagnostic value of the shoulder abduction test for evidence of cervical radiculopathy.

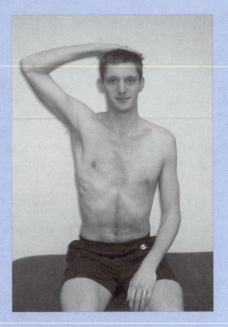

- Step One: The patient assumes a sitting position. The clinician assesses resting symptoms.
- Step Two: The patient actively places his or her arm on top of his or her head. The clinician then determines the presence or absence of the symptoms. It is unlikely that causative level of the cervical radiculopathy can be discriminated with this test.

**Figure 6.49**    The Shoulder Abduction Test

There are numerous other clinical special tests for the cervical spine. These tests have not been assessed for diagnostic value. Nonetheless, many of these tests may be beneficial in a manual therapist's examination of the patient's symptoms and are worth reporting. The following tests have been introduced within the literature but not specifically examined for diagnostic value.

## Sharp-Purser Test

The Sharp-Purser test is designed to assess upper cervical instability, specifically instability associated with disruption of the transverse ligament of the dens. Catyresse et al.[164] found that the Sharp-Purser test was not reliable for "feel" or valid for provocation of symptoms when testing hypermobility. In their study, the clinicians were unable to identify patients with congenital hypermobility in the upper cervical spine.

The test has been taught using two different procedures. Some advocate that a positive test is present if the head progresses posteriorly during testing. Another method suggested is if symptoms occur during forward flexion, then symptoms are relieved during posterior translation of the head. The original study by Sharp-Purser failed to define the procedure.

Although the test appears to demonstrate some utility, there is an element of risk associated with the procedure. If disruption of the transverse ligament is present, the passive migration of the axis anteriorly could place considerable pressure upon the spinal cord. Use of the Canadian C-spine rules may rule out the need of performing this test.

- Step One: The patient assumes a sitting position. The patient's head should be slightly flexed. The clinician assesses resting symptoms.
- Step Two: The clinician stands to the side of the patient and stabilizes the C2 spinous process using a pincer grasp.
- Step Three: Gently at first, the clinician applies a posterior translation force from the palm of the hand on the patient's forehead to a posterior direction. Symptoms are reassessed.
- Step Four: Symptoms are assessed for both degree of linear displacement (palpated) or symptom provocation.

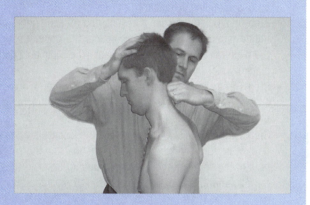

**Figure 6.50**  The Sharp-Purser Test

## Alar Ligament Stress Test

The Alar ligament stress test has long been advocated as a maneuver to assess the integrity of the Alar ligament. There are many iterations of the test but all have the same underlying philosophy. Because the Alar ligament controls axial rotation between the atlas and axis (i.e., right axial rotation is limited by the left Alar ligaments and vice versa), and because the ligament also controls excessive side flexion, both movements qualify for examination. During the test, if no rotation or side flexion is felt on the axis spinous process (C2), then it is assumed that damage has occurred to the Alar ligament. In normal situations, C2 attempts to move during side flexion and rotation. Both reproduction of symptoms and abnormal feel are considered positive.

- Step One: The patient assumes a sitting or supine position. The head is slightly flexed to engage further the Alar ligament. The clinician assesses resting symptoms.
- Step Two: The clinician stabilizes the C2 spinous process using a pincer grasp. A firm grip ensures appropriate assessment of movement.
- Step Three: Either side flexion or rotation is initiated. During these passive movements, the clinician attempts to feel movement of C2. A positive test is the failure to "feel" movement of the C2 process during side flexion and rotation.

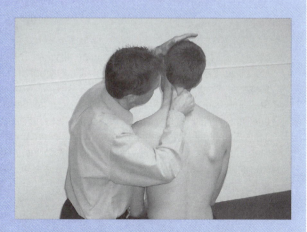

**Figure 6.51**  Alar Ligament Stress Test

## The Transverse Ligament of Atlas Test

The transverse ligament of atlas test also assesses the integrity of the transverse ligament. Essentially, this test is redundant to the Sharp-Purser test. Like the Sharp-Purser test, both movement and symptom provocation is the objective of this test. Because the anterior translation is focused on the C1 transverse processes, the test theoretically assesses excessive movement of C1 into the spinal canal. Additionally, because the transverse ligament functions to resist anterior shear and because failure to this ligament may result in symptoms such as dizziness, nausea, lip, face, or limb parasthesia, nystagmus, or any form of myelopathic symptoms, this test is crucial following a trauma to the cervical spine.

- Step One: The patient assumes a supine position. The clinician assesses resting symptoms.
- Step Two: Using a friction massage grip (digits 2 and 3 are held tightly together) the clinician contacts the posterior aspect of the bilateral C1 transverse processes. The clinician's palms are placed under the occiput of the patient.
- Step Three: The clinician then applies an anterior force to the C1 transverse processes, lifting the head as the force is applied. This position is held for 15–20 seconds.
- Step Four: If no symptoms occur, the clinician can apply a downward force on the patient's forehead using the anterior aspect of the shoulder to assess the superior aspect of the cruciform ligament. This position is held for 15–20 seconds.

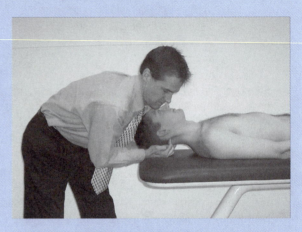

**Figure 6.52**    The Transverse Ligament of Atlas Test

## The Flexion-Rotation Test

The flexion-rotation test is a special clinical test designed to identify the presence of cervicogenic headache, specifically to implicate the upper cervical segments involved during rotation. Hall and Robinson[165] reported a sensitivity of 86% and a specificity of 100% in a two-sample comparison of patients with and without cervicogenic headache.

- Step One: The patient assumes a supine position. The clinician stands at the head of the patient. Resting symptoms are assessed.
- Step Two: The clinician first places the neck in full flexion. Second, the clinician applies a full rotational force to one of both sides. Symptoms are queried to determine if comparable.
- Step Three: The test is both a pain provocation test and a test for range-of-motion loss. If a loss of 10 degrees or greater is noted, the test is considered positive.

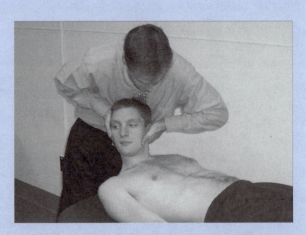

**Figure 6.53**    The Flexion-Rotation Test for Cervicogenic Headaches

## Summary

- There are two purposes of a clinical special test: (1) to provide the examiner with additional information regarding the nature of the condition and (2) to provide diagnostic value to a set of findings.
- Typically, palpation and muscle strength assessment provide additional data whereas clinical tests provide diagnostic information.
- The clinical special tests of Spurling's, shoulder abduction test, and the cervical distraction test have moderate diagnostic value.
- Many other clinical special tests have yet to be tested for diagnostic value.

# TREATMENT TECHNIQUES

The patient-response method endeavors to determine the behavior of the patient's pain and/or impairment by analyzing concordant movements and the response of the patient's pain to applied or repeated movements. The applied or repeated movements that positively or negatively alter the signs and symptoms of the patient deserve the highest priority for treatment selection[166,167] and should be similar in construct to the concordant examination movements. Examination methods that fail to elicit patient response may offer nominal or imprecise value, as do methods that focus solely on treatment decision making based on a single diagnostic label.[168]

With the exception of manipulation, which is not an examination procedure, the majority of active and passive treatment techniques are nearly identical to the examination procedures. In all cases of manual therapy treatment, there should be a direct mechanical relationship between the examination and treatment techniques selected.

In situations where the examination has failed to outline the appropriate treatment selection, a classification system may be useful. Classification allows large amounts of data to be broken down into common components and may improve the treatment outcome by homogeneity.[169] A recent proposed cervical classification tool outlines five classification groups for the cervical spine: (1) mobility, (2) centralization, (3) conditioning and increased exercise tolerance, (4) pain control, and (5) reduction of headache. Individuals that fail to respond to the provocation methods of the examination may fall within the third classification group and may benefit from a comprehensive strengthening program.

## Active Physiological Movements

Active physiological movements that consist of postural exercises or strengthening are plausible additions for treat-ment. Studies have shown some degree of success with implementation of an active exercise program[170], specifically those that focus on postural exercises[171,172] or strengthening.[173] Repeated neck retraction, a common intervention, has been shown to recover the H reflex amplitude, decompress cervical neural elements, and reduce cervical pain when compared against normal controls.[174] One common postural exercise is the prone cervical retraction technique, which is designed to incorporate a passive stretch during an active strengthening movement (Figure 6.54).

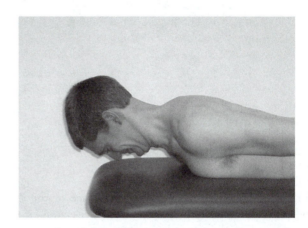

**Figure 6.54** Prone Cervical Retraction

Repeated chin retractions (Figure 6.55), such as those advocated by McKenzie, have demonstrated improvement in resting posture in asymptomatic subjects.[175] Additionally, active treatment mechanisms such as those proposed by McKenzie have resulted in comparative outcomes to general cervical strengthening and stretching exercises.[176] However, the theoretical reasoning behind why the "McKenzie-based" exercises work may be in question. Previously, McKenzie has postulated that selected movements allow reorientation of the nucleus within the cervical disc.[177] This movement of the nucleus is heralded as one of the mechanisms responsible for centralization of symptoms seen in patients with "derangement." Because the adult human does not have a gelatinous nucleus pulposus and since the annulus does not encircle the nucleus, a mechanism required for McKenzie's theoretical explanation, the McKenzie concept is inconsistent with anatomy[19] and, most likely, positive outcomes are based on some other explanative mechanism.

An active exercise program that focuses on the anterior craniocervical flexors has demonstrated excellent clinical utility during treatment of patients with cervicogenic headaches.[173,178,179] The exercises, performed in a supine position (Figure 6.56), target the deep neck flexors and the longus capitus and coli muscles. The specific protocol, devised by Jull[180], has demonstrated comparable outcomes to treatments that consist of manipulation and improved outcomes versus conventional medical care. Jull[180]

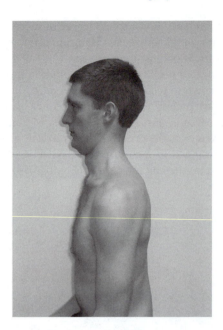

**Figure 6.55**    Sitting Chin Retractions

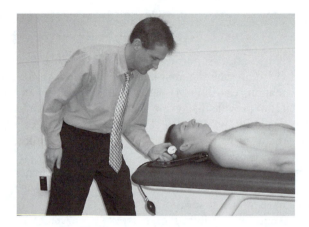

**Figure 6.56**    Supine Cervical Spine Stabilization Exercises

outlines that poor activation and endurance of the deep and postural supporting muscles of the neckshoulder girdle region, and deficits in kinesthesia are primary considerations in patients with cervicogenic headache.

## Passive Physiological Movements

Passive physiological stretching techniques have demonstrated strong association to range-of-motion gains in pa-

tients with neck dysfunction.[171,181] However, over time, when compared in isolation with active approaches, a passive physiological stretching program is less effective.[182] Subsequently, passive physiological exercises should be adjuncts to concurrent active strengthening programs that include active postural exercises.

All of the examination methods used previously are potential treatment techniques. For example, if a patient demonstrated concordant pain with restriction to the left during lateral side flexion, which benefited from repeated movements, a passive physiological treatment into side flexion is the treatment of choice. This concept is consistent throughout all planar movements.

### Suboccipital Distraction

Easing techniques are often used during occasions where the patient complains of pain or an irritable headache. Easing techniques may be helpful in reducing treatment soreness or reducing pain in a pain-dominant individual. One easing technique is the suboccipital distraction technique.

- Step One: The patient assumes a supine position with the head on the plinth. The resting symptoms of the patient are assessed.
- Step Two: Using all the fingertips in both hands from digits 2 through 5, the clinician cups the suboccipital region of the patient and supports the posterior skull.
- Step Three: The clinician provides a light distraction to the posterior skull.
- Step Four: The patient may perform extension-based isometric exercises for a hold relax stretch or allow a passive-specific treatment.
- Step Five: The patient is reassessed.

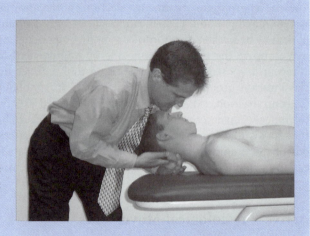

**Figure 6.57**    Suboccipital Distraction

## Passive Chin Retraction

A compliment to the active chin retraction technique is a passive technique. Since a passive physiological technique is designed to stretch beyond the ranges of an active method, this technique may provide a more vigorous stretch to the patient.

- Step One: The patient assumes a supine position. Assess the patient's resting symptoms.
- Step Two: Using the chin cradle grip, the clinician provides a retraction force to the patient's head.
- Step Three: The patient's condition is reassessed.

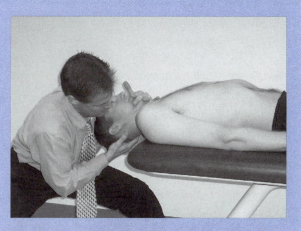

**Figure 6.58**    Chin Retraction with Overpressure

## Passive Accessory Movements

There is a moderate amount of evidence to support that passive accessory techniques provide an excitatory effect on sympathetic nervous system activity.[134,183,184] Mobilizations have produced skin temperature changes and an increase in skin conductivity.[185] Stimulation of the cervical spine has demonstrated upper extremity changes in pain response (pressure-pain), and a measurable sympathoexcitatory effect.[184,186] An excitatory effect on the sympathetic nervous system occurs concurrently with a reduction of hypoanalgesia and may parallel the effects of stimulation of the dorsal periaqueductal gray area of the midbrain, a process that has occurred in animal research.[187] Since mobilization does lead to a reduction of pain using the same procedures as those performed during examination, it makes sense to use the very mechanism that has been shown to be specific.

There is also evidence that cervical postero-anterior (PA) mobilizations are effective in reducing pain.[185] PAs helped to increase pain thresholds and led to significant reductions against controlled comparisons on a visual analog scale.[185] Treatment benefits were present during the treatment and over a 2-week period.[185]

The most commonly used treatment technique from a recent survey of manipulative physical therapists was the passive accessory intervertebral glide.[188] While detecting spinal accessory stiffness alone has not been shown to be consistently reliable,[189] several authors have suggested that palpating for pain accompanying stiffness is both reliable and valid.[112,129,190] Recently Jull et al.[190] demonstrated a very high degree of agreement among clinicians in isolating the painful cervical segment in patients with chronic cervicogenic headaches. The use of subjective responses while identifying stiffness through PA mobilization is consistently used in clinical situations, and reigns supreme over stiffness detection alone.

Lee et al.[113] reported that the movement of a PA subjects the patient to three point axial movements. Although these movements have been purported to produce isolated linear glides, significant axial or sagittal rotation is common through the movement application. This results in significant spinal bending under the application of PA loads, and variability in direction of the bend. Mobilization forces on the C5 processes resulted in extension at the C2-3 and C3-4 segments and flexion at the C7-T1 segments. Variability was found in the mid-cervical segments, which demonstrated both flexion and extension behavior.

Although the magnitude of intervertebral movements produced by mobilization was generally small, the forces applied at one spinous process produced not only movements at the target vertebra but also movements of the entire cervical spine. These findings are consistent with the findings of lower back–related research.[191,192] Based on these findings, it is imperative to acknowledge that PAs are recognized as a global mobilization process, not just a simple gliding of one vertebra upon another.

## CO-C1 Passive Mobilization for Headaches

A commonly used mobilization method for headaches targets the upper cervical structures of C0-1, C1-2, and C2-3. This method, first described by Maitland,[78] has been successful in a recent randomized trial that focused treatment to cervicogenic headaches.[173]

### CO-1 Cervicogenic Treatment

- Step One: The patient assumes a prone position. The patient's resting symptoms are assessed.
- Step Two: The clinician palpates the suboccipital region of the posterior skull. The ring finger should fall within a depression in this region. This is the area lying over the CO-1 joint.
- Step Three: A light pressure is applied using one thumb over the other. The clinician should press only to the first point of pain.
- Step Four: The clinician pushes beyond pain and the patient's symptoms are reassessed. If tolerated well, the clinician repeats the movements.
- Step Five: The patient's condition is reassessed.

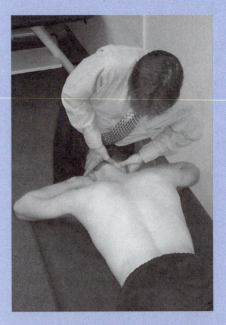

**Figure 6.59**   C0-1 Passive Accessory Treatment

### C2-3 Cervicogenic Treatment

- Step One: The patient assumes a prone position. The patient's resting symptoms are assessed.
- Step Two: Using his or her thumb, the clinician palpates the C2 spinous processes, moves the thumb just lateral to the spinous process, and pulls the muscles and soft tissue medial to expose the articular pillars.
- Step Three: The C2-3 segment is just lateral to the C2 spinous process. The clinician provides a light pressure using one thumb over the other. The clinician should press only to the first point of pain.
- Step Four: The clinician pushes beyond pain and the patient's symptoms are reassessed. If tolerable, repeat the movements.
- Step Five: The patient's condition is reassessed.

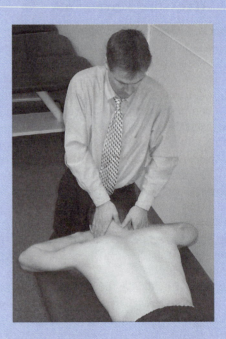

**Figure 6.60**   C2-3 Passive Accessory Treatment

## C1-2 Cervicogenic Treatment

- Step One: C1-2 mobilization involves a very similar process to C2-3. The patient assumes a prone position. The patient's resting symptoms are assessed.
- Step Two: Using his or her thumb, the clinician palpates the C2 spinous processes, moves the thumb just lateral to the spinous process, and pulls the muscles and soft tissue medial to expose the articular pillars.
- Step Three: While keeping the fingers on the C2-3 facet, the head is rotated to the same side of the facet (approximately 30 degrees). The rotation enhances the amount of movement that is applied through C1-2, but most likely does not eliminate all of the movement through C2-3. A light pressure is applied using one thumb over the other toward the patient's mouth. The clinician should press only to the first point of pain.
- Step Four: The clinician pushes beyond pain and the patient's symptoms are reassessed. If tolerated, the clinician should repeat the movements.
- Step Five: The patient's condition is reassessed.

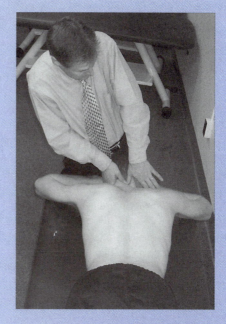

**Figure 6.61**   C1-2 Passive Accessory Treatment

If pain is concordant in any of the levels assessed, the treatment is isolated to those levels. Solid evidence exists that strengthening exercises in conjunction with mobilization is effective for reduction of pain in some headache patients.[64]

## Manually Assisted Movements

Manually assisted movements consist of muscle energy methods of patient-assisted stretching. Muscle energy techniques (METs) are a technique in manual therapy where the patient actively uses his or her muscles, on request, while maintaining a targeted preposition, against a distinctly executed counterforce.[193] PNF techniques make use of proprioceptive stimulus for strengthening or inhabitation of selected and targeted muscle groups.[194] Both are manually assisted methods and both have established benefit during manual therapy treatment. There are numerous different treatment techniques and this textbook only demonstrates a few.

## Upper Trapezius Stretching

Chronic forward head posture may lead to alterations of the anterior and selective posterior muscles such as the trapezius. One method designed to reduce pain and stiffness of the soft tissue regions of the spine is a lateral stretch.

- Step One: The patient assumes a supine position and the resting symptoms of the patient are assessed.
- Step Two: The clinician stabilizes the lower fibers of the trapezius by applying a downward pressure posterior to the clavicle.
- Step Three: The cervical spine is side flexed away and forward flexed to engage the trapezius fibers.
- Step Four: The patient may provide an isometric side flexion and extension contraction against the stretching force of the clinician.
- Step Five: The resting symptoms of the patient are reassessed.

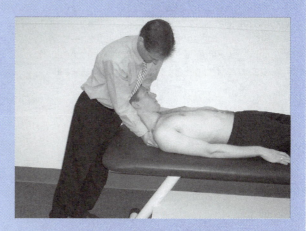

**Figure 6.62**   Upper Trapezius Stretching

## Side Flexion Physiological Glide

A lateral physiological glide is used to target structures other than the trapezius. A side flexion stretch may be helpful if the pain during the passive physiological examination was felt on the opposite side of the side flexion. One may also mobilize the lateral joint structures as well.

- Step One: The patient assumes a supine position and the resting symptoms of the patient are assessed.
- Step Two: The clinician stabilizes the lower fibers of the trapezius and the origin of the scalenes and lateral musculature by applying a downward pressure posterior-medial aspect of the neck.
- Step Three: The clinician provides a static stretch in the direction of side flexion away from the stabilization.
- Step Four: The patient may provide an isometric contraction against the clinician's stretch.
- Step Five: The resting symptoms of the patient are reassessed.

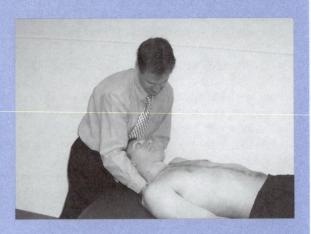

**Figure 6.63**    Lateral Flexion Stretching

## Chin Retraction with Overpressure

Chin retraction with compression of forehead is a technique used to reduce forward head. The technique is as follows.

- Step One: The patient assumes a supine position and the patient's resting symptoms are assessed.
- Step Two: Using the chin cradle grip, the clinician provides a retraction force to the patient's head.
- Step Three: The clinician may now add a downward stretch using one of two possible contact points. The clinician can provide a downward glide by providing a force downward through the forehead (pictured) using the anterior aspect of his or her shoulder, or may provide a downward force manually through the maxilla using the web space of the free hand.
- Step Four: The patient may apply a further downward force or a light upward force against the clinician's resistance.
- Step Five: The patient's condition is reassessed.

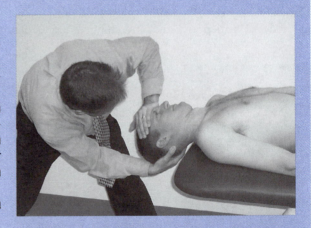

**Figure 6.64**    Chin Retraction with Compression of the Forehead

## Premanipulative Treatment

Manually assisted methods are also used to mobilize or manipulate segmental regions. One method includes the use of the premanipulative position and a manually assisted patient-generated response. The technique is as follows.

- Step One: The patient assumes a supine position. Resting symptoms are assessed.
- Step Two: The patient's neck is side glided toward an end point.
- Step Three: Using the lateral aspect of the first metacarpalphalangeal joint, the clinician provides a fulcrum force to the neck. The contact point should consist of the articular pillars or the transverse processes.
- Step Four: The patient's neck is side flexed to the level of the contact point. Since combined movements are often used when single plane movements are less sensitive, pain should not be as critical a consideration.
- Step Five: The patient's neck is rotated in the opposite direction as the side flexion, but not beyond.
- Step Six: The clinician should feel the neck "lock." The patient's condition should be reassessed, specifically for signs of VBI.
- Step Seven: The patient either rotates his or her head in the opposite direction of the prepositioning or side flexes his or her head in the opposite direction of the prepositioning. It is common to hear an audible with this technique.
- Step Eight: The patient's resting symptoms are reassessed.

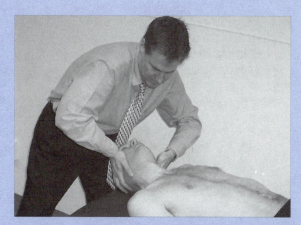

**Figure 6.65**    Manually Assisted Combined Movement

## Manipulation

Manipulation is a commonly used treatment technique used by 84.5% of the practicing respondents in a recent survey.[188] Although manipulation was used less frequently in the upper cervical spine when compared to the middle and lower regions (83.4%, 84.7%, and 98.3%, respectively), the technique still demonstrated a high frequency of use in all regions of the cervical spine.[195]

Manipulation techniques involve highly skilled psychomotor skills that require supervised practice.[195,196] Although the use of a textbook and didactic knowledge is helpful in understanding the components of manipulation, there is no substitute for safe practice and psychomotor learning in a well-organized environment.[196] This textbook is not designed to be a substitute for traditional laboratory-based learning.

Several different forms of manipulative treatments are used. Specific HVT techniques commonly included lateral flexion, longitudinal, postero-anterior (PA) thrust, transverse, and rotary techniques.[188] This textbook describes two different forms of manipulations, those that use the chin cradle grip and those that are "chin-free."

## Chin Cradle Maneuvers
## Longitudinal Distraction

One form of upper c-spine manipulation that targets the C0-1 segment is the C0-1 distraction maneuver. This technique may be useful in patients with upper cervicogenic headaches or unilateral pain and stiffness of origin in the upper c-spine. The following describes the technique procedure.

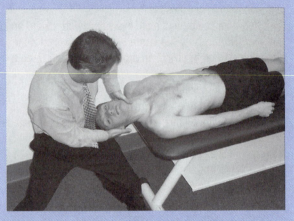

- Step One: The patient is positioned in supine with the head extended beyond the table to T2.
- Step Two: The head of the patient is prepositioned toward rotation.
- Step Three: The clinician applies a light distraction to the patient's head.
- Step Four: For a manipulation of the same region, the clinician uses a chin cradle grip and firmly holds the patient's head. The clinician stands to the same side of the patient's C0-1 that he or she wishes to treat.
- Step Five: The patient's head is rotated away from the treated segments, approximately 15–20 degrees.

**Figure 6.66**    Upper C-Spine C0-1 Distraction; Preposition in Rotation

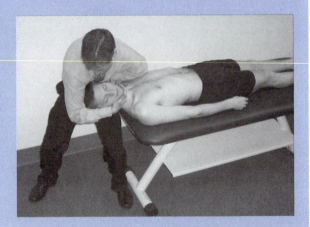

- Step Six: The radial aspect of the metacarpalphalangeal joint (the thrusting knuckle) is used to provide a traction force against the mastoid process.
- Step Seven: After several small oscillations, a longitudinal force is provided (traction) using a light thrust.
- Step Eight: The patient's condition is reassessed.

**Figure 6.67**    Upper C-Spine Manipulation

## Upper C-Spine Manipulation Using Translation

Upper cervical spine manipulation involves the greatest amount of risk of any manual therapy-based technique.[52] Therefore, it is crucial that careful screening has been performed and that the patient tolerates the position well prior to a manipulative thrust. This general technique, described below, most likely allows movement in the segments from C0-1 to C2-3, secondary to the anatomy of the structures.

- Step One: The patient is positioned in supine and the symptoms are assessed.
- Step Two: The patient's head is held in a chin cradle grip. To manipulate the right OA-AA region, the head should be held with the right cradle.
- Step Three: A translatory force is applied to the upper cervical spine (contact point is the left C2-3 transverse process). Simultaneously, a side flexion force (to the opposite direction as the translation) is applied.
- Step Four: The clinician provides a rotational force of approximately 45 degrees to the right. Allowing this quantity of rotation typically results in a "locking" of the upper cervical spine secondary to combined movements.
- Step Five: The patient's sagittal flexion and extension is modified to further "tighten" the position.
- Step Six: A light lateral translatory thrust is applied in the same translatory preposition used in Step Three.
- Step Seven: The patient's condition is reassessed.

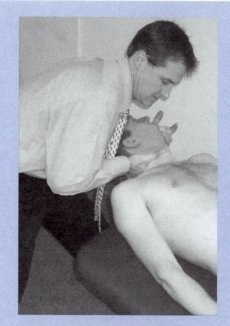

**Figure 6.68**    General Upper Cervical Spine Translational Manipulation

## Manipulation of the Mid and Lower Cervical Spine

The ability to lock the joint using apposition is clinically more the more cephalic the segments. Most likely, this is associated with the angulations of the facet joints, thus necessitating a small amount of extension during the thrust. Like the upper cervical spine, a comprehensive VBI assessment is essential prior to treatment.

- Step One: The patient is positioned in supine and the symptoms are assessed.
- Step Two: The patient's head is held in a chin cradle grip. To manipulate the left mid or lower cervical region, the head should be held with the right cradle. However, the determination of which side to manipulate is best selected using patient report of symptoms.
- Step Three: A translatory force is applied to the lower cervical spine (contact point is the isolated lower cervical transverse process or articular pillar). Simultaneously, a side flexion force (to the opposite direction as the translation) is applied.
- Step Four: The clinician provides a rotational force of approximately 10–20 degrees. The rotation should not go beyond the contact point of the side glide (thrusting knuckle). Allowing this quantity of rotation typically results in a "locking" of the mid or lower cervical spine secondary to combined movements.
- Step Five: The patient's sagittal flexion and extension is modified to further "tighten" the position. Extension tends to target the anterior capsule while flexion targets the posterior aspect of the capsule and is usually the best selection for the mid cervical region. Nonetheless, the technique does provide a general force to the complete region.
- Step Six: A light thrust is applied in the same translatory preposition used in Step Three.
- Step Seven: The patient's condition is reassessed.

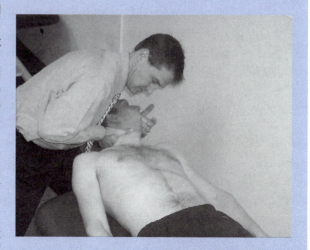

**Figure 6.69**    Chin-Cradle Manipulation of the Mid or Lower Cervical Spine

## Cervical Thoracic Junction Manipulation

The transition zone between the cervical and thoracic spine is difficult to access, secondary to a large amount of soft tissue structures that cover the area. Consequently, innovative methods are necessary to mobilize this particular region. The following describes a lower C-spine manipulative procedure in sitting.

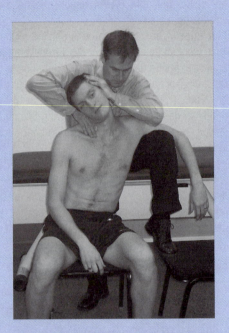

- Step One: The patient is seated with their back facing the clinician. Baseline symptoms are assessed.
- Step Two: The clinician stands or kneels directly behind the patient. The patient is positioned so that he or she leans back against the clinician.
- Step Three: If side flexion to a particular side is desired, one should place the opposite arm of the patient over the knee of the clinician.
- Step Four: The clinician places his or her palm on the zygomatic arch of the patient on the same side in which the patient is leaning on the clinician's leg.
- Step Five: A lateral force is applied using a thumb block to the spinous processes of the targeted level.
- Step Six: Using a simultaneous sequence, the clinician applies a lateral glide and a physiological glide to encourage spinal movement.
- Step Seven: The patient's symptoms are reassessed.

**Figure 6.70**    Lower C-Spine, Upper T-Spine Thrust

## Cervical Thoracic Junction Manipulation in Prone

A technically similar method that involves less psychomotor skill is performed in prone. The following procedure outlines the prone manipulative technique.

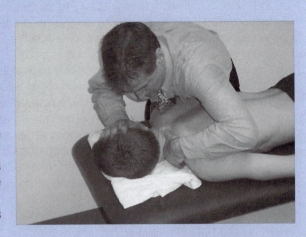

- Step One: The patient is positioned in prone. The head is rotated toward the direction the clinician desires to manipulate. A towel is placed under the patient's face to allow gliding on the plinth, and the patient's baseline symptoms are assessed.
- Step Two: A lateral block at the spinous process is used for stabilization of the desired segment. The clinician's thumb should engage the deepest aspect of spinous process, targeting the lamina's connection to the spinous process.
- Step Three: Using the palm of thd hand, the patient's head is prepositioned into extension, side flexion, and rotation to the opposite side.
- Step Four: At the "end point" of the preposition, a light thrust is provided by the clinician through the head of the patient.
- Step Five: The patient's symptoms are reassessed.

**Figure 6.71**    Prone Lower C-Spine, Upper Thoracic Thrust

## Thoracic Manipulation

Cleland et al.[197] have reported thoracic manipulation for improvements in the cervical spine. When compared against a "sham" manipulation to the thoracic spine, the thoracic manipulation group resulted in significant short term pain reduction using a VAS but no significance on the NDI.

- Step One: The patient assumes a supine position. Using an over- and under-crossing technique, the patient crosses his or her arms over the chest.
- Step Two: The clinician stands to the opposite side of the targeted segment. Using the arm furthest from the targeted side, the clinician gently pulls the patient into sidelying.
- Step Three: The clinician then leans over the patient and places the hand behind the patient's back just caudal to the targeted segment. The pistol grip allows the transverse processes to articulate with the thenar eminence and the folded digits of the clinician's hand.

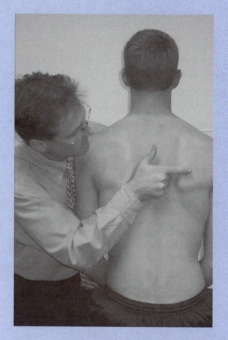

**Figure 6.72**  Thoracic Manipulation Using the Pistol Grip-Hand Placement

- Step Four: The patient is "scooped" into flexion (using his or her arms as a lever) and gently placed over the pistol hand of the clinician. Careful effort is made to keep the patient in flexion.
- Step Five: The clinician may further enhance the contact point on the patient's transverse process by pronating the wrist or ulnarly deviating the hand.
- Step Six: The clinician's thrust should be through the shaft of the humeri.

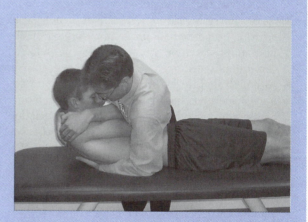

**Figure 6.73**  The Pistol Manipulation

## Traction

Manual traction is often used as an easing technique or a technique designed to decompress the cervical nerve root. Cervical traction has been shown to increase the blood flow to the neck musculature and positively affect the muscular activity.[198] Additionally, cervical traction may stimulate the receptors in the joints of the cervical spine, thus reducing pain.

## Cervical Traction

Traction is applicable for use in patients who exhibit a centralization or peripheralization of symptoms during selected examination movements.

- Step One: The patient lies supine. Resting symptoms are assessed.
- Step Two: The clinician uses a chin cradle grip with equal force anterior and posterior. If the patient demonstrates TMD or has dental work not conducive to compression, the posterior force using a towel may be beneficial.
- Step Three: The clinician supplies a light traction force of approximately 5–10 pounds. The patient's symptoms are assessed for change. The force is held for approximately 1 minute and the patient is reevaluated.
- Step Four: Force and time is modulated based on patient response. In most cases, it is not necessary to provide very high forces for traction. Light forces generally provide successful treatment outcomes. A towel can be used to increase the patient's comfort.

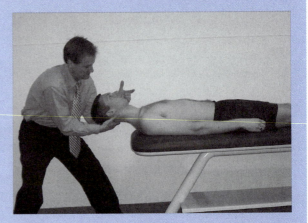

**Figure 6.74**    Cervical Distraction Using the Chin Cradle Grip

## *Summary*

- Strong association between examination and treatment should improve the outcome of a dedicated treatment program.
- Active physiological movements are beneficial in creating home exercise programs, working on abnormal posture, or strengthening the selected cervical musculature.
- Although slightly less effective than active physiological methods, passive physiological stretching techniques have demonstrated strong association to range-of-motion gains in patients with neck dysfunction.
- There is a moderate amount of evidence to support that manual therapy provides an excitatory effect on sympathetic nervous system activity, subsequently reducing pain levels in local and regional pain syndromes.

## Treatment Outcomes

Overall, there is moderate evidence that a treatment approach that consists of some element of orthopedic manual therapy is associated with a positive outcome.[199] Treatments elements such as mobilization and manipulation have functioned similarly when performed in isola-

tion[200] but exhibit stronger outcomes when combined with exercise[201] or some other form of intervention.[202,203]

Two studies found traction to exhibit useful outcomes in samples of patients with **cervical radiculopathy.** Joghataei et al.[204] reported that when traction was combined with electrotherapy and exercise there were improvements in upper extremity grip strength. Shakoor et al.[170] found a trend toward significance when traction was used in conjunction with neck strengthening exercises when compared to a control group, which received NSAIDs only.

In 1996, Hurwitz et al.[205] concluded in a systematic literature review that (1) mobilization provided short-term benefit for patients with acute neck pain, (2) manipulation was probably more effective than mobilization for patients with subacute or chronic neck problems, (3) both were more effective than conventional medical care, and (4) manipulation and mobilization were beneficial for cervicogenic headaches. In 2002, Hurwitz et al.[200] completed a large randomized clinical trial and discovered that outcomes of mobilization and manipulation were equally beneficial. Both groups reported mean reductions in pain and disability. In a 2004 Cochrane review of manipulation and mobilization for mechanical neck disorders, Gross et al.[201] suggested that mobilization and manipulation displayed similar outcomes but were not beneficial when performed alone on a heterogeneous group of patients. However, when combined with exercises both methods of treatment were beneficial for pain reduction and functional improvements in patients with or without cervicogenic headaches. Although Gross et al. reported there was insufficient evidence available to draw conclusions regarding patients with radiculopathy, two recent articles have demonstrated benefit using either indirect cervical mobilization methods[202] or selective mobilization of the nerve tissue.[206] Nonetheless, further research is required for definitive analysis.

Lastly, there is strong evidence to support the use of mobilization and manipulation combined with a targeted local musculature strengthening program for the neck.[64] One substantiated program is the cervical strengthening program suggested by Jull et al.[173] This program targets the anterior cervical deep flexors in a sequence of targeted progressive steps. Harris and colleagues[207] recently demonstrated differences in neck flexor endurance between subjects with and without neck pain, using the neck flexor endurance test. The test purportedly isolates the ability of the deep neck flexors for stability and endurance. The procedure was performed in supine and required the patient to statically hold his or her retracted neck approximately one inch above the plinth. The clinician times the patient's

hold time and determines their endurance. The procedure is similar to Jull et al. minus the use of a blood pressure cup to determine stabilization.

## Summary

- Overall, there is substantial evidence that a treatment approach that consists of some element of orthopedic manual therapy is associated with a positive outcome.
- Patient outcomes after treatment based on mobilization and manipulation are equally beneficial.
- When performed alone, mobilization and manipulation both provide some benefit; however, when combined with exercises both methods of treatment were beneficial for pain reduction and functional improvements in patients with or without cervicogenic headaches.

## Chapter Questions

1. Describe the responsibilities of the cervical intervertebral disc, the uncovertebral joints, and the zygopophyseal joints in stability and movement of the cervical spine.
2. Define the directional coupling pattern of the cervical spine and the importance of initiation of movement.
3. Indicate which spinal segments are most commonly associated with cervicogenic headaches and outline a treatment regimen.
4. Describe the subjective symptoms and patient examination findings associated with cervical instability, VBI, and whiplash.
5. Describe how combined movements of the cervical spine place greater force upon the elastic and/or inelastic aspects of a segment.

## References

1. Bonfort G, Evans R, Nelson B, Aker P, Goldsmith C, Vernon H. A randomized clinical trial of exercise and spinal manipulation for patients with chronic neck pain. *Spine.* 2001;26:788–799.
2. Linton SJ, Hellsing AL, Hallden K. A population-based study of spinal pain among 35-45-year-old individuals. Prevalence, sick leave, and health care use. *Spine.* 1998;23(13):1457–1463.
3. Linton SJ. The socioeconomic impact of chronic back pain: is anyone benefiting? *Pain.* 1998;75 (2-3):163–168.
4. Borghouts J, Janssen H, Koes B, Muris J, Metsemakers J, Bouter L. The management of chronic neck pain in general practice. A retrospective study. *Scand J Prim Health Care.* 1999;17(4):215–220.
5. Skargren EI, Carlsson PG, Oberg BE. One-year follow-up comparison of the cost and effectiveness of chiropractic and physiotherapy as primary management for back pain. Subgroup analysis, recurrence, and additional health care utilization. *Spine.* 1998; 23(17):1875–1883.
6. Makela M, Heliovaara M, Sievers K, Impivaara O, Knekt P, Aromaa A. Prevalence, determinants, and consequences of chronic neck pain in Finland. *Am J Epidemiol.* 1991;134:1356–1367.
7. Lagattuta F, Falco F. Assessment and treatment of cervical spine disorders. In: Braddom (ed) *Physical medicine and rehabilitation.* Philadelphia; Saunders: 2000.
8. Malanga GA: The diagnosis and treatment of cervical radiculopathy. *Med Sci Sports Exerc.*1997;29 (7 Suppl):S236–245.
9. Penning L. Normal movements of the cervical spine. *Am J Roentgenology.* 1978;130:317–326.

10. Leone A, Cerase A, Colosito C, Lauro L, Puca A, Marano P. Occipital Condylar Fractures: A Review. *Radiology*. 2000;216:635–644.

11. Dean NA, Mitchell BS. Anatomic relation between the nuchal ligament (ligamentum nuchae) and the spinal dura mater in the craniocervical region. *Clin Anat*. 2002;15(3):182–185.

12. White A, Panjabi M. *Clinical biomechanics of the spine*. Philadelphia; J.B. Lippincott Co: 1990.

13. Dvorak J, Schneider E, Saldinger P, Rahn B. Biomechanics of the craniocervical region: the Alar and transverse ligaments. *J Orthop Res*. 1988;6(3): 452–461.

14. Lewis H. *Gray's anatomy*. 20th ed. Philadelphia; Lea & Friberger: 2001.

15. Panjabi M. The stabilizing system of the spine. Part I. Function, dysfunction, adaptation, and enhancement. *J Spinal Disord*. 1992;5:383–389.

16. Lysell E. Motion in the cervical spine. An experimental study on autopsy specimens. *Acta Orthop Scand*. 1969;Suppl 123:1+.

17. Bogduk N. Functional and applied anatomy of the cervical spine. In: Grant R. *Physical therapy of the cervical and thoracic spine*. 3rd ed. New York; Churchill Livingstone: 2002.

18. Mercer S, Bogduk N. The ligaments and annulus fibrosus of human adult cervical intervertebral discs. *Spine*. 1999;24(7):619–626.

19. Mercer SR, Jull GA. Morphology of the cervical intervertebral disc: implications for McKenzie's model of the disc derangement syndrome. *Man Ther*. 2000; 1(2):76–81.

20. Bogduk N, Mercer S. Biomechanics of the cervical spine. 1: Normal kinematics. *Clin Biomech*. 2000;15: 633–648.

21. Russell SM, Benjamin V. The anterior surgical approach to the cervical spine for intervertebral disc disease. *Neurosurgery*. 2004;54(5):1144–1149.

22. McAfee PC, Cunningham B, Dmitriev A, Hu N, Woo Kim S, Cappuccino A, Pimenta L. Cervical disc replacement-porous coated motion prosthesis: a comparative biomechanical analysis showing the key role of the posterior longitudinal ligament. *Spine*. 2003;28(20):S176–185.

23. Williams P, Warwick R, Dyson M, Bannister L. *Gray's anatomy*. 37th ed. Edinburgh; Churchill Livingstone: 1989.

24. Pal GP, Routal RV, Saggu SK. The orientation of the articular facets of the zygopophyseal joints at the cervical and upper thoracic region. *J Anat*. 2001;198 (Pt 4):431–441.

25. Penning L, Tondury G (Abstract). Enststehung, Bau and Funktion der meniskoiden Strukturen in den Halswirbelgelenken. *Z Orthop* 1964;1:14.

26. Dvorak J. Epidemiology, physical examination, and neurodiagnostics. *Spine*. 1998;23:2663–2672.

27. Inami S, Kaneoka K, Hayashi K, Ochiai N. Types of synovial fold in the cervical facet joint. *J Orthop Sci*. 2000;5(5):475–480.

28. Sherk H. Disorders of the cervical spine. *Clin Orthop*. 1999;(359):2–3.

29. Chen TY, Crawford NR, Sonntag VK, Dickman CA. Biomechanical effects of progressive anterior cervical decompression. *Spine*. 2001;1;26(1):6–13.

30. Bergmark A. Stability of the lumbar spine. A study in mechanical engineering. *Acta Orthop Scand Suppl*. 1989;230:1–54.

31. Falla D. Unraveling the complexity of muscle impairment in chronic neck pain. *Man Ther* 2004;9(3): 125–133.

32. Jull G, Barrett C, Magee R, Ho P. Further clinical clarification of the muscle dysfunction in cervical headache. *Cephalalgia*. 1999;19(3):179–185.

33. Russell S, Vallo B. Posterior surgical approach to the cervical neural foramen for intervertebral disc disease. *Neurosurgery*. 2004;54(3):662–665.

34. Trott PH, Pearcy MJ, Ruston SA, Fulton I, Brien C. Three-dimensional analysis of active cervical motion: the effect of age and gender. *Clin Biomech*. 1996;11(4):201–206.

35. Haynes MJ, Edmondston S. Accuracy and reliability of a new, protractor-based neck goniometer. *J Manipulative Physiol Ther*. 2002;25(9):579–586.

36. Antonaci F, Ghirmai S, Bono G, Nappi G. Current methods for cervical spine movement evaluation: a review. *Clin Exp Rheumatol*. 2000;18(2 Suppl 19): S45–52.

37. Nilsson N, Hartvigsen J, Christensen HW. Normal ranges of passive cervical motion for women and men 20-60 years old. *J Manipulative Physiol Ther*. 1996;19(5):306–309.

38. Youdas JW, Carey JR, Garrett TR. Reliability of measurements of cervical spine range of motion—comparison of three methods. *Phys Ther*. 1991;71(2): 98–104.

39. Panjabi M, Oda T, Crisco J, Dvorak J, Grob D. Posture affects motion coupling patterns of the upper cervical spine. *J Orthop Research*. 1993;11: 525–536.

40. Iai H, Hideshige M, Goto S, Takahashi K, Yamagata M, Tamaki T. Three-dimensional motion analysis of the upper cervical spine during axial rotation. *Spine*. 1993;18:2388–2392.

41. Mimura M, Hideshige M, Watanbe T, Takahashi K, Yamagata M, Tamaki T. Three-dimensional motion analysis of the cervical spine with special reference to axial rotation. *Spine*. 1989;14:1135–1139.

42. Ishii T, Mukai Y, Hosono N, Sakaura H, Nakajima Y, Sato Y, Sugamoto K, Yoshikawa H. Kinematics of the upper cervical spine in rotation. *Spine*. 2004;29: 139–144.

43. Panjabi M, Summers D, Pelker R, Videman T, Friedlaender G, Southwick W. Three-dimensional

load-displacement curves due to forces on the cervical spine. *J Orthop Research*. 1986;4:152–161.

44. Panjabi MM, Crisco JJ, Vasavada A, Oda T, Cholewicki J, Nibu K, Shin E. Mechanical properties of the human cervical spine as shown by three-dimensional load-displacement curves. *Spine*. 2001; 26(24):2692–2700.

45. Cook C. Lumbar Coupling biomechanics—A literature review. *J Manual Manipulative Ther*. 2003;11(3): 137–145.

46. Harrison D, Harrison D, Troyanovich S. Three-dimensional spinal coupling mechanics: Part one. *J Manipulative Physiol Ther*. 1998;21(2):101–113.

47. Olin T, Olsson T, Selvik G, Willner S. Kinematic analysis of experimentally provoked scoliosis in pigs with Roentgen stereophotogrammetry. *Acta Radiologica*. 1976;1(1):107–127.

48. Rab G, Chao E. Verification of roentgenographic landmarks in the lumbar spine. *Spine* 1977;2:287–293.

49. Stokes I, Medlicott P, Wilder D. Measurement of movement in painful intervertebral joints. *Medical and Biological Engineering and Computing*. 1980; 18:694–700.

50. Fryette H. *The principles of Osteopathic technique*. Carmel, CA; Academy of Applied Osteopathy: 1954.

51. Grieve G. *Common vertebral joint problems*. 2nd ed. Edinburgh; Churchill Livingstone: 1988.

52. Di Fabio RP. Manipulation of the cervical spine: risks and benefits. *Phys Ther*. 1999;79(1):50–65.

53. Reiter MF, Boden SD. Inflammatory disorders of the cervical spine. *Spine*. 1998;23:2755–2766.

54. Cook C, Brismee JM, Sizer P. Suggested factors associated with clinical cervical spine instability: A Delphi study of physical therapists. *Phys Ther*. 2005; 85:895–906.

55. Pietrobon R, Coeytaux R, Carey T, Richardson W, DeVellis R. Standard scales for measurement of functional outcome for cervical pain or dysfunction. *Spine*. 2002;27:515–522.

56. Ackelman B, Lindgren U. Validity and reliability of a modified version of the neck disability index. *J Rehabil Med*. 2002;34:284–287.

57. Vernon H. The Neck disability index: patient assessment and outcome monitoring in whiplash. *J Musculoskel Pain*. 1996;4:95–104.

58. Wheeler A, Goolkasian P, Baird A, Darden B. Development of the Neck Pain and Disability Scale: item analysis, face and criterion-repeated validity. *Spine*. 1999;24:1290–1299.

59. Abdulwahab S. Treatment based on H-reflexes testing improves disability status in patients with cervical radiculopathy. *Int J Rehabil Res*. 1999;22: 207–214.

60. Jette D, Jette A. Physical therapy and health outcomes in patients with spinal impairments. *Phys Ther*. 1996;76:930–941.

61. Marchiori D, Henderson C. A cross-sectional study correlating cervical radiographic degenerative findings to pain and disability. *Spine*. 1996;21: 2747–2751.

62. Ernst E. Cerbrovascular complications associated with spinal manipulation. *Physical Therapy Reviews*. 2004;9:5–15.

63. Barker WH, Howard VJ, Howard G, Toole JF. Effect of contralateral occlusion on long-term efficacy of endarterectomy in the asymptomatic carotid atherosclerosis study (ACAS). ACAS Investigators. *Stroke*. 2000;10:2330–2334.

64. Gross AR, Kay T, Hondras M, Goldsmith C, Haines T, Peloso P, Kennedy C, Hoving J. Manual therapy for mechanical neck disorders: a systematic review. *Man Ther*. 2002;7(3):131–149.

65. Mann T, Refshauge KM. Causes of complications from cervical spine manipulation. *Aust J Physiotherapy*. 2001;47(4):255–266.

66. McKechnie B. Vertebrobasilar arterial insufficiency. Part I: presenting symptoms. *Dynamic Chiropractic*. 1994;(10).

67. McKechnie B. Vertebrobasilar arterial insufficiency. Part II: neurological examination findings in cases of vertebrobasilar infarct. *Dynamic Chiropractic*. 1994; 12(13).

68. Lincoln J. Case report. Clinical instability of the upper cervical spine. *Man Ther*. 2000;5(1):41–46.

69. Panjabi MM, Oxland TR, Parks EH. Quantitative anatomy of cervical spine ligaments. Part I. Upper cervical spine. *J Spinal Disord*. 1991;4(3):270–276.

70. Dvorak J, Antinnes JA, Panjabi M, Loustalot D, Bonomo M. Age and gender related normal motion of the cervical spine. *Spine*. 1992;17(10 Suppl): S393–398.

71. Rothwell DM, Bondy SJ, Williams JI. Chiropractic manipulation and stroke: a population-based case-control study. *Stroke*. 2001;32(5):1054–1060.

72. Arnold C, Bourassa R, Langer T, Stoneham G. Doppler studies evaluating the effect of a physical therapy screening protocol on vertebral artery blood flow. *Man Ther*. 2004;9(1):13–21.

73. Johnson C, Grant R, Dansie B, Taylor J, Spyropolous P. Measurement of blood flow in the vertebral artery using colour duplex Doppler ultrasound: establishment of the reliability of selected parameters. *Man Ther*. 2000;5(1):21–29.

74. Schneider PA, Rossman ME, Bernstein EF, Ringelstein EB, Torem S, Otis SM. Noninvasive evaluation of vertebrobasilar insufficiency. *J Ultrasound Med*. 1991;10(7):373–379.

75. Licht PB, Christensen HW, Hojgaard P, Marving J. Vertebral artery flow and spinal manipulation: a randomized, controlled and observer-blinded study. *J Manipulative Physiol Ther*. 1998;21(3): 141–144.

76. Refshauge KM. Rotation: a valid premanipulative dizziness test? Does it predict safe manipulation? *J Manipulative Physiol Ther.* 1994;17(1):15–19.

77. Rivett DA, Sharples KJ, Milburn PD. Effect of pre-manipulative tests on vertebral artery and internal carotid artery blood flow: a pilot study. *J Manipulative Physiol Ther.* 1999;22(6):368–375.

78. Maitland GD. *Maitland's vertebral manipulation.* 6th ed. London; Butterworth-Heinemann: 2001.

79. Grant R. Vertebral artery testing—the Australian Physiotherapy Association Protocol after 6 years. *Man Ther.* 1996;1(3):149–153.

80. Zaina C, Grant R, Johnson C, Dansie B, Taylor J, Spyropolous P. The effect of cervical rotation on blood flow in the contralateral vertebral artery. *Man Ther.* 2003;8(2):103–109.

81. Grant R. *Physical therapy of the cervical and thoracic spine.* 3rd ed. New York; Churchill Livingstone: 2002.

82. Magarey ME, Rebbeck T, Coughlan B, Grimmer K, Rivett DA, Refshauge K. Pre-manipulative testing of the cervical spine review, revision and new clinical guidelines. *Man Ther.* 2004;9(2):95–108.

83. Fischer RP. Cervical radiographic evaluation of alert patients following blunt trauma. *Ann Emerg Med.* 1984;13:905–907.

84. Fedorak C, Ashworth N, Marshall J, Paull H. Reliability of the visual assessment of cervical and lumbar lordosis: how good are we? *Spine.* 2003;28(16):1857–1859.

85. Makofsky H. The influence of forward head posture on dental occlusion. *Cranio.* 2000;18:30–39.

86. Visscher C, De Boer W, Lobbezoo F, Habets L, Naeije M. Is there a relationship between head posture and craniomandibular pain? *J Oral Rehabilitation.* 2002;29:1030–1036.

87. Michelotti A, Manzo P, Farella M, Martina R. (abstract) Occlusion and posture: is there evidence of correlation? *Minerva Stomatol.* 1999;48:525–534.

88. Nicolakis P, Nicolakis M, Piehslinger E, Ebenbichler G, Vachuda M, Kirtley C, Fialka-Moser V. Relationship between craniomandibular disorders and poor posture. *Cranio.* 2000;18:106–112.

89. Santander H, Miralles R, Perez J, Valenzuela S, Ravera M, Ormeno G, Villegas R. Effects of head and neck inclination on bilateral sternocleidomastiod EMG activity in healthy subjects and in patients with myogenic cranio-cervical mandibular dysfunction. *Cranio.* 2000;18:181–191.

90. Wright E, Domenech M, Fischer J. Usefulness of posture training for patients with temporo-mandibular disorders. *J Am Dent Assoc.* 2000;131:202–210.

91. Watson DH, Trott PH. Cervical headache: an investigation of natural head posture and upper cervical flexor muscle performance. *Cephalalgia.* 1993;13(4):272–284.

92. Marcus D, Scharff L, Mercer S, Turk D. Musculoskeletal abnormalities in chronic headache: A controlled comparison of headache diagnostic groups. *Headache.* 1998;39:21–27.

93. Werne S. Spontaneous atlas dislocation. *Acta Orthopaedica Scandinavica.* 1955;25:32–43.

94. Herzka A, Sponseller P, Pyeritz R. Atlantoaxial rotatory subluxation in patients with Marfan's syndrome. A report of three cases. *Spine.* 2000;15:524–526.

95. Muhle C, Busichoff L, Weinert D, Lindner V, Falliner A, Maier C, Ahn J, Séller M, Resnick D. Exacerbated pain in cervical radiculopathy at axial rotation, flexion, extension, and coupled motions of the cervical spine: evaluation by kinematic magnetic resonance imaging. *Invest Radiol.* 1998;33:279–288.

96. Niere KR, Torney SK. Clinicians' perceptions of minor cervical instability. *Man Ther.* 2004;9(3):144–150.

97. Paley D, Gillespie R. Chronic repetitive unrecognized flexion injury of the cervical spine (high jumper's neck). *Am J Sports Med.* 1986;14:92–95.

98. Olsen K, Joder D. Diagnosis and treatment of cervical spine clinical instability. *J Orthop Sports Phys Ther.* 2001;31(4):194–206.

99. Lestini W, Wiesel S. The pathogenesis of cervical spondylosis. *Clin Orthop.* 1989;239:69–93.

100. Montazem A. Secondary tinnitus as a symptom of instability of the upper cervical spine: operative management. *Int Tinnitus J* 2000;6(2):130–133.

101. Niere K, Selvaratnam P. The cervical region. In Zuluaga et al., *Sports physiotherapy. Applied science and practice.* Melbourne; Churchill Livingstone: 1995.

102. O'Sullivan P, Burnett A, Alexander F, Gadsdon K, Logiudice J, Miller D. Quirke H. Lumbar repositioning deficit in specific a low back pain population. *Spine.* 2003;28:1074–1079.

103. Klein G, Mannion A, Panjabi M, Dvorak J. Trapped in the neutral zone: another symptom of whiplash-associated disorder? *Eur Spine J.* 2001;10(2):141–148.

104. Emery SE. Cervical spondylotic myelopathy: diagnosis and treatment. *J Am Acad Orthop Surg.* 2001;9(6):376–388.

105. McNamara RM, Heine E, Esposito B. Cervical spine injury and radiography in alert, high-risk patients. *J Emerg Med.* 1990;8:177–182.

106. McKee TR, Tinkoff G, Rhodes M. Asymptomatic occult cervical spine fracture: case report and review of the literature. *J Trauma.* 1990;30:623–626.

107. Gbaanador GBM, Fruin AH, Taylon C. Role of routine emergency cervical radiography in head trauma. *Am J Surg.* 1986;52:643–648.

108. Bayless P, Ray VG. Incidence of cervical spine injuries in association with blunt head trauma. *Am J Emerg Med.* 1989;7:139–142.

109. Neifeld GL, Keene JG, Hevesy G, Leikin J, Proust A, Thisted RA. Cervical injury in head trauma. *J Emerg Med.* 1988;6:203–207.

110. Vandemark RM. Radiology of the cervical spine in trauma patients: practice pitfalls and recommendations for improving efficiency and communication. *AJR.* 1990;155:465–472.

111. Bandiera G, Stiell C, Wells G, Clement C, De Maio V, Vandemheen K, Greenberg G, Lesiuk H, Brison R, Cass D, Dreyer J, Eisenhauer M, MacPhail I, McKnight R, Morrison L, Reardon M, Schull M, Worthington J. Canadian C-Spine and CT Head Study Group, The Canadian C-Spine rule performs better than unstructured physician judgment, *Annals Emergency Medicine.* 2003;42:395–402.

112. Sandmark H, Nisell R. Validity of five common manual neck pain provoking tests. *Scand J Rehabil Med.* 1995;27(3):131–136.

113. Lee RY, McGregor AH, Bull AM, Wragg P. Dynamic response of the cervical spine to posteroanterior mobilisation. *Clin Biomech.* 2005;20(2):228–231.

114. Sterling M, Jull G, Carlsson Y, Crommert L. Are cervical physical outcome measures influenced by the presence of symptomatology? *Physiother Res Int.* 2002;7(3):113–121.

115. Yelland M. Back, chest and abdominal pain. How good are spinal signs at identifying musculoskeletal causes of back, chest or abdominal pain? *Aust Fam Physician.* 2001;30:980–912.

116. Patla C, Paris S. Reliability of interpretation of the Paris classification of normal end feel for elbow flexion and extension. *J Manual Manipulative Ther.* 1993;1:60–66.

117. Hayes W, Petersen C, Falconer J. An examination of Cyriax's passive motion tests with patients having osteoarthritis of the knee including commentary by Twomey LT with author response. *Phys Ther.* 1994;74:697–708.

118. Olson K, Paris S, Spohr C, Gorniak G. Radiographic assessment and reliability study of the craniovertebral sidebending test. *J Manual Manipulative Ther.* 1998;6:87–96.

119. Chesworth B, MacDermid J, Roth J, Patterson SD. Movement diagram and "end-feel" reliability when measuring passive lateral rotation of the shoulder in patients with shoulder pathology. *Phys Ther.* 1998;78:593–601.

120. Cooperman J, Riddle D, Rothstein J. Reliability and validity of judgments of the integrity of the anterior cruciate ligament of the knee using the Lachman's test. *Phys Ther.* 1990;70:225–233.

121. Petersen C, Hayes K. Construct validity of Cyriax's selective tension examination: association of end-feels with pain at the knee and shoulder. *J Orthop Sports Phys Ther.* 2000;30:512–527.

122. Hall T, Robinson K. The flexion-rotation test and active cervical mobility—a comparative measurement study in cervicogenic headache. *Man Ther.* 2004;9(4):197–202.

123. Tong HC, Haig AJ, Yamakawa K. The Spurling test and cervical radiculopathy. *Spine.* 2002;27(2): 156–159.

124. Fjellner A, Bexander C, Faleij R, Strender LE. Interexaminer reliability in physical examination of the cervical spine. *J Manipulative Physiol Ther.* 1999;22 (8):511–516.

125. Haas M, Groupp E, Panzer D, Partna L, Lumsden S, Aickin M. Efficacy of cervical endplay assessment as an indicator for spinal manipulation. *Spine.* 2003; 28(11):1091–1096.

126. Childs J. Risk associated with the failure to offer manipulation for patients with low back pain. Platform Presentation. American Academy of Orthopaedic Manual Physical Therapists Conference. Louisville, KY. 2004.

127. Cleland J, Childs J, McRae M, Palmer J. Immediate effects of thoracic spine manipulation in patients with neck pain: a randomized clinical trial. Platform Presentation. American Academy of Orthopaedic Manual Physical Therapists Conference. Louisville, KY. 2004.

128. Hartman L. *Handbook of osteopathic technique.* 2nd ed. San Diego, CA; Singular Pub Group: 1985.

129. Jull G, Bogduk N, Marsland A. The accuracy of manual diagnosis for cervical zygopophyseal joint pain syndromes. *Med J Aust.* 1988;148(5):233–236.

130. Jull G. Treleaven J. Versace G. Manual examination: is pain provocation a major cue for spinal dysfunction? *Aust J Physiotherapy.* 1994;40(3):159–165.

131. Matyas T, Bach T. The reliability of selected techniques in clinical arthrometrics. *Aust J Physiotherapy.* 1985;31:175–199.

132. Maher C, Latimer J. Pain or resistance-the manual therapists' dilemma. *Aust J Physiotherapy.* 1992;38: 257–260.

133. Anson E, Cook C, Comacho C et al. The use of education in the improvement in finding R1 in the lumbar spine. *J Manual Manipulative Ther.* 2003;11 (4):204–212.

134. Vicenzino B, Collins D, Wright A. An investigation of the interrelationship between manipulative therapy-induced hypoalgesia and sympathoexcitation. *J Manipulative Physiol Ther.* 1998;21:448–453.

135. Vicenzino B, Collins D, Wright A. The initial effects of a cervical spine manipulative physiotherapy treatment on the pain and dysfunction of lateral epicondylalgia. *Pain.* 1996;68:69–74.

136. Wright A, Vicenzino B. Cervical mobilization techniques, sympathetic nervous system effects, and their relationship to analgesia. In: Shacklock M, (ed). *Moving in on pain.* Melbourne; Butterworth Heinemann: 1995.

137. Maigne R. Diagnosis and treatment of pain or vertebral origin. *A manual medicine approach.* Balitimore; Williams and Wilkins: 1996.

138. De Laat A, Meuleman H, Stevens A, Verbeke G. Correlation between cervical spine and temporomandibular disorders. *Clin Oral Investig.* 1998;2(2): 54–57.

139. Humphreys B, Delahaye M, Peterson C. An investigation into the validity of cervical spine motion palpation using subjects with congenital block vertebrae as a 'gold standard'. *BMC Musculoskeletal Disorder.* 2004;5:19–25.

140. Wainner R, Fritz J, Irrgang J, Boninger M, Delitto A, Allison S. Reliability and diagnostic accuracy of the clinical examination and patient self-report measures for cervical radiculopathy. *Spine.* 2003;28: 52–62.

141. Davidson R, Dunn E, Metzmaker J. The shoulder abduction test in the diagnosis of radicular pain in cervical extradural compression monomradiculopathies. *Spine.* 1981;6:441–446.

142. Yoss R, Corbin K, MacCarty C, Love J. Significance of symptoms and signs in localization of involved root in cervical disc protrusion. *Neurology.* 1957;7 (10):673–683.

143. Lauder T, Dillingham T, Andary M, Kumar S, Pezzin L, Stephens R. Predicting electrodiagnostic outcome in patients with upper limb symptoms: are the history and physical examination helpful? *Arch Phys Med Rehabil.* 2000;81:436–441.

144. Hong C, Lee S, Lum P. Cervical radiculopathy: clinical, radiographic and EMG findings. *Orthop Rev.* 1986;15:433–439.

145. Partanen J, Partanen K, Oikarinen H, Niemitukia L, Hernesniemi J. Preoperative electro-neuromyography and myelography in cervical root compression. *Electromyogr Clin Neurophysiol.* 1991;31:21–26.

146. Rezasoltani A, Ahmadi A, Jafarigol A, Vihko V. The reliability of measuring neck muscle strength with a neck muscle force measurement device. *J Phys Ther Sci.* 2003;15:7–12.

147. Silverman JL, Rodriques AA, Agre JC. Quantitative cervical flexor strength in healthy subjects and in subjects with mechanical neck pain. *Arch Phys Med Rehabil.* 1991;72:679–681.

148. Ylinen J, Ruuska J. Clinical use of neck isometric strength measurement in rehabilitation. *Arch Phys Med Rehabil.* 1993;74:425–430.

149. Semmes R, Murphy F. The syndrome of unilateral rupture of the sixth cervical intervertebral. *JAMA.* 1943;121:1209–1214.

150. Michelsen J, Mixter W. Pain and disability of shoulder and pain due to herniation of the nucleus pulposis of cervical intervertebral disks. *N Engl J Med.* 1944;231:279–287.

151. Spurling R, Scoville W. Lateral rupture of the cervical intervertebral discs. *Surg Gyencol Obstet.* 1944;78: 350–358.

152. Waylonis G. Electromyographic findings in chronic cervical radicular syndromes. *Arch Phys Med Rehabil.* 1968;49:407–412.

153. Yoss R, Corbin K, MacCarty C, Love J. Significance of symptoms and signs in localization of involved root in cervical disc protrusion. *Neurology.* 1957; 7(10):673–683.

154. Lauder T, Dillingham T, Andary M, Kumar S, Pezzin L, Stephens R. Predicting electrodiagnostic outcome in patients with upper limb symptoms: are the history and physical examination helpful? *Arch Phys Med Rehabil.* 2000;81:436–441.

155. Hong C, Lee S, Lum P. Cervical radiculopathy: clinical, radiographic and EMG findings. *Orthop Rev.* 1986;15:433–439.

156. Nygaard O, Mellgren S. The function of sensory nerve fibers in lumbar radiculopathy: Use of quantitative sensory testing gin the exploration of different populations of nerve fibers and dermatomes. *Spine.* 1998;23:348–352.

157. Zwart J, Sand T, Unsgaard G. Warm and cold thresholds in patients with unilateral sciatica: C-fibers are more severely affected than A-delta fibers. *Acta Neurol Scand.* 1998;97:41–45.

158. Mosek A, Yarnitsky D, Korczyn A, Niv D. The assessment of radiating low back pain by thermal sensory testing. *Eur J Pain.* 2001;5:347–351.

159. Schiff E, Eisenberg E. Can quantitative sensory testing predict the outcome of epidural steroid injections in sciatica? A preliminary study. *Anesth Analg* 2003:97:828–832.

160. Viikari-Juntura E, Porras M, Laasonen EM. Validity of clinical tests in the diagnosis of root compression in cervical disc disease. *Spine.* 1989;14(3):253–257.

161. Kleinrensink GJ, Stoeckart R, Vleeming A, Snijders CJ, Mulder PG. Mechanical tension in the median nerve. The effects of joint positions. *Clin Biomech.* 1995;10(5):240–244.

162. Butler D. *Mobilsation of the nervous system.* Melbourne; Churchill Livingston: 1991.

163. McGee D. *Orthopedic physical assessment.* 4th ed. Philadelphia; Saunders: 2002.

164. Cattrysse E, Swinkels R, Oostendorp R, Duquet W. Upper cervical instability: are clinical tests reliable? *Man Ther.* 1997;2(2):91–97.

165. Hall T, Robinson K. The flexion-rotation test and active cervical mobility—A comparative measurement study in cervicogenic headache. *Man Ther.* 2004;9:197–202.

166. Maitland GD. *Peripheral manipulation* 3rd ed. London; Butterworth-Heinemann: 1986.

167. Edmondston SJ, Allison GT, Gregg CD, Purden SM, Svansson GR, Watson AE. Effect of position on the posteroanterior stiffness of the lumbar spine. *Man Ther.* 1998;3(1):21–26.

168. Trott P. Management of selected cervical syndromes. In: Grant R. *Physical therapy of the cervical and thoracic spine.* 3rd ed. New York; Churchill Livingstone: 2002.

169. Childs J, Fritz J, Piva S, Whitman J. Proposal of a classification system for patients with neck pain. *J Orthop Sports Phys Ther.* 2004;34:686–700.

170. Shakoor M, Ahmed M, Kibria G, Khan A, Mian M, Hasan S, Nahar S, Hossian M. (abstract). Effects of cervical traction and exercise therapy in cervical spondylosis. *Bangladesh Med Res Counc Bull.* 2002; 28:61–69.

171. Harrison D, Cailliet R, Betz J, Haas J, Harrison D, Janik T, Holland B, Conservative methods of reducing lateral translation postures of the head: A non-randomized clinical control trial. *J Rehabil Res Dev.* 2004;41:631–639.

172. Grant R, Jull G, Spencer T. Active stabilizing training for screen based keyboard operators—A single case study. *Aust J Physiotherapy.* 1997;43:235–242.

173. Jull G, Trott P, Potter H, Zito G, Niere K, Shirley D, Emberson J, Marschner I, Richardson C. A randomized controlled trial of exercise and manipulative therapy for cervicogenic headache. *Spine.* 2002; 27:1835–1843.

174. Abdulwahab S, Sabbahi M. Neck retractions, cervical root decompression, and radicular pain. *J Orthop Sports Phys Ther.* 2000;30:4–12.

175. Pearson N, Walmsley R. Trial into the effects of repeated neck retractions in normal subjects. *Spine.* 1995;20:1245–1250.

176. Clare H, Adams R, Maher C. A systematic review of efficacy of McKenzie therapy for spinal pain. *Aust J Physiotherapy.* 2004;50:209–216.

177. McKenzie R. The cervical and thoracic spine. *Mechanical diagnosis and therapy.* Waikanae; Spinal Publications: 1990.

178. O'Leary S, Falla D, Jull G. Recent advances in therapeutic exercise for the neck: implications for patients with head and neck pain. *Aust Endod J.* 2003;29:138–142.

179. Stanton W, Jull G. Cervicogenic headache: Locus of control and success of treatment. *Headache.* 2003;43: 956–961.

180. Jull G. Management of cervicogenic headaches. In: Grant R. *Physical therapy of the cervical and thoracic spine.* 3rd ed. New York; Churchill Livingstone: 2002.

181. Swank A, Funk D, Durham M, Roberts S. Adding weights to stretching exercise increases passive range of motion for healthy elderly. *J Strength Cond Res.* 2003;17:374–378.

182. Levoska S, Keinanen-Kiukaanniemi S. Active or passive physiotherapy for occupational cervicobrachial disorders? A comparison of two treatment methods with a 1-year follow-up. *Arch Phys Med Rehabil.* 1993;74:425–430.

183. Vicenzino B, Collins D, Wright A. Sudomotor changes induced by neural mobilization techniques in asymptomatic subjects. *J Manual Manipulative Ther.* 1994;2:66–74.

184. Simon R, Vicenzino B, Wright A. The influence of an anteroposterior accessory glide of the glenohumeral joint on measures of peripheral sympathetic nervous system function in the upper limb. *Man Ther.* 1997;2(1):18–23.

185. Solly S. Cervical postero-anterior mobilization: A brief review of evidence of physiological and pain relieving effects. *Physical Therapy Reviews.* 2004;9: 182–187.

186. Vicenzino B, Paungmali A, Buratowski S, Wright A. Specific manipulative therapy treatment for chronic lateral epicondylalgia produces uniquely characteristic hypoalgesia. *Man Ther.* 2001;6:205–212.

187. Lovick T. Interactions between descending pathways from the dorsal and ventrolateral periaqueductal gray matter in the rat. In: Depaulis A, Bandler R. (eds) *The midbrain periaqueductal gray matter.* Plenum Press, New York: 1991.

188. Magarey ME, Rebbeck T, Coughlan B, Grimmer K, Rivett DA, Refshauge K. Pre-manipulative testing of the cervical spine review, revision and new clinical guidelines. *Man Ther.* 2004;9(2):95–108.

189. Boline PD, Haas M, Meyer JJ, Kassak K, Nelson C, Keating JC. Interexaminer reliability of eight evaluative dimensions of lumbar segmental abnormality: Part II. *J Manipulative Physiol Ther.* 1993;16(6): 363–374.

190. Jull G, Zito G, Trott P, Potter H, Shirley D. Interexaminer reliability to detect painful cervical joint dysfunction. *Aust J Physiotherapy.* 1997;43: 125–129.

191. Lee R, Evans J. An in-vivo study of the intervertebral movements produced by posteroanterior mobilisation. *Clin Biomech.* 1997;12:400–408.

192. McGregor A, Wragg P, Gedroyc W. Can interventional MRI provide an insight into the mechanics of a posterior–anterior mobilisation? *Clin Biomech.* 2001;16, 926–929.

193. Goodridge JP. Muscle energy technique: definition, explanation, methods of procedure. *J Am Osteopath Assoc.* 1981;81(4):249–254.

194. Ferber R, Osternig L, Gravelle D. Effect of PNF stretch techniques on knee flexor muscle EMG activity in older adults. *J Electromyography. Kinesiology.* 2002;12:391–397.

195. Triano JJ, Rogers CM, Combs S, Potts D, Sorrels K. Quantitative feedback versus standard training for cervical and thoracic manipulation. *J Manipulative Physiol Ther.* 2003;26(3):131–138.

196. Triano JJ, Rogers CM, Combs S, Potts D, Sorrels K. Developing skilled performance of lumbar spine manipulation. *J Manipulative Physiol Ther.* 2002;25(6):353–361.

197. Cleland J, Childs J, McRae M, Palmer J, Stowell T. Immediate effects of thoracic manipulation in patients with neck pain: A randomized clinical trial. *Man Ther.* 2005;10:127–135.

198. Hiraoka K, Nagata A. Modulation of the flexor carpi radialis reflex induced by cervical traction. *J Phys Ther Sci.* 1998;10:41–45.

199. Sarigiovannis P, Hollins B. Effectiveness of manual therapy in the treatment of non-specific neck pain: A review. *Physical Therapy Reviews.* 2005;10:35–50.

200. Hurwitz EL, Morgenstern H, Harber P, Kominski GF, Belin TR, Yu F, Adams AH. A randomized trial of medical care with and without physical therapy and chiropractic care with and without physical modalities for patients with low back pain: 6-month follow-up outcomes from the UCLA low back pain study. *Spine.* 2002;27(20):2193–2204.

201. Gross AR, Hoving JL, Haines TA, Goldsmith CH, Kay T, Aker P, Bronfort G. A Cochrane review of manipulation and mobilization for mechanical neck disorders. *Spine.* 2004;29(14):1541–1548.

202. Cleland JA, Whitman JM, Fritz JM. Effectiveness of manual physical therapy to the cervical spine in the management of lateral epicondylalgia: a retrospective analysis. *J Orthop Sports Phys Ther.* 2004;34(11):713–722.

203. Giles LG, Muller R. Chronic spinal pain: a randomized clinical trial comparing medication, acupuncture, and spinal manipulation. *Spine.* 2003;28(14):1490–1502.

204. Joghataei MT, Arab AM, Khaksar H. The effect of cervical traction combined with conventional therapy on grip strength on patients with cervical radiculopathy. *Clin Rehabil.* 2004;18(8):879–887.

205. Hurwitz EL, Aker PD, Adams AH, Meeker WC, Shekelle PG. Manipulation and mobilization of the cervical spine. A systematic review of the literature. *Spine.* 1996;21(15):1746–1759.

206. Allison GT, Nagy BM, Hall T. A randomized clinical trial of manual therapy for cervico-brachial pain syndrome—a pilot study. *Man Ther.* 2002;7(2):95–102.

207. Harris K, Heer D, Roy T, Santos D, Whitman J, Wainner R. Reliability of a measurement of neck flexor muscle endurance. *Phys Ther.* 2005;85:1349–1355.

# 7

# Manual Therapy
# of the Temporomandibular Joint

## Objectives

- Understand the prevalence of temporomandibular disorders (TMD) and the percentage of those that seek medical attention in the general population.
- Understand the normal and pathological kinematics associated with temporomandibular joint (TMJ) movement.
- Recognize the patient subjective characteristics associated with TMD.

- Understand the pertinent cervical and TMJ clinical examination features.
- Recognize the techniques of treatment that have yielded the highest success in the literature.

## PREVALENCE

**Temporomandibular disorders** (TMD) is the umbrella term used to describe a clinical disorder associated with the extraarticular and intraarticular aspects of the temporomandibular joint (TMJ) and corresponding masticatory muscle systems.[1] *The International Association for the Study of Pain* defines TMD as "aching in the muscles of mastication, sometimes with occasional brief severe pain on chewing, often associated with restricted jaw movement and clicking or popping sounds."[2] One or more of the following generally manifest temporomandibular disorders: (1) joint sounds, (2) limitations of joint movements, (3) muscle tenderness, (4) joint tenderness, and (5) pain just anterior to the **auricular canal.**[3,4]

It is suspected that up to 50–75% of the general population have experienced at least one bout of unilateral TMD and at least 33% have reported at least one continuing persistent symptom.[5–9] Dao and LeResche[10] re-

ported that 8–15% of women develop chronic symptoms associated with TMD compared to 3–10% of men. TMD tends to increase with age,[11] although only approximately 5% of the general population with symptoms will pursue medical care for the condition.[12] TMD tends to affect women more often than men,[13] specifically women over the age of 50.[14] Younger women age 20–40 are most likely to report TMD symptoms; the least likely are adolescents and elderly men.[13] Some have suggested a relationship between hormones in women and TMD, although this relationship is not absolute.[13]

The causes of TMD are still debated, although it is suspected that a major contributor is repeated jaw clinching and grinding associated with stress.[15] In addition to creation of TMD problems, stress is considered a prime factor in maintenance and amplification of the symptoms. One significant problem associated with TMD is that the condition is multifactorial and is generally recognized as a physical, psychological, and functional disorder.[15]

## Summary

- TMD is a condition associated with pain, joint sounds, joint tenderness, and decreased mobility of the temporomandibular joint.
- Symptoms associated with TMD are very common in the lay population but only approximately 5% of individuals seek medical attention for these symptoms.
- Stress and related phenomena are related to TMD.

# ANATOMY

The TMJ is actually two separate (right and left) but similar joints and is a freely mobile articulation. The TMJ consists of the condyle of the mandible and the squamous portion of the temporal bone of the skull (Figure 7.1).[16] Both mandible condyles project vertically for articulation with the temporal bone and assist in creating congruency between the two structures.

## The Articular Disc

The **articular disc** of the TMJ separates the joint into an upper and lower compartment and during nonpathologic circumstances does not communicate.[16] The disc (Figure 7.2) is biconcave and is made of flexible, dense collagenous connective tissue. Both the anterior and posterior aspects of the disc are innervated, the posterior more extensively.[17] The posterior aspect is thicker than the anterior and the central aspect is thinner than both peripheral regions. The disc is attached to the lateral and medial poles of the mandibular condyle, which allows movements in an anterior and posterior direction. During aging, the disc is less flexible and thickens throughout the structure. The disc is responsible for reoccurring clicking and popping sounds, specifically during improper movement or during instability.[18]

## Intraarticular Region

The **intraarticular region** (Figure 7.3) that lies posterior to the articular disc is commonly referred to as the **retrodiscal area**.[19] This highly innervated region contains synovial fluid, a synovial membrane, blood vessels, nerves, loose connective tissue, fat, and ligaments.[20] The retrodiscal region demonstrates poor tolerance to constant load or tensile stresses[19] that occur during overstretch. Overstretching generally manifests during excessive mouth opening or compression, potentially a consequence of trauma. Trauma or overstretching may lead to inflammation of the retrodiscal region and is frequently a cause of persistent TMD symptoms.[19] Nonetheless, this region does require frequent loading and unloading for nutrition, a requirement that is generally fulfilled during chewing movements and daily mandible motion.

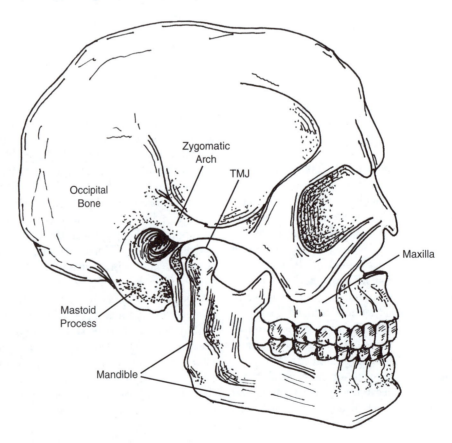

**Figure 7.1**   The Mandible and the Squamous Portion of the Temporal Bone

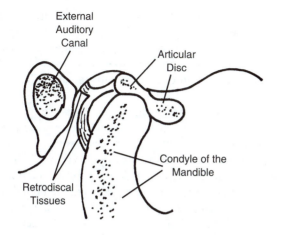

**Figure 7.2**    The Articular Disc of the TMJ

## Ligaments

Several ligaments serve to reduce movement of the TMJ. The TMJ ligament extends from the lateral joint capsule as a thickening of the capsule, the sphenomandibular ligament extends from the greater wing of the sphenoid to the mandible, and the stylomandibular ligament extends from the styloid process to the mandible.[16]

## Muscles

Three muscles are responsible for jaw closing: the temporalis, the powerful masseter, and the medial pterygoid. Several smaller muscles contribute to jaw opening including the lateral pterygoid, the geniohyoid, the genioglossus, the anterior bellies of the digastric, and the mylohyoid muscles.[16] Protrusion is accomplished through contraction of the lateral and medial pterygoids and retraction is a function of temporalis (posterior fiber) contraction.[19] Lateral movements are a consequence of alternative contraction of the medial and lateral pterygoids.

## BIOMECHANICS

During normal opening kinematics of the TMJ, the condyle of the mandible, which normally is suspended from the concave articular fossa by joint capsule and ligaments, rolls posteriorly on the articular disc then glides forward (with the disc) within the articular fossa.[16] Subsequently, the condyle rolls and slides up to 6–9 mm in opposite directions while concurrently providing a stretch on the posterior–superior anchoring structures.[19] The disc has free motion in anterior and posterior directions but moves very little in the directions of medial to lateral (Figure 7.4).

For achievement of maximal mouth opening, angular rotation must be greater than angular swing.[21] If condylar

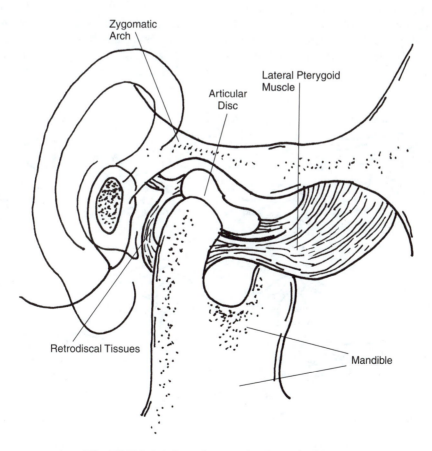

**Figure 7.3**    The TMJ Joint Capsule, Ligaments, and Intraarticular Region

## Summary

- The TMJ is created by the bony articulation of the mandibular condyle and the squamous portion of the temporal bone.
- A mobile, biconcave disc separates the TMJ into an upper and lower compartment.
- Several ligaments contribute to movement control. These ligaments are sometimes injured during compressive and tension-related dysfunction.
- The primary muscles associated with closure of the jaw include the masseter and the medial pterygoid.
- The primary muscles associated with opening of the jaw include the lateral pterygoid, the geniohyoid, the genioglossus, the anterior bellies of the digastric, and the mylohyoid muscles.

movement occurred without subsequent roll, the condyle would move posteriorly and impinge structures. The passive restraint associated with the sphenomandibular ligament provides the necessary mechanism for stability of the jaw.[21]

The loose- and closed-packed positions of the TMJ are currently debated. Rocabado[22] suggested that the closed-packed position of the jaw is during full mouth opening whereas others suggest variations of mouth opening. The loose-packed position is generally suspected to consist of slight retraction of the jaw with tongue placement near the roofline of the mouth.

Normal range of mouth opening is both age and gender dependent. Gallagher et al.[23] reported that men range from 41 to 44 mm of mouth opening (ages 16 to 65+) whereas women range from 39 to 43 mm (ages 15 to 65+). Mouth opening declines steadily with age and is less in individuals who report TMD.[23]

Pathological movement may cause excessive loading or tension to the retrodiscal structures. Damage may exacerbate the potential of anterior disc displacement, which is the most problematic intraarticular dysfunction.[19] When the disc fails to reduce accordingly during condylar motion, the condyle pushes the disc anteriorly down the temporal articular surface during the process of mouth opening (Figure 7.5).[19] This action further stretches the retrodiscal tissue until the disc pops loose of the condyle, causing an audible click.

## Summary

- During normal kinematics of the TMJ the condyle of the mandible, which normally is suspended from the concave articular fossa by joint capsule and ligaments, rolls posteriorly on the articular disc then glides forward (with the disc) within the articular fossa.
- Pathological kinematics involves the failure of the disc to reduce accordingly during condylar motion. In essence, the condyle pushes the disc anteriorly down the temporal articular surface during the process of mouth opening and the condyle moves posterior to compress the retrodiscal structures.

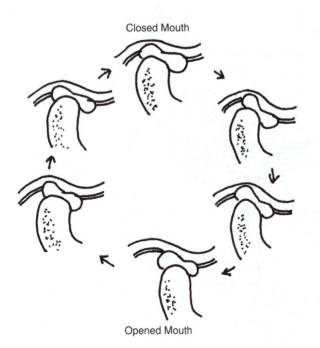
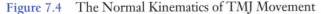

**Figure 7.4**   The Normal Kinematics of TMJ Movement

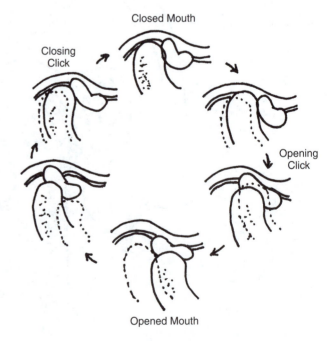

**Figure 7.5**   Pathological Movement of the TMJ

# ASSESSMENT AND DIAGNOSIS

## Subjective Considerations

The primary patient subjective complaints associated with TMD include one or more of the following: joint sounds, limitation of jaw movement, muscle tenderness, and pain in the periauricular region.[24] Others have reported symptoms such as bruxism (teeth grinding), sensitive teeth, and burning mouth symptoms associated with TMD.[14] Any of these findings should be evaluated during a carefully constructed patient history.

Because concurrent symptoms with pain of cervical spine origin may exist with TMD, further questioning should reflect pain provocations associated with the cervical spine.[25] Conditions such as radiculopathy and myelopathy are most likely of cervical spine origin since they are commonly associated with nerve root or spinal cord compression. Additionally, pain that occurs near the end of a day, during sleep, or during cervical movements may be associated with the cervical spine and should be carefully evaluated.

## *Psychosocial Factors*

Since psychosocial factors are considered common covariates in the cause and contribution of TMD, a careful examination of selected psychosocial factors is suggested. Wright et al.[15] reported that high-risk patients with TMD were more likely to have anxiety disorders and were four times more likely to exhibit a personality disorder such as avoidant, dependent, or obsessive–compulsive traits. Those with high-risk TMD also were more depressed and reported higher pain levels than controlled subjects. Rantala et al.[26] acknowledged the influence of somatization in patients with TMD, noting the concurrence of TMD symptoms and myofascial complaints of pain. Lastly, Ahlberg et al.[27] reported that smoking and high reported stress levels were associated with concurrent higher report of pain compared to controls, thus necessitating smoking cessation and stress rehabilitation.

## *Functional Assessment Tools*

### *TMD Disability Index*

The TMD Disability Index was created in 1997 and involves 10 functionally related questions associated with TMD.[28] The scale is a self-report, disease-specific instrument with five possible selections for each question, each with increasing severity. At present, the TMD Disability Index has not been validated, thus the reliability, validity, and responsiveness is unknown.

### *Beck Depression Scale*

The Beck Depression Inventory (BDI) is a 21-item questionnaire that demonstrates high content validity differentiating depressed from nondepressed individuals, good internal consistency,[29] the ability to detect negative attitudes toward self, performance impairment, and somatic disturbances, as well as a general factor of depression.[30] Generally, values over 40 are considered significant for depression and may potentially identify personality disorders.[31] The BDI is not a specific tool for TMD, but is an effective tool to measure the common comorbidity of depression.

### *Anxiety Questionnaire*

The Anxiety Sensitivity Scale (ASI)[32] is a 16-item self-report questionnaire designed to assess the construct of anxiety sensitivity: the dispositional tendency to fear the somatic and cognitive symptoms of anxiety due to a belief that these symptoms may be dangerous or harmful. Each item is rated on a 5-point Likert scale ranging from 0 (very little) to 4 (very much). The ASI is the most widely used measure of the anxiety sensitivity construct, and the instrument's psychometric properties and predictive validity have been well established.[33] The ASI may consist of anywhere from a single factor to four factors depending on the sample in which the factor analysis was run.[34] At present, this scale and others have not been validated for patients with TMD.

## *Summary*

- Common patient subjective complaints associated with TMD include joint sounds, limitation of jaw movement, muscle tenderness, pain in the periauricular region, bruxism, sensitive teeth, and burning mouth.
- Several psychosocial co-contributors are present in TMD including anxiety, depression, personality disorders, and stress.
- The use of a depression scale, anxiety scale, and TMD Disability Index may improve the ability to measure covariates and function. None of these scales have been validated specifically for the TMD population.

## Objective/Physical Examination

### *Diagnosis*

At present there is no true undeniable "criterion standard" for detection of TMD.[35] Comparison with MRI is purportedly the most accurate method for identification of disc impairments[36] and osteoarthritis, but yields little value in detecting pain of myofascial origin.

Selected clinical tests have shown merit in identifying patients with significant symptoms associated with TMD. Four tests—passive maximal mouth opening, palpation of the TMJ and masticatory muscles, TMJ joint play, and TMJ compression—were significantly associated with patient report of pain in the TMD.[37] Others have advocated the use of palpation but suggest that active maximal mouth opening yields comparable value with passive movements.[38] Including joint noises with the previously suggested categories may improve the capability of identifying an intraarticular disorder.[39] All the clinical criteria exhibit similar fair to moderate reliability whether performed by a physical therapist, dentist, or surgeon.[40] Because TMD can be both extraarticular and intraarticular, no one test stands out as a significantly strong predictor for TMD.

Roberts et al.[41] suggest that clinical findings are not discriminatory enough to identify patients with a variety of dysfunctions associated with TMD. Others agree, indicating that clinicians are poor at discriminating between conditions such as osteoarthritis and internal derangement and whether the presence of an anteriorly translated disc exists.[42,43] The trend within the literature suggests that clinicians are effective in identifying the presence of TMD but lack the discrimination to identify the origin and type of dysfunction.

## Observation

### Posture

Several studies have suggested a relationship of posture to TMD.[44-47] Others have suggested no or poor relationships between posture and TMD.[48,49] Most postural dysfunctions are associated with concurrent forward head and elevated trapezius tension.[50,51] Forward head and corresponding muscle activity negatively influences masticatory function,[44] thus potentially placing subjects at risk for muscle strain and tension to the masticatory system. Friction and colleagues[52] identified 85% of subjects with TMJ to have forward head posture, thus elevating the risk of masticatory dysfunction.

### Resting Position of the Teeth

During observation, assessment of the resting position of the teeth (Figure 7.6) may assist the clinician in determining if the patient is predisposed to TMD. Conditions such as overbites, underbites, and other dental abnormalities may alter the bite and function of the temporomandibular joint.

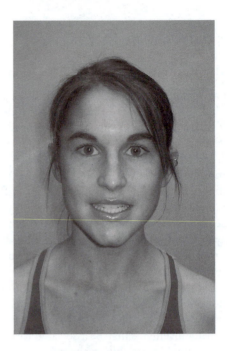

**Figure 7.7**   Normal Symmetry of Bite at Rest

### Symmetry of Movement

Observation of symmetry of jaw movement (Figure 7.7), bite, and facial muscle composition may also provide useful information. Most individuals with TMD have overactive muscles of mastication and may demonstrate hypertrophy of the masseter. Asymmetric bites may alarm the clinician to internal derangements during moving of the jaw.

> ## Summary
>
> - There is no single criterion standard for TMD.
> - Selected clinical tests such as passive maximal mouth opening, palpation of the TMJ and masticatory muscles, TMJ joint play, and TMJ compression were significantly associated with patient report of pain in the TMD have been associated with appropriate diagnosis of TMD.
> - Observations such as asymmetries of teeth, jaw movement, muscle hypertrophy, and posture may yield useful information when examining TMD.

# Clinical Examination

## Active Physiological Movements

### Cervical Spine

There is significant overlap between pain associated with TMD and cervicogenic pain.[25,53] Because of this, it is necessary to perform a cervical screen to identify the potential contribution or pain in isolation of the cervical spine.

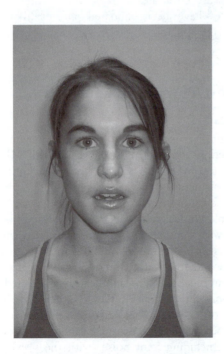

**Figure 7.6**   Normal Resting Position of the Teeth

Cervicogenic pain may arise from a number of causes including trauma,[24] posture,[44] and degenerative changes. Since posture of the cervical spine and related muscular spasm can increase the risk for muscle strain and tension to the masticatory system, it is essential to rule out the presence of a cervical disorder prior to evaluation of the temporomandibular joint.

The reader is suggested to refer back to Chapter 6, specifically the active physiological examination of the cervical spine. Of the cervical physiological movements, cervical rotation may yield the most influential findings during examination. Braun and Schiffman[54] reported that cervical rotation and flexion and extension measures of mobility were useful predictors to determine masticatory muscle tenderness. In addition to rotation, active physiological movements such as extension, flexion, and side flexion with overpressure are necessary to determine the contribution of the cervical spine to the presenting patient symptoms.

## Examination of the Temporomandibular Joint

The clinical examination is the most important diagnostic component of evaluation of TMJ pain.[16] The clinical examination is directed toward assessment of symmetry of motion and reproduction of pain during the movement

## Summary

- An appropriate examination of the cervical spine is necessary to "rule out" cervical involvement and to determine if contribution from the cervical spine is prominent.
- The movements of active physiological rotation and to a lesser extent flexion and extension are associated with increased masseter pain.

cycle. Pain with active and passive movements may identify retrodiscal structures as the source of symptoms since these structures are tensioned or compressed during movement. Selection of the appropriate treatment modality (i.e., stretching, strengthening, or physical agents) hedges on the findings of the clinical evaluation.[16]

## Active Movements of a Nondisplaced Disc

All four active movements of depression, protrusion, and medial and lateral translation may stress the posterior–superior ligamentous structures. These motions should be assessed for pain production and asymmetry of movement.

### Depression (Mouth Closing Measurement of Deviation)

Depression involves the closing of the mouth, incorporating contact between the upper and lower teeth (if present) of the patient.

- Step One: Resting symptoms are assessed.
- Step Two: The clinician instructs the patient to bite down hard.
- Step Three: If necessary, with a gloved hand, the clinician views the bite formation for symmetry.
- Step Four: The patient is queried regarding production of concordant symptoms.

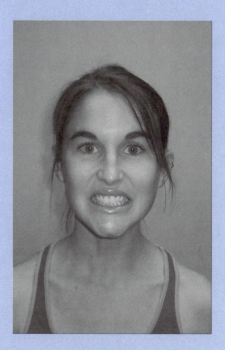

**Figure 7.8**    TMJ Depression

## Protrusion

**Protrusion** involves the anterior displacement of the lower jaw and subsequent unloading of retrodiscal tissues.

- Step One: Resting symptoms are assessed.
- Step Two: The clinician instructs the patient to stick his or her chin outward as far as they can. The clinician may be required to demonstrate the movement for the patient.
- Step Three: The clinician views the bite formation for symmetry.
- Step Four: The patient is queried regarding production of concordant symptoms.

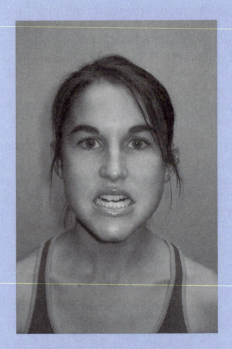

**Figure 7.9**    TMJ Protrusion

- Step Five: With a gloved hand, the clinician measures the protrusive displacement of the patient.

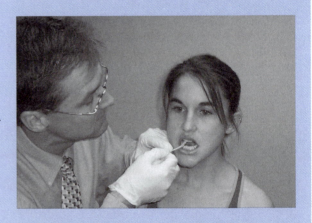

**Figure 7.10**    TMJ Protrusion: Measurement

## Medial Translation and Lateral Translation

Medial and lateral translation involves the medial and lateral movement of the lower jaw with respect to the maxilla.

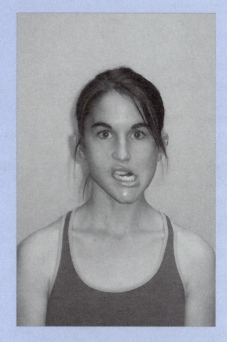

- Step One: Resting symptoms are assessed.
- Step Two: The clinician instructs the patient to translate his or her jaw as far as they can to the left.
- Step Three: The clinician views the bite formation for symmetry.
- Step Four: The patient is queried regarding production of concordant symptoms.

**Figure 7.11**    TMJ Medial and Lateral Translation

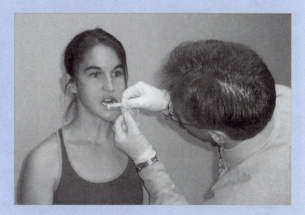

- Step Five: Using a gloved hand, the clinician measures the translation using the landmarks of the front two bottom and top teeth.
- Step Six: The process is repeated in the opposite direction (right).

**Figure 7.12**    TMJ Medial and Lateral Translation: Measurement

## Mouth Opening (Measurement)

Masumi et al.[55] reported that differences in mouth opening were not discriminatory enough to identify a selected type of TMD, indicating that all forms of TMD demonstrate restrictions in maximal mouth opening. The sphenomandibular ligament provides the necessary mechanism for stability of the jaw and may be painful at end ranges of mouth opening (without disc involvement) or during forced retrusion.[21]

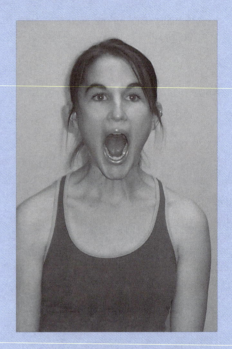

- Step One: Resting symptoms are assessed.
- Step Two: The clinician instructs the patient to open his or her mouth as wide as possible.
- Step Three: With a gloved hand, the clinician views the bite formation for symmetry by moving the lips away from the teeth.
- Step Four: The patient is queried regarding production of concordant symptoms.

**Figure 7.13**     TMJ Maximal Mouth Opening

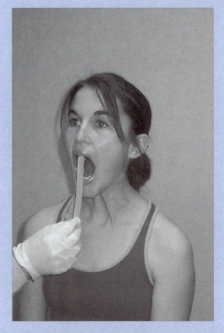

- Step Five: The patient is evaluated for symmetry during opening.

**Figure 7.14**     TMJ Maximal Mouth Opening: Assessment of Symmetry

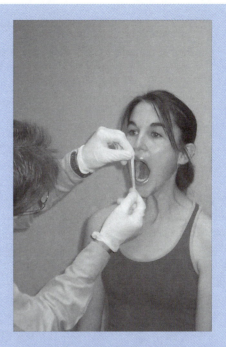

**Figure 7.15** TMJ Maximal Mouth Opening: Measurement

- Step Six: Using a gloved hand, the clinician measures the distance of mouth opening by using the bottom of the top teeth and the top of the bottom teeth as the landmarks.

- Step Seven: If the movement reproduces the patient's symptoms, auscultation of the TMJ is necessary to determine the presence of a click.

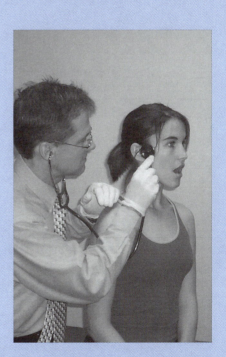

**Figure 7.16** Auscultation of the TMJ

## Lower Jaw Retrusion

**Retrusion** involves an anterior-to-posterior movement of the lower jaw with respect to the stationary maxilla. Retrusion can compress retrodiscal tissues.

- Step One: Resting symptoms are assessed.
- Step Two: The clinician instructs the patient to retract his or her lower jaw as posteriorly as possible.
- Step Three: The clinician views the bite formation for symmetry.
- Step Four: The patient is queried regarding production of concordant symptoms.

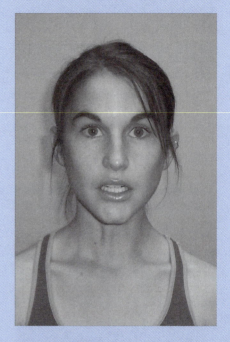

**Figure 7.17**    TMJ Retrusion

- Step Five: Using a gloved hand, the clinician measures the retrusion by using the bottom of the top teeth and the top of the bottom teeth as the landmarks.

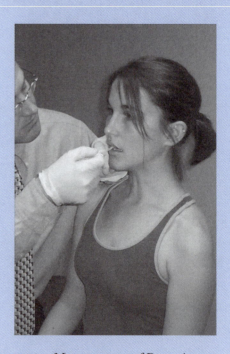

**Figure 7.18**    Measurement of Retrusion

## *Active Movements of a Displaced Disc*

With an anteriorly displaced disc, the superior–posterior structures and the sphenomandibular ligament are compressed or stretched by the condyle during movement.[19] Because of this, active and passive movement may yield differences in findings. Protraction will stretch retrodiscal tissue and may reproduce pain similar to end range pain. During full mouth opening an audible repositioning is generally noticeable as the condyle slips posteriorly to the disc.[19] Reducing cranial compression reduces the likelihood of repositioning and can be accomplished by placing a device such as a gauge between the molars of the patient prior to mouth opening.[19] This reduces the cranial compression during opening.

## Passive Movements

All four passive movements of depression, protrusion, and medial and lateral translation may stress the posterior–superior ligamentous structures. In most cases, the findings associated with passive range of movement should replicate the findings of the active examination.[19] Conditions associated with myofascial pain may be less painful and demonstrate less articular dysfunction during passive movement than active. Truelove et al.[56] suggest that differences of 5 millimeters between active and passive movements are indicative of muscular dysfunction and may represent a myofascial disorder.

## *Passive Accessory Tests*

Although the movement of the TMJ is not purely linear, passive accessory movements may be helpful in identifying that the TMJ is the origin of the pain.[37]

## *Summary*

- Several TMJ specific movements require examination to determine the movement associated with TMD.
- Measurement of maximal mouth opening, protrusion, and retrusion may be a useful method to determine dysfunction and to measure progress.
- The presence of a displaced disc may yield different active examination findings and warrant careful attention. Typically, disc displacement is associated with pain during full mouth opening and a clicking noise.

### Caudal Glide

A caudal glide may place tension on contractile and noncontractile tissues and is a purported treatment method for contractile relaxation and pain control.

- Step One: Resting symptoms are assessed.
- Step Two: Using a gloved hand, the clinician places his or her thumb inside the mouth of the patient. The thumb lies parallel on the top of the teeth and flush to the posterior–inferior molars of the patient. This technique should not be performed if the patient has false teeth or no molars.
- Step Three: The clinician applies a caudal distraction and repeats the movement several times to examine a trend if concordant.
- Step Four: The patient is queried for reproduction of the concordant sign and the behavior of the reproduction.

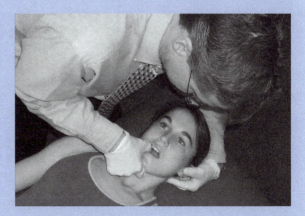

**Figure 7.19** Caudal Glide

## Anterior Glide

Like the caudal glide, an anterior glide may be useful to determine if a treatment consisting of repeated anterior movements is useful in reducing contractile tension and myofascial pain.

- Step One: Resting symptoms are assessed.
- Step Two: Using a gloved hand, the clinician places his or her thumb inside the mouth of the patient. The thumb hooks the bottom teeth at the incisor and four front teeth.
- Step Three: The clinician applies an anterior distraction and repeats the movement several times to examine a trend if concordant.
- Step Four: The patient is queried for reproduction of the concordant sign and the behavior of the reproduction.

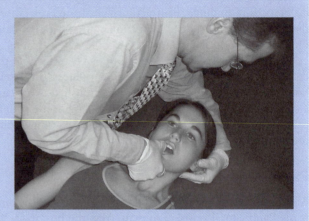

**Figure 7.20**    Anterior Glide

Hesse et al.[18] reported that joint play movements are beneficial in identifying the presence of a TMJ dysfunction. The following techniques allow joint play assessment and concurrent palpation through the auricular canal. The examination is required bilaterally for comparison of mobility.

## Posterior–Anterior Mobilization

- Step One: The patient assumes a sidelying position. Resting symptoms are assessed.
- Step Two: With one thumb, the clinician palpates the posterior aspect of the condyle of the mandible. The first finger of the opposite hand is placed in the auricular canal to palpate movement.
- Step Three: Using a light to progressively more heavy force, the clinician applies a posterior-to-anterior movement to the condyle. The finger of the opposite hand palpates for movement.
- Step Four: The patient is queried for reproduction of the concordant sign and the behavior of the reproduction.

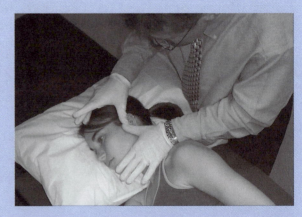

**Figure 7.21**    PA of Condyle on Temporal Bone-Sidelying

## Anterior–Posterior Mobilization

- Step One: The patient assumes a sidelying position. Resting symptoms are assessed.
- Step Two: With one thumb, the clinician palpates the anterior aspect of the condyle of the mandible. The first finger of the opposite hand is placed in the auricular canal to palpate movement.
- Step Three: Using a light to progressively more heavy force, the clinician applies an anterior-to-posterior movement to the condyle. The finger of the opposite hand palpates for movement.
- Step Four: The patient is queried for reproduction of the concordant sign and the behavior of the reproduction.

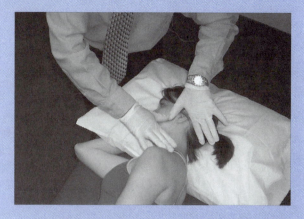

**Figure 7.22**  AP of Condyle on Temporal Bone-Sidelying

## Combined Passive Movements

During passive opening of the dysfunctional jaw, the condyles are often displaced superiorly placing both tension and compression forces on the ligamentous structures and retrodiscal region. Combining a caudal displacement by placing an inferior force as closely to the TMJ as possible reduces the risk of compressing and abnormally tensioning these structures. This requires a combined passive movement in order to adequately examine the passive physiological and accessory movements of the jaw.

## Ventrocaudal Translation

A ventrocaudal translation more accurately mimics the actual movement of the TMJ and may reduce the compression of selected tissues that was present during a passive accessory and was not relieved during repeated movements. The posterior–superior structures are stressed during ventrocaudal translation with a slight caudal orientation.

- Step One: The patient assumes a supine position. Resting symptoms are assessed.
- Step Two: Using a gloved hand, the clinician places his or her thumb inside the mouth of the patient. The thumb lies parallel and on top of the teeth and flush to the posterior–inferior molars of the patient. This technique should not be performed if the patient has false teeth or no molars.
- Step Three: The ventrocaudal translation requires a combined caudal glide concurrently with a ventral or anterior glide. The movement allows a decompressive force of the condyle to the temporal bone.
- Step Four: The patient is queried for reproduction of the concordant sign and the behavior of the reproduction.

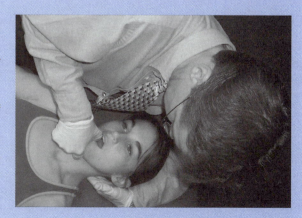

**Figure 7.23**  Ventrocaudal Translation

### Caudal–Retrusive Glide

Perform a concurrent caudal and retrusion glide (AP) if symptoms were reproduced slightly during active retrusion. If caudal glide and retrusion are implemented, both the superior–posterior structures and the sphenomandibular ligament are compressed.[19]

- Step One: The patient assumes a supine position. Resting symptoms are assessed.
- Step Two: Using a gloved hand, the clinician places his or her thumb inside the mouth of the patient. The thumb lies parallel and on top of the teeth and flush to the posterior–inferior molars of the patient. This technique should not be performed if the patient has false teeth or no molars.
- Step Three: The caudal–retrusive glide requires a combined caudal glide concurrently with a posterior glide or retrusion movement. The movement allows a decompressive force of the superior–anterior structures in the retrodiscal region.
- Step Four: The patient is queried for reproduction of the concordant sign and the behavior of the reproduction.

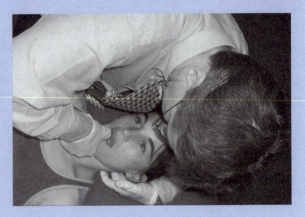

**Figure 7.24**    Caudal Glide and Retrusion

### Summary

- Selected passive movements place tension on targeted structures and may be useful in identifying the origin of the movement dysfunction.
- Combined passive movements are affective in provoking tissues in a biomechanically normal position.
- Some of the other passive movements may cause pain by placing tension or compression on tissues by moving into a plane that doesn't normally occur during jaw excursion.

## Clinical Special Tests

Essentially, the diagnostic value of the majority of special tests for TMD remains unknown. Visscher et al.[57] compared overlapping tests of TMD and the cervical spine to identify the best distinguishing maneuvers for use during an examination. They reported that the highest pain intensities reported for TMD were palpation followed by dynamic/static tests, pain on passive movements, and finally pain during active movements.[57] Some studies have measured the diagnostic value of selected clinical findings and special tests for diagnosing TMD. Two studies involve opening amplitude,[58] anterior/vertical ratio,[59] and palpation.[58]

### Opening Amplitude

Dworkin et al.[58] measured the likelihood of TMD based on opening amplitude. The authors used a mandatory cutoff point of <35 mm for men and <30 mm for women. The reported sensitivity for men was 21.6% and the specificity was 97.8%. For women, the sensitivity was similar at 21.8% and a specificity of 97.5%. The +LR ratio for opening amplitude was 9.8 and 8.7, respectively.

### Anterior/Vertical Ratio

A palpatory and radiographic technique known as the anterior/vertical ratio has been used to identify TMD conditions associated with anterior disc displacement. Gateno et al.[60] found that when compared to controls, patients with anterior disc displacement demonstrate 2.4 times the displacement of the posterior condyles (thus presenting a higher anterior/vertical ratio). Feine and Hutchins[59] reported a sensitivity of 86% and a specificity of 30% using a cutoff ratio of 1–2. Their reported +LR was only 1.23.

### Palpation

Palpation is recognized as an essential criterion for identifying the likelihood of TMD. Dworkin et al.[58] investigated the presence of audible phenomena during palpation and tested the diagnostic value of this finding. The investigators reported a sensitivity of 43% and a specificity of 75% for the digital palpation of a click (+LR = 1.72; sensitivity of 8% and a specificity of 92% for the digital palpation of crepitus (+LR = 1.0); sensitivity of 6% and a specificity of 99% for the presence of grating (+LR = 6.0); and sensitivity of 57% and a specificity of 66% for the presence of any sounds (+LR = 1.67). Of the sounds, the presence of grating appears to demonstrate the highest diagnostic value during assessment.

Pain with palpation at baseline is an excellent predictor for the necessity of conservative treatment and has been advocated as a useful diagnostic tool for presence of myofascial, internal derangement, and/or osteoarthritis.[37,61] However, palpation does not have the capacity to identify disparate conditions.[62]

### Helkimo Di Index

The Helkimo Di index was created in 1974 by Helkimo[61] and is an index that combines anamnestic and clinical dysfunction criteria. The anamnestic movements consist of measurement of mandibular opening, overbite, protrusive movement, and measurement of deviation. Palpation is used to measure tenderness in the masseter, temporalis, and medial pterygoids. The lateral pterygoid is measured against resistance for recreation of symptoms. Based on the clinical scores a rating of I, II, or III is provided. It is generally accepted that the Helkimo Di index provides useful information, although the evaluative properties of the index are not as discriminatory as a thorough, comprehensive assessment with appropriate use of diagnostic tests.[63,64]

### *Manual Muscle Testing*

Contractile structures are often painful during conditions associated with myofascial pain.[56] By testing the selected muscular actions, the examiner may be able to identify painful movements or coordination problems during activation.

## *Summary*

- Selected special tests exhibit diagnostic value in assessing TMD.
- Maximal mouth opening exhibits the highest diagnostic value in diagnosing TMD.
- Palpation for noise yields disparate diagnostic value during assessment.
- The Helkimo Di index yields uncertain diagnostic value and may only be an extension of a good examination.
- Manual muscle testing may be an effective way of diagnosing a myofascial disorder, although the diagnostic value remains uncertain.

## Resisted Opening

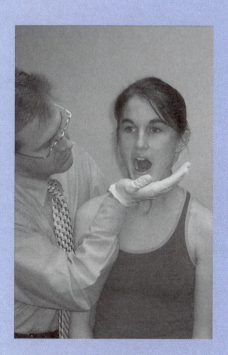

- Step One: The patient is placed in a sitting position. The head is carefully positioned in proper alignment. The mouth is prepositioned in a closed position, with neutral protrusion or retrusion. Resting symptoms are assessed.
- Step Two: The clinician places a comfortable but firm grip on the mandible of the patient.
- Step Three: The patient is instructed to open his or her mouth against the resistance of the clinician. Symptoms are reassessed.

**Figure 7.25**    Resisted Opening

## Resisted Closing

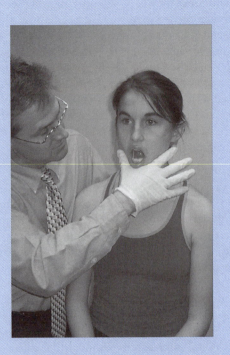

- Step One: The patient is placed in a sitting position. The head is carefully positioned in proper alignment. The mouth is prepositioned in opening. Resting symptoms are assessed.
- Step Two: The clinician places a comfortable but firm grip on the mandible of the patient.
- Step Three: The patient is instructed to bite downward against the resistance of the clinician. Symptoms are reassessed.

**Figure 7.26**    Resisted Closing

## Resisted Medial and Lateral Excursion

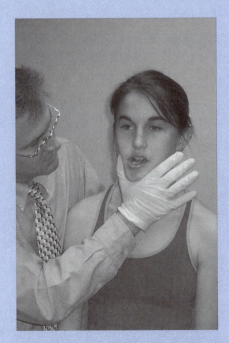

- Step One: The patient is placed in a sitting position. The head is carefully positioned in proper alignment. Resting symptoms are assessed.
- Step Two: The clinician places a comfortable but firm grip on the mandible of the patient.
- Step Three: The patient is instructed to perform a lateral excursion to a directed side. Symptoms are reassessed.
- Step Four: The process is repeated for the opposite side.

**Figure 7.27**    Resisted Medial and Lateral Excursion

# TREATMENT TECHNIQUES

## Treatment Philosophy

The treatment philosophy for TMD is no different from that advocated within this textbook. The patient-response model requires a careful evaluation of pain-provoking movements and a diligent understanding of the cause and effect of repeated movements, positions, or stability exercises. Like shoulder pathology, a TMD may exhibit unidirectional hypermobility. Mobilizing in the appropriate direction may reduce the tendency of the jaw to displace during mouth opening and may further promote normalized movement. When assessing TMD it is imperative that the clinician distill what "form" of dysfunction he or she is treating in order to more effectively target the concordant sign. Careful examination is necessary because it is apparent that patients with TMD do not spontaneously recover over time and multiple forms of treatments have demonstrated improvement over no intervention.[65]

Like cervical disorders, TMD may best be categorized into classification groups. Truelove[56] offers a classification system that is further reduced into three major categories: (1) internal derangement, (2) degenerative and/or inflammatory conditions, and (3) myofascial conditions (Table 7.1).

### Internal Derangement

The term "internal disc derangement" is often used to describe the altered biomechanics of the TMJ. Traditionally, internal disc derangement is diagnosed when clicking is prevalent, intermittent bouts of locking occur, and a reduction in mouth opening is prominent during passive and active assessment.[56] Early conditions of internal disc derangement involve disc displacement with reduction. A disc displacement occurs when the normally superior disc displaces, typically anterior, so that the concave aspect of the disc is anterior and no longer congruent with the convex aspect of the condyle. A disc displacement with reduction refers to a disc that is displaced in the closed-mouth position but assumes a normal position relative to the condyle with jaw opening. A disc displacement without reduction refers to a disc that is displaced at all mandibular positions and does not reduce during opening or closing of the jaw. It has been suggested that a disc displacement without reduction is a consequential condition associated with long-term disc displacement with reduction.[66] Further evidence to support this hypothesis is provided by Sener and Akganlu,[67] who found that there were no differences in MRI characteristics between an anterior disc displacement with and without reduction or degenerative tendencies between the two disorders.

A disc displacement with perforation refers to a disc that is displaced and damaged. Disc perforation may occur from abnormal stress and poor articulation during movement that can lead to degeneration and break down over time. There are no distinctive criteria associated with disc perforation.[56]

### Degenerative and or Inflammatory Conditions

Degenerative conditions include symptoms such as pain in the joint during palpation, function, and passive opening.[56] Several different categories may fall within the realm of degeneration including capsulitis/synovitis, sprain/strain, degenerative joint disease, and arthritis.[56]

### Myofascial Conditions

Myofascial conditions are associated with orofacial pain and are typically quantified during palpation of the muscle

**TABLE 7.1    Characteristics of TMD Classifications (Adapted from Truelove et al.[56])**

| Classification | Included Diagnoses | Clinical Symptoms |
|---|---|---|
| Myofascial pain | 1. Myalgia Type I<br>2. Myalgia Type II<br>3. Myofascial pain dysfunction | • Orofacial pain<br>• Muscle pain with palpation<br>• Greater pain with active opening and closing than with passive opening and closing |
| Internal derangement | 1. Disc displacement with reduction<br>2. Disc displacement without reduction<br>3. Perforation of the posterior ligament or disc | • Click in the TMJ during ROM<br>• Click in the TMJ during lateral excursion<br>• < 35 mm of mouth opening<br>• No significant difference between active and passive opening |
| Degenerative and or inflammatory conditions | 1. Capsulitis<br>2. Synovitis<br>3. Sprain/strain<br>4. Arthritis<br>5. Arthralgia | • Pain in the joint during palpation<br>• Pain in the joint during function<br>• Pain in the joint during assisted opening<br>• Possible history of trauma (sprain/strain)<br>• Pain on right and left excursions |

sites (two or more sites) and greater movement during passive movement than active movement.

## Differentiation of Pain from Cervical Contribution

In normal conditions, the resting position of the jaw requires minimal muscular contraction and places little stress in intraarticular structures.[21] This relaxed position is associated with normal postural positioning of the head, neck, and jaw. Krause[21] suggests that the amount of time spent in this position is therapeutic to the patient and should be sought as an intervention. Since forward head and abnormal cervical position can affect the resting activity of the TMJ, postural training has merit during treatment of TMJ dysfunction, specifically when reduction of mouth opening is an issue.[68]

In the cervical chapter, several postural exercises were presented. These exercises were both active and passively oriented and involved techniques to provide normal posture. Studies have shown some degree of success with implementation of an active exercise program,[69] specifically those that focus on postural exercises[70,71] or strengthening.[72] One common postural exercise is the prone cervical retraction technique, which is designed to incorporate a passive stretch during an active strengthening movement.

Repeated chin retractions, such as those advocated by McKenzie, have demonstrated improvement in resting posture in asymptomatic subjects.[73] Additionally, postural exercises such as those discussed in the thoracic chapter may be useful for postural improvement. The exercises in Figures 7.28–7.31 are analogous to those presented by Wright et al.[44] in their successful intervention.

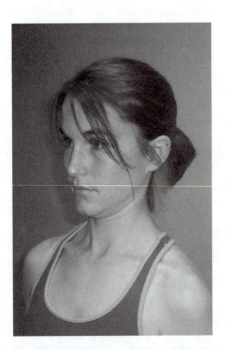

**Figure 7.28**   Chin Retractions

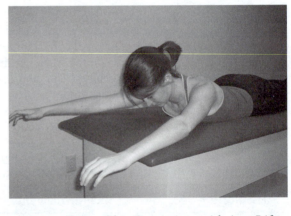

**Figure 7.29**   Prone Chin Retractions with Arm Lifts

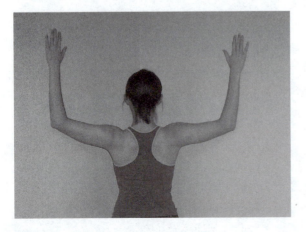

**Figure 7.30**   Thoracic Corner Stretch

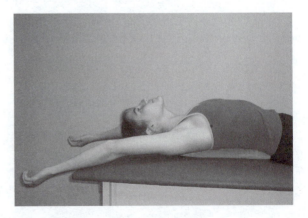

**Figure 7.31**   Supine Upper Back Stretches

## Internal Derangement

Internal derangement often refers to a nonhomogeneous set of symptoms that are associated with improper TMJ movement. Treatment of internal derangement, specifically the use of mobilization, has been successful in reducing the anterior displacement of a disc[74,75] and yields higher outcomes than no intervention.[76]

### Caudal Glide

- Step One: Resting symptoms as assessed.
- Step Two: Using a gloved hand, the clinician places his or her thumb inside the mouth of the patient. The thumb lies parallel to the top of the teeth and flush to the posterior–inferior molars of the patient. This technique should not be performed if the patient has false teeth or no molars.
- Step Three: The clinician applies a caudal distraction and repeats the movement several times to examine a trend if concordant.
- Step Four: The patient is queried for reproduction of the concordant sign and the behavior of the reproduction.

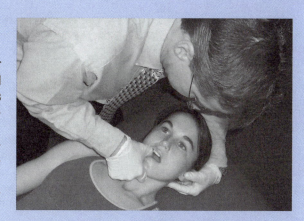

**Figure 7.32**    Caudal Glide

### Anterior Glide

- Step One: Resting symptoms are assessed.
- Step Two: Using a gloved hand, the clinician places his or her thumb inside the mouth of the patient. The thumb hooks the bottom teeth at the incisor and four front teeth.
- Step Three: The clinician applies an anterior distraction and repeats the movement several times to examine a trend if concordant.
- Step Four: The patient is queried for reproduction of the concordant sign and the behavior of the reproduction.

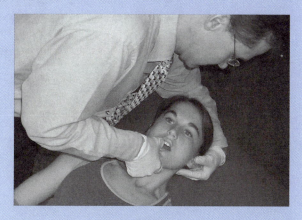

**Figure 7.33**    Anterior Glide

## Ventrocaudal Translation

- **Step One:** The patient assumes a supine position. Resting symptoms as assessed.
- **Step Two:** Using a gloved hand, the clinician places his or her thumb inside the mouth of the patient. The thumb lies parallel to the top of the teeth and flush to the posterior–inferior molars of the patient. This technique should not be performed if the patient has false teeth or no molars.
- **Step Three:** The ventrocaudal translation requires a combined caudal glide concurrently with a ventral or anterior glide. The movement allows a decompressive force of the condyle to the temporal bone.
- **Step Four:** The patient is queried for reproduction of the concordant sign and the behavior of the reproduction.

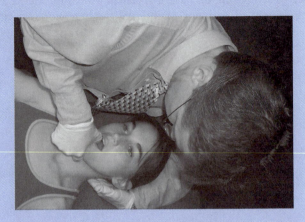

**Figure 7.34**    Ventrocaudal Translation

Therapeutic exercise has shown benefit on a patient population of anterior disc displacement with reduction. Yoda et al.[77] demonstrated that exercise that also consisted of selected mobilization and stretching was successful enough to reduce the risk of surgery and lowered the requirement for splint therapy. Similar findings have also been recorded for internal derangement conditions treated by mobilization, posture, and exercises postoperatively.[78]

Pain-free strengthening and coordination exercises should be performed with careful attention for prevention of clicking and displacement. Both isometric and isotonic exercises are helpful in building coordination during movement.

## Resisted Opening (Isometric)

- **Step One:** The patient is placed in a sitting position. The head is carefully positioned in proper alignment. The mouth is prepositioned in a closed position, with neutral protrusion or retrusion.
- **Step Two:** The patient is instructed to perform a comfortable but firm grip on his or her mandible. The objective of the exercise is a static hold.
- **Step Three:** The patient is instructed to open his or her mouth against the resistance of his or her own hand.
- **Step Four:** The hold and repetitions are dependent upon the goal of the exercise.

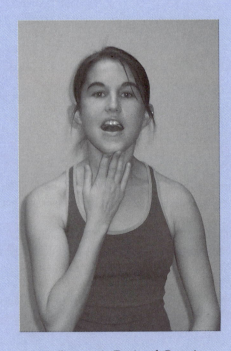

**Figure 7.35**    Isometric Resisted Opening

## Resisted Opening (Isotonic)

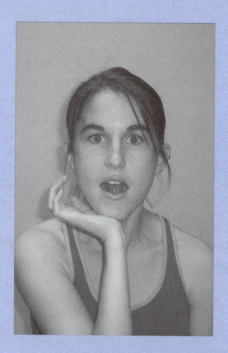

- Step One: The patient is placed in a sitting position. The head is carefully positioned in proper alignment. The mouth is prepositioned in a closed position, with neutral protrusion or retrusion.
- Step Two: The patient is instructed to perform a comfortable but firm grip on his or her mandible. The objective of the exercise is the application of enough force that allows repeated movements.
- Step Three: The patient is instructed to open his or her mouth against the resistance of his or her own hand.
- Step Four: The hold and repetitions are dependent upon the goal of the exercise.

**Figure 7.36**    Isotonic Opening with Resistence

## Resisted Closing (Isometric)

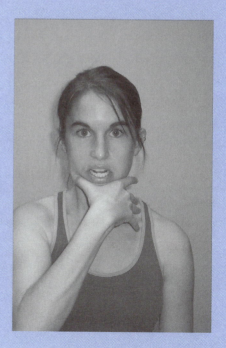

- Step One: The patient is placed in a sitting position. The head is carefully positioned in proper alignment. The mouth is prepositioned in opening. Resting symptoms are assessed.
- Step Two: The patient is instructed to perform a comfortable but firm grip on his or her mandible. The objective of the exercise is a static hold.
- Step Three: The patient is instructed to bite downward against the resistance of his or her own hand.

**Figure 7.37**    Isometric Resisted Closing

## Resisted Closing (Isotonic)

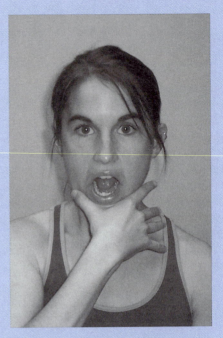

- Step One: The patient is placed in a sitting position. The head is carefully positioned in proper alignment. The mouth is prepositioned in an open position, with neutral protrusion or retrusion.
- Step Two: The patient is instructed to perform a comfortable but firm grip on his or her mandible. The objective of the exercise is the application of enough force that allows repeated movements.
- Step Three: The patient is instructed to close his or her mouth against the resistance of his or her own hand.
- Step Four: The hold and repetitions are dependent upon the goal of the exercise.

**Figure 7.38**    Isotonic Closing Exercises

## Resisted Medial and Lateral Excursion (Isometric)

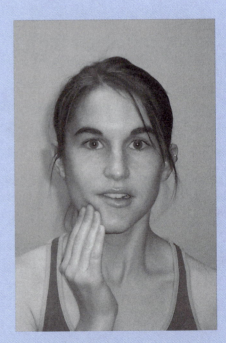

- Step One: The patient is placed in a sitting position. The head is carefully positioned in proper alignment. Resting symptoms are assessed.
- Step Two: The patient places a comfortable but firm grip on his or her mandible.
- Step Three: The patient is instructed to perform a lateral excursion to a directed side and is directed to apply resistance from his or her own hand.
- Step Four: The process is repeated for the opposite side.

**Figure 7.39**    Isometric Medial and Lateral Excursion

**Resisted Medial and Lateral Excursion (Isotonic)**

- Step One: The patient is placed in a sitting position. The head is carefully positioned in proper alignment. The mouth is prepositioned in an open position, with neutral protrusion or retrusion.
- Step Two: The patient is instructed to perform a comfortable but firm grip on his or her mandible. The objective of the exercise is the application of enough force that allows repeated movements.
- Step Three: The patient is instructed to move his or her mouth laterally against the resistance of his or her own hand.
- Step Four: The hold and repetitions are dependent upon the goal of the exercise.
- Step Five: The process is repeated for the opposite side.

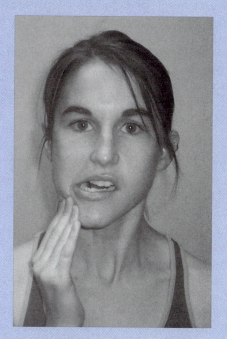

**Figure 7.40**    Isotonic Medial and Lateral Translation

## Treating Myofascial Pain

Treating myofascial pain is generally performed with night splints, postural improvements, rest, and modalities.[79] However, mobilization techniques designed to reduce pain may be appropriate[80] when this dysfunction is encountered, specifically those designed to assist in allowing a nonpainful resting position.[81] Physical therapy treatment of myofascial conditions, which consisted of massage, ultrasound, and muscle stretching, was as effective as counseling.[82] In another study, some patients reported complete abolishment of pain with improvement levels higher than those reported in the no-treatment control group.[83]

## Treating Inflammation

Inflammation may be present specifically if movements such as passive and active opening at full range or retrusion reproduce symptoms. Passive movements during mobilization including passive (Figure 7.41) and repetitive stretching have been associated with chemical changes that reduce pain and improve appropriate collagen remodeling.[84] When compared with a control group those who received manual therapy techniques and postural control improved significantly over those on a waiting list with no treatment.[83] Long-term results demonstrated the positive outcomes continued comparatively even after 3 years' removal from care.[85]

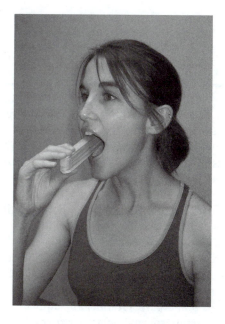

**Figure 7.41**    Stretch Sticks for Passive Stretching

## Summary

- Treatment of TMD follows the patient-response method format but may benefit from further subcategorization into classification models.
- Manual therapy methods may be helpful when performed in conjunction with other rehabilitative methods.

# TREATMENT OUTCOMES

There is a paucity of well-designed clinical trials that report the benefit of a manual therapy rehabilitative intervention for TMD. The majority of trials have reported the outcomes of pharmacological or splint-related interventions. Although physical therapy has been commonly associated with significantly better outcomes than a pragmatic intervention, the physical therapy intervention has varied widely among studies.

Frequently, interventions ranged among the use of ultrasound, exercise, diathermy, home education, and stretching.[86] Of these interventions exercise, with the addition of selected mobilization and stretching methods, has the most documented merit, having demonstrated the ability

to reduce the risk of surgery and intensity of need for splint therapy.[77,78] Evidence for the benefit of an upper-quarter postural treatment is present as well. Wright et al.[44] performed general posture stretching exercises that targeted the thoracic and cervical spine on a group of 60 patients with TMD. After 4 weeks, the patients were reexamined for changes in symptoms and found statistically significant changes when compared to the normal intervention control group.

Otherwise, the majority of manual therapy studies for TMD have included case reports or series. Future clinical trials are necessary to distill further the benefit of manual therapy for the temporomandibular joint.

## Summary

- Numerous studies advocate the use of manual therapy, postural exercises, stretching, and modalities in the treatment of various forms of TMD. The majority of these studies are case reports.
- Exercise, combined with mobilization and stretching, yields positive outcomes for TMD. Postural exercise targeted to the upper quarter has demonstrated clinical utility as well.

## Chapter Questions

1. Please describe the role of the retrodiscal tissue toward the pathology of the temporomandibular joint.
2. Describe the documented relationship between cervical posture, cervical impairment, and the presence of TMD.
3. Describe the three primary classifications of TMD and outline how treatment varies between each classification.
4. Outline the mechanism of which the patient-response method is applied for assessment and treatment of patients with applicable TMD.

## References

1. Gross A, Haines T, Thomson A, Goldsmith C, McIntosh J. Diagnostic tests for temporomandibular disorders: an assessment of the methodological quality of research reviews. *Man Ther.* 1996;1:250–257.
2. Merksey H, Bogduk N. *Classification of chronic pain.* Seattle; IASP Press: 1994.
3. Clark G, Seligman D, Solberg W. Guidelines for the examination and diagnosis of temporomandibular disorders. *J Craniomandib Disord Facial Oral Pain.* 1989; 3:(1):7–14.
4. Dworkin S, LeResche L, DeRouen T. Assessing clinical signs of temporomandibular disorders: reliability of clinical examiners. *J Prosthet Dent.* 1990;63(5):574–579.
5. Rugh J, Solberg W. Oral health status in the United States. Temporomandibular disorders. *J Dent Educ.* 1985;49:398–406.
6. Schiffman E, Friction J. Epidemiology of TMJ and craniofacial pain. In Friction JR, Kroening R, Hathaway K (eds). *TMJ and craniofacial pain: diagnosis and management.* St. Louis; IEA Publications: 1988.
7. Solberg WK. Temporomandibular disorders: management of problems associated with inflammation, chronic hypomobility, and deformity. *Br Dent J.* 1986; 160(12):421–428.
8. Schiffman EL, Friction JR, Haley DP, Shapiro BL. The prevalence and treatment needs of subjects with temporomandibular disorders. *J Am Dent Assoc.* 1990; 120(3):295–303.
9. Nassif NJ, Al-Salleeh F, Al-Admawi M. The prevalence and treatment needs of symptoms and signs of temporomandibular disorders among young adult males. *J Oral Rehabil.* 2003;30(9):944–950.

10. Dao T, LeResche L. Gender differences in pain. *J Orofac Pain*. 2000;14:169–194.

11. Behrents RG, White RA. TMJ research: responsibility and risk. *Am J Orthod Dentofacial Orthop*. 1992; 101(1):1–3.

12. Dimitroulis G. Temporomandibular disorders: a clinical update. *Br Med J*. 1998;317:190–194.

13. Warren M, Fried J. Temporomandibular disorders and hormones in women. *Cells Tissues Organs*. 2001; 169:187–192.

14. Johansson A, Unell L, Carlsson G, Soderfeldt B, Halling A. *J Orofac Pain*. 2003;17:29–35.

15. Wright A, Gatchel R, Wildenstein L, Riggs R, Buschang P, Ellis E. Biopsychosocial differences between high-risk and low-risk patients with acute TMD related pain. *JADA*. 2004;135(4):474–483.

16. Katzburg R, Westesson PL. *Diagnosis of the temporomandibular joint*. Philadelphia; WB Saunders Co: 1993.

17. Eggelton T, Langton D. Clinical anatomy of the TMJ complex. In: Krause S. *Clinics in physical therapy: Temporomandibular disorders*. New York; Churchill Livingstone: 1994.

18. Hesse J, Naeije M. Biomechanics of the TMJ. In: Krause S. *Clinics in physical therapy: Temporomandibular disorders*. New York; Churchill Livingstone: 1994.

19. Langendoen J, Muller J, Jull G. Retrodiscal tissue of the temporomandibular joint: clinical anatomy and its role in diagnosis and treatment of arthropathies. *Man Ther*. 1997;2:191–198.

20. Bertolucci L. The trilogy of the triad of O'Donohugue in the knee and its analogy to the TMJ derangement. *J Craniomandibular Pract*. 1990;8:264–270.

21. Krause S. Physical therapy management of TMD. In: Krause S. *Clinics in physical therapy: Temporomandibular disorders*. New York; Churchill Livingstone: 1994.

22. Rocabado M. Arthrokinematics of the temporomandibular joint. *Dental Clin North Am*. 1983;27: 573–594.

23. Gallagher C, Gallagher V, Whelton H, Cronin M. The normal range of mouth opening in an Irish population. *J Oral Rehabil*. 2004;31:110–116.

24. Benoit P. History and physical examination for TMD. In: Krause S. *Clinics in physical therapy: Temporomandibular disorders*. New York; Churchill Livingstone: 1994.

25. Visscher CM, Lobbezoo F, de Boer W, van der Zaag J, Naeije M. Prevalence of cervical spinal pain in craniomandibular pain patients. *Eur J Oral Sci*. 2001; 109:76–80.

26. Rantala M, Ahlberg J, Suvinen T, Savolainen A, Kononen M. Chronic myofascial pain, disk displacement with reduction and psychosocial factors in Finnish non-patients. *Acta Odontol Scand*. 2004;62:293–297.

27. Ahlberg J, Savolainen A, Rantala M, Lindholm H, Kononen M. Reported bruxism and biopsychosocial symptoms: a longitudinal study. *Community Dent Oral Epidemiol*. 2004;32:307–311.

28. Steigerwald D, Maher J. The Steigwald/Maher TMD disability questionnaire. *Today's Chiropractic*. 1997; July–August:86–91.

29. Beck A, Steer R, Garbin M. Psychometric properties of the Beck Depression Inventory: Twenty-five years of evaluation. *Clinical Psychology Review*. 1988;8(1): 77–100.

30. Brown C, Schulberg H, Madonia J. (Assessing depression in primary care practice with the Beck Depression Inventory and the Hamilton Rating Scale for Depression. *Psychological Assessment*. 1995;7(1):59–65.

31. Groth-Marnat G. *The handbook of psychological assessment*. 2nd ed. New York; John Wiley & Sons: 1990.

32. Reiss S, Peterson R, Gursey D, McNally R. Anxiety sensitivity, anxiety frequency, and the prediction of fearfulness. *Behav Res Ther*. 1986;24:1–8.

33. Peterson R, Plehn K. Measuring anxiety sensitivity. In: S. Taylor, Editor, *Anxiety sensitivity: Theory, research, and treatment of the fear of anxiety*. Hillsdale, NJ; Erlbaum: 1999.

34. Rodriguez BF, Bruce SE, Pagano ME, Spencer MA, Keller MB. Factor structure and stability of the Anxiety Sensitivity Index in a longitudinal study of anxiety disorder patients. *Behav Res Ther*. 2004;42(1):79–91.

35. Emshoff R, Brandlmaier I, Bosch R, Gerhard S, Rudisch A, Bertram S. Validation of the clinical diagnostic criteria for temporomandibular disorders for the diagnostic subgroup—disc derangement with reduction. *J Oral Rehabil*. 2002;29(12):1139–1145.

36. Tasaki MM, Westesson PL. Temporomandibular joint: diagnostic accuracy with sagittal and coronal MR imaging. *Radiology*. 1993;186(3):723–729.

37. Hesse J, van Loon L, Maeije M. Subjective pain report and the outcome of several orthopaedic tests in craniomandibular disorder patients with recent pain complaints. *J Oral Rehabil*. 1997;24:483–489.

38. Lobbezoo-Scholte AM, Steenks MH, Faber JA, Bosman F. Diagnostic value of orthopedic tests in patients with temporomandibular disorders. *J Dent Res*. 1993;72(10):1443–1453.

39. Lobbezoo-Scholte AM, de Wijer A, Steenks MH, Bosman F. Inter-examiner reliability of six orthopaedic tests in diagnostic subgroups of craniomandibular disorders. *J Oral Rehabil*. 1994;21(3): 273–285.

40. de Wijer A, Lobbezoo-Scholte AM, Steenks MH, Bosman F. Reliability of clinical findings in temporomandibular disorders. *J Orofac Pain*. 1995;9(2):181–191.

41. Roberts C, Katzberg RW, Tallents RH, Espeland MA, Handelman SL. The clinical predictability of internal derangements of the temporomandibular joint. *Oral Surg Oral Med Oral Pathol*. 1991;71(4):412–414.

42. Emshoff R, Innerhofer K, Rudisch A, Bertram S. Relationship between temporomandibular joint pain and magnetic resonance imaging findings of internal derangement. *Int J Oral Maxillofac Surg*. 2001;30(2): 118–122.

43. Yatani H, Minakuchi H, Matsuka Y, Fujisawa T, Yamashita A. The long-term effect of occlusal therapy on self-administered treatment outcomes of TMD. *J Orofac Pain.* 1998;12(1):75–88.

44. Wright E, Domenech M, Fischer J. Usefulness of posture training for patients with temporomandibular disorders. *JADA.* 2000;131:202–210.

45. Gonzalez H, Manns A. Forward head posture: its structural and functional influence on the stomatognathic system, a conceptual study. *Cranio.* 1996;14:71–80.

46. Austin D. Special considerations in orofacial pain and headache. *Dent Clin North Am.* 1997;41:325–339.

47. Braun B. Postural differences between asymptomatic men and women and craniofacial pain patients. *Arch Phys Med Rehabil* 1991;72:653–656.

48. Hackney J, Bade D, Clawson A. Relationship between forward head posture and diagnosed internal derangement of the temporomandibular joint. *J Orofac Pain.* 1993;7:386–390.

49. Darlow L, Pesco J, Greenberg M. The relationship of posture to myofascial pain dysfunction syndrome. *J Am Dent Assoc.* 1987;114:73–75.

50. Enwemeka C, Bonet I, Ingle J, Prudhithumrong S, Ogbahon F, Gbenedio N. Postural correction in persons with neck pain. Part II. Integrated electromyography of the upper trapezius in three simulated neck positions. *J Orthop Sports Phys Ther.* 1986;8:240–242.

51. Schuldt K, Ekholm J, Harms-Ringdahl K, Nemeth G, Arborelius U. Effects of changes in sitting work posture on static neck and shoulder muscle activity. *Ergonomics.* 1986;29:1525–1537.

52. Friction JR, Hathaway KM, Bromaghim C. Interdisciplinary management of patients with TMJ and craniofacial pain: characteristics and outcome. *J Craniomandib Disord.* 1987;1(2):115–122.

53. Evcik D, Aksoy O. Correlation of temporomandibular joint pathologies, neck pain, and postural differences. *J Phys Ther Sci.* 2000;12:97–100.

54. Braun B, Schiffman E. The validity and predictive value of four assessment instruments for evaluation of the cervical and stomatognathic systems. *J Craniomandib Disord.* 1991;5:239–244.

55. Masumi S, Kim Y, Clark G. The value of maximum jaw motion measurements for distinguishing between common temporomandibular disorder subgroups. *Oral Surg Med Oral Pathol Oral Radiol Endod.* 2002;93:552–559.

56. Truelove E, Sommers E, LeReshce L, Dworkin S, von Korff M. Clinical diagnostic criteria for TMD. New classification permits multiple diagnoses. *J Am Dent Assoc.* 1992;123:47–54.

57. Visscher C, Lobbezoo F, de Boer W, van der Zaag J, Verheij J, Naeije M. Clinical tests in distinguishing between persons with or without craniomandibular or cervical spinal pain complaints. *Eur J Oral Sci.* 2000; 108:475–483.

58. Dworkin SF, Huggins KH, LeResche L, Von Korff M, Howard J, Truelove E, Sommers E. Epidemiology of signs and symptoms in temporomandibular disorders: clinical signs in cases and controls. *J Am Dent Assoc.* 1990;120(3):273–281.

59. Feine J, Hutchins M, Lund J. An evaluation of the criteria used to diagnose mandibular dysfunction with the manidibular kinesiograph. *J Prosthet Dent.* 1988; 60(3):374–380.

60. Gateno J. Closed lock of the temporomandibular joint. *Tex Dent J.* 1994;111:32–35.

61. Helkimo M. Studies on function and dysfunction of the masticatory system. II. Index for anamnestic and clinical dysfunction and occlusal state. *Swedish Med J.* 1974;67:101–121.

62. Kirveskari P. Prediction for demand for treatment of temporomandibular disorders. *J Oral Rehabil.* 2001; 28:572–575.

63. van der Weele L, Dibbets J. Helkimo's index: a scale or just a set of symptoms? *J Oral Rehabil.* 1987;14: 229–237.

64. Otuyemi OD, Owotade FJ, Ugboko VI, Ndukwe KC, Olusile OA. Prevalence of signs and symptoms of temporomandibular disorders in young Nigerian adults. *J Orthod.* 2000;27(1):61–65.

65. Brown D, Gaudet E. Temporomandibular disorder treatment outcomes: second report of a large-scale prospective clinical study. *Cranio.* 2002;20:244–253.

66. Nitzan DW, Dolwick MF. An alternative explanation for the genesis of closed-lock symptoms in the internal derangement process. *J Oral Maxillofac Surg.* 1991;49(8):810–815.

67. Sener S, Akganlu F. MRI characteristics of anterior disc displacement with and without reduction. *Dentomaxillofac Radiol.* 2004;33(4):245–252.

68. Komiyama O, Kawara M, Arai M, Asano T, Kobayashi K. Posture correction as part of behavioral therapy in treatment of myofascial pain with limited opening. *J Oral Rehabil.* 1999;26(5):428–435.

69. Shakoor M, Ahmed M, Kibria G, Khan A, Mian M, Hasan S, Nahar S, Hossian M. (abstract). Effects of cervical traction and exercise therapy in cervical spondylosis. *Bangladesh Med Res Counc Bull.* 2002;28:61–69.

70. Harrison D, Cailliet R, Betz J, Haas J, Harrison D, Janik T, Holland B, Conservative methods of reducing lateral translation postures of the head: A nonrandomized clinical control trial. *J Rehabil Res Dev.* 2004; 41:631–639.

71. Grant R, Jull G, Spencer T. Active stabilizing training for screen based keyboard operators—a single case study. *Aust J Physiotherapy.* 1997;43:235–242.

72. Jull G, Trott P, Potter H, Zito G, Niere K, Shirley D, Emberson J, Marschner I, Richardson C. A ran-

domized controlled trial of exercise and manipulative therapy for cervicogenic headache. *Spine*. 2002;27: 1835–1843.

73. Pearson N, Walmsley R. Trial into the effects of repeated neck retractions in normal subjects. *Spine*. 1995;20:1245–1250.

74. Babadag M, Sahin M, Gorgun S. Pre- and posttreatment analysis of clinical symptoms of patients with temporomandibular disorders. *Quintessence Int*. 2004; 35:811–814.

75. Cleland J, Palmer J. Effectiveness of manual physical therapy, therapeutic exercise, and patient education on bilateral disc displacement without reduction of the temporomandibular joint: A single case design. *J Orthop Sports Phys Ther*. 2004;34:535–545.

76. Nicolakis P, Erdogmus B, Kopf A, Ebenbichler G, Kollmitzer J, Piehslinger E, Fialka-Moser V. Effectiveness of exercise therapy in patients with internal derangement of the temporomandibular joint. *J Oral Rehabil*. 2001;28:1158–1164.

77. Yoda T, Sakamoto I, Imai H, Honma Y, Shinjo Y, Takano A, Tuskahara H, Morita S, Miyamura J, Yoda Y, Sasaki Y, Tomizuka K, Takato Y. A randomized controlled trial of therapeutic exercise for clicking due to disk anterior displacement with reduction in the temporomandibular joint. *Cranio*. 2003;21:10–16.

78. Oh D, Kim K, Lee G. The effect of physiotherapy on post-temporomandibular joint surgery patients. *J Oral Rehabil*. 2002;29:441–446.

79. Nicolakis P, Erdogmus B, Kropf A, Nicolakis M, Piehslinger E, Fialka-Moser V. Effectiveness of exercise therapy in patients with myofascial pain dysfunction syndrome. *J Oral Rehabil*. 2002;29:362–368.

80. Friedman MH. The hypomobile temporomandibular joint. *Gen Dent*.1997;45(3):282–285.

81. Deodata F, Cristiano S, Trusendi R, Giorgetti R. A functional approach to the TMJ disorders. *Prog Orthod*. 2003;4:20–37.

82. De Laat A, Stappaerts K, Papy S. Counseling and physical therapy as treatment for myofascial pain of the masticatory system. *J Orofac Pain*. 2003;17:42–49.

83. Nicolakis P, Burak E, Kollmitzer J, Kopf A, Piehslinger E, Wiesinger G, Fialka-Moser V. An investigation of the effectiveness of exercise and manual therapy in treating symptoms of TMJ osteoarthritis. *Cranio*. 2001;19:26–32.

84. Sambajon V, Cillo J, Gassner R, Buckley M. The effects of mechanical strain on synovial fibroblasts. *J Oral Maxillofac Surg*. 2003;61:707–712.

85. Nicolakis P, Erdogmus CB, Kollmitzer J, Kerschan-Schindl K, Sengstbratl M, Nuhr M, Crevenna R, Fialka-Moser V. Long-term outcome after treatment of temporomandibular joint osteoarthritis with exercise and manual therapy. *Cranio*. 2002;20(1):23–27.

86. Gray R, Quayle AA, Hall CA, Schofield MA. Physiotherapy in the treatment of temporomandibular joint disorders: a comparative study of four treatment methods. *Br Dent J*. 1994;176:257–261.

# 8

# Manual Therapy of the Thoracic Spine

## Objectives

- Identify the pertinent structure and biomechanics of the thoracic spine.
- Demonstrate the appropriate and valid thoracic spine examination sequence.
- Identify plausible mobilization and manual therapy treatment techniques for the thoracic spine and rib cage.
- Discuss the effect of mobilization and manual therapy on recovery for patients with thoracic impairments in randomized trials.

## PREVALENCE

As a whole, the thoracic spine is woefully understudied and may be best divided into three separate and related regions: the upper, mid-, and lower thoracic spine. It is apparent that the lower thoracic spine (thoracolumbar) is the most frequently injured region of the spine.[1] What is less apparent is the injury rate of other regions such as the mid and upper thoracic spine. The overall size of the thoracic spine permits a number of nonrelated disorders, some of which are more prevalent to selected regions (i.e., upper, middle, or lower).

The most common injuries of the thoracic spine include compression fractures, burst fractures, flexion-distraction, and fracture-dislocation injuries,[2] conditions that are more likely to occur in the mid- and lower thoracic regions. The mid thoracic region is beset frequently with idiopathic and acquired pathologies such as extreme **kyphosis** or **scoliosis**.[3] Although scoliosis is considered an adolescent-dominated disorder, a recent study has demonstrated 32–68% of the geriatric population (average age 70.5 years) does demonstrate scoliosis-related dysfunction.[4]

Conditions such as a thoracic herniated disc are rare, accounting for less than 0.2–5.0% of all intervertebral disc injuries.[5,6] Only one patient in a million suffers an intervertebral thoracic disc herniation, typically initiated with nonspecific pain and only rarely presenting with sensory and motor losses.[7] There is a natural narrowing of the spinal canal at T6, increasing the risk of cord compression from disc herniation at that level.

### Summary

- The thoracic spine may best be divided into the upper, mid-, and lower thoracic spine.
- Thoracic-specific pathologies are less prevalent than other musculoskeletal regions.
- Idiopathic and occasionally traumatic injuries such as kyphosis, scoliosis, or compression fractures are common in the lower and mid-thoracic spine.
- Disc-related injuries are not common in the thoracic spine, accounting for only 0.2–5% of all spinal intervertebral injuries.

## ANATOMY

The thoracic spine is unique from the cervical and lumbar spine because of the size and extent of the region and the articulations with the rib cage (Figure 8.1). The articulation with the rib cage leads to regional variations in movement patterns and function.[8] The upper thoracic spine mimics the movement and, to some extent, the anatomy of the cervical spine and the lower thoracic vertebra mimics the lumbar spine.

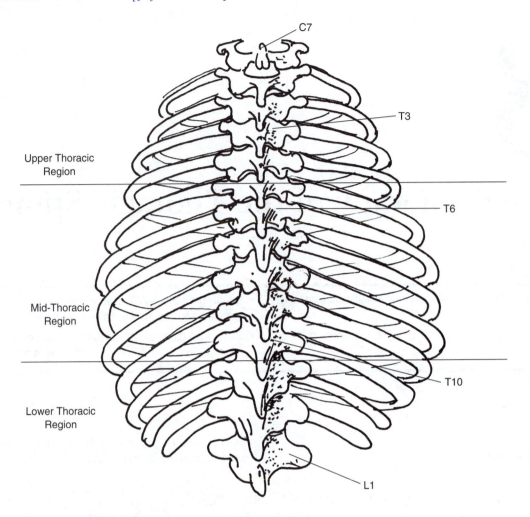

**Figure 8.1**    The Three Regions of the Thoracic Spine

## Osseous Structures

The thoracic vertebra can be subdivided anterior to posterior into three specific regions (Figure 8.2): the body, the pedicles, and the posterior structures such as the transverse and spinous processes.[9] Joint articulations occur at the body of the vertebra and at the posterior structures.

The thoracic vertebral body is primarily made of cancellous bone and progressively is wider from the upper thoracic segments to the lower segments.[10] Each thoracic vertebra demonstrates a concavity within the horizontal plane that may reduce the tendency for disc herniation.[11] The inclination of the end plates remains constant throughout the thoracic spine even though the posterior height of the vertebral body increases slightly with caudal progression.[10]

Kothe et al.[9] reported that the average pedicle height demonstrated greater variability in the lower thoracic spine than in the middle thoracic spine. The pedicle is a complex three-dimensional structure that is filled mostly with cancellous bone (62–79%) for structural rigidity. The outer cortical shell showed different thicknesses throughout its perimeter and variations in trabeculae at disparate levels.

The posterior structures include the transverse processes and the articulations, the facets, and the spinous processes. The spinous processes angle inferiorly and progressively from the upper thoracic spine to the mid- to lower tho-

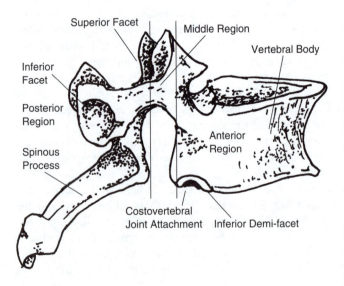

**Figure 8.2**    Typical Thoracic Vertebra

racic spine. The transverse process angle posteriorly and provide the contact points for the facets.[10]

The ribs are long, thin bones that are commonly fractured during trauma to the thoracic region[12] and connect to the thoracic spine anteriorly and posteriorly. Each rib has a convex head that articulates with the concave facets of the vertebral body (**costovertebral joint**) and transverse processes of the thoracic spine (**costotransverse joint**). The anterior connection is called the costo-sternal attachment and identifies the two separate articulations of the sternum to the costal cartilage and the costal cartilage to the rib. The anterior articulation is a flattened, concave depression.

### The Intervertebral Disc

The intervertebral disc plays a major role in movement control of the thoracic spine, a much more significant role than the posterior structures.[13] With respect to height, the disc in the thoracic spine demonstrates less height in ratio to the vertebral body than the cervical and lumbar spines.[14] Additionally, the thoracic disc has a relatively small nucleus pulposis.[15]

It is expected that the compliance of the thoracic disc is lost much earlier than the cervical or lumbar disc.[13] Disc space narrowing is common from the third decade of life and disc degeneration, osteophytes, and subsequent degenerative changes are frequent findings in the mid-thoracic segment.[16]

With respect to intradiscal pressures, Polga et al.[17] found that the positions of standing upright with 10-kg weights in each arm display the highest pressure versus other positions such as prone lying, sidelying, sitting with and without flexion, and other variations of standing including twisting.

### Joints

There are variations in the zygopophyseal joints (facets) throughout the length of the thoracic spine (Figure 8.3). In general, the superior facets face anteriorly, but are not completely aligned in the frontal plane.[18] This angulation is reduced as the thoracic spine descends, culminating at T12. At T12, the facets have a similar orientation to those of the lumbar spine.[18]

The facet architecture changes throughout the upper, mid, and lower thoracic segments. In the mid-thoracic region, the superior and inferior articular processes are curved in both the transverse and sagittal planes, thus permitting multidirectional movement.[19,20] However, the facet architecture does not dictate or guide a specific, directional coupling movement of the mid-thoracic region.

Within the transverse plane, the superior facet demonstrates near sagittal angulation as compared to inferior facet.[18] In the coronal plane the sagittal angulation of the superior facets demonstrates a steeper degree with respect to the inferior facets.[18]

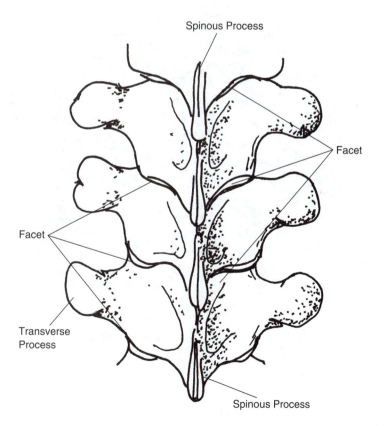

**Figure 8.3**   Zygopophyseal Joints of the Thoracic Spine

Each facet demonstrates fibrous annular menisci, which may originate medially from the ligamentum flavum or laterally from the joint capsule.[21] These meniscal folds are hypothesized as the culprits during an acute thoracic facet lock.[22] Additionally, each facet demonstrates asymmetry from right to left at nearly all levels.[18] This may produce abnormalities in range of motion between the right and the left, although in most case the differences are small.[23]

## Rib Cage Joints

There are three primary joints associated with the rib cage: the costovertebral joints, the costotransverse joints, and the costo-sternal joints (Figure 8.4). The costovertebral joint is formed by a convex rib head with two adjacent vertebral bodies, superiorly and inferiorly. The concave inferior costal demi facet of the superior vertebral body and the concave superior costal construction of the inferior vertebral body provide a synovial attachment to the rib head. The rib head articulates with the lateral aspect of the intervertebral disc in addition to the two separate vertebral connections. The joint has two synovial cavities separated by an intraarticular ligament.[19] This joint also houses meniscoids that may be involved during acute costovertebral pain.[24]

Peculiarities regarding the costovertebral joint exist throughout the thoracic spine, specifically the facet orientation for the articulation of the costovertebral joint. The first thoracic vertebra has an articular facet for the head of the first rib and a demi facet for the upper half of the head of the second rib, yet the 9th vertebra occasionally has no demi facets below that participate in the articulation with the head of the 10th rib.[20]

The 11th vertebra has large articular facets that are located on the pedicles of the vertebra. At the 10th vertebra, the orientation of the vertebral body changes and mimics that of the lumbar spine.[25] The transverse processes shorten and have no articular facet to interface with the rib. The 12th vertebra is similar to the 11th except that the facet orientation is further sagittal, thus mimicking the biomechanical inclination of the lumbar spine.[25]

The costotransverse joint is formed by articulation of the rib tubercle and thoracic vertebral transverse process (Figure 8.5). The articulation of the ribs with the transverse processes yields two synovial capsules, one above and one below articulations with an interarticular ligament that provides stability.[25] The costotransverse joint is highly integrated with vertebral body movement and typically moves in sequence with the vertebral movement.

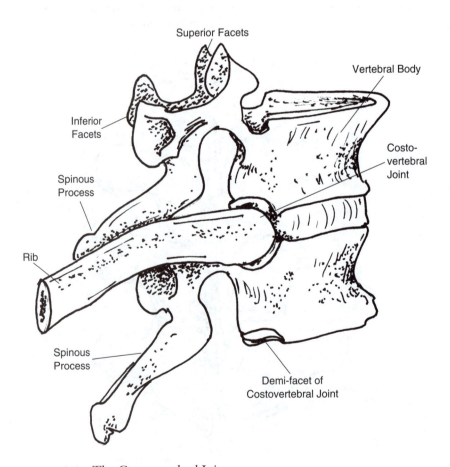

**Figure 8.4** The Costovertebral Joint

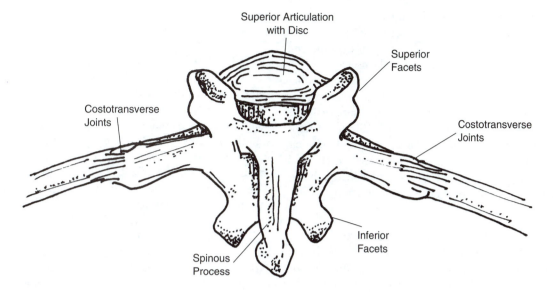

**Figure 8.5**   The Costotransverse Joint Attachment

The width of the anterior cartilage gives rise to two separate anterior costo-sternal attachments. The first, the costo-sternal attachment, consists of the costal cartilage and the articulation of the sternum. The second, the costo-rib connection, includes the anterior head of the rib to the flattened, concave depression of the costo-cartilage.[25]

## Ligaments

Several ligaments contribute to the thoracic spine structure and function. These ligaments are best divided into anterior, lateral, and posterior structures.[11] The anterior ligaments consist of the anterior longitudinal ligament and the sternocostal ligaments.[11]

The anterior longitudinal ligament (ALL), one of the strongest ligaments of the body, runs the length of the spine, originating from the cervical atlas and finally blending into the periosteum of the sacrum. This ligament lies on the posterior of the body whereas the sternocostal ligaments comprise the anterior aspect of the body.

The sternocostal ligament is a broad membranous band that originates from the anterior and posterior aspect of the sternal cartilage of the upper ribs and inserts to the posterior surfaces of the sternum. The interarticular sternocostal ligament attaches one rib to another with the fibrocartilage and the connection to the manubrium.

The lateral costotransverse ligaments are subdivided into three ligaments: the superior costotransverse ligament, the middle costotransverse ligament, and the lateral costotransverse ligament.[25] The superior costotransverse ligament originates on the border of the transverse process and inserts on the upper border of the neck and angle of the rib. The middle costotransverse ligament originates between the neck of the rib and inserts on the transverse process at the same level. The lateral costo-transverse ligament originates from the lateral aspect of the transverse process and inserts on the adjacent rib. The intertransverse ligament is only well formed within the lumbar region and occasionally demonstrates attachments in the lower thoracic spine. The ligaments prevent excessive movements of side flexion and rotation.[11]

The posterior ligaments include the posterior longitudinal ligament, the ligamentum flavum, the interspinous ligament, and the supraspinous ligament. The posterior longitudinal ligament descends along the posterior surfaces of the thoracic vertebra and discs to the insertion point in the sacrum.[11,26] The ligamentum flavum ligaments are paired (right and left) ligaments that insert upward into the anterior lower third of the vertebral lamina at the level above and originate on the posterior upper third of the lamina below. The elastic, yellow-colored ligament forms the posterior wall of the vertebral canal and assist in preventing the synovial capsule and menisci from entrapment into the facet joints.[11,25,26] The interspinous ligament runs from each spinous process and controls the movements of flexion. The radiate ligament connects the anterior portion of each rib with the bodies of the two adjacent vertebrae and the intervertebral fibrocartilage between the vertebrae. Lastly, the supraspinous ligament is composed of a bundle of fibrous tissue that courses over the tips of each spinous process inserting in the lumbar region at L3-4.[25,26]

## The Nervous System

Within the thoracic spine, the **sympathetic nervous system** plays an important part in pain autoregulation and perception. There are 12 sympathetic ganglia within the thoracic region. The thoracolumbar sympathetic fibers arise from the dorso-lateral region of the anterior column of the gray matter of the spinal cord and pass with the anterior roots of all the thoracic and the upper two or three lumbar spinal nerves.[25] Some of the fibers connect with the sympathetic trunk, enter the white rami, and eventually progress to the prevertebral plexuses.

The sympathetic nervous system is responsible for dilation of the bronchi and pupils as well as other organ-specific responses. Documented evidence supports the benefit of modulation of pain and remarkably has a non-localized effect. Stimulation of the cervical and thoracic spine has demonstrated upper extremity changes in pain response, (pressure-pain), and a measurable sympathoexcitatory effect[27–29] that can lead to pain reduction.

## Muscles

The paraspinal muscles of the thoracic spine are responsible for both trunk and upper extremity movements and are a common source of injury and pain. Several studies[30–32] have found that back extensor strength was negatively correlated with degree of kyphosis, suggesting that strengthening the thoracic spine should reduce the angle of kyphosis. Additionally, strengthening of the thoracic spinal musculature also improves scapular dynamics and positively alters the scapulohumeral rhythm.[31]

## Summary

- The osseous structures of the thoracic spine include the vertebral body and corresponding right and left ribs.
- The thoracic vertebra can be subdivided anterior to posterior into three specific regions: the body, the pedicles, and the posterior structures such as the transverse and spinous processes.
- The thoracic intervertebral disc has less height in comparison to the vertebral body as compared to the cervical and lumbar spine.
- The ribs attach in three joints (costovertebral, costotransverse, and costo-sternal) and are long, thin bones with four primary planes.
- The facets of the spine face anteriorly and within the transverse plane; the superior facet demonstrates near sagittal angulation as compared to the inferior facet.
- The ligaments of the thoracic spine help reduce spine displacement along with the stability provided by the rib cage.
- A notable component of the nervous system in the thoracic spine is the contribution of the sympathetic nervous system. This system may affect visceral structures as well as joints in the periphery.
- The muscles of the thoracic spine contribute not only to thoracic stability but also to stability of the shoulder girdle.

# Biomechanics

## Range of Motion

According to White and Panjabi,[33] the combined flexion and extension range of motion in the thoracic spine is bimodal, superior to inferior. The upper thoracic spine demonstrates a combined 3–5 degrees of flexion or extension that is reduced to 2–7 degrees at T5 to T6 and further increases to 6–20 degrees at T12 to L1. Overall, greater range of motion is available in flexion than in extension. The combined side flexion of the thoracic spine is also bimodal, with approximately 5 degrees of motion in the upper thoracic region slipping to 3–10 for the levels of T7 to T11 than progressing to 5–10 at T12-L1. Lastly, combined rotation is purported to be 14 degrees at T1-2, which progressively declines to 2–3 degrees combined at T12-L1, mimicking the movement available in the lumbar spine.

## Stabilization

Generally, within the thoracic spine the inferior articular facets face backward slightly downward and medially and the superior facets are nearly flat and are directed backward as well.[20] This alignment, combined with the contribution of the costovertebral and costotransverse joints and ligamentous structures, results in significant stability within the thoracic spine.[20]

The stability and coordination of movement of the thoracic spine is significantly enhanced and altered by the rib cage.[13] The contribution of the rib cage may increase the load capacity of the spine by three times the normal amount.[13,26] Removal of the rib cage demonstrated pronounced increases in the neutral zone motions of the thoracic spine and resection of the costovertebral joints significantly altered the ranges of motion such as lateral flexion and rotation of the thoracic spine.[34]

The thoracolumbar spine is able to tolerate compressive loads of up to 975 Newtons. This preload can occur without damage or instability if applied in the sagittal plane along the natural curvature of the spine through estimated centers of rotation.[35] The spine was found to be least flexible and demonstrated less range of motion during axial compression.[36]

## Coupled Movement

Coupling characteristics of the thoracic spine are location dependent. The upper thoracic spine tends to couple using the same side flexion and rotation (ipsilaterally) pattern as the lower cervical spine.[33] The coupling pattern in the mid-thoracic spine demonstrates variability.[33,36,37] The lower thoracic spine generally mimics the pattern of the lumbar spine[33] and that pattern is inconsistent.[38]

There are several reasons for this phenomenon. First, rotation is greatest in the mid-thoracic region[13] and this rotation may often occur in isolation of side flexion or sagittal movements.[36] Second, instability may lead to abnormal coupling patterns specifically adjacent to spinal fusions.[33]

White and Panjabi[33] identified T4 as the initial site of variability in coupling. This region to L1 has demonstrated variability in coupling patterns but the most attention has been given to T4 to T8. Lee[19] identifies the kinematic process of right-side flexion during left lateral translation and the coupling of anterior rotation of the left rib during right initiation of vertebral rotation and posterior rotation of the right rib. During physiological flexion, the ribs rotate superiorly with respect to the transverse process. During extension, the opposite occurs, with inferior rotation of the rib with respect to the transverse process.[19]

During conditions such as scoliosis, it is normal to see the spinous processes reflect toward the convexity of the rotation; or side flexion and rotation that occurs to the same side. This pattern is highly consistent in the upper thoracic spine, predominates in the mid- and lower thoracic spine, but does demonstrate variability.[36]

## Summary

- Generally, thoracic spine range of motion is similar but bimodal. The range of motion declines near the mid-thoracic region but increases caudal and cephalic to the mid-thoracic segments.
- The thoracic spine is very stable, receiving stability contributions from the ligaments, the joints of the rib cage, and the rib cage structure.
- Coupling of the lumbar spine is location dependent. Generally, the upper thoracic spine couples with the lower cervical spine consistently. The mid-thoracic region demonstrates variable coupling and the lower thoracic region tends to couple with the upper lumbar spine that is also variable.

# ASSESSMENT AND DIAGNOSIS

Differentiation of musculoskeletal pain for that of visceral origin is necessary for proper treatment identification.[39] There are several potential pain generators within the thoracic spine including the vertebral disc, the vertebrae, dura mater, longitudinal ligaments, the posterior thoracic muscles, the costotransverse joints, and the zygopophyseal joints.[40] Testicular pain has been linked to lower thoracic dysfunction.[41] Headaches have been associated with a dysfunction to T4.[42] **Costochondral** deformities may mimic a submucosal gastric tumor.[43] Furthermore, the lower thoracic segments often refer pain that mimics lumbar spine origin.[44]

The thoracic region houses numerous visceral organs that can refer pain that mimics musculoskeletal origin.[39] Chest pain can be from the heart, abdominal organs, musculoskeletal tissue, psychogenic generators, or selected disease processes.[45–47] In addition, musculoskeletal struc-

tures can mimic pain of visceral origin as well. Hypertonic saline injections in normal volunteers into the thoracic interspinous muscles and ligaments can produce local or referred pain to the anterior aspect of the chest that mimics heart pain.[40]

Differentiation is necessary to avoid misdiagnosis of an individual during the initial screen. Many patients with noncardiac chest pain have anterior chest tenderness to palpation that is absent in control groups without chest pain; however, reproduction of the pain by palpation alone is only found in some of the patients.[48] The location of the complaint of pain cannot with certainty be used as a guide to determine the location of source since the thoracic pain generators can refer pain to multiple areas of the body.[40] Adler[49] suggests the use of pain reproduction methods to differentiate musculoskeletal and psychogenic phenomena based on two principles: (1) the ability to reproduce or reduce the pain and (2) selective change in the motoric action of the subject.

## Summary

- Pain generators of the thoracic spine include both musculoskeletal and visceral origins.
- Differentiation of pain is necessary. It is recommended that pain reproduction is mandatory prior to treatment secondary to the risks of underlying pain of visceral origin.

## Subjective Considerations

### Psychosocial Factors

Like the psychosocial factors associated with lumbar spine pain, similar factors may contribute to recovery for the thoracic spine. These psychosocial factors include abnormalities in pain perception, job-related intricacies, psychological dysfunction, social support challenges, and disability perceptions. It is imperative to note that factors that increase one's risk for injury may not increase one's risk for poor prognosis.[50] A challenge to the rehabilitation clinician is that many thoracolumbar injuries that are intrinsically pathologically similar involving similar treatment interventions often result in a wide range of outcomes.[50]

### Functional Assessment Tools

Few if any scales are unique to the thoracic region. Typically, researchers utilize the same functional scales identified for the lumbar spine. The *Functional Rating Index* (FRI) has been used in the cervical, thoracic, and lumbar spine to analyze functional impairment and has demonstrated good psychometric properties. Like most functional scales, the FRI is a self-report scale that utilizes similar constructs from the *Oswestry Disability Index* (ODI) and *Neck Disability*

*Index* (NDI) scales.[51] The FRI is a 10-item questionnaire, seven of which are represented in the NDI and nine of which are covered within the ODI. Each item of the FRI has five possible Likert-type answers arranged in a scale from 0 to 4. To obtain an overall score on the questionnaire, the clinician is required to add the point values for each of the items answered by the patient. The maximum score is 40. The FRI is easy to administer, seems to have satisfactory validity and reliability, and may be useful in geriatric assessment of individuals with spinal disorders.[52] The FRI has been shown to be responsive for changes in spinal impairments and only takes approximately 78 seconds for administration and completion.[53] The minimally important difference has been reported as 8.4, indicating a change of 8.4 in the overall scoring results in a significant outcome change for the patient.[51]

# Summary

- Patients with pain from the thoracic spine are expected to be affected from similar psychosocial factors as patients with lumbar spine origin.
- No functional scales are specific for the thoracic spine. The Functional Rating Index may be a useful unidimensional disability index for the thoracic spine that can carry over to the cervical and lumbar spines.

## Objective/Physical Examination

### *Observation*

#### *Posture*

In standing posture, the line of gravity passes anteriorly to the thoracic spine, creating a moment that increases thoracic kyphosis.[13] Both passive and active force function to prevent excessive kyphosis; the deep paraspinal musculature is constantly active, thus functioning to stabilize the posture.[54] Nonetheless, the morphology of the thoracic spine is highly related to the resting length of an individual's posture and most likely contributes more to postural parameters than any other component.[55]

Increased thoracic kyphosis is a common finding among the general population, a dysfunction that purportedly may lead to musculature weakness, arthrological pain and stiffness, and alteration of mechanoreceptors.[55] Janda described a postural phenomenon called "upper crossed syndrome," a sequence of adaptive changes associated with forward head posture, shortened pectoralis major and minor, upper trapezius, levator scapula, and sternocleidomastoid musculature and lengthened middle and lower trapezius, serratus anterior, rhomboids, and deep neck musculature (Figure 8.6).[56] Generally, patients with upper crossed syndrome exhibit increases in thoracic kyphosis.[56] Forward head and thoracic kyphosis are directly related and may contribute to myofascial pain syndromes and de-

creased pain thresholds.[57] Resting muscle posture most likely does influence cervico-thoracic posture. Ironically, although postural abnormalities are often treated as a cause of thoracic pain, little quantitative evidence exists to directly correlate pain and postural dysfunction.[13,58]

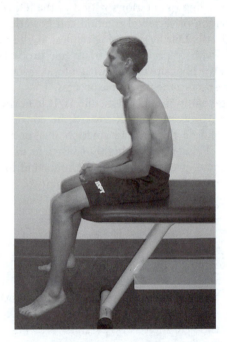

**Figure 8.6**    Poor Thoracic Posture-Upper Crossed Syndrome

Postural changes are common in patients with osteoporosis, often contributing to vertebral compression fractures that result in wedging and compression of the vertebrae.[59] Compression fractures can lead to physiological changes in posture, most commonly kyphosis and potentially scoliosis.[59] Postural kyphosis alters the shape and function of the rib cage by increasing the anterior–posterior diameter, thus altering the respiratory capacity of the individual.[59] Two studies have suggested that thoracic kyphosis changes above 50 degrees may lead to balance disturbances.[60,61]

Scoliosis may be functional or structural and is common in younger individuals or individuals who have experienced a trauma.[62] Structural scoliosis is considered a loss of flexibility in the thoracic spine that does not resolve passively or actively.[63] Functional scoliosis retains a functional normal range but exhibits lateral curvature that is adaptive or "functionally required" for external commands.[63]

#### *Introspection*

Older patients often exhibit dysfunctions associated with compression fractures or postural abnormalities. Women especially are susceptible to osteoporosis and postural changes associated with increased kyphosis, insidious and traumatic in nature.[60] Younger individuals and older patients, specifically after degenerative changes, may exhibit structural scoliosis.[4] Shoulder dysfunction may be associated with posture or weak scapular muscles.

## *Summary*

- Postural problems, typically associated with kyphosis, are common dysfunctions within the postural spine.
- Poor posture is not directly correlated with thoracic spine pain.
- Scoliosis is typically associated with younger individuals but may be present in older patients.

# CLINICAL EXAMINATION

## Active Physiological Movements

Isolating active physiological movement to the thoracic spine is challenging. In all forms of movement, the cervical and lumbar spines will contribute to motion and may require clearing. Within the following descriptions, subtle tips regarding positioning may best emphasize movements to improve the focus on the thoracic spine.

### Active Flexion

Because many elderly patients assume a slight flexed thoracic posture as a position of comfort, end range active movements may be beneficial to assess. If a patient exhibits pertinent pretest signs of a potential compression fracture, the performance of active flexion and specifically flexion with overpressure are contraindicated. A careful history and assessment of risk factors may helpfully outline the risk of this procedure.

- Step One: The patient sits in a straddled position to stabilize the pelvis. Resting symptoms are assessed.
- Step Two: The patient is instructed to move toward flexion by pulling his or her elbows toward the groin. The patient is instructed to move only to the first point of pain. Pain is assessed to determine if concordant.
- Step Three: The patient is instructed to move beyond the first point of pain toward end range. After a sustained hold or repeated movements, the concordant movement is again reassessed.

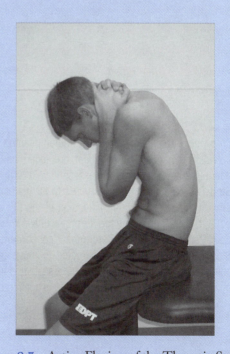

**Figure 8.7**   Active Flexion of the Thoracic Spine

*(continued)*

- Step Four: If the patient demonstrates pain-free movement, an overpressure is applied by pulling the elbows into flexion and placing the lumbar region into flexion.

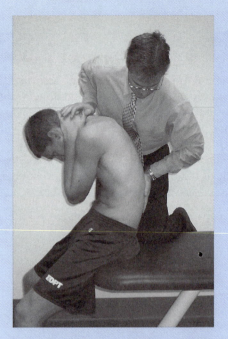

Figure 8.8    Overpressure of Flexion of the Thoracic Spine

## Active Extension

Individuals lose extension for a number of reasons including degenerative changes. Subsequently, it is important to determine the outcome of repeated movement near end range of extension or a sustained hold prior to administering this approach as a home program or an in-house treatment based on visual postural changes.

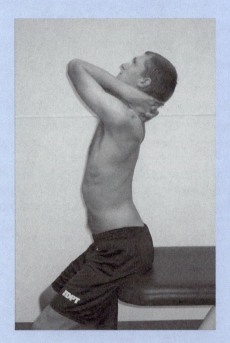

- Step One: The patient sits in a straddled position to stabilize the pelvis. The hands of the patient are laced behind his or her head. Resting symptoms are assessed.
- Step Two: The patient is instructed to lift his or her elbows up toward the sky, promoting extension of the thoracic spine. The patient is further instructed to move only to the first point of pain. Pain is assessed to determine if concordant.
- Step Three: The patient is instructed to move beyond the first point of pain toward end range. After a sustained hold or repeated movements, the concordant movement is again reassessed.

Figure 8.9    Active Extension of the Thoracic Spine

- Step Four: If the patient demonstrates pain-free movement, an overpressure is applied by pulling up on the elbows toward the ceiling while stabilizing the thoracic spine into extension with the opposite hand.

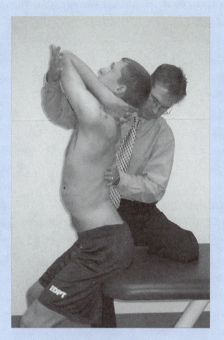

Figure 8.10    Overpressure of Extension of the Thoracic Spine

## Active Side Flexion

Active side flexion is generally coupled in the upper and lower thoracic regions but is often isolated in the mid-thoracic region. It is helpful to view the side flexion from the posterior of the patient to determine the curvature of side flexion, especially in the mid-thoracic region.

- Step One: The patient sits in a straddled position to stabilize the pelvis. Resting symptoms are assessed. The elbows of the patient are flexed to his or her side and the fingers are laced and placed behind the head.
- Step Two: The patient is instructed to move toward side flexion by moving one elbow toward his or her pelvis in a curvilinear movement. The patient is instructed to move only to the first point of pain. Pain is assessed to determine if concordant.
- Step Three: The patient is instructed to move beyond the first point of pain toward end range. After a sustained hold or repeated movements, the concordant movement is again reassessed.

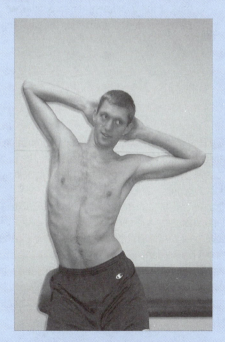

Figure 8.11    Active Side Flexion of the Thoracic Spine

(continued)

- Step Four: If the patient demonstrates pain-free movement, an overpressure is applied by pulling the patient into further side flexion using a handgrip near the axilla of the patient.
- Step Five: The procedure is repeated on the opposite side.

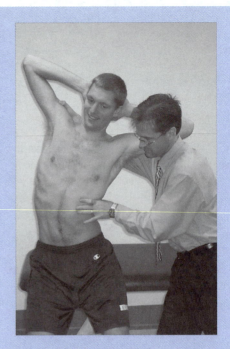

**Figure 8.12**    Overpressure of Side Flexion of the Thoracic Spine

## Active Rotation

Rotation in the upper and lower thoracic spine is coupled but often is not in the mid-thoracic region. In order to promote full rotation of the upper thoracic spine, cervical rotation toward end range is necessary. If the movement demonstrates pain, it is important to differentiate the cervical and thoracic spine using isolated rotation tests for each segment.

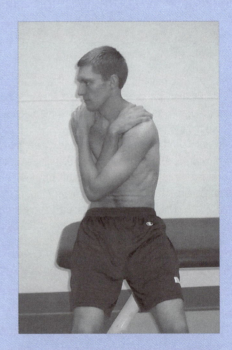

- Step One: The patient sits in a straddled position to stabilize the pelvis. Resting symptoms are assessed. The patient's arms are crossed over his or her chest but the thoracic spine remains in slight flexion.
- Step Two: The patient is instructed to rotate in a horizontal plane, including the cervical spine. The patient is instructed to move only to the first point of pain. Pain is assessed to determine if concordant.
- Step Three: The patient is instructed to move beyond the first point of pain toward end range. After a sustained hold or repeated movements, the concordant movement is again reassessed.

**Figure 8.13**    Active Rotation of the Thoracic Spine

- Step Four: If the patient demonstrates pain-free movement, an overpressure is applied by pulling the elbows into further rotation and emphasizing the movement at the posterior of the patient.
- Step Five: The procedure is repeated on the opposite side.

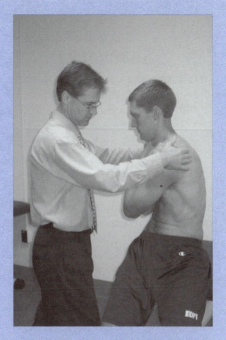

**Figure 8.14**  Overpressure of Rotation of the Thoracic Spine

## Bilateral–Unilateral Shoulder Flexion

It has been suggested that end range shoulder dysfunction may be associated with restrictions in the upper thoracic spine.[64] Unilateral shoulder flexion toward end range requires unilateral upper thoracic side flexion and rotation to the same side as the arm elevation.[64] Restrictions are evident in two fashions: (1) the arm is typically restricted from full flexion and (2) the thoracic spine side flexes away from the elevated arm in an attempt to compensate for the restriction.

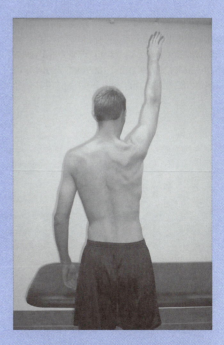

- Step One: The patient stands. Resting symptoms are assessed.
- Step Two: The patient is instructed to lift one arm as high into flexion as possible. The clinician remains behind the patient to view the thoracic movement.
- Step Three: The procedure is repeated on the opposite side.

**Figure 8.15**  Example of Restricted Upper Thoracic Rotation

## Summary

- To differentiate the concordant, thoracic active physiological movements may require separate clearing of the cervical or lumbar spine movements.
- Repeated flexion or overpressure is contraindicated on an older patient with a history of osteoporosis.
- It is necessary to evaluate the effect of sustained movement or repeated movements during concordant findings to determine the potential effect of treatment within that movement.

## Passive Movements

### Passive Physiological Tests

For many clinicians, the passive physiological movements can be performed simultaneously during active physiological movements. The passive movements occur after the active range when the clinician takes up the slack of the remaining unoccupied range of motion. Some clinicians choose to perform the passive physiological movements in isolation to adjust the forces and repeated passive movements to determine potential treatment choices.

**Passive Flexion**

- Step One: Flexion is applied by pulling the elbows into flexion and placing the lumbar region into flexion.
- Step Two: Flexion can be emphasized by pushing the targeted region either up with the movement of the ribs or against the movements of the ribs with the palm of the hand.

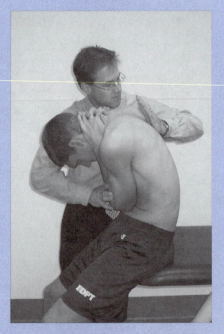

**Figure 8.16**   Passive Flexion of the Thoracic Spine

## Passive Extension

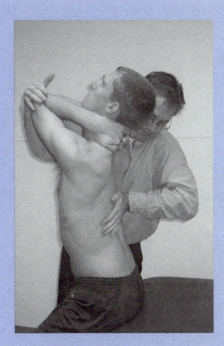

- Step One: Passive extension is applied by pulling up on the elbows into extension while stabilizing the thoracic spine into extension with the opposite hand.
- Step Two: Extension can be emphasized by pushing the targeted region either up against the movement of the ribs or downward with the movement of the ribs with the palm of the hand.

**Figure 8.17**    Overpressure of Extension of the Thoracic Spine

## Passive Physiological Rotation

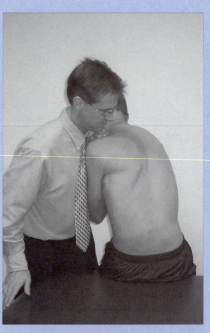

- Step One: Passive rotation is applied by pulling the elbows into further rotation and emphasizing the movement at the posterior of the patient.

**Figure 8.18**    Passive Physiological Rotation of the Thoracic Spine

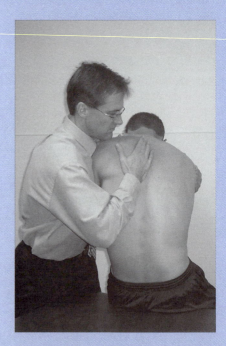

- Step Two: The clinician can emphasize the location of the rotation posteriorly by providing additional force with the palm of his or her hand, emphasizing the bulk of the rotation at that region.
- Step Three: For emphasis on the rib motion, the clinician should supply a superior force on the ribs opposite of the direction of rotation and an inferior force on the ribs in the direction of the rotation.[19]
- Step Four: The procedure is repeated on the opposite side.

**Figure 8.19**    Physiological Rotation with Emphasis

**Passive Physiological Side Flexion**

- Step One: Passive physiological side flexion is applied by pulling the patient into further side flexion using a handgrip near the axilla of the patient.

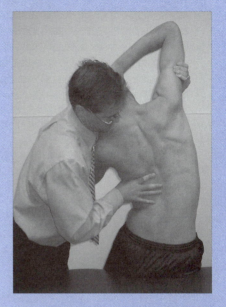

**Figure 8.20**    Overpressure of Side Flexion of the Thoracic Spine

- Step Two: Like rotation, the movement can be emphasized by pushing the targeted region with the palm of the hand.
- Step Three: For emphasis on the rib motion during side flexion, the clinician should place an inferior force on the ribs in the direction of the side flexion, understanding that movements may be variable at the mid-thoracic spine.[19]
- Step Four: The procedure is repeated on the opposite side.

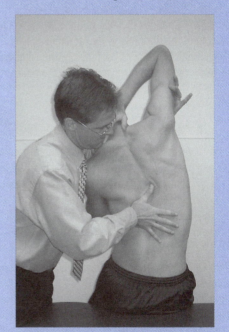

**Figure 8.21**    Side Flexion with Emphasis

## Passive Accessory Tests

Passive accessory movements can be subdivided into two forms, provocation-based and plane-based. Provocation-based movements are performed to identify the causal segment with subsequent treatment directed to the cause. Plane-based movements that theoretically move the segment allow movement within the facet's axial plane and are generally less painful during application. In the thoracic spine, plane-based movements are difficult to perform without incorporating combined movements (accessory and physiological movements). True planar movement in the thoracic spine requires alterations in mobilization angles depending on the region of the thoracic spine and the movement of distraction into flexion and may best be performed when combined with other movements.

## Central Posterior Anterior (CPA)

Assessment of a CPA is part of a normal thoracic examination.[13] A CPA performed directly posterior to anterior is a provocation-based movement. Stiffness of a CPA is effected by many factors including the level of the assessed vertebra (cephalic has greater stiffness than caudal segments)[13] and the rigidity of the rib cage.[65] Because the spinous processes of the thoracic spine are angled inferiorly, a PA motion to the thoracic spine may promote extension of the specific segment, similar to the force placed on a pump handle while drawing water.

- Step One: The patient assumes a prone lying position. Resting symptoms are assessed.
- Step Two: The clinician palpates the targeted level, feeling for the first thoracic spinous processes. This segment is localized first by finding C6 and working caudally. C6 disappears (moves posterior to anterior) during passive extension while C7 stays pronounced.
- Step Three: The clinician applies a PA force to the first point of reported pain. Pain is assessed to determine if concordant. This process is continued at all thoracic segments or is focused on those segments based on the detailed history.
- Step Four: Movement and force is applied beyond the first point of pain toward end range. Sustained holds or repeated movements that affect the concordant sign are utilized to determine potential treatment selection.
- Step Five: Changes of angle of pressure may alter the report of symptoms of the patient. By targeting movements more caudally, cranially, medially, or laterally, the clinician may more effectively reproduce the symptoms of the patient.

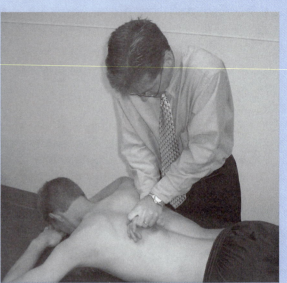

**Figure 8.22**    Central Posterior Anterior to Facet

## Unilateral Posterior Anterior (UPA)

Assessment of a UPA is part of a normal thoracic examination.[13] A UPA is a provocation-based movement. Provocation-based accessory movements are applied perpendicular to the facet planes causing compression of the segments. The facets lie just lateral to the spinous processes (albeit at different levels). The facets can be palpated in thin-framed individuals as a valley or deficit within the boney architecture.

### UPA to the Facet

- Step One: The patient assumes a prone lying position. Resting symptoms are assessed.
- Step Two: The clinician palpates the targeted level, feeling for the deficit just lateral to the spinous processes.
- Step Three: The clinician applies a PA force to the first point of reported pain. Pain is assessed to determine if concordant. This process is continued at all thoracic segments or is focused on those segments based on the detailed history.
- Step Four: Movement and force is applied beyond the first point of pain toward end range. Sustained holds or repeated movements that affect the concordant sign are utilized to determine potential treatment selection.
- Step Five: Changes of angle of pressure may alter the report of symptoms of the patient. By targeting movements more caudally, cranially, medially, or laterally, the clinician may more effectively reproduce the symptoms of the patient.
- Step Six: The process is repeated on the opposite side.

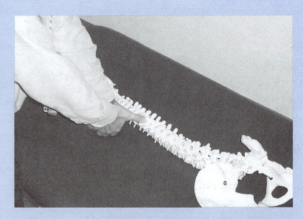

**Figure 8.23**    Unilateral Posterior Anterior to the Facet

## Unilateral Posterior Anterior (UPA) to the Costotransverse Joint

A unilateral PA of the costotransverse joint requires the identification of the joint articulation lateral to the midline of the thoracic spine. The articulation is both inferior and superior to the rib attachment. The elevated portion laterally is the distal end of the transverse process.

- Step One: The patient assumes a prone lying position. Resting symptoms are assessed.
- Step Two: The clinician palpates the targeted level, feeling for the raised region approximately two thumbs' width lateral to the spinous processes.
- Step Three: The clinician applies a PA force to the first point of reported pain. Pain is assessed to determine if concordant. This process is continued at all thoracic segments or is focused on those segments based on the detailed history.
- Step Four: Movement and force is applied beyond the first point of pain toward end range. Sustained holds or repeated movements that affect the concordant sign are utilized to determine potential treatment selection.
- Step Five: Changes of angle of pressure may alter the report of symptoms of the patient. By targeting movements more caudally, cranially, medially, or laterally, the clinician may more effectively reproduce the symptoms of the patient.
- Step Six: The process is repeated on the opposite side.

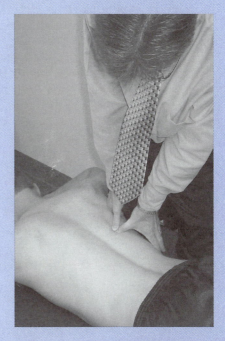

**Figure 8.24** Unilateral Posterior Anterior to the Costotransverse Joint

## Transverse Glides

Transverse glides are common methods that apply a lateral glide to the spinous processes of the spine. These techniques are also provocation-based procedures. The technique is also commonly used in examination and treatment and has been well studied for its neurophysiologic affects.[28,29]

- Step One: The patient is positioned in prone or sidelying, and the neck is placed in neutral.
- Step Two: The clinician palpates the T1 spinous process using the tips of the thumb. Using one thumb pad, the clinician applies a very broad and deep contact to the side of the spinous process, applying more force on the base of the spinous than the posterior tip.
- Step Three: The clinician then aligns the forearm so that it is parallel to the force to the spinous process and pushes to the first point of reported pain. Concordant pain is assessed.
- Step Four: The clinician then pushes beyond the first point of pain toward end range, reassesses pain and quality of movement, and checks for splinting or muscle spasm. Concordant pain is assessed.
- Step Five: Passive repeated movements are performed at end range. Changes in pain level or determination if the pain is concordant are performed.
- Step Six: The process is repeated on each spinous process to T12 to identify the concordant segment.
- Step Seven: Repeat the process on the opposite side.

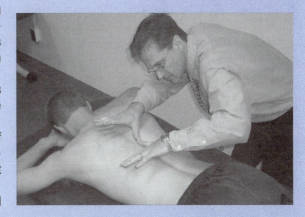

**Figure 8.25** Transverse Glide of Thoracic Spinous Process

## Anterior Posterior (AP) Mobilizations

An AP mobilization is a provocation-based examination technique. The assessment of an anterior posterior accessory motion at the sternum does demonstrate greater flexibility than a similar PA assessment to the facets or costovertebral joints.[13] Isolated rib movement is opposite of the movement posterior to the spine with extension-producing cephalic rotation of the joint and flexion-producing caudal rotation.[66]

A condition known as costochondritis may produce isolated pain directed at the two rib–sternal attachments. This is a common cause of chest-wall pain that mimics a cardiac response. This condition is occasionally reported as Tietze's syndrome and frequently occurs over the fourth to sixth ribs.[67]

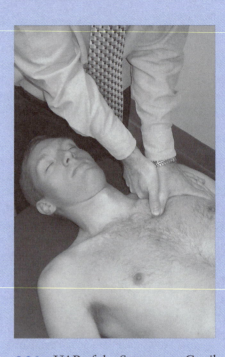

**Figure 8.26**    UAP of the Sternum to Cartilage

- Step One: The patient assumes a supine position. Resting symptoms are assessed.
- Step Two: The clinician palpates the targeted level. To assess the connection of the sternum to the cartilage the clinician should palpate joint line just lateral to the sternum on ribs 3 to 8. To assess the ribs' connection to the cartilage the clinician may need to palpate laterally, approximately 2 inches from the sternum toward the angular connection of the rib.
- Step Three: The clinician applies an AP force to the first point of reported pain. Pain is assessed to determine if concordant.
- Step Four: Movement and force is applied beyond the first point of pain toward end range. Sustained holds or repeated movements that affect the concordant sign are utilized to determine potential treatment selection.
- Step Five: As with the posterior anterior movements, changes of angle of pressure may alter the report of symptoms of the patient.

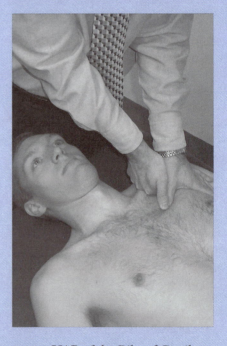

**Figure 8.27**    UAP of the Ribs of Cartilage

## Combined Passive Movements

The size of the thoracic spine and the complexity of movements often require the use of combined movements to determine the actual concordant sign. Potentially combined movements may include a combination of or the isolated movement of any of the active physiological motions, passive physiological movements concurrently during passive accessory, provocation, or plane-based glides.

### Accessory Glide with Rotation

- Step One: The patient sits at the edge of the plinth. Resting symptoms are assessed.
- Step Two: The clinician rotates the patient into rotation while loading. Special effort should be made not to engage end-range rotation.
- Step Three: At the desired rotation (concordant position), the clinician applies a transverse glide into the rotation to the first point of reported pain. Pain is assessed to determine if concordant. The clinician may also choose to apply a posterior anterior force, central or unilateral.

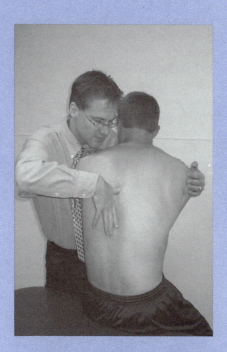

**Figure 8.28**    Unilateral PA during Preposition of Rotation

- Step Four: Movement and force is applied beyond the first point of pain toward end range. Sustained holds or repeated movements that affect the concordant sign are utilized to determine potential treatment selection.
- Step Five: As with the posterior–anterior movements, changes of compression force may alter the report of symptoms of the patient.

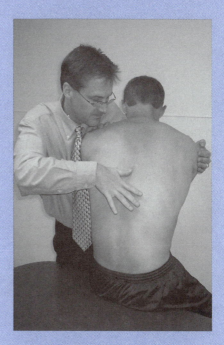

**Figure 8.29**    Physiological Rotation with Transverse Glide

## Rotation and Side Flexion

Rotation and side flexion can be integrated for a combined procedural assessment.

- Step One: The patient sits at the edge of the plinth. Resting symptoms are assessed.
- Step Two: The clinician rotates the patient into rotation while loading. Special effort should be made not to engage end-range rotation.
- Step Three: At the desired rotation (concordant position), the clinician applies a passive physiological side flexion force to the first point of reported pain. Pain is assessed to determine if concordant.
- Step Four: Movement and force is applied beyond the first point of pain toward end range. Sustained holds or repeated movements that affect the concordant sign are utilized to determine potential treatment selection.

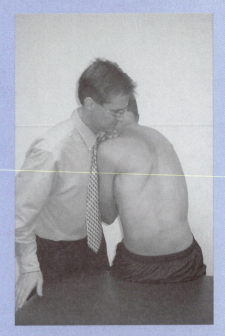

**Figure 8.30**  Ccombined Physiological Rotation and Side Flexion

## Extension with a Posterior–Anterior Mobilization

Extension and a posterior–anterior force may be useful in identifying patients who may benefit from postural treatment. During extension, the ribs rotate caudally during facet closure. The clinician may choose to work opposite of the rib movement or with the rib movement to enhance extension motion.

- Step One: The patient sits at the edge of the plinth. Resting symptoms are assessed.
- Step Two: The clinician extends the patient into the desired pre-extension position.
- Step Three: At the desired preposition of extension (concordant position), the clinician can apply either a superiorly based or an inferiorly based force to the ribs and facets. The clinician must modulate the force with the first point of reported pain. Pain is assessed to determine if concordant.
- Step Four: Movement and force is applied beyond the first point of pain toward end range. Sustained holds or repeated movements that affect the concordant sign are utilized to determine potential treatment selection.

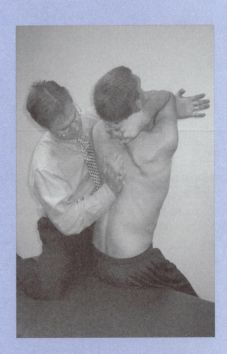

**Figure 8.31**  Passive Physiological Extension with a PA Force

## Summary

- Passive physiological movements are often integrated with active physiological movements of the thoracic spine.
- Passive accessory movements require the careful separate examination of the facet joints and the costotransverse joints, both of which may be the pain generator of the thoracic spine.
- Combined movements can be used to further isolate a movement dysfunction.

## Clinical Special Tests

Unlike the cervical spine or shoulder, there are minimal clinical special tests for the thoracic spine, nearly none of which has been studied for diagnostic accuracy. Thus, only a few of the special tests of the thoracic spine are presented here.

### Palpation

Christensen et al.[68] reported the reliability of sitting motion palpation, prone motion palpation, and paraspinal palpation for tenderness. Using an expanded and more liberal definition of agreement, the pooled kappa values were 0.59 to 0.77 overall. Love and Brodeur[69] found poor interrater reliability but good intrarater reliability by chiropractic students in detecting hypomobility of the thoracic spine.

Haas et al.[70] advocated the use of end range palpation for detection of rotation stiffness as a decision-making tool for a manipulative procedure. Their study outlined the clinical effectiveness after isolating the restricted movement during palpation and subsequent manipulation. Lewis et al.[71] reported the benefit of surface palpation for location of the scapula as well as the use of the position of the scapula to determine thoracic landmarks such as the lower border of the scapula (T12).

### Manual Muscle Testing

Frese reported low interrater reliability when testing middle and inferior trapezius strength.[72] Paraspinal strength testing is also poorly quantified and has been presented numerous ways within the literature. Empirically, strength assessment of the paraspinal muscles should yield useful information since passive and active stabilization forces are required to prevent excessive kyphosis. Within the thoracic spine, the deep paraspinal musculature is constantly active functioning to stabilize the posture, a process that differs from the lumbar spine.[54]

## Thoracic Slump

The thoracic slump is a variation of the (lumbar) slump sit test originally introduced by Maitland.[73] Like the lumbar slump, the thoracic slump is positive when tension on a nerve root is painful, specifically during the onset of discogenic pain. Similar to the lumbar spine, a positive finding may implicate a primary disc herniation, degenerative disc, irritation of the posterior longitudinal ligament,[74] or a chronic nerve root adhesion. Additionally, a positive test requires (1) asymmetrical reproduction of the concordant sign, (2) the same report of concordant pain, and (3) sensitization (e.g., movement from a distal or proximal area that engages the tension of the nerve root should increase the symptoms).[75] At present, there are no studies that have measured the diagnostic utility of the thoracic slump test.

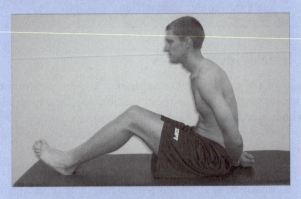

- Step One: The patient assumes a long sitting position with the knees bent approximately 45 degrees. The hands are placed behind the back to allow therapist maneuvering. Resting symptoms are assessed.

**Figure 8.32**    Starting Position of the Thoracic Slump Test

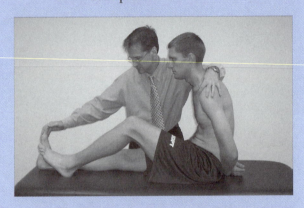

- Step Two: The clinician loads the patient over the shoulders. Resting symptoms are assessed.
- Step Three: The patient is instructed to flex the lower cervical spine and extend the upper cervical spine. The clinician may add overpressure to the movement. Resting symptoms are assessed.

**Figure 8.33**    Prepositioning of the Thoracic Slump Test

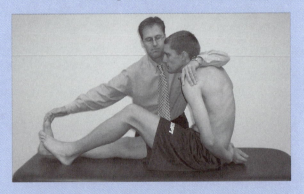

- Step Four: The clinician then passively moves the lower extremity on the concordant side into extension and the ankle into dorsiflexion. Resting symptoms are again assessed.
- Step Five: The clinician can then add side flexion to the right or the left and/or rotation to the right or left to engage further the dural tissue. Symptoms are further assessed to determine the concordant nature.
- Step Six: In addition, patients may extend both knees or perform upper limb tension movements during this examination.

**Figure 8.34**    End Positioning of the Thoracic Slump Test

## Cervical Thoracic Differentiation

Because the upper thoracic spine mimics the biomechanical movement of the lower cervical spine, movements of the cervical spine originate pain that is causal to the upper thoracic spine. To differentiate structures, a simple rotation test is beneficial, especially if rotation elicits the concordant movement of the patient.

- Step One: The patient assumes a sitting position. Resting symptoms are assessed.
- Step Two: The patient is instructed to rotate toward end range in order to reproduce the concordant movement. This movement produces both cervical and thoracic rotation.

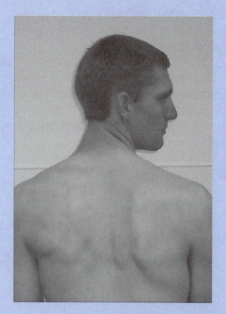

**Figure 8.35**   Preposition of Full End Range Rotation

- Step Three: At the end range, the clinician applies a transverse glide to the spinous process toward the direction the spinous process moves during rotation (opposite of the vertebral body movement) at the cervico-thoracic junction.

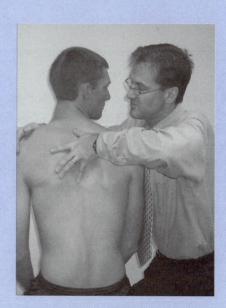

**Figure 8.36**   Blocking the Rotation of the Thoracic Spine

*(continued)*

- Step Four: The patient is instructed to derotate the cervical spine while the clinician maintains the hold of the thoracic spine in rotation.
- Step Five: If symptoms are eliminated during derotation of the cervical spine, the symptoms are of cervical spine origin. If symptoms maintain during derotation of the cervical spine, the symptoms are of thoracic origin.
- Step Six: This method only displays utility if rotation produces the concordant sign of the patient.

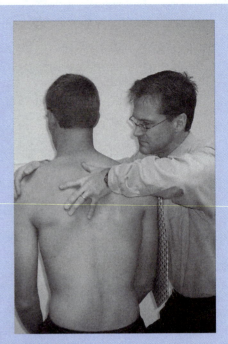

**Figure 8.37**    The Cervical Thoracic Rotation Clinical Special Test

## Summary

- There are few special tests of the thoracic spine, none of which has been validated for diagnostic accuracy.
- The thoracic slump test may be useful to rule out the presence of a herniated disc prior to manipulation.
- The cervical-thoracic rotation test may be useful in differentiating the origin of symptoms of the cervico-thoracic spine.

# TREATMENT TECHNIQUES

## For Posture

Renno et al.[59] have demonstrated improvements in thoracic posture in a mixed treatment program that consisted of stretching, strengthening, and respiratory work. Mostly, however, conservative postural treatment consisting of similar treatments to the above mentioned has included populations of patients with thoracic outlet syndrome or other characterized disorders. Although understudied, there does seem to be a consistency toward the benefit of stretching and strengthening exercises for the thoracic spine. These techniques may be passive or therapist administered.

## Passive Stretches

The following passive approaches adopt the same principle for pain reduction and postural improvement associated with stretching discussed in Chapter 1. Stretches should be limited to patient tolerance with hold times of 15–20 seconds or to tolerance.

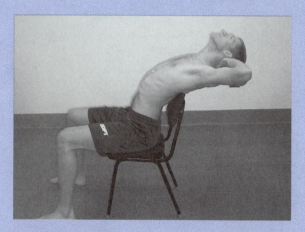

**Figure 8.38**    Thoracic Extension in Sitting

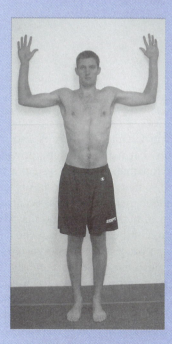

**Figure 8.39**    Wall Angle Stretches

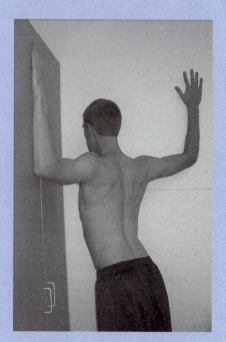

**Figure 8.40**    Corner Stretches for Upper Thoracic Mobility

## Therapist Administered

The therapist-administered techniques are useful if the patient does not tolerate mobilization or manipulation and serve as a strong adjunct to strengthening exercises.

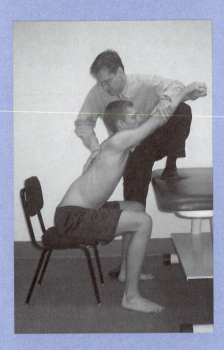

**Figure 8.41**    Seated Mid-Thoracic Stretch

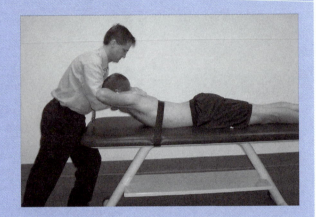

**Figure 8.42**    Prone Mid-Thoracic Stretch

### *Use of Tape for Posture*

Taping for posture has been used as a kinematic trigger for patients with habitually poor posture. No studies were found to analyze the effectiveness. Taping is designed to deload the nociceptive processing in order to alter neurophysiologic pain perception. O'Leary et al.[76] demonstrated that deloading tape does not alter pain perception during application. However, although pain perception was not altered, the benefit of taping may be postural. The benefits may best be described as kinesthetic, providing the patient with cueing for posture and stability.

## Mobilization

Detection of stiffness of the rib cage is significantly altered by the rib cage during a PA.[65] Additionally, if the patient has a variable amount of air within the lungs, compression will demonstrate variability. This necessitates the importance of pain response during assessment as well as detection of stiffness.

As discussed in Chapter 1, there is also moderate evidence to support that manual therapy provides an excitatory effect on sympathetic nervous system activity[28,29,77,78] and the thoracic spine is no exception. An excitatory effect on the sympathetic nervous system occurs concurrently with a reduction of hypoanalgesia and may parallel the effects of stimulation of the dorsal periaqueductal gray matter of the midbrain, a process that has occurred in animal research.[79,80] Documented evidence supports the benefit of modulation of pain and remarkably has a nonlocalized effect. Wright[81] outlines that hypoalgesia and sympathoexcitation are correlated, suggesting that individuals who exhibit the most change in pain perception also exhibit the most change in sympathetic nervous system function.

Like the cervical spine mobilizations, those used during the examination may yield potential treatment choices if positive results were found with sustained or repeated movements. The techniques of the PA, AP (of the costosternal joints), the transverse glide, and the UPA may be effective in modulating pain and stiffness.

## Mobilization of the First Rib

Although controversial and without appropriate investigation, the first rib may be the culprit in thoracic outlet syndrome. Thoracic outlet syndrome is a combination of symptoms in which cervico-brachial nerve-related pain occurs because of compression or traction. Theoretically, elevation of the first rib may lead to entrapment or injury of the nerve.

- Step One: The patient is placed in a supine position. Resting symptoms are assessed.
- Step Two: The first rib is palpated posteriorly using the following landmark identification. First, the clinician drops caudally just below the mastoid process. This should identify the landmark of the first rib.
- Step Three: The clinician places the patient's head in side flexion to the same side and rotation away. This reduces the stress of the scalene muscles on the first rib and allows the rib to "drop" during mobilization.
- Step Four: The force of the mobilization is toward the anterior, contralateral hip (ASIS). As with all mobilizations, the force is modulated based on positive patient response.

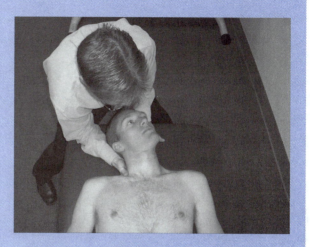

**Figure 8.43**   Mobilization of the First Rib

## *Manipulation*

Ross et al.[82] reported that the location of a thoracic manipulation is less specific than previously assessed. Slightly over 50% of thoracic joint manipulations resulted in a cavitation at the targeted level. Typical errors in segmental manipulation of nearly 3.5 cm from the desired target were recorded. Bereznick et al.[83] acknowledged a similar problem during the use of a "screw" manipulation identifying that the skin friction tension was not helpful in allowing a clinician to target the manipulation at a selected vector.

Selection of manipulation over mobilization is based on clinical reasoning. Manipulation may be effective for those patients who are not irritable, have limited relative or no absolute contraindications, and for those that have demonstrated benefit in the past. Unfortunately, little data are available on clinical predictive rules for selecting manipulation over mobilization. Since manipulation does not provide the luxury of an examination-based outcome (i.e., use of repeated or sustained holds to outline the potential response), the results of a manipulation are essentially unknown.

### *Manipulation of the Cervical-Thoracic Junction*

The cervical-thoracic junction is a stable region solidified by the connection of the ribs to the cervical-like upper thoracic segments. The procedures of the techniques effective in the cervical spine are inappropriate in the upper thoracic secondary to the inability to perform the necessary handholds.

## Distraction Manipulation of the Upper Thoracic Segments

The upper thoracic facets tilt anteriorly, decreasing the likelihood of a gapping during an AP manipulation procedure. Consequently, an effective technique that produces facet sliding can be performed in sitting if the flexion of the upper thoracic region is maintained throughout the process.

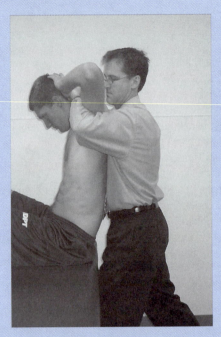

- Step One: The patient sits at the edge of the plinth. The arms are wrapped behind the head and the fingers are interlaced.
- Step Two: The clinician stands behind the patient and inserts his or her forearms anteriorly to the humerus and posterior to the forearm of the patient. The clinician then grips the thumbs of the patient with his or her hands.
- Step Three: The patient is placed in further flexion and encouraged to relax.
- Step Four: The clinician increases the stability of the arm-to-arm grip by pulling outward into external rotation. Gently rocking the patient side to side may also assist in relaxing the patient.
- Step Five: The manipulation force is anterior and upward. Careful attention is required to avoid an extension movement of the patient's thoracic spine.

**Figure 8.44**    Distraction Manipulation of the Upper Thoracic Segments

## Prone Cervico-Thoracic (CT) Junction Manipulation

The prone CT junction manipulation is a method that is effective in targeting segments C7 to T2. Less force is required for the manipulation and for smaller clinicians, the prone CT junction manipulation is relatively easy to administer.

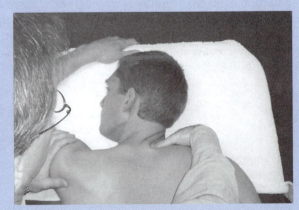

- Step One: The patient lies in a prone position. The head is rotated away from the targeted side of the manipulation. The arm that is on the side that the head is rotated is placed in shoulder abduction and elbow flexion.
- Step Two: The clinician leans over the patient caudal to the head. Using the thumb, the clinician blocks the spinous process caudal to the targeted joint.

**Figure 8.45**    The Spinous Process Blocking Method

- Step Three: The clinician then places the palm of his or her hand on the patient's zygomatic arch and applies a superior diagonal force into side flexion and extension.
- Step Four: At the perceived end point, the clinician applies a thrust into the extended side flexion position.

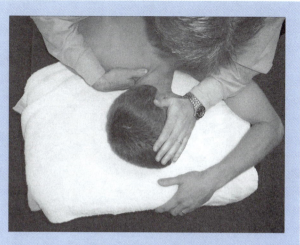

**Figure 8.46**    Prone CT Junction Manipulation

## The Pistol Manipulation

Cleland et al.[27] also found strength gains of the inferior trapezius with thoracic manipulation versus a sham technique. The pistol technique used may be responsible for improvement of thoracic extension, a physiological movement that has been linked to improvements in shoulder flexion.[84]

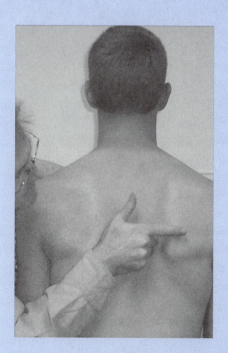

- Step One: The patient assumes a supine position. Using an over and under crossing technique, the patient crosses his or her arms over the chest.
- Step Two: The clinician stands to the opposite side of the targeted segment. Using the arm furthest from the targeted side, the clinician gently pulls the patient into sidelying.
- Step Three: The clinician then leans over the patient and places the hand behind the patient's back just caudal to the targeted segment. The pistol grip (pictured) allows the transverse processes to articulate with the thenar eminence and the knuckle of the clinician's hand.

**Figure 8.47**    The Pistol Grip

*(continued)*

- Step Four: The patient is "scooped" into flexion (using his or her arms as a lever) and gently placed over the pistol hand of the clinician. Careful effort is made to keep the patient in flexion.
- Step Five: The clinician may further enhance the contact point on the patient's transverse process by pronating the wrist or ulnarly deviating the hand.
- Step Six: The clinician's thrust should be through the shaft of the humeri with careful maintenance of the position of flexion of the trunk.

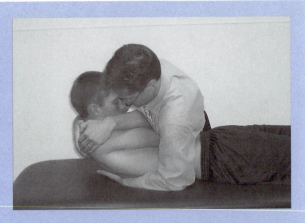

**Figure 8.48**   The Pistol Manipulation

Two adjustments can be made with the Pistol manipulation to target the upper and lower thoracic spines. For the upper thoracic spine, pulling the thoracic spine into extension (by pulling caudally on the transverse processes) rearranges the facet planes toward the horizontal and improves the likelihood of a manipulation.

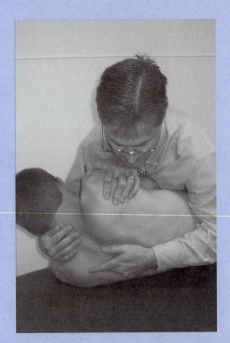

**Figure 8.49**   Adjustment for the Upper Thoracic Spine

For the lower thoracic spine, pushing the thoracic spine into flexion (by pushing cranially on the transverse processes) re-arranges the facet planes toward the horizontal and improves the likelihood of a successful manipulation.

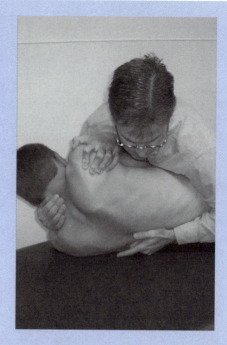

**Figure 8.50**   Adjustment for the Lower Thoracic Spine

## The Screw Manipulation

Maitland describes a manipulative technique in which the transverse processes are forced into a posterior-to-anterior direction. Chiropractors average 462–482 Newtons of force during a thoracic screw manipulation technique, producing this peak force in approximately 120 milliseconds.[85] Others have reported peak thrust values of over 1,100 Newtons with a thoracic screw thrust, albeit shorter periods of peak output.[86] Prior to administration, the clinician should review the contraindications to manipulation in Chapter 5.

- Step One: The patient lies in a prone position.
- Step Two: The clinician identifies the targeted guilty segment with the concordant application of a UPA.
- Step Three: The clinician identifies the direction of the manipulation by applying a lateral stress (transverse force) to adjacent spinous process to determine the painful and stiff segment. For example, if a UPA of the T5 facet on the right produced the concordant sign, and a transverse glide of the spinous process to the right and a transverse process of the spinous process of T6 to the left caused similar pain, then the hand placement by the clinician would be one pisiform on the right transverse process of T5 and one pisiform on the left transverse process of T6.

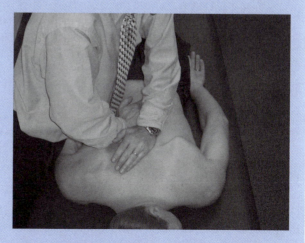

**Figure 8.51**   Hand Placement for the Screw Manipulation

*(continued)*

- Step Four: The clinician then preloads the tissue and takes up the slack.
- Step Five: The thrust occurs directly toward the patient once the patient completely exhales his or her respiratory volume.

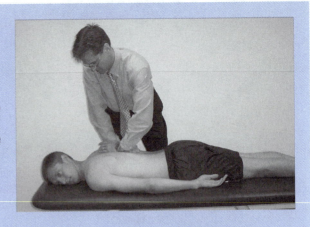

**Figure 8.52**    The Screw Manipulation

## The Costotransverse Manipulation

The costotransverse manipulation is a general manipulation that is often effective on the lower costotransverse joints of the thoracic spine.

- Step One: The patient lies in a prone position.
- Step Two: The clinician stabilizes the costotransverse joint with the palm of one hand while lifting upward on the ASIS of the ipsilateral side.
- Step Three: The clinician rotates the ASIS upward until movement is felt at the stabilized costotransverse joint.
- Step Four: The ASIS is pulled further upward (into contralateral rotation) until an anterior-to-posterior directed force is felt by the clinician at the costotransverse joint. At that point, a downward thrust is applied to the costotransverse joint.

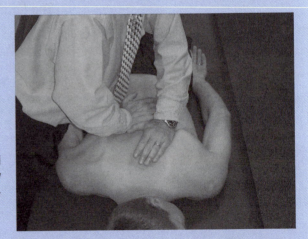

**Figure 8.53**    Costotransverse Manipulation

## *Combined Movements*

Combined movements are often required to move within the plane of the facet. Because the thoracic segments face inferiorly and anteriorly, facet movement is curvilinear and will often slide during opening and closing. Gapping occurs when the joint is opened using a perpendicular-directed force.

## Facet Joint Gapping

The mobilization of a locked thoracic facet has been reported by Horton. Using a postural mobilization along the axis and plane of the facet may open the facet and decrease the impingement of the miscode.

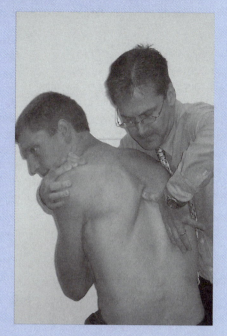

- Step One: The patient assumes a sitting position. The patient's arms are crossed in front of the body so that the clinician may use the arms as a lever to position the thoracic spine.
- Step Two: The clinician pulls the arms into flexion and rotation to the opposite side of the facet dysfunction. This movement serves to "open" the thoracic facet on the targeted side.
- Step Three: The clinician then applies a superior-to-anterior directed force along the plane of the facet. This motion theoretically creates traction to the facet to enhance an opening moment.
- Step Four: The clinician may apply a static hold, a muscle energy technique, or oscillations in this position.

**Figure 8.54**   Mobilization of a Locked Thoracic Facet

## Combined Rotation and Accessory Movements with Slump Testing

The combined rotation and accessory movement during slump testing is an effective way to target the dural signs of the patient.

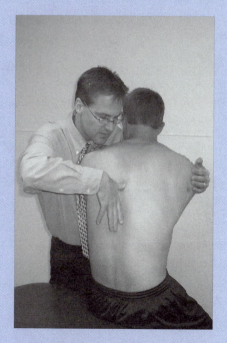

- Step One: The patient assumes a long sitting position with the knees bent approximately 60 degrees. The hands are placed behind the back to allow therapist maneuvering. Resting symptoms are assessed.
- Step Two: The clinician loads the patient over the shoulders. Resting symptoms are assessed.
- Step Three: The patient is instructed to flex the lower cervical spine and extend the upper cervical spine. The clinician may add overpressure to the movement. The following techniques are especially beneficial if the patient's dural symptoms are reproduced at this point.
- Step Four: The clinician passively moves the patient into rotation while continuingly maintaining the load. Special effort should be made not to engage end-range rotation.
- Step Five: At the desired rotation (concordant position), the clinician applies a transverse glide into the rotation to the first point of reported pain. Pain is assessed to determine if concordant. The clinician may also choose to apply a posterior–anterior force, central or unilateral.
- Step Six: Movement and force is applied beyond the first point of pain toward end range. Sustained holds or repeated movements that affect the concordant sign are utilized to determine potential treatment selection.
- Step Seven: As with the posterior–anterior movements, changes of compression force may alter the report of symptoms of the patient.

**Figure 8.55**   Unilateral PA During Preposition of Rotation

## Rotation and Side Flexion

Rotation and side flexion combines two passive physiological techniques for assessment.

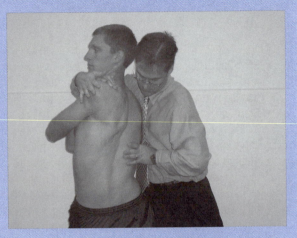

- Step One: The patient sits at the edge of the plinth. Resting symptoms are assessed.
- Step Two: The clinician passively moves the patient into rotation while loading. Special effort should be made not to engage end-range rotation.
- Step Three: At the desired rotation (concordant position), the clinician applies a passive physiological side flexion force to the first point of reported pain. Pain is assessed to determine if concordant.
- Step Four: Movement and force is applied beyond the first point of pain toward end range. Sustained holds or repeated movements that affect the concordant sign are utilized to determine potential treatment selection.

**Figure 8.56**  Combined Physiological Rotation and Side Flexion

## Extension with a Posterior–Anterior Mobilization

Extension and a posterior–anterior force may be useful in identifying patients who may benefit from postural treatment. During extension, the ribs rotate caudally during facet closure. The clinician may choose to work opposite of the rib movement or with the rib movement to enhance extension motion.

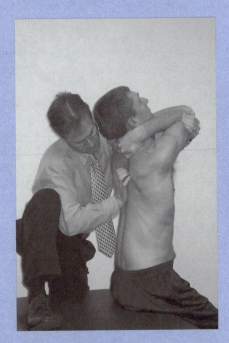

- Step One: The patient sits at the edge of the plinth. Resting symptoms are assessed.
- Step Two: The clinician extends the patient into the desired pre-extension position.
- Step Three: At the desired preposition of extension (concordant position), the clinician can apply either a superiorly based or an inferiorly based force to the ribs and facets. The clinician must modulate the force with the first point of reported pain. Pain is assessed to determine if concordant.
- Step Four: Movement and force is applied beyond the first point of pain toward end range. Sustained holds or repeated movements that affect the concordant sign are utilized to determine potential treatment selection.

**Figure 8.57**  Passive Physiological Extension with a PA Force

## Summary

- Passive stretches may be beneficial for postural correction or as an adjunct for pain modulation techniques.
- Passive mobilization techniques are selected based on patient response.
- Mobilization of the first rib is designed to decrease pain associated with thoracic outlet syndrome.
- Manipulation may be effective for reduction of pain and stiffness.
- Manipulation is selected based on clinical reasoning. At present, no clinical prediction rules are present to determine when to select manipulation versus mobilization.
- Combined techniques may be necessary for mobilization along the plane of the facet.

control and promote the decreased risk associated with thoracic versus cervical manipulation as additive benefit.[87] The idea of treating the upper thoracic quadrant, creating overflow to the shoulder and neck, seems to have strong merit. Another study by Savolainen et al.[88] found similar results in the treatment of shoulder neck pain when thoracic manipulation was compared to an active exercise approach. Four thoracic manipulations were more effective than an active exercise program at 6 and 12 months.

Like mobilization, few studies have investigated the benefit of treating the thoracic spine with manipulation. Schiller[89] performed a small randomized controlled trial including 30 subjects and found benefit over subtherapeutic ultrasound. However, this trial was very small and used subjects that were younger and were followed for a very short time. Additionally, subjects were not classified into similar groups. Further investigation is needed to determine the scientific merit of manual therapy to the thoracic spine. Results appear promising, but at this time, little direction is provided for the practitioner.

# TREATMENT OUTCOMES

Overall, few studies have investigated the benefits of manual therapy on the thoracic spine. Studies have outlined the effectiveness of mobilization for treatment of thoracic disorders in case studies[16,39] and have reported positive benefit. Others have reported that mobilization and manipulation leads to increases in lower thoracic strength when compared to controls such as sham manipulation.[27,55] At this time, no studies had evaluated the effectiveness of mobilization of the thoracic spine in a well-designed randomized clinical trial.

Cleland et al. advocate the benefit of spinal manipulation of the thoracic spine for treatment of cervical pain. The authors outlined positive outcomes versus a sham

## Summary

- Thoracic mobilization and manipulation are advocated in single case study designs.
- There appears to be merit and benefit in treating the cervical spine and/or shoulder with thoracic manipulation.
- Only one study has been performed that randomized patients with a thoracic spine injury into comparison groups. More research is needed to determine the benefit of manual therapy of the thoracic spine.

# Chapter Questions

1. Describe the facet orientation of the thoracic spine. How does the facet orientation and the contribution of the rib cage affect the stability of the thoracic spine?
2. Describe the coupling pattern of the thoracic spine. Does this coupling pattern change throughout the thoracic spine?
3. Identify the specific characteristics of the thoracic spine examination that are unique. How does fine-tuning selected movement in the thoracic spine assist in improving data collection during treatment? Describe methods of this process.
4. Compare and contrast the biomechanical constructs behind mobilization and manipulation of the thoracic spine.
5. Describe the literature associated with thoracic spine outcomes with manual therapy.

# References

1. Tawackoli W, Marco R, Liebschner MA. The effect of compressive axial preload on the flexibility of the thoracolumbar spine. *Spine.* 2004;29(9):988–993.

2. Singh K, Vaccaro AR, Eichenbaum MD, Fitzhenry LN. The surgical management of thoracolumbar injuries. *J Spinal Cord Med.* 2004;27(2):95–101.

3. White AA, Panjabi MM, Thomas CL. The clinical biomechanics of kyphotic deformities. *Clin Orthop.* 1977; 128:8–17.

4. Schwab F, Dubey A, Gamez L, El Fegouri AB, Hwang K, Pagala M, Farcy JP. Adult scoliosis: prevalence, SF-36, and nutritional parameters in an elderly volunteer population. *Spine.* 2005;30(9):1082–1085.

5. Benson M, Burnes D. The clinical syndromes and surgical treatments of thoracic intervertebral disc prolapse. *J Bone Jnt Surg.* 1975;8:457–471.

6. Stone J, Lichtor T, Banerjee S. Intradural thoracic disc herniation. *Spine.* 1994;19:1281–1284.

7. Wilke A, Wolf U, Lageard P, Griss P. Thoracic disc herniation: a diagnostic challenge. *Man Ther.* 2000;5: 181–184.

8. Willems JM, Jull G, Ng J. An in-vivo study of the primary and coupled rotations of the thoracic spine. *Clin Biomech.* 1996;11:311–316.

9. Kothe R, O'Holleran JD, Liu W, Panjabi MM. Internal architecture of the thoracic pedicle. An anatomic study. *Spine.* 1996;21(3):264–270.

10. Panjabi MM, Takata K, Goel V, Federico D, Oxland T, Duranceau J, Krag M. Thoracic human vertebrae. Quantitative three-dimensional anatomy. *Spine.* 1991; 16(8):888–901.

11. Panjabi MM, Hausfeld J, White A. A biomechanical study of the ligamentous stability of the thoracic spine in man. *Acta Orthop Scand.* 1981;52:315–326.

12. Karmakar MK, Chui PT, Joynt GM, Ho AM. Thoracic paravertebral block for management of pain associated with multiple fractured ribs in patients with concomitant lumbar spinal trauma. *Reg Anesth Pain Med.* 2001;26(2):169–173.

13. Edmondston SJ, Singer KP. Thoracic spine: anatomical and biomechanical considerations for manual therapy. *Man Ther.* 1997;2(3):132–143.

14. Kapandji I. *The Physiology of the joints. Vol. 3. The trunk and the vertebral column.* 2nd ed. London; Churchill Livingstone: 1978.

15. Galante JO. Tensile properties of the human lumbar annulus fibrosis. *Acta Orthop Scand.* 1967;Suppl 100: 1–91.

16. Horton SJ. Acute locked thoracic spine: treatment with a modified SNAG. *Man Ther.* 2002;7:103–107.

17. Polga DJ, Beaubien BP, Kallemeier PM, Schellhad KP, Lew WD, Buttermann GR, Wood KB. Measurement of in vivo intradiscal pressure in healthy thoracic intervertebral discs. *Spine.* 2004;29(12): 1320–1324.

18. Masharawi Y, Rothschild B, Dar G, Peleg S, Robinson D, Been E, Hershkovitz I. Facet orientation in the thoracolumbar spine. *Spine.* 2004;29:1755–1763.

19. Lee D. Rotational instability of the mid thoracic spine: assessment and management. *Man Ther.* 1996; 1:234–241.

20. White AA, Panjabi MM. *Clinical biomechanics of the spine.* Philadelphia; JB Lippincott: 1975.

21. Bogduk N, Engle R. The menisci of the lumbar zygopophyseal joints. A review of their anatomy and clinical significance. *Spine.* 1984;9:454–460.

22. Bogduk N, Jull G. (abstract). The theoretical pathology of acute locked back: A basis for manipulative therapy. *Man Med.* 1990;1:78–82.

23. Boszczyk B, Boszczyk A, Putz R, Buttner A, Benjamin M, Milz S. An immunohistochemical study of the dorsal capsule of the lumbar and thoracic facet joints. *Spine.* 2001;26(15):E338–343.

24. Erwin WM, Jackson PC, Homonko D. Innervation of the human intercostals joint: Implications for clinical back pain syndromes. *J Manip Physiol Ther.* 2000;23: 395–403.

25. Williams P, Bannister L. In: Berry M, Collins P. Dyson M, Dussek J, Ferguson M (eds) *Gray's Anatomy.* 38th ed. Churchill Livingstone, Edinburgh: 1995.

26. Andriacchi T, Shultz A, Belytschko T, Galante J. A model for studies of mechanical interactions between the human spine and rib cage. *J Biomech.* 1974;7: 497–507.

27. Cleland J, Selleck B, Stowell T, Browne L, Alberini S, St. Cyr H, Caron T. Short-term Effect of Thoracic Manipulation on Lower Trapezius Muscle Strength. *J Man Manip Ther.* 2004;12(2):82–90.

28. Vicenzino B, Paungmali A, Buratowski S, Wright A. Specific manipulative therapy treatment for chronic lateral epicondylalgia produces uniquely characteristic hypoalgesia. *Man Ther.* 2001;6:205–212.

29. Simon R, Vicenzino B, Wright A. The influence of an anteroposterior accessory glide of the glenohumeral joint on measures of peripheral sympathetic nervous system function in the upper limb. *Man Ther.* 1997; 2(1):18–23.

30. Sinaki M, Itoi E, Rogers JW, Bergstralh EJ, Wahner HW. Correlation of back extensor strength with thoracic kyphosis and lumbar lordosis in estrogen-deficient women. *Am J Phys Med Rehabil.* 1996;75(5):370–374.

31. Wang CH, McClure P, Pratt NE, Nobilini R. Stretching and strengthening exercises: their effect on three-dimensional scapular kinematics. *Arch Phys Med Rehabil.* 1999;80(8):923–929.

32. Itoi E, Sinaki M. Effect of back-strengthening exercise on posture in healthy women 49 to 65 years of age. *Mayo Clin Proc.* 1994;69(11):1054–1059.

33. White AA, Panjabi MM. *Clinical Biomechanics of the Spine.* 2nd ed. Philadelphia; JB Lippincott: 1990.

34. Oda I, Abumi K, Cunningham B, Kaneda K, McAfee PC. An in vitro human cadaveric study investigating the biomechanical properties of the thoracic spine. *Spine.* 2002;27(3):E64–70.

35. Tawackoli W, Marco R, Liebschner MA. The effect of compressive axial preload on the flexibility of the thoracolumbar spine. *Spine.* 2004;29(9):988–993.

36. Panjabi MM, Brand RA, White AA III. Mechanical properties of the human thoracic spine as shown by three-dimensional load-displacement curves. *J Bone Joint Surg Am.* 1976;58(5):642–652.

37. Buchalter D, Parnianpour M, Viola K, Nordin M, Kahanovitz N. Three-dimensional spinal motion measurements. Part 1: A technique for examining posture and functional spinal motion. *Spinal Disord.* 1988;1(4):279–283.

38. Cook C. Lumbar Coupling biomechanics-A literature review. *J Man Manip Ther.* 2003;11(3):137–145.

39. McRae M, Cleland J. Differential diagnosis and treatment of upper thoracic pain: A case study. *J Man Manip Ther.* 2003;11:43–48.

40. Bogduk N. Innervation and pain patterns of the cervical spine. In: Grant R. *Physical therapy of the cervical and thoracic spine.* 3rd ed. New York; Churchill Livingstone: 2002.

41. Doubleday KL, Kulig K, Landel R. Treatment of testicular pain using conservative management of the thoracolumbar spine: a case report. *Arch Phys Med Rehabil.* 2003;84(12):1903–1905.

42. DeFranca GG, Levine LJ. The T4 syndrome. *J Manipulative Physiol Ther.* 1995;18(1):34–37.

43. Mergener K, Brandabur JJ. Costochondral deformity masquerading as a submucosal gastric tumor. *Endoscopy.* 2003;35(3):255.

44. Feinstein B, Langton JBK, Jameson RM, Schiller F. Experiments on referred pain from deep somatic tissues. *J Bone Jnt Surg.* 1954;36:981–987.

45. Jinno T, Tago M, Yoshida H, Yamane M. (abstract). Case of thoracoabdominal aortic aneurysm complicated with Buerger's disease. *Kyobu Geka.* 2001;54: 1121–1124.

46. Hubbard J. The differential diagnosis of chest pain. *Nurs Times.* 2002;98(50):30–31.

47. Hamberg J, Lindahl O. Angina pectoris symptoms caused by thoracic spine disorders. Clinical examination and treatment. *Acta Med Scand Suppl.* 1981;644:84–86.

48. Wise CM, Semble EL, Dalton CB. Musculoskeletal chest wall syndromes in patients with noncardiac chest pain: a study of 100 patients. *Arch Phys Med Rehabil.* 1992;73(2):147–149.

49. Adler R. The differentiation of organic and psychogenic pain. *Pain.* 1981;10(2):249–252.

50. Crook J, Milner R, Schultz IZ, Stringer B. Determinants of occupational disability following a low back injury: a critical review of the literature. *J Occup Rehabil.* 2002;12(4):277–295.

51. Childs MJ, Piva SR. Psychometric properties of the functional rating index in patients with low back pain. *Eur Spine J.* 2005.

52. Bayar B, Bayar K, Yakut E, Yakut Y. Reliability and validity of the Functional Rating Index in older people with low back pain: preliminary report. *Aging Clin Exp Res.* 2004;16(1):49–52.

53. Feise RJ, Michael Menke J. Functional rating index: a new valid and reliable instrument to measure the magnitude of clinical change in spinal conditions. *Spine.* 2001;26(1):78–86.

54. Moore KL. Muscles and ligaments of the back. In Singer KP, Giles LF (eds). *Clinical anatomy and management of low back pain.* Oxford; Butterworth-Heinemann: 1997.

55. Liebler E, Tufano-Coors L, Douris P, Makofsky H, McKenna R, Michels C, Rattray S. The effect of thoracic spine mobilization on lower trapezius strength testing. *J Man Manip Ther.* 2001;9:207–212.

56. Janda V. Muscles and motor control in cerviogenic disorders: assessment and management. In: Grant R. *Physical therapy of the cervical and thoracic spine.* 3rd ed. New York; Churchill Livingstone: 2002.

57. Christie HJ, Kumar S, Warren SA. Postural aberrations in low back pain. *Arch Phys Med Rehabil.* 1995; 76:218–224.

58. Refshauge KM, Goodsell M, Lee M. The relationship between surface contour and vertebral body measures of upper spine curvature. *Spine.* 1994;19(19): 2180–2185.

59. Renno A, Granito R, Driusso P, Costa D, Oishi J. Effects of an exercise program on respiratory function, posture, and on quality of life in osteoporotic women: a pilot study. *Physiotherapy.* 2005;91:113–118.

60. Cook C. The Relationship between posture and balance disturbances in women with osteoporosis. *Physical and Occupational Therapy in Geriatrics.*2003;20 (3):37–50.

61. Woodhull-McNeal AP. Changes in posture and balance with age. *Aging* (Milano). 1992;4(3):219–225.

62. White AA III, Panjabi MM. The clinical biomechanics of scoliosis. *Clin Orthop Relat Res.* 1976;(118): 100–112.

63. Hawes M. The use of exercises in the treatment of scoliosis: an evidence-based critical review of the literature. *Ped Rehabilitation.* 2003;6:171–182.

64. Theodoridis D, Ruston S. The effect of shoulder movements on thoracic spine 3D motion. *Clin Biomech* (Bristol, Avon). 2002;17(5):418–421.

65. Chansirinukor W, Lee M, Latimer J. Contribution of ribcage movement to thoracolumbar posteroanterior stiffness. *J Manipulative Physiol Ther.* 2003;26(3): 176–183.

66. Lee D. Biomechanics of the thorax. . In: Grant R. *Physical therapy of the cervical and thoracic spine.* 3rd ed. New York; Churchill Livingstone: 2002.

67. Freeston J, Karim Z, Lindsay K, Gough A. Can early diagnosis and management of costochondritis reduce acute chest pain admissions? *J Rheumatol.* 2004;31 (11):2269–2271.

68. Christensen HW, Vach W, Vach K, Manniche C, Haghfelt T, Hartvigsen L, Hoilund-Carlsen PF. Palpation of the upper thoracic spine: an observer reliability study. *J Manipulative Physiol Ther.* 2002;25(5): 285–292.

69. Love RM, Brodeur RR. Inter- and intra-examiner reliability of motion palpation for the thoracolumbar spine. *J Manipulative Physiol Ther.* 1987;10(1):1–4.

70. Haas M, Panzer D, Peterson D, Raphael R. Short-term responsiveness of manual thoracic end-play assessment to spinal manipulation: a randomized controlled trial of construct validity. *J Manip Physiol Ther.* 1995;18:582–589.

71. Lewis J, Green A, Reichard Z, Wright C. Scapular position: the validity of skin surface palpation. *Man Ther.* 2002;7(1):26–30.

72. Frese E, Brown M, Norton BJ. Clinical reliability of manual muscle testing. Middle trapezius and gluteus medius muscles. *Phys Ther.* 1987;67(7):1072–1076.

73. Maitland GD. *Maitland's vertebral manipulation.* 6th ed. London; Butterworth-Heinemann: 2001.

74. Sizer P. The clinical utility of the straight leg and slump sit test. American Academy of Orthopedic Manual Physical Therapists. Louisville, KY. 2004.

75. Butler D. *Mobilization of the nervous system.* Edinburgh; Churchill Livingstone: 1991.

76. O'Leary S, Carroll R, Mellor A, Vicenzino S. The effect of soft tissue deloading tape on thoracic spine pressure pain thresholds in asymptomatic subjects. *Man Ther.* 2002;7:150–153.

77. Vicenzino B, Collins D, Wright A. Sudomotor changes induced by neural mobilization techniques in asymptomatic subjects. *J Manual Manip Ther.* 1994;2: 66–74.

78. Vicenzino B, Collins D, Wright A. An investigation of the interrelationship between manipulative therapy-induced hypoalgesia and sympathoexcitation. *J Manipulative Physiol Ther.* 1998;21:448–453.

79. Wright A. Pain-relieving effects of cervical manual therapy. In. Grant R. *Physical therapy of the cervical and thoracic spine.* 3rd ed. New York; Churchill Livingston: 2002.

80. Lovick T. Interactions between descending pathways from the dorsal and ventrolateral periaqueductal gray matter in the rat. In: Depaulis A, Bandler R. (eds) *The midbrain periaqueductal gray matter.* New York; Plenum Press: 1991.

81. Wright A. Recent concepts in the neurophysiology of pain. *Man Ther.* 1999;4:196–202.

82. Ross JK, Bereznick D, McGill S. Determining cavitation location during lumbar and thoracic spinal manipulation. *Spine.* 2004;29:1452–1457.

83. Bereznick DE, Ross JK, McGill SM. The frictional properties at the thoracic skin-fascia interface: implications in spine manipulation. *Clin Biomech* (Bristol, Avon). 2002;17(4):297–303.

84. Crawford HJ, Jull GA. The influence of thoracic posture and movement of range of arm elevation. *Physiother Theory Pract.* 1993;9:143–149.

85. Forand D, Drover J, Suleman Z, Symons B, Herzog W. The forces applied by female and male chiropractors during thoracic spinal manipulation. *J Manipulative Physiol Ther.* 2004;27(1):49–56.

86. Kirstukas SJ, Backman JA. Physician-applied contact pressure and table force response during unilateral thoracic manipulation. *J Manipulative Physiol Ther.* 1999;22(5):269–279.

87. Cleland JA, Childs JD, McRae M, Palmer JA, Stowell T. Immediate effects of thoracic manipulation in patients with neck pain: a randomized clinical trial. *Man Ther.* 2005;10(2):127–135.

88. Savolainen A, Ahlberg J, Nummila H, Nissinen M. Active or passive treatment for neck-shoulder pain in occupational health care? A randomized controlled trial. *Occup Med* (Lond). 2004;54(6):422–424.

89. Schiller L. Effectiveness of spinal manipulative therapy in the treatment of mechanical thoracic spine pain: a pilot randomized clinical trial. *J Manipulative Physiol Ther.* 2001;24(6):394–401.

# 9

# Manual Therapy of the Shoulder Complex

CHAD E. COOK AND ERIC J. HEGEDUS

## Objectives

- Identify the pertinent structure and biomechanics of the shoulder complex.
- Demonstrate the appropriate and valid shoulder examination sequence.
- Identify plausible mobilization and manual therapy treatment techniques for the shoulder complex.
- Discuss the effect of mobilization and manual therapy on recovery for shoulder-related dysfunction.

## PREVALENCE

In a study in the Netherlands, slightly over one-fifth of the general population reported constant shoulder pain.[1] Studies performed in Great Britain and Scandinavian countries yielded similar numbers.[2] Slightly over 50% of individuals will report shoulder pain at least once per year, which progresses to a lifetime prevalence in approximately 10% of cases.[3] Bongers[2] reported that nearly 50% of those with shoulder pain consult his or her family physician and despite this, half of those still report shoulder problems after one full year. In Sweden, 21% of all disability payments are associated with shoulder injuries.[4] About half of shoulder problems resolve within 6 months of injury[4], while another 40% continue to languish for up to 1 year.

The relatively high prevalence rate for shoulder injuries is associated with the large degree of range of motion at the shoulder and the incidence of dislocation and other forms of instability-related trauma.[5] Risk factors associated with shoulder injury include working with the arms above the shoulders, working with vibratory devices, repetitive movements, pushing and pulling activities, and carrying heavy loads.[1] Sporting and recreational activities that require repetitive overhead activities such as swimming, throwing, and weightlifting also predispose the shoulder to injury.

### Summary

- Shoulder pain is a common occurrence, affecting up to 50% of all individuals at some point within their lifetime.
- The high prevalence of shoulder pain is most likely associated with the demands of mobility and subsequent stability of the shoulder joint.
- Overhead activities predispose an individual to shoulder pain.

## ANATOMY

### Osseous Elements

The shoulder complex includes the articulations of the humerus, the clavicle, the scapula, and the posterior surface of the ribs. The humerus is a long bone that forms the articulations of the glenohumeral joint proximally (with the scapula) and the humeral ulnar joint and humeral radial joint distally (with the ulna and radius, respectively). The head of the humerus is semi-circular in shape and is directed cephalically, medially, and slightly posteriorly and is covered with smooth hyaline cartilage. The head articulates with the glenoid cavity of the scapula, a fossa that is much smaller than the diameter of the humeral head. The planar orientation of the head of the humerus and the glenoid fossa, a ball-and-socket relationship, allows for substantial range of motion for the shoulder specifically when compared to the ball-and-socket coxafemoral joint. The glenoid cavity is further deepened by the contributions of the **labrum,** which is a fibrocartilaginous structure that consists of a confluence of ligaments and capsular attachments.[6]

The anatomical neck of the humerus lies distal to the articulating head of the humerus. The anatomical neck is obliquely directed and is represented by a narrow groove separating the head of the humerus from the lesser and greater tubercles. The anatomical neck is the attachment site of the articular capsule of the glenohumeral joint and the corresponding glenohumeral ligaments.

Two prominent features of the humerus are the greater and lesser tubercles. The greater tubercle is positioned lateral to the head of the humerus and lesser tubercle. The greater tubercle provides a site of insertion to the supraspinatus, infraspinatus, and the teres minor. The lesser tubercle provides the insertion of the tendon of the subscapularis and lies medially and inferior to the head of the humerus. The greater and lesser tubercles are separated by the bicipital groove in which the long head of the biceps brachii lies.[7] The pectoral ridge extends from the greater tubercle along the medial edge of the bone and is the insertion site of the pectoralis major. The deltoid ridge extends from the greater tubercle along the lateral edge of the humerus and is the broad insertion site for the deltoid muscle group. Caudal to the greater and lesser tubercle is the surgical neck of the humerus. The surgical neck is narrower than the proximal humerus and is a common site of fractures.

The clavicle (Figure 9.1) contributes to the anterior and superior aspect of the glenohumeral articulation. The clavicle lies horizontally on the anterior aspect of the chest wall and articulates medially with the manubrium sterni, and laterally with the acromion of the scapula. The clavicle has been compared to a "crank" because it contains a double curve.[8] Several muscles, including the deltoid, the trapezius, and the pectoralis major, have important attachments to the clavicle.[8]

The lateral aspect of the clavicle, the area that articulates with the acromion of the scapula, is generally concave with a roughened attachment for the acromioclavicular (AC) ligaments. The AC joint is generally oriented laterally and posteriorly, although variations do exist.[9] The superior AC ligaments are better defined and thicker than the inferior AC ligaments and attach in the roughened region of the distal clavicle.[8] Damage to the joint can lead to a variety of abnormal movements including increased superior excursion and abnormalities in rotation.[10]

The scapula forms the posterior and superior aspect of the shoulder glenohumeral articulation. The concave ventral surface of the scapula (Figure 9.2) creates a pseudo-articulation with the thorax. The stabilization of the concave surface to the thorax is performed by the complex interaction of several muscles that stabilize the joint during static and dynamic actions.[11] The dorsal surface (Figure 9.3) is divided into a superior and inferior section by the spine of the scapula. The inferior section houses the origination of the infraspinatus, and teres minor and

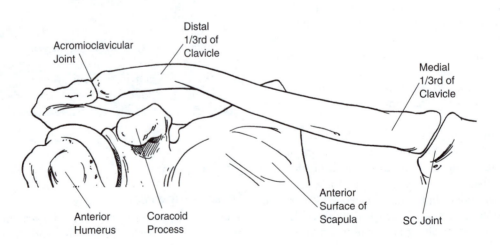

**Figure 9.1**    The Clavicle

major, while the superior section is the origination of the supraspinatus.[7] The acromion forms as a projection from the spine of the scapula and overhangs the glenoid cavity. The medial border of the acromion articulates with the lateral aspect of the clavicle and is convex in shape (Figure 9.4). Studies have suggested that the acromion takes several different shapes that may predispose the individual to impingement-related problems.[12,13] Bigliani and Morrison[14] identified three types of acromion shapes based on the grade of the anterior slope at the distal aspect. The third type (Type III), which has a hooked slope, is frequently seen in patients with impingement syndrome[15,16] and rotator cuff tears.[14]

## Summary

- The shoulder complex includes the articulations of the humerus, the clavicle, the scapula, and the posterior surface of the ribs.
- The clavicle and the scapula are important osseous structures that provide origination sites for many of the shoulder muscles. The design of these structures promotes movement.
- Selected prominences of the scapula such as the acromion may contribute to conditions such as impingement.

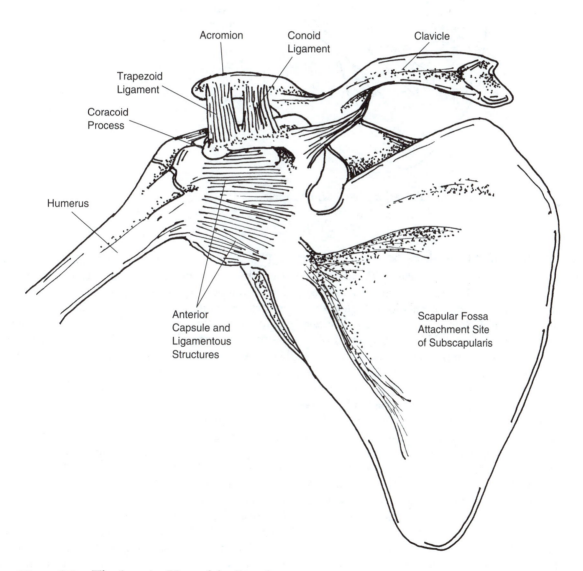

**Figure 9.2**   The Anterior View of the Scapula

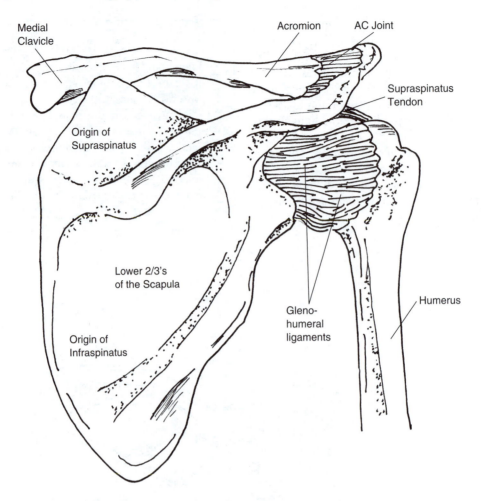

**Figure 9.3**    The Posterior View of the Scapula

## Joints of the Shoulder Complex

There are four distinct joints that make up the shoulder complex: the **glenohumeral, acromioclavicular, sterno-clavicular** and **scapulothoracic** articulations (Figure 9.5). The most notable joint is the glenohumeral articulation. The glenohumeral joint is a multiaxial ball-and-socket joint that faces slightly anterior and superiorly. The scapula and clavicle form the socket of the joint, and the humeral head that fits within the socket. The relative size of the humeral head in comparison to the glenoid fossa results in poor congruency of articular surfaces. The surface area of the humeral head is 1.5 to 3 times greater than its articulating surface of the glenoid fossa,[17] further contributing to the intrinsic mobility of the shoulder.[18]

The AC joint includes the distal or lateral end of the clavicle and the medial margin of the acromion of the scapula. Between the distal or lateral end of the clavicle and the medial margin of the acromion of the scapula lies an articular disc, although this disc is occasionally absent in some individuals.[8] The disc frequently divides the joint into two cavities.

The joint is housed in an articular capsule that is strengthened by the superior and inferior AC ligaments.[7] The acromioclavicular joint capsule controls anterior and posterior stability of the AC joint whereas the trapezoid maintains posterior stability.[19] The primary function of the AC joint is to maintain the biomechanical association between the clavicle and the scapula and to allow the scapula to gain additional range of rotation on the thorax in the latter stages of upper limb elevation.

The sternoclavicular (SC) joint (Figure 9.6) is a synovial sellar joint.[20] The SC joint maintains osseous contact of the upper limb to the axial skeleton, while both contributing to mobility and stability. Because the SC is incongruous and contributes to an unstable osseous joint, a fibrocartilage disc is engaged to enhance stability. The disc functions as a hinge during clavicular movement.[21] The disc also functions to decrease compression forces during shoulder function.[21] Three significant ligaments assist stability and control limits of motion during shoulder elevation. The costoclavicular ligament limits elevation and superior glide of the clavicle[20] whereas the

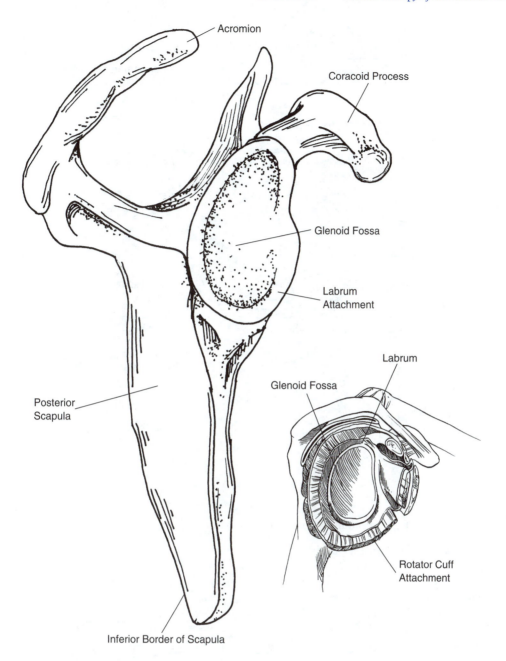

**Figure 9.4**    The Lateral Aspect of the Scapula

anterior sternoclavicular ligament controls anterior migration of medial clavicular movement. The interclavicular ligament connects the two SC joints across the upper border of the manubrium. This very stable complex is responsible for less than 1% of shoulder complex–related injuries.[22]

The scapulothoracic (ST) joint does not contain a capsule or synovial tissue, thus the joint is classified as a physiological joint versus a synovial joint.[23] The parameters of stability of the ST joint are maintained by the closed chain mechanism at the acromioclavicular joint (AC), the sternoclavicular joint (SC), and the numerous muscle attachments to the scapula.[20]

With the ST joint, disassociated movement with respect to the AC, SC, and GH joint is unlikely. Additionally, secondary to the atmospheric pressure and the numerous forces that act upon the ST joint, single planes of motion are more aptly defined as an associated movement with the AC and SC.[20] The ST joint is instrumental during the movement of scapulothoracic rhythm.

Several orthrokinematic/planar motions exist at the glenohumeral joint. These movements include external rotation, internal rotation, flexion, abduction, adduction, horizontal adduction, horizontal abduction, and extension. These plane-based movements technically do not move

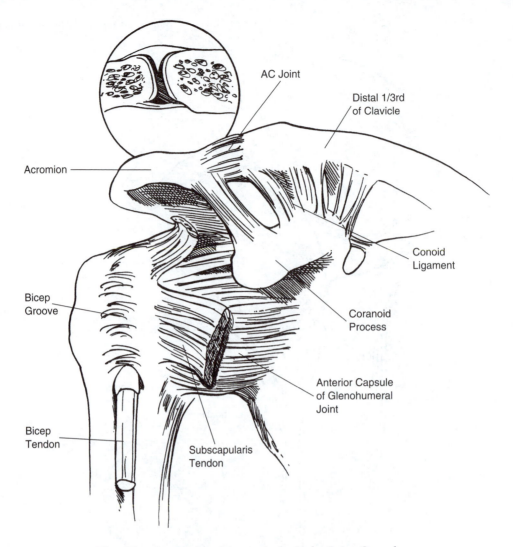

**Figure 9.5**    The Glenohumeral and Acromioclavicular Joint Complex

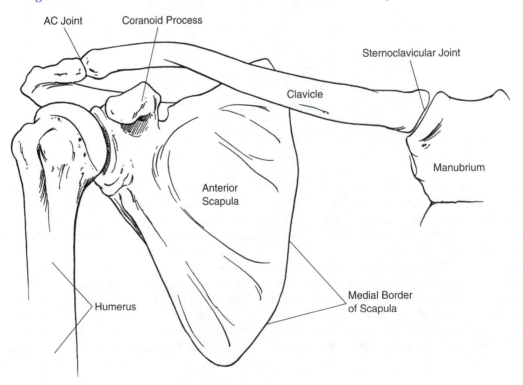

**Figure 9.6**    The Sternoclavicular Joint

within the true plane of the glenohumeral joint. The true plane of movement of the glenohumeral joint may best be observed in the plane of the scapula. Movement within the scapular plane, known as scaption, results in a combined osteokinematic movement of flexion and abduction. This movement is in both the coronal and sagittal planes. Scaption is hypothesized to represent the most clinical, significant-length tension relationship of the elevators and rotators of the shoulder.[24] However, selected studies demonstrate the external rotators are the only shoulder musculature that benefits from greater torque when placed in the scaption plane.[25–27]

Another notable component of scaption is the presence of greater joint congruency in the scaption plane.[24] This allows for capsular relaxation of fibers in a nonimpaired shoulder and less potential for impingement of structures during movement.[24]

involves the careful combination of the movements of glenohumeral, ST, AC, and SC and varies with age.

Historically, manual therapists have used two distinct biomechanical principles in the examination and treatment of the shoulder complex: (1) the **convex–concave** rule and (2) Cyriax's capsular pattern. MacConail[29] first described the convex–concave theory of arthrokinematic motion. This theory asserts that the joint surface geometry dictates the accessory movement pattern during physiological movement.[30] Examination and treatment is guided by the joint geometry and variations are considered either abnormal or inappropriate. In the shoulder, evidence to support this theory is poor. Numerous studies indicate that the glenohumeral joint does not always move as a ball-and-socket joint, but occasionally displays translatory-only movements during pathology.[30–32] Because of this, it appears that the selection of a technique that focuses on a specific direction based solely on the convex–concave rule may not yield values any better than the antagonistic direction at the shoulder.[33,34]

Cyriax initially proposed that pathology in the shoulder results in range-of-motion loss in proportional patterns based on a ratio.[35] He used this ratio to differentiate between losses of motion secondary to bony, muscle, or capsular changes. His hierarchical-based capsular pattern was external rotation limited more than abduction limited more than internal rotation, proportionally. Several studies have identified variability of a capsular pattern of the shoulder[36–39] and subsequently the use of this biomechanical principle may yield little value.

## Summary

- There are four distinct joints that make up the shoulder complex: the glenohumeral, acromioclavicular, sternoclavicular, and scapulothoracic articulations.
- The primary function of the glenohumeral joint is to allow mobility of the humerus by providing a very precariously unstable connection.
- The primary function of the AC joint is to maintain the biomechanical association between the clavicle and the scapula and to allow the scapula to gain additional range of rotation on the thorax in the latter stages of upper limb elevation.
- The primary function of the SC joint is to maintain osseous contact of the upper limb to the axial skeleton, while both contributing to mobility and stability.
- The clavicle and the scapula are important osseous structures that provide origination sites for many of the shoulder muscles. The design of these structures promotes movement.
- The scapulothoracic (ST) joint does not contain a capsule or synovial tissue but does supply a muscle contact with the thoracic region.

## Summary

- The glenohumeral joint has six degrees of freedom that consist of three rotations and three translations.
- There is limited evidence to support the existence of a definitive capsular pattern for a shoulder dysfunction.
- There is limited evidence to support that the shoulder exhibits an accessory and physiological relationship as explained by the capsular pattern.
- Nearly all biomechanical movement of the shoulder involves the concurrent movements of all four regional joints.

# BIOMECHANICS

## Glenohumeral Range of Motion

The glenohumeral joint has six degrees of freedom, which consist of three rotations and three translations.[28] Glenohumeral movement is significantly affected by the interaction of passive and active structures that are further altered by pathology. Normal shoulder range of motion

## Scapulohumeral Rhythm

**Scapulohumeral rhythm** (SHR) (Figure 9.7) is a three-dimensional movement of scapular and glenohumeral kinematics.[28] Scapulohumeral rhythm is nonlinear with inconsistent ratios associated with gender, speed, and angles.[40] With asymptomatic subjects, the scapula generally

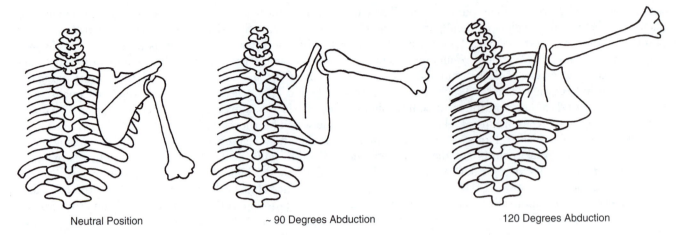

| Neutral Position | ~ 90 Degrees Abduction | 120 Degrees Abduction |

**Figure 9.7**    The Scapulohumeral Rhythm Sequence

moves into upward rotation, external rotation, and posterior tilting during glenohumeral elevation.[28] The first 30 degrees of SHR is primarily associated with glenohumeral movement with simultaneous movement of the glenohumeral and scapulothoracic joints after 30 degrees of shoulder elevation.

Overall, the SHR is typically a 2-to-1 ratio within the Y-axis of scapulohumeral movement, although others have reported differences in this ratio.[40,41] McClure[42] reported that an average of 50 degrees of scapular upward rotation occurs during arm elevation, along with 24 degrees of external rotation and 30 degrees of posterior tilting. There is movement within the X and Z axes as well, the Z-axes promoting more or similar scapular movement to glenohumeral motion.[43]

Capsuloligamentous structures within the glenohumeral joint may also affect the scapulohumeral rhythm. A tight posterior capsule, which has a profound effect on the glenohumeral joint, may also have an adverse effect on the scapulohumeral rhythm. Warner et al.[44] proposed that due to a tight capsule and the resultant decreased glenohumeral motion, the scapulothoracic joint must substitute motion in order for the individual to perform the required overhead task. In their study, 100% of the subjects with impingement syndromes had scapulothoracic asymmetries. It has been demonstrated that the scapulothoracic movement is altered in subjects with impingement syndrome and suggested that this alteration may be a contributor to impingement.[45]

The benefit of assessment of SHR lies in the optimum positioning of the GH head in the glenoid fossa.[46] Optimal positioning allows optimal net reaction forces of the shoulder stabilizers. When the scapula moves appropriately throughout the range of GH movement, the joint can sustain maximal force production through a larger portion of the range of motion.

## Summary

- Scapulohumeral rhythm (SHR) is a three-dimensional movement of scapular and glenohumeral kinematics.
- Although the SHR is variable across individuals, generally the movement is associated with two parts glenohumeral motion to one part scapular motion.
- Abnormalities in SHR are commonly associated with impairments such as impingement syndrome.
- Scapulohumeral rhythm is designed to improve the position of the humeral head within the glenoid fossa.

### *Acromioclavicular Range of Motion*

Normal acromioclavicular motion works synergistically with scapulohumeral movement to increase joint stability.[10] Although nearly 40–50 degrees of clavicle rotation occurs during arm elevation, only 5–8 degrees of movement occurs specifically at the AC since the clavicle moves synergistically with the scapula.[8]

### *Sternoclavicular Range of Motion*

Like the AC, the SC is a synovial joint but has 3 degrees of freedom. The SC moves with elevation–depression and protraction–retraction of the clavicle. During normal shoulder elevation, the SC moves approximately 30–35 degrees. The majority of SC movement occurs in the first 90 degrees of arm movement with a ratio of 4 degrees of SC movement for every 10 degrees of glenohumeral movement.[8]

## Summary

- Although nearly 40–50 degrees of rotation of the clavicle occurs during shoulder elevation only 5–8 degrees of motion is required at the AC joint.
- During shoulder elevation, the SC moves approximately 30–35 degrees.

## Passive Stabilization

Normally, the shoulder sacrifices passive stability for gains in mobility. The passive stabilizers of the shoulder include the bony, cartilaginous, capsular, and ligamentous structures.[46]

*Capsule and ligaments.* The capsuloligamentous complex includes multiple integrated ligaments and capsule.[46] The glenohumeral ligaments are thickenings of the joint capsule and vary in size and laxity from person to person.[17] The shoulder capsule has about twice the surface area of the humeral head and allows for generous range of motion and laxity.[6] In resting positions of the arm such as mid ranges of motion, the capsular ligaments are generally lax, and the dynamic restraints and negative pressure of the joint produce most of the glenohumeral joint stability by compressing the humeral head into the glenoid. A negative pressure within the joint supplies a small element of passive stability.[47] However, at more extreme positions the capsuloligamentous structures control excessive translations in the joint (Table 9.1).[6]

It is well known that selected aspects of the capsuloligamentous complex can be impaired, thus limiting motion at disparate ranges. The anterior capsule is reinforced by the superior glenohumeral (SGHL), middle glenohumeral (MGHL), and inferior glenohumeral complex (Figure 9.8).[34]

The inferior glenohumeral ligament (IGHLC) has a variable representation; in some cases the ligament is three distinct components: a thick anterior band, a less prominent posterior band, and a thin interposed pouch; in others it is only one.[34] The origination of the IGHLC is the anterior glenoid rim and labrum and the insertion is inferior to the MGHL along the inferior margin of the humeral articular surface and anatomic neck.[6] A competent IGHLC is the primary static stabilizer during arm abduction of 45–90 degrees and external rotation.[46] The IGHLC has the ability to stretch extensively prior to rupture.[46] The IGHLC resembles a hammock that supports the humeral head during abduction and external rotation of the arm.[6] During abduction and extension, the thick anterior band restricts anterior and posterior translation. During the combined movement of abduction and flexion, the posterior band of the IGHLC is the primary stabilizer.[6] Additionally, sectioning of the coracohumeral ligament increases the likelihood of posterior subluxation.[5]

The MGHL is variable as well and is not present in 30% of individuals.[6] The function of the MGHL is to limit anterior translation of the humeral head during 45 degrees of abduction. Furthermore, during adduction, the MGHL limits external rotation and inferior translation.[44]

The superior glenohumeral ligament (SGHL) originates from the anterior superior glenoid of the scapula and inserts at the proximal surface of the lesser tubercle.[6]

**TABLE 9.1   Physiological Structures Responsible for Glenohumeral Stabilization**

| Structure | Movement Resistance | References |
|---|---|---|
| Superior glenohumeral ligament | Extension rotation at 0 degrees of abduction | Terry et al.[100] |
| Medial glenohumeral ligament | Extension rotation at 0–90 degrees of abduction | Turkel et al.[169]; Terry et al.[100] |
| Anterior band of the inferior glenohumeral ligament | External rotation at 90 degrees of abduction | O'Brien et al.[142] |
| Inferior glenohumeral ligament | Internal rotation at 70–90 degrees of abduction<br>External rotation at 70 degrees of abduction | O'Brien et al.[142]<br>Terry et al.[100] |
| Posterior capsule | Internal rotation through full range of abduction | Ovensen and Nielson[170] |
| Inferior posterior capsule | Internal rotation at 70 degrees of abduction | Terry et al.[100] |
| Superior and middle posterior capsule | Internal rotation at 0 degrees of abduction | Terry et al.[100] |

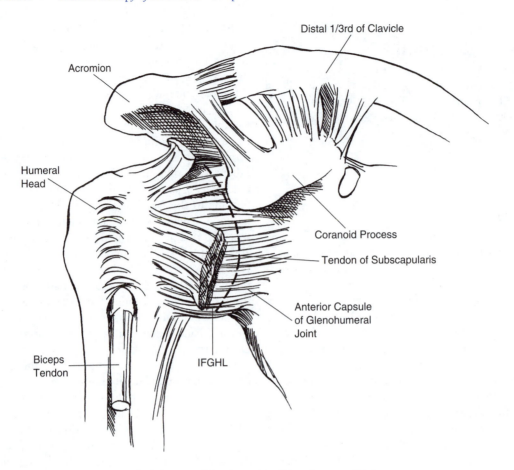

**Figure 9.8**    Passive Stabilizers of the Anterior Glenohumeral Joint

The ligament runs parallel with the coracohumeral ligament and collectively limits inferior translation and external rotation during adduction and posterior translation during flexion, adduction, and internal rotation.[48] When stiff, this ligament limits passive and active movement of external rotation and flexion.

The posterior capsule begins superior to the posterior band of the inferior glenohumeral ligament and is extremely thin. Joint stiffness associated with a tight posterior capsule is associated with altered SHR and impingement syndrome.[28] Tightness in the posterior capsule leads to a superior and anterior migration of the humeral head during passive[34] and active flexion[49] and internal rotation.[34] It is believed that this tightening of the posterior capsule is a result of fibrosis due to chronic inflammation of the posterior capsule.[50,51]

Due to the abnormal kinematics created by a tight posterior capsule, restoration of normal tissue length is recommended in rehabilitation of conditions such as impingement syndrome.[51–53] Techniques designed to improve the mobility of the capsule such as joint mobilization are required and have been shown to decrease joint stiffness.[54,55] It is believed that this is due to the plastic deformation and resulting increased length of connective tissue brought about by selectively stressing the pathological tissue during mobilization.[56]

Passive structures responsible for stabilization of the AC include the joint capsule, the trapezoid, and conoid ligaments. The joint capsule of the AC is very thin and is significantly supported by ligaments.[8] The superior AC ligament significantly affects the stabilization of the distal clavicle during rotation.[8] The inferior AC ligament is often indistinguishable from the capsule and the contribution of this ligament to stability is not completely known.[8] Fukuda et al.[19] noted that the conoid ligament was the most significant contributor of stability during anterior and superior translation. The conoid is often disrupted during marked superior translation of the clavicle with respect to the scapula.[8] Ironically, the conoid ligament inserts more medially on men than women, potentially increasing the anterior and posterior movement of the clavicle to the scapula, though data does not exist to support this.[8] Additionally, soft tissue at the AC joint functions synergistically to provide joint stability in all planes of movement.[10]

Passive structures responsible for the SC include costoclavicular ligaments, which stabilize during elevation and rotation of the clavicle, and the interclavicular ligaments, which stabilize the clavicle with the SC capsule and sternum. Although the joint structure (diarthrodial, saddletype joint) is inherently flexible, the joint is one of the least dislocated in the body.[8] The SC also has an intraar-

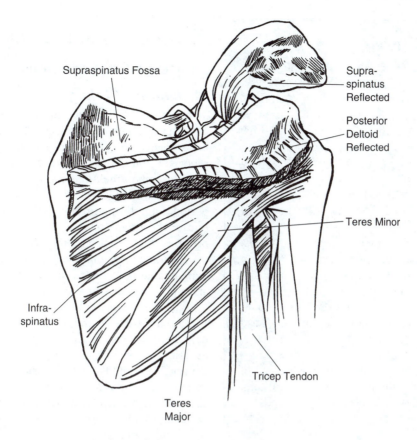

Supraspinatus Fossa

Supra-
spinatus
Reflected

Posterior
Deltoid
Reflected

Teres Minor

Infra-
spinatus

Tricep Tendon

Teres
Major

**Figure 9.9**    Active Stabilizers of the Posterior Glenohumeral Joint

ticular disc that allows complex rotational motion similar to movement available in a ball-and-socket joint. Passive stabilization of the joint through surgery is rarely successful since the majority of surgeries result in a loosening of the hardware placed within the joint.[8]

## Active Stabilization

The active stabilizers of the shoulder include all of the muscles of the shoulder.[46] Poor muscle and motoric control leads to impairments in dynamic stability of the shoulder. Passively, the capsuloligamentous structures contribute to glenohumeral stability, yet on their own, they are poor stabilizers.[57] Unlike other joint stabilizers, active muscle contraction of the glenohumeral joint comprises the principal stabilization of the shoulder, specifically during dynamic motion.[58,59] Co-contraction of the rotator cuff musculature is designed to translate the humerus to the center of the glenoid.[60]

The supraspinatus is active during elevation of the arm, specifically at the early ranges of motion and after 90 degrees of elevation.[57] Rupture of the supraspinatus can cause anterior and superior translation of the humeral head.[46] Together with the deltoid, the majority of elevation of the arm is associated with this muscle. Collectively with all of the rotator cuff musculature, the head of the

humerus is compressed into the glenoid fossa and further stabilized during movement.[46]

Active contraction of the infraspinatus and teres minor (Figure 9.9) reduce anterior–superior translation and produce active external range of motion.[57] The infraspinatus assists in pulling the humeral head inferiorly during elevation and works complimentarily with the supraspinatus. The combined contraction of the infraspinatus and the subscapularis increases the compression of the head of the humerus during arm elevation and is an essential element of a force couple.

The subscapularis functions in a dual role providing anterior stability (reducing anterior translation of the humerus) and caudal depression of the humeral head.[57] Uncontrolled humeral translation increases dramatically during reduced rotator cuff activity.[61] Normally, this uncontrolled translation is countered by the subscapularis.[60] Inflammation and constant pressure of the humeral head on the anterior capsule may inhibit the action of the subscapularis muscle, leading to further anterior laxity problems.

When stability of the shoulder is compromised, the humeral head will typically migrate anteriorly with rotator cuff activity generally the opposite of the tightness of the capsule (usually posterior).[34] In some cases, however, such as subacromial impingement, the humeral head may translate superiorly rather than anteriorly or posteriorly.[62]

## Summary

- The capsuloligamentous complex includes multiple integrated ligaments and capsule.
- The inferior glenohumeral ligament (IGHLC) has a variable representation; in some cases the ligament is three distinct components: a thick anterior band, a less prominent posterior band, and a thin interposed pouch; in others it is only one.
- The middle glenohumeral ligament (MGHL) is variable as well and is not present in 30% of patients.
- The superior glenohumeral ligament (SGHL) limits inferior translation and external rotation during adduction and posterior translation during flexion, adduction, and internal rotation.
- Tightness in the posterior capsule leads to a superior and anterior migration of the humeral head during passive and active flexion and internal rotation.
- Passive structures responsible for stabilization of the AC include the joint capsule, the trapezoid, and conoid ligaments. The joint capsule of the AC is very thin and is significantly supported by ligaments.
- Passive structures responsible for the SC include the costoclavicular ligament, which stabilizes during elevation and rotation of the clavicle, and the interclavicular ligaments, which stabilize the clavicle with the SC capsule and sternum.

## Summary

- Active stabilizers of the shoulder include the rotator cuff muscles. They are the principle structures associated with dynamic control of the shoulder.
- The supraspinatus is active during elevation of the arm specifically at the early ranges of motion and after 90 degrees of elevation. Rupture of the supraspinatus can cause anterior and superior translation of the humeral head.
- The infraspinatus and teres minor reduce anterioinferior translation and produce active external range of motion.
- The subscapularis functions in a dual role providing anterior stability (reducing anterior translation of the humerus) and caudal depression of the humeral head.

# ASSESSMENT AND DIAGNOSIS

## Subjective Considerations

### Mechanism of Injury

The incident of injury is helpful in identifying the type of shoulder dysfunction. For example, pain during a fall may be associated with AC joint pain specifically if the patient reports a concordant movement across the body. Additionally, pain in the AC is common when heavy items such as a backpack are carried over the shoulder for a long time period. Pain during progressive overhead activity may implicate the rotator cuff just as pain during selected arm postures that implicate impingement may warrant investigation of flexibility and strength assessment. Lastly, patients that report a "dead arm" sensation in the acceleration phase of throwing may have instability.[63]

The age of the individual may prove noteworthy as well. Older patients are more likely to experience rotator cuff injuries[64] just as younger patients are more likely to experience instability.[65] Capsulitis restrictions are more common in middle-aged females and less common in younger individuals.[65] External factors associated with shoulder pain such as cervical somatic referred pain or radiculopathy are more common in patients aged 45 and older and less common in younger individuals.[65]

### Psychosocial Issues

A relationship between selected psychosocial factors and shoulder pain among workers has been suggested in several studies.[66–68] Although the relationship is not nearly as strong as the relationship between psychosocial factors and low back pain, selected factors are consistently identified as covariates of pain or determinants of chronicity. Those factors include burnout,[66] mild and severe depression,[66] inability to express one's symptoms well,[66] high job demands or stress,[67–69] and low pain threshold.[67] Others have reported that the influence of psychosocial factors are not nearly as prevalent as physiological requirements such as repetitive work, suggesting that the actual contribution of psychosocial factors remains unknown.[70,71]

### Functional Impairment Scales

The Disability of the Arm, Shoulder, and Hand Instrument (DASH) is a relative region-specific outcome instrument that measures self-rated upper-extremity disability and symptoms. The questionnaire was designed to measure a number of conditions associated with activities of daily living that affect the shoulder, elbow, wrist, and hand.[72] The DASH has been validated on populations of shoulder-, elbow-, wrist-, and hand-related dysfunction.[73] The DASH consists of a 30-item disability/symptom scale, scored zero (no disability) to 100, and was originally introduced by the American Academy of Orthopedic Surgeons in collaboration with a number of other organizations.[74]

The Shoulder Pain and Disability Scale (SPADI) is a non-disease-specific, region-specific questionnaire. The SPADI is a 13-question pain-related disability questionnaire that is designed to take 3 minutes to complete.[75] The scale uses five visual analog scales to measure pain and eight visual analog scales to measure the function at the shoulder.[76] The sum of the pain index VAS is divided by 55 and then multiplied by 100 to provide the overall score. Furthermore, the sum of the functional index VAS is divided by eight then multiplied by 100 to reach the final score. By adding the two values, the complete score is provided. Bot et al.[77] found unidimensionality of the instrument, although it claims to measure two dimensions. Test–retest scores range from 0.64 to 0.66 and the internal consistency ranges from 0.86 to 0.95.[75] The scale has demonstrated content, construct, and discriminant validity in past studies.[78,79]

The American Shoulder and Elbow Surgeons Standardized Shoulder Assessment Form (ASES) is a non-disease-specific, region-specific questionnaire. The scale has two sections, a patient report form and a surgeon report form. There are two dimensions associated with the patient report form, pain and function.[80] Pain is evaluated using a 10 cm VAS whereas function is assessed using a 4-point Likert scale for level of difficulty. The scale takes anywhere from 3–4 minutes to complete.[80] Test–retest reliability was approximately 0.84 while the internal consistency was 0.86.[75] The scale has demonstrated content, construct, and discriminate validity.[81] The scale is responsive and has been tested on surgical and nonsurgical patients.[81]

## Differential Diagnosis

A careful patient history will improve the identification of potential red flags for shoulder dysfunction. The presence of a red flag does not isolate the likelihood of a serious

## Summary

- The mechanism of injury may help distill the type of pathology of the shoulder.
- Trauma is generally associated with a rotator cuff tear, an AC injury, or a labral tear. Degeneration is associated with impingement, rotator cuff weakness, and capsulitis.
- Although likely not as significant as physiological factors, psychosocial factors may affect the recovery rate of patients with a shoulder-related injury.
- Two scales, the SPADI and the DASH, are frequently used for conservative functional assessment of the shoulder. The dimensionality of the DASH is unknown and the SPADI is unidimensional.

pathology; however, special care is suggested if these factors exist. Many of the reported red flags are similar to those identified in Chapter 5 (Table 9.2).

Multiple structures can refer pain to the shoulder region.[82–84] Subsequently, it is essential that the manual therapist understand these structures to recognize the potential guilty pain generator. Most commonly, cervical spine lesions can cause secondary shoulder symptoms or referred pain to the shoulder.[65] Additionally, it is common to see shoulder structures that refer pain proximally to the cervical region misdiagnosed as cervical pain.[85] It is essential to rule out the contribution of the cervical spine for shoulder pain by using overpressures or a brief cervical examination.

Shoulder pain can occasionally be the initial manifestation of a serious pathology. Structures such as the lung, pancreas, aortic artery, and liver may refer pain to the shoulder. Pain associated with extrinsic factors is not reproduced during mechanical movements and may not

**TABLE 9.2    Red Flags for Shoulder Impairment**

| Red Flag | Relationship |
|---|---|
| Age > 50 | Increased risk of rotator cuff tear and other serious pathologies |
| Night pain | Increased risk of serious pathology such as tumor |
| Weight loss | Increased risk of cancer or autoimmune dysfunction |
| Fever | Increased risk for systemic infection |
| Pain unrelated to activity | Increased risk for referred pain from a visceral source |
| Pain not relieved by rest | Increased risk for referred pain from a visceral source |
| History of smoking | Increase risk for lung cancer and referred pain associated with cancer |
| Previous history of cancer | Increase risk for referral of pain and/or metastatis |
| Cardiac risk factors | MI may refer pain to the left shoulder |
| Pleuritic pain | Increased risk for Pancoast tumor |

**LE 9.3    Extrinsic Causes of Shoulder Pain**

| Type | Source |
|---|---|
| Neurologic | Cervical radiculopathy |
| | Upper trunk brachial plexopathy |
| | Neurologic amyotrophy |
| | Focal mononeuropathy |
| | Muscular dystrophy |
| Cardiovascular | Cardiac ischemia |
| | Thoracic outlet syndrome |
| | Aortic disease |
| | Axillary thrombosis |
| Pulmonary | Upper lobe pneumonia |
| | Pulmonary embolism |
| | Pneumothorax |
| | Pneumoperitoneum |
| Malignancy | Pancoast tumor |
| | Metastatic cancer |
| Abdominal | Biliary disease |
| | Hepatic disease |
| | Pancreatitis |
| | Splenic injury |
| | Perforated viscus |

## Summary
- Several non-shoulder-related physical structures can refer pain to the shoulder. Differentiation is required for accurate treatment.
- The cervical spine may refer pain to the shoulder and structures such as the lung, pancreas, aortic artery, and liver may refer pain to the shoulder.

## Objective/Physical Examination

### Observation

Asymmetry is often used erroneously to determine pathology in a shoulder. Some degree of asymmetry in a shoulder is normal and does not indicate the presence of pathology.[63] Priest and Nagel[87] found that hand dominance often leads to a lower (depressed) dominant shoulder and hypertrophy of the musculature on the ipsilateral side. However, gross atrophy may be an indicator of spinal accessory nerve or long thoracic nerve entrapment and is essential to evaluate.

Altered humeral head position, specifically anterior displacement, may predispose an individual to shoulder pain and dysfunction.[88,89] Anterior displacement is a common problem and is generally associated with a tight posterior capsule.[57]

### Posture

Chronic posture associated with rounded shoulders will also initiate anterior translation. Weiser et al.[90] demonstrated an increase in anterior translation of the glenohumeral joint, resulting in excessive strain on the inferior glenohumeral ligament in simulated scapular protraction. The authors believed that chronic protraction results in an anterior glenohumeral instability due to overstretching of the anterior capsule.

Taping for posture does not increase the muscle activity for scapular muscles but is effective in reducing a passive load on the anterior structures that are impinged.[91] Additionally, increasing the mobility of the anterior shoulder structures may improve the resting position of the scapula, potentially improving the scapular and glenohumeral kinematics.[28]

Cervicothoracic posture can significantly influence the position and mobility of the scapula. Forward head may reduce the available range of motion of shoulder flexion[92] (Figure 9.10) whereas upper thoracic flexion may limit unilateral upper shoulder abduction and flexion.[93] Thoracic kyphosis is also associated with decreased shoulder flexion[94,95] and a reduction of force generation at the glenohumeral joint.[94]

decrease with appropriate rest.[63] Patients with an insidious onset but intractable pain may exhibit symptoms caused from external structures outside the shoulder (Table 9.3).

In some cases, functional shoulder loss outweighs pain as the most concordant problem. Thus, it is necessary to identify specific movement-related dysfunctions that may assist in identifying a particular disorder.[86] If scapular winging is prominent during arm elevation, a serratus anterior or trapezius dysfunction should be expected. Furthermore, it is necessary to determine if recent trauma or a viral illness may have contributed to dysfunction of the long thoracic nerve. If the patient demonstrates breaking during movements and the inability to externally rotate the arm upon command, one should suspect the possibility of a rotator cuff tear or suprascapular nerve entrapment. When pain radiates below the elbow the clinician should always clear the cervical spine, although referred pain from the rotator cuff is not abnormal. If pain occurs during throwing or if a "dead arm" is present after using the arm, one should suspect instability. If pain occurs with clicking, the labrum may be involved. Lastly, if pain is worse while lying on the shoulder during sleeping, impingement may be present. Although these are generalized guidelines, these guidelines may be effective in further isolating the disorder.

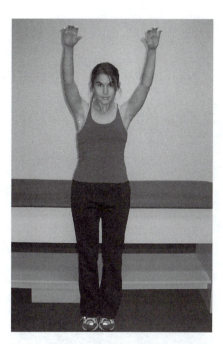

**Figure 9.10**    Active Elevation With and Without Poor Cervicothoracic Posture

## Summary

- Asymmetry is often erroneously used to determine pathology in a shoulder, specifically, since some degree of asymmetry in a shoulder is normal and does not indicate the presence of pathology.
- An anteriorly translated humeral head is common in shoulder pathology.
- Although treatment for postural abnormalities may not be directly related to shoulder recovery, improvements in shoulder range of motion and scapular position are common when posture is addressed.

# CLINICAL EXAMINATION

## Active Physiological Movements

Range-of-motion losses associated with pathology can occur in all planes of motion.[96] Cyriax initially promoted the concept of a pattern of loss in patients with capsuloligamentous dysfunction, or a "capsular pattern." Cyriax[97] proposed that the shoulder capsular pattern was external rotation, followed by abduction then internal rotation. This suggests that external rotation should demonstrate the most loss of range during a pathology, followed by abduction then internal rotation.[97] Treatments are often based on the assumption of a capsular pattern and Cyriax's capsular pattern has been the basis for clinical treatment for some time,[39] however, there is little evidence to support this assumption.

Rundquist et al.[38] reported that significant variability in capsular patterns were present in patients with idiopathic loss of range of motion, a pattern that changed when shoulder abduction was incorporated. In 2003 Rundquist et al.[39] and in 2004 Mitsch et al.[36] discovered variability in the capsular pattern in patients diagnosed with adhesive capsulitis of the shoulder and suggested that the theory of a single capsular pattern lacks evidence.

Most likely, the variability of a capsular pattern is explained by the different contributions of the capsule and ligaments during movement of the shoulder. As discussed in the biomechanics section, movements such as abduction can alter the contribution of the shoulder ligaments and may place selective tension on disparate aspects of the capsule. Because damage or injury can be isolated to a specific aspect of the capsule, it is intuitive to assume that different injuries will yield variations in range-of-motion loss.

Shoulder restrictions may result in a drift during active range of motion toward the plane of the scaption, specifically during shoulder flexion and abduction.[98] Commonly, this manifests as an anteriorly displaced humerus.

### Bilateral Shoulder Flexion

Bilateral shoulder flexion is beneficial in determining symmetry of movement and assessing scapulohumeral rhythm. Symmetrical movement requires a balance of muscle control and compliant passive structures.[57] The primary contributors to symmetrical movement include the force couple movements of the rotator cuff for the glenohumeral joint, force coupled movement of the serratus anterior and trapezius for the scapulothoracic joint.[24,62]

Pain is important to identify during movement because pain has been shown to inhibit the contribution of the serratus anterior and the lower fibers of the trapezius. With inhibition of these two critical muscles, movements near and above 90 degrees of elevation are significantly altered. The scapula should move congruently with the thorax, with slight internal rotation and a medial glide.[99] Pain might cause abnormal scapular elevation, lateral translation, and AC joint separation.

*(continued)*

- Step One: The patient stands in the targeted posture. Baseline symptoms are evaluated.
- Step Two: The patient is requested to raise both arms together. The clinician should carefully evaluate movement for symmetry and appropriate sequencing.
- Step Three: The patient is requested to lower both arms together. The clinician should carefully evaluate movement for symmetry and appropriate sequencing.

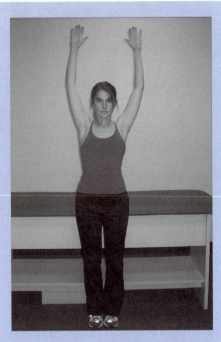

**Figure 9.11**    Bilateral Active Physiological Shoulder Flexion

## Unilateral Shoulder Flexion

It is common to see overactivity of the scapular elevators during active shoulder flexion.[98] Typically, with active range of movements, the noninvolved shoulder is evaluated first.

- Step One: The patient stands in the targeted posture. Baseline symptoms are evaluated.
- Step Two: The patient is requested to raise the arm to the first point of pain (if present). Movement height and quality are evaluated.
- Step Three: The patient is requested to raise the arm past the first point of pain (if present) toward end range. Pain is again evaluated and compared to the initial point of pain.
- Step Four: The patient is requested to perform repeated movements near the end range to determine the behavior of the pain.

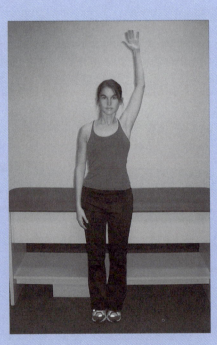

**Figure 9.12**    Unilateral Active Physiological Shoulder Flexion

- Step Five: If no pain was reproduced during the movement, an overpressure is performed to the patient.
- Step Six: The motion is repeated on the other side.

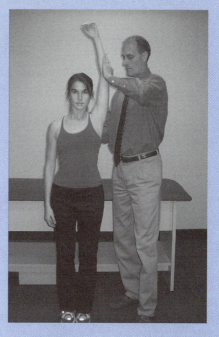

**Figure 9.13**   Unilateral Active Physiological Shoulder Flexion with Overpressure

## Bilateral Shoulder Abduction

Bilateral shoulder abduction is beneficial to analyze. As with shoulder flexion, the appropriate force couple contractions of the shoulder musculature are required for symmetry and stability. One common problem seen during pain and/or rotator cuff dysfunction is the rapid dropping of the arm during 70–110 degrees of shoulder abduction. At this position, the force required for control of the humerus in eccentric contraction is the highest and if weakness or pain is present during this position the arm will rapidly drop.

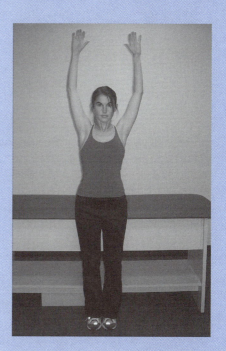

- Step One: The patient stands in the targeted posture. Baseline symptoms are assessed.
- Step Two: The patient is requested to raise both arms together. The clinician should carefully evaluate movement for symmetry and appropriate sequencing.
- Step Three: The patient is requested to lower both arms together. The clinician should carefully evaluate movement for symmetry and appropriate sequencing.

**Figure 9.14**   Bilateral Active Physiological Shoulder Abduction

## Unilateral Shoulder Abduction

Shoulder abduction is most limited by the medial glenohumeral ligament. Typically, with active range of movements, the noninvolved shoulder is evaluated first; however, this is at the discretion of the clinician.

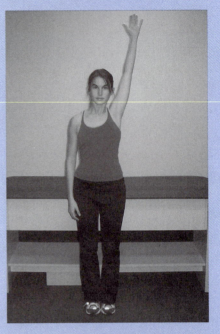

- Step One: The patient stands in the targeted posture. Baseline symptoms are evaluated.
- Step Two: The patient is requested to raise the arm to his or her side, to the first point of pain (if present). Movement height and quality are evaluated.
- Step Three: The patient is requested to raise the arm to his or her side past the first point of pain (if present) toward end range. Pain is again evaluated and compared to the initial point of pain.
- Step Four: The patient is requested to perform repeated movements near the end range to determine the behavior of the pain.

**Figure 9.15**   Active Physiological Shoulder Abduction

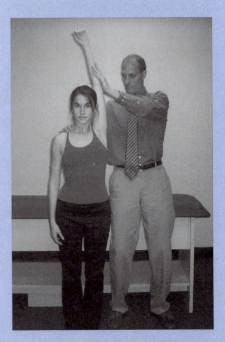

- Step Five: If no pain was reproduced during the movement, an overpressure is performed to the patient.
- Step Six: The motion is repeated on the other side.

**Figure 9.16**   Active Physiological Shoulder Abduction with Overpressure

## Individual Extension

Isolated active extension is an effective method to determine the passive mobility of the biceps tendon and may be useful in determining if the humerus is anterior in the joint cavity versus near midpoint in nonpathological shoulders.

- Step One: The patient stands in the targeted posture. Baseline symptoms are evaluated.
- Step Two: The patient is requested to move his or her arm backward to the first point of pain (if present). Movement distance and quality are evaluated.
- Step Three: The patient is requested to move beyond the first point of pain near end range. Pain is reassessed.
- Step Four: The patient is requested to perform repeated movements at the end range or the available range.
- Step Five: If no pain is present, an overpressure is applied to clear the joint. The complete procedure is repeated on the opposite side.

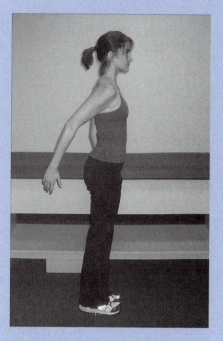

**Figure 9.17**   Active Physiological Shoulder Extension

## Horizontal Adduction

Isolated horizontal adduction is an effective movement to test the flexibility of the posterior capsule. To engage the posterior capsule further, internal rotation can be added as a combined movement.

- Step One: The patient stands in the targeted posture. Baseline symptoms are evaluated.
- Step Two: The patient is requested to move his or her arm across his or her body in an attempt to place the hand on the opposite shoulder. The patient is instructed to identify the first point of pain (if present). Movement distance and quality are evaluated.
- Step Three: The patient is requested to move beyond the first point of pain near end range. Pain is reassessed.
- Step Four: The patient is requested to perform repeated movements at the end range or the available range.
- Step Five: If no pain is present an overpressure is applied to clear the joint. The complete procedure is repeated on the opposite side.

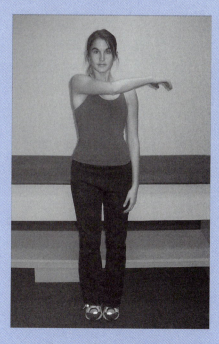

**Figure 9.18**   Active Physiological Shoulder Horizontal Adduction

## *Functional Active Shoulder Movements*

### Bilateral External Rotation

Bilateral external rotation at 90 degrees places a greater stress on the inferior capsular structures than external rotation when the arm is placed at the side.[100] It may be conducive to measure lateral rotation in both positions, although a passive physiological assessment will provide more specific information as to the position of the impairment.

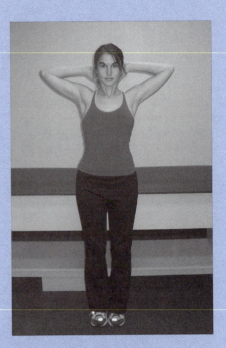

- Step One: The patient stands in the targeted posture. Baseline symptoms are evaluated.
- Step Two: The patient is directed to raise both arms and lace the hands behind the head. Symptoms are assessed if concordant.

**Figure 9.19**    Functional Abduction and External Rotation

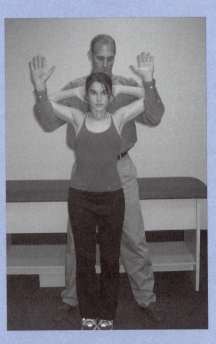

- Step Three: If no pain is present, the patient may require overpressure. Overpressure is applied by gently pulling back on the elbows while behind the patient. Overpressure can occur to one or both arms at the same time.

**Figure 9.20**    Functional Abduction and External Rotation with Overpressure

## D2 Flexion

The D2 Flexion posture provides a number of functional movement analyses. First, this posture may provide nerve root irritation at end range.[101] Second, this movement is often painful and apprehensive in subjects with anterior instability of the shoulder. Lastly, this functional movement is required in various sporting activities and may determine a guilty movement that is otherwise difficult to distill in a conventional examination.

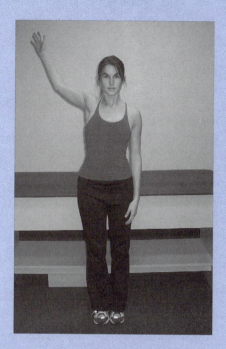

- Step One: The patient stands in the targeted posture. Baseline symptoms are evaluated.
- Step Two: The patient is directed to raise a single arm in a combined movement of flexion, abduction, external rotation, with forearm supination and wrist extension. Symptoms are assessed if concordant.
- Step Three: The procedure is repeated on the opposite side.

**Figure 9.21**    D2 Flexion Position

## Bilateral Internal Rotation/Extension and Adduction

The combined movement of internal rotation, extension, and adduction is a global movement to determine the mobility of numerous structures of the shoulder. Limitations of range may be associated with tightness of the posterior capsule, irritation of the biceps tendon, capsulitis and tenderness of the anterior capsule, and a number of other causes. It is essential to further the examination using passive movements to isolate tightness or lack of stability during the assessment of the individual movements.

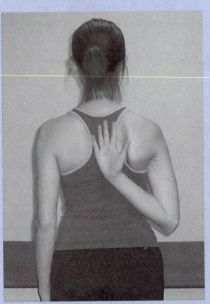

- Step One: The patient stands in the targeted posture. Baseline symptoms are evaluated.
- Step Two: Starting with the uninvolved side first, the patient is instructed to lift his or her arm behind his or her back as high as they can reach.
- Step Three: The clinician uses his or her finger to identify the height reached.
- Step Four: The patient is instructed to perform the activity on the opposite symptomatic side.
- Step Five: The maximum heights are compared for symmetry.

**Figure 9.22**    IR, Extension, and Adduction

## Apley's Scratch Test

Apley's maneuver is useful in assessing functional shoulder range of motion in the combined movements of abduction and external rotation and abduction and internal rotation.[102] The test is functional because the movements are required during daily activities such as don and doffing shirts and undergarments, combing the hair, and hygiene activities.

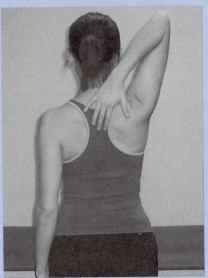

- Step One: The patient stands in the targeted posture. Baseline symptoms are evaluated.
- Step Two: Starting with the uninvolved side first, the patient is instructed to reach behind his or her head and touch the opposite shoulder blade.

**Figure 9.23**    Abduction and External Rotation

- Step Three: The patient is then instructed to reach behind his or her back and reach the same aspect of the opposite shoulder blade now moving with the involved side.
- Step Four: The motion is repeated on the opposite side and assessed for the concordant sign.

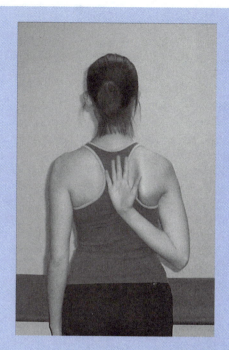

**Figure 9.24**    Adduction and Internal Rotation

## Summary

- Active physiological patterns of motion such as the capsular pattern do not demonstrate validity at the shoulder. Shoulder impairments often demonstrate variable patterns of range-of-motion loss.
- Functional movements are beneficial to determine where in the active range of motion individuals report concordant signs.

## Passive Movements

### Passive Physiological

Passive physiological stretching is beneficial in increasing planar range of motion and translation of the glenohumeral joint. Passive movement patterns may or may not provide beneficial information in isolating causal structures. Selected movements are indicative of isolated pathology, although the ability to classify these pathologies is only fair to moderate.[103]

The use of combined movements is essential in the shoulder since there are a variety of ranges and thousands of potential degrees of motion with the joint. Additionally,

selected standards of the shoulder such as the loose-packed and close-packed position are variable and questionable.[104] Consequently, the following procedures are considered base positions for assessing the passive physiological movements of the shoulder. Any modification of these positions is warranted if the modification finds the concordant movement of that patient.

#### Passive End Feel for the Shoulder

Cyriax proposed a verbal classification scheme called "end feel" to describe the passive resistance of end range passive movement in a joint.[97] End feel is described in terms of resistance and pain expressed by the patient. For the shoulder, physical therapists determining end feel have demonstrated moderate agreement for resistance and substantial agreement for pain in a study by Chesworth et al.[105] Hayes and Peterson[106] reported substantial intra- and interrater reliability for shoulder abduction, adduction, and internal and external rotation.[107] End feel appears to be a reliable and useful method for determining resistance of the shoulder.[105] Abnormal end feels are more likely to be associated with a pain response than normal end feels.[107] Since a capsular pattern demonstrates poor validity and because clinicians often make decisions associated with mobilization or stretching based on end feel assessment, agreement is an essential aspect for treatment decision making.

## Shoulder Flexion

Passive shoulder flexion may be painful during anterior impingement or in isolated cases of capsulitis or shoulder restriction associated with a rotator cuff tear. Shoulder flexion is most limited by the medial glenohumeral ligament.

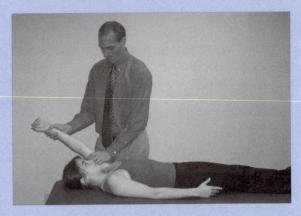

- Step One: The patient is placed at 0 degrees of shoulder flexion and internal/external rotation. Resting symptoms are evaluated.
- Step Two: The clinician first addresses the noninvolved extremity. The patient is instructed to report the first incidence of pain during passive movement. Slowly, the clinician elevates the upper extremity into flexion. The ROM is recorded at the first reported incidence of pain. Pain is evaluated to determine if concordant.
- Step Three: The clinician passively moves the shoulder beyond the first point of pain (if present) toward end range. End feel of the shoulder end range is evaluated.
- Step Four: The process is repeated for the opposite involved side.

**Figure 9.25**   Passive Shoulder Flexion

## Shoulder Abduction

Passive shoulder abduction may implicate restrictions of the capsule or impingement of the subacromial space. Additionally, significant capsular restrictions may be present if scapular movement occurs concurrently with glenohumeral movement during the first 30 degrees of abduction.

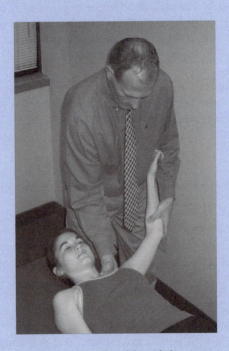

- Step One: The patient is placed at 0 degrees of shoulder abduction and internal/external rotation. Resting symptoms are evaluated.
- Step Two: The clinician first addresses the noninvolved extremity. Slowly, the clinician elevates the upper extremity into abduction. The patient is instructed to report the first incidence of pain during passive movement. The ROM is recorded at the first reported incidence of pain. Pain is evaluated to determine if concordant.
- Step Three: The clinician passively moves the shoulder beyond the first point of pain (if present) toward end range. End feel of the shoulder end range is evaluated.
- Step Four: The process is repeated for the opposite involved side.

**Figure 9.26**   Passive Shoulder Abduction

## Shoulder External Rotation

Passive assessment of external rotation requires examination in different degrees of abduction to investigate fully the capsuloligamentous complex of the shoulder. The superior glenohumeral ligament is tensioned during external rotation at 0 degrees of abduction. The middle glenohumeral ligament is tensioned during the gradual increase in ranges of 0–90 degrees of abduction. The inferior glenohumeral ligament is tensioned during passive external rotation at 90 degrees or more of abduction. The direct relationship between passive external rotation and translatory glide and vice versa is well supported in the literature. Mihata et al.[108] found that external rotation stretching led to improvements in anterior, inferior, and anterior–posterior glide on cadaveric specimens. Excessive stretching leads to elongation of the anterior band of the inferior glenohumeral ligament. For careful evaluation of external rotation, the movement should be tested at 0, 45, and 90 degrees.

Typically, IR and ER requires stabilization of the anterior shoulder to reduce a false improvement in range of motion. This is accomplished by the clinician using his or her forearm, to block the anterior aspect of the shoulder, thus preventing compensatory movement. The hand of the same arm cups the elbow to provide a pivot point.

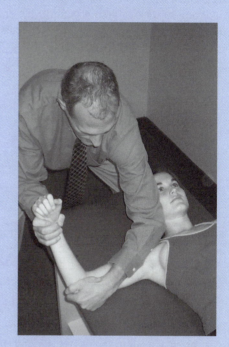

- Step One: The patient is placed in supine. When the involved extremity is tested, the shoulder is placed in zero degrees of abduction. Slowly, the clinician passively rotates the upper extremity into external rotation. The patient is instructed to report the first incidence of pain during passive movement. The ROM is recorded at the first reported incidence of pain. Pain is evaluated to determine if concordant.

**Figure 9.27**  Stabilization Procedure for External Rotation

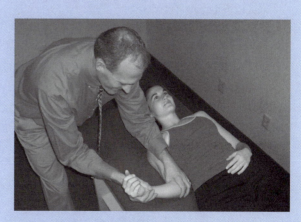

- Step Two: The clinician passively moves the affected shoulder beyond the first point of pain (if present) toward end range. End feel of the shoulder end range is evaluated.

**Figure 9.28**  External Rotation at 0 Degrees of Abduction

*(continued)*

- Step Three: The shoulder is moved to approximately 45 degrees of abduction.
- Step Four: The clinician first addresses the noninvolved extremity. Slowly, the clinician passively rotates the upper extremity into external rotation. The patient is instructed to report the first incidence of pain during passive movement. The ROM is recorded at the first reported incidence of pain. Pain is evaluated to determine if concordant.
- Step Five: The clinician passively moves the shoulder beyond the first point of pain (if present) toward end range. End feel of the shoulder end range is evaluated.

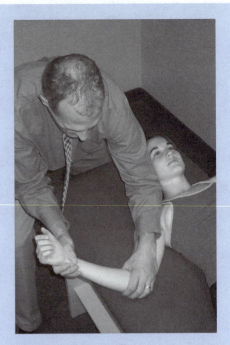

**Figure 9.29**    External Rotation at 45 Degrees of Abduction

- Step Six: The shoulder is placed in abduction at 90 degrees. Using his or her forearm, the clinician blocks the anterior aspect of the shoulder to prevent compensatory movement. The hand of the same arm cups the elbow to provide a pivot point. Baseline symptoms are evaluated.
- Step Seven: The clinician first addresses the noninvolved extremity. Slowly, the clinician passively rotates the upper extremity into external rotation. The patient is instructed to report the first incidence of pain during passive movement. The ROM is recorded at the first reported incidence of pain. Pain is evaluated to determine if concordant.
- Step Eight: The clinician passively moves the shoulder beyond the first point of pain (if present) toward end range. End feel of the shoulder end range is evaluated.
- Step Nine: The procedure is repeated for all three external rotation examinations on the opposite side.

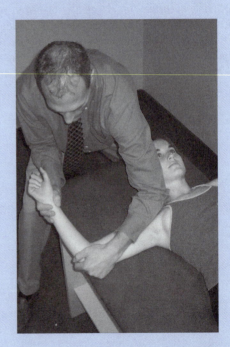

**Figure 9.30**    External Rotation at 90 Degrees of Abduction

# Shoulder Passive Physiological Internal Rotation

Internal rotation can be assessed with the arm at the side or at 70–90 degrees of abduction or flexion. In all cases, the posterior capsule limits the allocation of movement but other structures may be indicated if pain is concordant in one movement and not another. Internal rotation during shoulder flexion places stress on the anterior structures of the shoulder and may be painful in asymptomatic shoulders. At 70–90 degrees, the inferior glenohumeral ligament is engaged and if restricted may limit movement. Furthermore, tightness in the inferior posterior capsule may restrict internal rotation at approximately 70 degrees of abduction.

## Internal Rotation at 0 Degrees of Abduction

- Step One: The patient is placed in supine. The elbow is flexed to 90 degrees and the shoulder is placed at 0 degrees of abduction. Using his or her forearm, the clinician blocks the anterior aspect of the shoulder to prevent compensatory movement. The hand of the same arm cups the elbow to provide a pivot point. Baseline symptoms are evaluated.
- Step Two: Slowly, the clinician passively rotates the upper extremity into internal rotation. The patient is instructed to report the first incidence of pain during passive movement. The ROM is recorded at the first reported incidence of pain. Pain is evaluated to determine if concordant.
- Step Three: The clinician passively moves the shoulder beyond the first point of pain (if present) toward end range. End feel of the shoulder end range is evaluated.

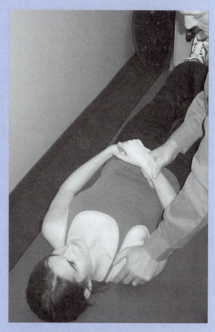

**Figure 9.31**  Internal Rotation at 0 Degrees of Abduction

## Internal Rotation at 70–90 Degrees of Abduction

- Step One: The patient is placed in supine. The elbow is flexed to 90 degrees and the shoulder is placed at 70–90 degrees of abduction. Using his or her forearm, the clinician blocks the anterior aspect of the shoulder to prevent compensatory movement. The hand of the same arm cups the elbow to provide a pivot point. Baseline symptoms are evaluated.
- Step Two: The clinician first addresses the noninvolved extremity. Slowly, the clinician passively rotates the upper extremity into internal rotation. The patient is instructed to report the first incidence of pain during passive movement. The ROM is recorded at the first reported incidence of pain. Pain is evaluated to determine if concordant.
- Step Three: The clinician passively moves the shoulder beyond the first point of pain (if present) toward end range. End feel of the shoulder end range is evaluated.
- Step Four: The procedure is repeated for the opposite involved side.

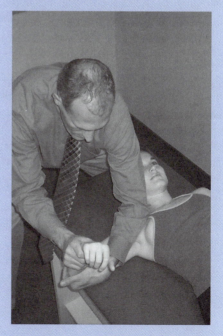

**Figure 9.32**  Internal Rotation at 0 Degrees of Abduction

## Shoulder Horizontal Adduction

The passive movement of horizontal adduction may be limited due to tightness in the posterior capsule, pain in the anterior structures of the glenohumeral joint (anterior impingement syndrome), or secondary to pain in the AC joint. Passive horizontal adduction with internal rotation of the glenohumeral joint may further engage the posterior capsule and may be necessary to ascertain fully the limitation (if present). It is essential to query the patient regarding the location of the pain, whether the pain is concordant, and to determine the potential reasons why the movement is painful.

### Horizontal Adduction with Neutral Rotation

- Step One: The patient is placed in supine. The clinician stands to the side of the extremity evaluated. Using the cephalic hand, the clinician stabilizes the lateral border of the scapula. The opposite hand holds the elbow and functions to move the patient's extremity. Baseline symptoms are evaluated.
- Step Two: The clinician first addresses the noninvolved extremity. The patient is instructed to report the first incidence of pain during passive movement. The ROM is recorded at the first reported incidence of pain. Pain is evaluated to determine if concordant.
- Step Three: The clinician passively moves the shoulder beyond the first point of pain (if present) toward end range.

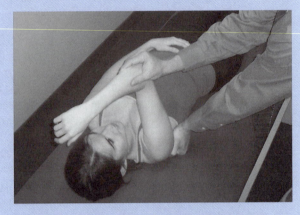

**Figure 9.33**   Horizontal Adduction at Neutral

### Horizontal Adduction with 45–70 Degrees of Internal Rotation

- Step One: The patient is placed in supine. The clinician stands to the side of the extremity evaluated. Using the cephalic hand, the clinician stabilizes the lateral border of the scapula. The opposite hand holds the elbow and functions to move the patient's extremity. Baseline symptoms are evaluated.
- Step Two: The clinician passively internally rotates the extremity at the elbow. Baseline symptoms are evaluated.
- Step Three: The clinician first addresses the noninvolved extremity. The patient is instructed to report the first incidence of pain during passive movement. The ROM is recorded at the first reported incidence of pain. Pain is evaluated to determine if concordant.
- Step Four: The clinician passively moves the shoulder beyond the first point of pain (if present) toward end range.
- Step Five: The process is repeated on the involved, opposite side.

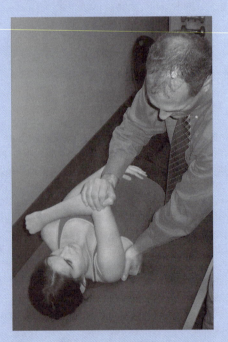

**Figure 9.34**   Horizontal Adduction with Pre-positioned Internal Rotation

## Shoulder Passive Extension

Shoulder extension may be limited if the anterior structures of the shoulder are restricted.

- Step One: The patient is placed in supine. Resting symptoms are assessed. The patient is placed lateral to the edge of the table to allow the shoulder to clear the side of table during extension.
- Step Two: The clinician first addresses the noninvolved extremity. The patient is instructed to report the first incidence of pain during passive movement. The clinician passively moves the shoulder into extension. The ROM is recorded at the first reported incidence of pain. Pain is evaluated to determine if concordant.
- Step Three: The clinician passively moves the shoulder beyond the first point of pain (if present) toward end range.
- Step Four: The process is repeated on the involved, opposite side.

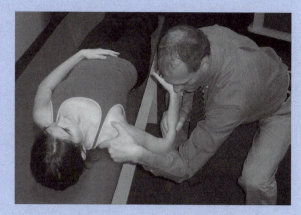

**Figure 9.35**    Passive Physiological Extension

## Summary

- End feel and the first point of resistance are reliable concepts within the shoulder.
- Because different capsuloligamentous components are responsible for resisting movements at different ranges, it is important to test movements such as external rotation at variable degrees of flexion and abduction.
- Combining movements to increase the tension within the capsuloligamentous region may be necessary to isolate the concordant sign.

## Passive Accessory Movements

Prepositioning of the humerus anteriorly or posteriorly in the joint is common during pathology to the shoulder. Harryman et al.[34] suggested that this phenomenon is associated with asymmetric tightening of the capsule, which results in translation of the humeral head in the opposite direction of the limited capsule. Subsequently, a tight posterior capsule would lead to a prepositioning of translation anteriorly in the joint, vice versa for a tight anterior capsule.

Joint mobilization techniques are beneficial for shoulder patients and preferable to physiological stretching because the movements provide a precise stretch to the restricted aspect of the capsule (when prepositioned in the restricted position) with less subsequent pain, less force, and less compression on painful structures.[109–111] Conroy and Hayes outline that joint mobilizations are effective in reducing pain and edema, through selective stretching of causative structures.[111] Selective stretching requires the administration of the appropriate force, in the targeted and appropriate direction, performed over a period of time.[112]

End range mobilizations have long been advocated for improvement of range of motion by many authors.[113,114] However, end ranges of motion do limit the amount of translation of the humeral head.[115,116] Most notably, PA translation decreases during a prepositioning of external rotation of the shoulder. However, AP translation is not decreased with a preposition of internal rotation of the shoulder.[115] Hsu and colleagues[116] reported that more displacement occurs during a PA glide than AP in a preposition of abduction. End range mobilizations do lead to multidirectional improvements in range of motion for patients with adhesive capsulitis[117] and are appropriate for stiffness-dominant patients.

## Glenohumeral Posterior–Anterior Glide

A PA glide in a loose-packed position may not be helpful in improving range of motion for restriction abduction and/or external rotation.[116] A PA glide is equally effective for improving abduction as an AP when the humerus is placed in an end range position.[116] A PA glide does lead to neurophysiologic changes such as increased conductivity for the complete upper limb.[118]

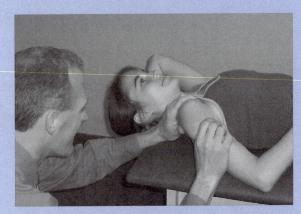

**Figure 9.36**    Starting Position for the PA for Pain Control

### PA for Pain Control
- Step One: The patient is placed in supine. The patient's hands are draped across his or her stomach. Resting symptoms are assessed.
- Step Two: The clinician uses both thumbs to contact the posterior aspect of the humerus of the patient. The fingers rest gently on the anterior surface of the patient's shoulder.

- Step Three: Using a sequential movement and the side of the plinth as a lever, the clinician gently applies force posterior to anterior and then pulls downward on the humeral head.
- Step Four: The patient's resting symptoms are reassessed.

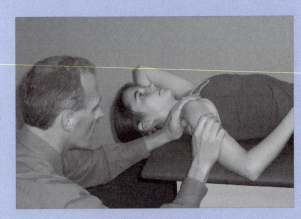

**Figure 9.37**    PA for Pain Relief

**PA for Range-of-Motion Gains**

- Step One: The patient is placed in prone. Resting symptoms are assessed.
- Step Two: The clinician uses the palm of his or her hand to contact the posterior aspect of the shoulder. The shoulder is elevated (flexion or abduction) to the limit of the patient.
- Step Three: The clinician performs a PA mobilization at the limitation of the patient. External and internal rotation is prepositioned to further the effects of the end range mobilization.
- Step Four: The patient's resting symptoms and range of motion are reassessed.

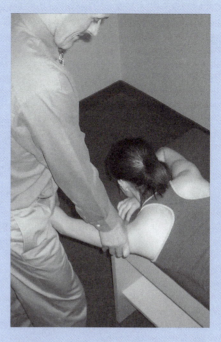

**Figure 9.38**   Prone PA for Range-of-Motion Gains

## Glenohumeral Anterior–Posterior Glide

An AP glide in a loose-packed position may not be helpful in improving range of motion for abduction and/or internal rotation specifically if internal rotation is limited near end range.[116] In a neutral position the middle posterior capsule limits AP translation whereas in a preposition of abduction, the middle and inferior posterior capsule limits movement.[119,120]

Mobilization to improve shoulder flexion/abduction is most appropriately performed at end range[116] and since the majority of shoulder pathologies lead to anterior migration of the humeral head, an anterior-to-posterior glide may be best. Conroy and Hayes[111] performed mobilizations at mid range and theorized that the lack of benefit may be associated with the inability to engage the capsule appropriately at this range.

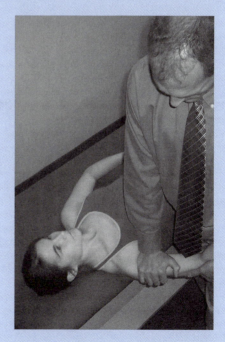

- Step One: The patient is placed in supine. Resting symptoms are assessed.
- Step Two: The clinician moves the patient's shoulder to the first point of pain. If pain occurs before the onset of stiffness, the mobilization should be performed at that range using less intense force.

**Figure 9.39**   Mobilization at Early AP Ranges

*(continued)*

- Step Three: If stiffness is encountered concurrently or before pain, more aggressive mobilization at that range is beneficial.
- Step Four: Reassess the movement restriction of the patient.

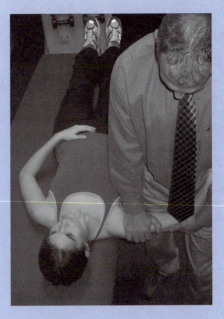

**Figure 9.40** End Range AP Mobilization

## Glenohumeral Shoulder Traction

Techniques such as traction do not lead to joint separation with the arm placed at the side near the supposed loose-packed position or during a closed-packed position. Neither position demonstrated differences in distraction amounts.[104] Subsequently, traction-based mobilization will primarily demonstrate benefit for a patient with pain as the primary disorder.

- Step One: The patient is placed in supine. Resting symptoms are assessed.
- Step Two: The clinician moves the patient's shoulder to the first point of pain. The clinician should back away from the range of pain and perform the traction mobilization at that point.
- Step Three: The clinician should reevaluate the resting pain level of the patient.

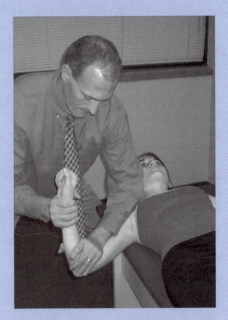

**Figure 9.41** Traction Mobilization for Pain Reduction

## Glenohumeral Inferior (Caudal) Glide

Hsu et al.[33] reported improvements in mobility of cadaveric tissue when an inferior glide was applied to the shoulder at the end or near end range of abduction. These techniques were effective for abduction mobility gains and were more effective than similar mobilization performed at 40 degrees of abduction (non–end range).

- Step One: The patient is placed in supine. Resting symptoms are assessed.
- Step Two: The clinician moves the patient's shoulder to the first point of pain. If pain occurs before the onset of stiffness, the mobilization should be performed at that range using less intense force.

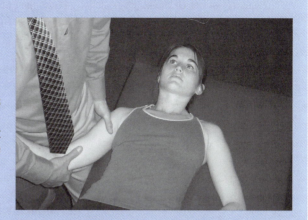

**Figure 9.42**    Mobilization at Early Ranges of Inferior Glide

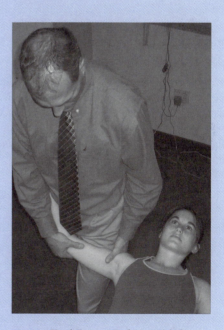

- Step Three: If stiffness is encountered concurrently or before pain, aggressive mobilization at that range is beneficial. For patients who tolerate aggressive mobilization and who demonstrate significant range limitations, end range mobilization may be necessary.
- Step Four: Reassess the movement restriction of the patient.

**Figure 9.43**    End Range Inferior Glide Mobilization

## Acromioclavicular PA Glide

The acromioclavicular joint translates posterior to anterior during scapular retraction.

- Step One: The patient assumes a supine position. The clinician places his or her thumb in the posterior V notch (just posterior to the medial aspect of the AC joint).
- Step Two: The clinician applies a PA glide to the AC in an attempt to reproduce symptoms.
- Step Three: If concordant, the clinician may apply treatment using this technique and can adjust the position of the scapular to sensitize the movement.

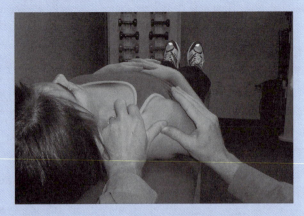

**Figure 9.44**   Acromioclavicular PA Mobilization

## Acromioclavicular Inferior Glide

The clavicle moves inferiorly on the scapular (acromial) contact during arm elevation.

- Step One: The patient assumes a supine position. The clinician places his or her thumb on the superior surface just medial to the AC joint (clavicular contact).
- Step Two: The clinician applies an inferior glide to the AC in an attempt to reproduce symptoms.

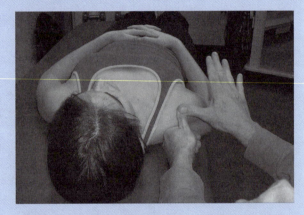

**Figure 9.45**   Acromioclavicular Inferior Mobilization

- Step Three: If concordant, the clinician may apply treatment using this technique, and can adjust the position of the scapula to sensitize the movement.

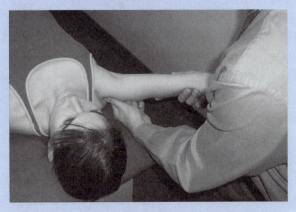

**Figure 9.46**   Preposition of the Shoulder to Enhance the Inferior Glide of the AC Joint

## Acromioclavicular AP Glide

The clavicle moves posteriorly on the acromion during protraction and abduction of the scapula.

- Step One: The patient assumes a supine position. The clinician places his or her thumb anterior on the V notch (just anterior to the medial aspect of the AC joint).
- Step Two: The clinician applies an AP glide to the AC in an attempt to reproduce symptoms.
- Step Three: If concordant, the clinician may apply treatment using this technique and can adjust the position of the scapula to sensitize the movement.

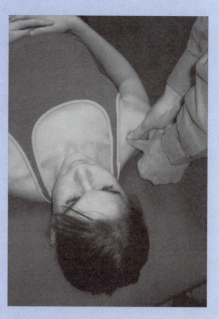

**Figure 9.47**   Anterior-Posterior Mobilization of the AC Joint

## Sternoclavicular Inferior Glide

The clavicle moves inferiorly with respect to the sternum during arm elevation. The motion involves both inferior translation and upward rotation.

- Step One: The patient assumes a supine position. The clinician places his or her thumb superior to the SC joint, lateral to the actual joint space.
- Step Two: The clinician applies an inferior glide to the SC in an attempt to reproduce symptoms.
- Step Three: If concordant, the clinician may apply treatment using this technique and can adjust the position arm (greater or less arm elevation) to sensitize the movement.

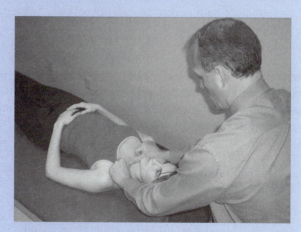

**Figure 9.48**   Inferior Glide of the Sternoclavicular Joint

## *Summary*

- Passive accessory movements are most appropriately assessed at early, mid and end ranges.
- Because most pathologies cause an anterior migration of the humeral head, an AP force may exhibit the most sensitivity as the concordant sign.
- End range accessory motions may be more beneficial in improving range of motion at the shoulder.

## Clinical Special Tests

A useful clinical special test should help the examiner distinguish between disorders with symptoms that closely mimic each other. The tests are performed to shed additional light when the examiner is still unsure of the diagnosis after taking a thorough history and performance of active physiological motion, passive physiological motion, and accessory motion. Palpation, muscle strength assessment, and physical examination tests (special tests) can be helpful in this elucidating role. Essentially, the clinical special test should be confirmatory in nature.

### *Palpation*

Numerous authors have reported the benefit of palpation in the diagnostic process. Wolf and Agrawal[121] and Lyons and Tomlinson[122] described the accuracy of transdeltoid palpation (the *Rent Test*) in detecting full thickness rotator cuff tears. Palpation over the acromioclavicular (AC) joint was found to be highly sensitive, though not specific, in detecting AC joint pathology.[123] Palpation over the cervical spine may reproduce shoulder symptoms if the cause of the shoulder pain is cervical radiculopathy.[65] Subacromial impingement often hurts directly over the shoulder joint at the connection of the C4-5 dermatome.[65] Osteoarthritis is typically painful directly on the joint line of the patient. Anterior impingement is often painful directly over the acromion but caution must be used during this assessment because any condition that causes anterior migration of the humeral head (and most conditions do cause this) will place pressure on the anterior soft tissue structures and will be painful. A patient with rotator cuff weakness will often report pain over the upper trapezius but not the posterior cervical spine.[65]

### *Muscle Testing*

Kelly et al.[124] used EMG to determine the optimal test to isolate each rotator cuff muscle during the motions of elevation, internal rotation, and external rotation. They defined the optimal test as one with good test–retest reliability with maximum muscle activation while minimizing synergist activation and positional pain. The optimal supraspinatus test was the "full can," arms elevated to 90 degrees in the scapular plane with thumbs facing up. Testing the supraspinatus in the "empty can" position, which is 90 degrees of elevation in the scapular plane, with full internal shoulder rotation is a specific but not a sensitive test, useful only in ruling in subacromial impingement.

Although less investigated, selected positions may also improve the contractile capacity of the infraspinatus. According to Kelly et al.[124], the infraspinatus was best tested with the patient's elbow at the side and flexed to 90 degrees, and the shoulder in 45 degrees of internal rotation.

Kelly et al.[124] found that "giving way" due to weakness or pain was a specific but not sensitive test, useful in ruling in subacromial impingement. Subscapularis was tested optimally, with the patient's arm behind his or her low back and lifted off of the low back. The optimal test position of the teres minor muscle has not been as rigorously studied but the suggested position to isolate this muscle is with the patient in supine resisting an internal rotation force.[126] The best position in which to evaluate rotator cuff co-contraction is where the fibers of the relevant muscles are optimally aligned to achieve relocation of the humeral head in the scapular plane.[127]

### *Clinical Special Tests*

Clinical special tests are designed to provide diagnostic value to a set of findings. This is accomplished by providing discriminatory power for ruling in and ruling out a disorder. There are multitudes of clinical special tests for the shoulder, many of which have been studied for diagnostic value but in studies of mediocre design. The following tests have been examined for diagnostic value.

### *Clinical Special Tests for Impingement*

The amount of purported tests for impingement is astounding. A preponderance of studies has used poor reference standards for comparison or has displayed only poor to fair diagnostic values. Comprehensively, there are mixed findings on which impingement tests yield diagnostic value in ruling in or out a disorder. Some tests demonstrate greater specificity than sensitivity whereas others appear to be more sensitive than specific. When used judiciously, special tests for impingement may add some value to the conclusion of impingement; however, the findings provide little assistance in treatment.

## Neer Test—Impingement

The *Neer* test was described by Neer in 1983.[128] The test is designed to identify impingement of soft tissue in the shoulder between the humeral head and the anterior acromion. Table 9.4 (p. 261) outlines the diagnostic values of the Neer test, the accuracy of which has since been studied in various pathologies including subacromial bursitis and rotator cuff tears.

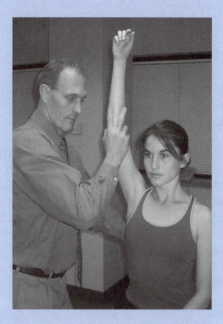

- Step One: The patient is seated while the clinician stands to the side of the involved shoulder.
- Step Two: The clinician raises the patient's arm into flexion with one hand while the other hand stabilizes the scapula.
- Step Three: The clinician applies forced flexion toward end range in an attempt to reproduce the shoulder pain. If concordant shoulder pain is present, the test is positive.
- Step Four: As originally described, the test was completed by injecting 10 mL of xylocaine beneath the anterior acromion to assess the elimination of pain. A positive test is the elimination of pain with injection.

**Figure 9.49**   The Neer Impingement Test

## Hawkins–Kennedy Test—Impingement

The *Hawkins–Kennedy* test was described by Hawkins and Kennedy in 1980.[129] The test was designed to identify impingement of soft tissue in the shoulder between the greater tuberosity of the humeral head and the coracoacromial ligament. Table 9.4 outlines the diagnostic values of the *Hawkins–Kennedy* test, the accuracy of which has since been studied in various pathologies including subacromial bursitis and rotator cuff tears.

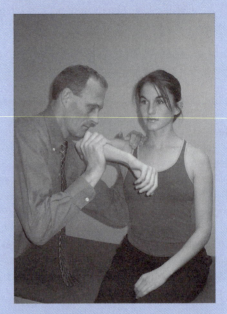

- Step One: The patient is seated while the clinician stands anteriorly to the involved shoulder.
- Step Two: The clinician first raises the patient's arm into approximately 90 degrees of shoulder flexion or abduction with one hand while the other hand stabilizes the scapula (typically superiorly).
- Step Three: The clinician applies forced humeral internal rotation in an attempt to reproduce the concordant shoulder pain. If concordant shoulder pain is present, the test is positive.

**Figure 9.50**   The Hawkins–Kennedy Test of Impingement

## Painful Arc Test—Impingement

The *Painful Arc* test was described by Kessel and Watson in 1977.[130] The test is designed to identify impingement "in the subacromial region" versus an AC joint pathology. Table 9.4 outlines the diagnostic values of the *Painful Arc* test.

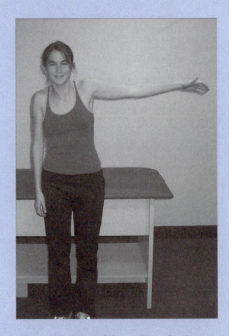

- Step One: The patient is standing. The clinician faces the patient to observe shoulder motion.
- Step Two: The patient is instructed to actively abduct the involved shoulder.
- Step Three: A positive test is indicated by patient report of concordant pain in the 60- to 120-degree range. Pain outside of this range is considered a negative test. Pain that increases in severity as the arm reaches 180 degrees is indicative of "a disorder of the acromioclavicular joint."

**Figure 9.51**   The Painful Arc Test for Impingement

## Cross-Body Adduction Test—Impingement

The *Cross-Body Adduction Impingement* test was originally described by McLaughlin in 1951.[131] The test compresses the greater tuberosity of the humeral head against the coracoid process and the coracoacromial ligament. Table 9.4 outlines the diagnostic values of the *Cross-Body Adduction Impingement* test.

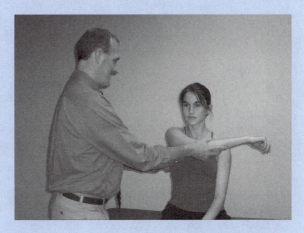

- Step One: The patient assumes a sitting position. The patient is instructed to elevate the arm to 90 degrees of shoulder flexion.
- Step Two: The clinician stands in front of the patient and horizontally adducts the patient's arm to end range maintaining the flexion at the shoulder.
- Step Three: If shoulder pain is present, the test is positive.

**Figure 9.52**   The Cross-Body Adduction Test for Impingement

## Speed's (Biceps Tension) Test—Impingement

*Speed's* test was originated by Speed in 1952 and first reported in published literature in 1966.[132] The test was originally used to detect biceps tenosynovitis but has been applied to other pathologies of the shoulder including impingement and labral tears. Table 9.4 outlines the diagnostic values of *Speed's* test.

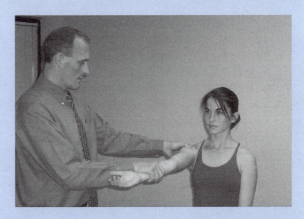

- Step One: The patient assumes a standing position. The patient is instructed to extend his or her elbow and fully supinates the forearm.
- Step Two: The clinician, standing in front of the patient, resists shoulder flexion from 0 to 60 degrees.
- Step Three: If the patient localizes concordant pain to the bicipital groove, the test is positive.

**Figure 9.53**   Speed's Test for Impingement

## Yergason's Test for Impingement

*Yergason's* test was first described in 1931.[133] The test was originally used to detect degeneration of the long head of the biceps and/or biceps tenosynovitis, but has been applied to other pathologies of the shoulder including impingement and labral tears. Table 9.4 outlines the diagnostic values of *Yergason's* test for Impingement.

- Step One: The patient may sit or stand. The clinician stands in front of the patient.
- Step Two: The patient's elbow is flexed to 90 degrees and the forearm is pronated while maintaining the upper arm at the side.
- Step Three: The patient is instructed to supinate his or her forearm, while the clinician concurrently resists forearm supination at the wrist.
- Step Three: If the patient localizes concordant pain to the bicipital groove, the test is positive.

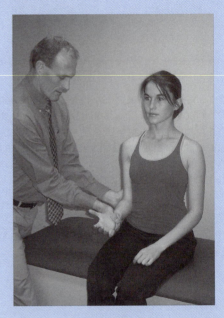

**Figure 9.54**   Yergason's Test for Impingement

## Internal Rotation Resistance Stress Test (IRRST) for Impingement

The *IRRST* was originally described by Zaslav in 2001.[134] The test purportedly differentiates between subacromial impingement (outlet impingement) and intraarticular impingement (internal impingement/secondary impingement). Table 9.4 outlines the diagnostic values of the *IRRST* for impingement.

- Step One: The patient is instructed to stand. The clinician stands behind the patient.
- Step Two: The clinician places the patient's shoulder in 90 degrees of abduction and 80 degrees of external rotation.
- Step Three: The clinician applies manual resistance to the wrist, first to test isometric external rotation and then to test isometric internal rotation.
- Step Four: The clinician compares the results of this isometric test. If internal rotation strength is weaker than external rotation, the IRRST test is considered positive and the patient purportedly has internal impingement.

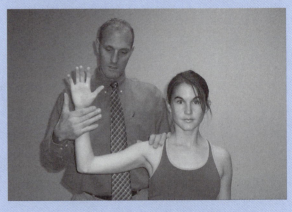

**Figure 9.55**   The Internal Rotation Stress Test for Impingement

## The Posterior Impingement Sign for Impingement

The *Posterior Impingement Sign* was originally described by Meister et al. in 2004.[135] The test purportedly detects articular side tears of the rotator cuff and/or posterior labrum from posterior–superior glenoid impingement. Table 9.4 outlines the diagnostic values of the *Posterior Impingement Sign*.

- Step One: The patient assumes a supine position with his or her arms to the side.
- Step Two: The clinician, positioned beside the patient's involved extremity, concurrently places the patient's shoulder in 90–110 degrees of abduction, 10–15 degrees of extension, and maximum external rotation.
- Step Three: A positive sign is indicated by recreation of the patient's concordant symptoms and/or a report of concordant pain deep within the posterior aspect of the shoulder.

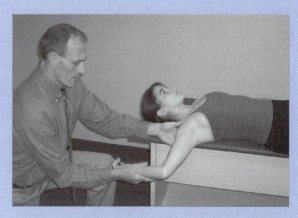

**Figure 9.56**   The Posterior Impingement Sign

**TABLE 9.4**   Shoulder Clinical Special Tests for Impingement: Diagnostic Values

| Author (Study) | Test | Sensitivity | Specificity | +LR | −LR | Criterion Standard |
|---|---|---|---|---|---|---|
| MacDonald et al.[171] | Neer test | 75 | 48 | 1.44 | 0.52 | Arthroscopy |
| Park et al.[125] | Neer test | 68 | 69 | 2.19 | 0.46 | Arthroscopy |
| Calis et al.[172] | Neer | 89 | 31 | 1.28 | 0.35 | Subacromial injection |
| MacDonald et al.[171] | Hawkins–Kennedy test | 92 | 44 | 1.64 | 0.18 | Arthroscopy |
| Park et al.[125] | Hawkins–Kennedy | 72 | 66 | 2.11 | 0.42 | Arthroscopy |
| Calis et al.[172] | Hawkins–Kennedy | 92 | 25 | 1.22 | 0.32 | Subacromial injection |
| Park et al.[125] | Painful Arc | 74 | 81 | 3.89 | 0.32 | Arthroscopy |
| Calis et al.[172] | Painful Arc | 33 | 81 | 1.73 | 0.82 | Subacromial injection |
| Park et al.[125] | Cross-body Adduction | 23 | 82 | 1.27 | 0.93 | Arthroscopy |
| Calis et al.[172] | Cross-body Adduction | 82 | 28 | 1.13 | 0.64 | Subacromial injection |
| Park et al.[125] | Speed's Test | 38 | 83 | 2.23 | 0.74 | Arthroscopy |
| Calis et al.[172] | Speed's Test | 69 | 56 | 1.56 | 0.55 | Subacromial injection |
| Meister et al.[135] | Posterior Impingement | 76 | 85 | 5.06 | 0.28 | Arthroscopy |
| Calis et al.[172] | Yergason's Test | 37 | 86 | 2.64 | 0.73 | Subacromial injection |
| Zaslav[134] | Internal Rotation Stress Test | 88 | 96 | 22 | 0.12 | Arthroscopy |
| Calis et al.[172,171] | Drop-arm | 8 | 97 | 2.66 | 0.94 | Subacromial injection |
| Itoi[140] | Empty can | 63 | 55 | 1.4 | 0.67 | MRI |
| Itoi[140] | Full can | 66 | 64 | 1.83 | 0.53 | MRI |

## *Clinical Special Tests for Rotator Cuff Dysfunction/Tear*

Comprehensively, most clinical special tests for rotator cuff tear or dysfunction provide better diagnostic values than impingement tests. They may reflect the most specific dysfunction associated with a rotator cuff tear versus impingement (which is a cluster of occasionally dissimilar findings). Rotator cuff specific tests generally demonstrate good specificity and resulting diagnostic values that may assist the clinician in improving the selection of a treatment.

### Lift-Off Test—Subscapularis Tear

The *Lift-Off* test was described by Gerber and Krushell in 1991.[136] The test is designed to identify a full-thickness tear of the subscapularis tendon. Table 9.5 (p. 266) outlines the diagnostic values of the *Lift-Off* test.

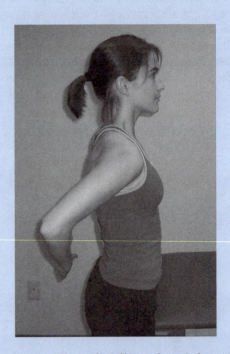

- Step One: The patient assumes a standing position. His or her arms are placed at the sides.
- Step Two: The patient is instructed to place the dorsum of the hand on his or her low back at the waist level. The patient is then instructed to lift the dorsum of the hand from his or her back.
- Step Three: A positive test is indicated by inability of the patient to lift his or her hand off of his or her back.

**Figure 9.57**    The Lift-Off Test for a Subscapularis Tear

## Modified Lift-Off Test/Internal Rotation Lag Sign (IRLS)—Subscapularis Tear

The *Modified Lift-Off/Internal Rotation Lag* test was described by Gerber et al.[137] and Hertel et al.[138] in 1996. The test is designed to identify a tear of the subscapularis tendon. Table 9.5 outlines the diagnostic value of the Modified Lift-off test.

- Step One: The patient assumes a seated position on a stool or a chair without arms. The clinician stands behind the patient.
- Step Two: The clinician places the arm of the patient behind their lower back at the waist level.
- Step Three: The clinician lifts the dorsum of the patient's hand away from his or her lower back into shoulder internal rotation and extension. The patient is instructed to hold the hand away from his or her lower back.
- Step Four: The clinician releases the patient's arm and records the degree of movement of the hand toward the lower back.
- Step Five: A full-thickness tear is indicated by inability of the patient to keep his or her hand off of the back and a partial thickness tear is indicated by the patient's hand moving more than 5 degrees toward the lower back but not touching the lower back.

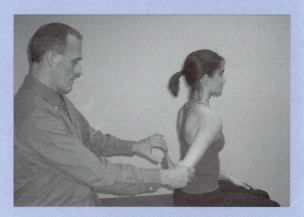

**Figure 9.58**    The Modified Lift-Off/Internal Rotation Lag Test

## Modified Belly Press Test—Subscapularis Tear

The *Modified Belly Press* test was described by Gerber et al. in 1996.[137] The test is designed to identify a full-thickness tear of the subscapularis tendon in a patient who cannot achieve the behind-the-back position required for the *Lift-Off* and *Modified Lift-Off* tests. Table 9.5 outlines the diagnostic value of the *Modified Belly Press* test.

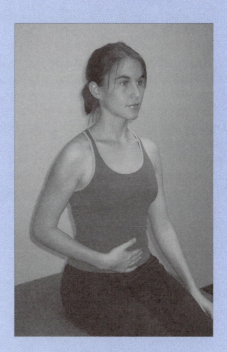

- Step One: The patient is seated with the palm of the hand on his or her stomach and his or her elbow flexed and in front of his or her body.
- Step Two: The patient presses into his or her stomach with his or her hand by extending the shoulder and attempts to keep the elbow in front of his or her body.
- Step Three: A positive test is indicated by inability of the patient to keep the elbow in front of his or her body.

**Figure 9.59**    The Belly Press Test

## Empty Can/Supraspinatus Test—Supraspinatus Tear

The *Empty Can/Supraspinatus* test was described by Jobe and Jobe in 1983.[139] The test is designed to identify a weakness due to a supraspinatus tendon tear or pain due to rotator cuff impingement. Table 9.5 outlines the diagnostic value of the *Empty Can/Supraspinatus* test.

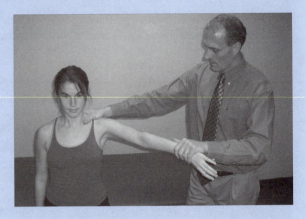

- Step One: The patient is standing with arms elevated to 90 degrees in the scapular plane (scaption) with the shoulders in full internal rotation (thumbs facing the floor). The clinician stands anteriorly to the patient.
- Step Two: The clinician applies an adduction force bilaterally while the patient resists this force.
- Step Three: A positive test is indicated by weakness of the involved side compared to the uninvolved side (supraspinatus tear) or pain in the involved shoulder (impingement) or both.

**Figure 9.60**    The Empty Can/Supraspinatus Test

## Full Can Test—Supraspinatus Tear

The *Full Can* test was described by Jobe and Jobe in 1983.[139] The test is designed to identify a weakness in the supraspinatus tendon. Itoi et al.[140] later studied the ability of the full can to detect a supraspinatus tear and impingement. Table 9.5 outlines the diagnostic value of the *Full Can* test.

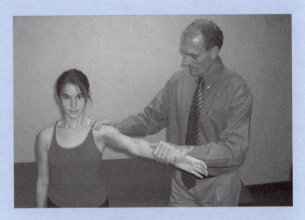

- Step One: The patient is standing with arms elevated to 90 degrees in the scapular plane (scaption) with the shoulders in 45 degrees of internal rotation (thumbs facing the ceiling). The clinician stands anteriorly to the patient.
- Step Two: The clinician applies an adduction force bilaterally while the patient resists this force.
- Step Three: A positive test is indicated by weakness of the involved side compared to the uninvolved side (supraspinatus tear) or pain in the involved shoulder (impingement) or both.

**Figure 9.61**    The Full Can Test for a Supraspinatus Tear and Impingement

## External Rotation Lag Sign (ERLS)—Supraspinatus/Infraspinatus Tear

The modified ERLS was described by Hertel et al. in 1996.[138] The test is designed to identify a small tear of the supraspinatus/ infraspinatus tendons with a lag of 5 degrees or a larger tear of these tendons with a greater-than-5-degree lag. Table 9.5 outlines the diagnostic values of the ERLS.

- Step One: The patient assumes a sitting position. The clinician stands behind the patient.
- Step Two: The clinician grasps one of the patient's wrists with one hand and the elbow of the patient with the other.
- Step Three: The clinician places the patient's shoulder in 20 degrees of elevation in the scapular plane (scaption) and near end range of external rotation with the elbow flexed to 90 degrees. The clinician then releases the patient's arm.
- Step Four: A positive test is identified by the inability of the patient to keep his or her shoulder positioned in external rotation.
- Step Five: A small tear of the supraspinatus/infraspinatus tendons is indicated by the patient "lagging" into internal rotation by 5 degrees. A larger tear is identified by the patient's shoulder "lagging" into more than 5 degrees of internal rotation.

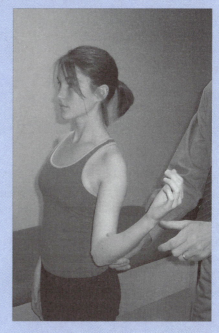

**Figure 9.62**  The External Rotation Lag Sign (ERLS) for a Supraspinatus/ Infraspinatus Tear

## Drop-Arm Test—Supraspinatus Tear

The *Drop-Arm* test was described by Moseley in 1960[141] and reportedly detects a tear in the rotator cuff. Table 9.5 outlines the diagnostic value of the *Drop-Arm* test.

- Step One: The patient assumes a sitting position. The clinician stands behind the patient.
- Step Two: The clinician elevates the patient's arm to 90 degrees of abduction.
- Step Three: The clinician releases the patient's arm with instructions for the patient to lower the arm to his or her side slowly and deliberately.
- Step Four: A positive test is indicated by the inability of the patient to slowly lower the arm and/or letting the arm "drop" rapidly.

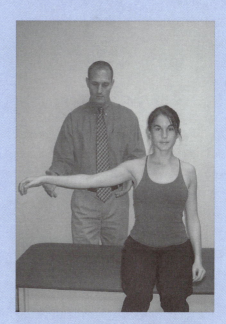

**Figure 9.63**  The Drop-Arm-Supraspinatus Test

## Drop Sign—Subscapularis Tear

The *Drop Sign* was described by Hertel et al. in 1996.[138] The test is designed to "assess the function of the infraspinatus." Table 9.5 outlines the diagnostic values of the *Drop Sign*.

- Step One: The patient assumes a sitting position. The clinician stands behind the patient.
- Step Two: With one hand, the clinician grasps the patient's wrist; with the other, the clinician grasps the patient's elbow.
- Step Three: The clinician places the patient's shoulder in 90 degrees of abduction and near end range of external rotation with the elbow flexed to 90 degrees.
- Step Four: The clinician releases the patient's wrist.
- Step Five: The clinician records the degree of movement of the shoulder back into internal rotation.

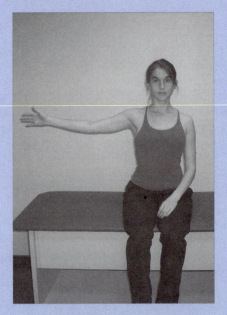

**Figure 9.64**    The Drop Sign for a Supraspinatus Tear

**TABLE 9.5**    Clinical Special Tests for Rotator Cuff Integrity: Diagnostic Values

| Author (Study) | Test | Sensitivity | Specificity | +LR | −LR | Criterion Standard |
|---|---|---|---|---|---|---|
| Wolf & Agrawal[121] | Rent test | 96 | 97 | 32 | 0.04 | Arthroscopy |
| Lyons & Tomlinson[122] | Rent test | 91 | 75 | 3.64 | 0.12 | Surgery |
| MacDonald et al.[171] | Neer test | 83 | 51 | 1.69 | 0.33 | Arthroscopy |
| MacDonald et al.[171] | Hawkins-Kennedy Test | 88 | 43 | 1.54 | 0.27 | Arthroscopy |
| Gerber & Krushell[136] | Lift-off | 89 | 98 | 44.5 | 0.11 | Arthroscopy |
| Hertel et al.[138] | Lift-off | 62 | 100 | NA | NA | Open or arthroscopic surgery |
| Gerber et al.[137] | Modified Lift-off/Internal Rotation Lag (IRLS) | ND | ND | ND | ND | Surgery |
| Hertel et al.[138] | IRLS | 97 | 96 | 24.25 | 0.03 | Open or arthroscopic surgery |
| Itoi[140] | Empty can | 77 | 68 | 2.40 | 0.33 | MRI |
| Itoi[140] | Full can | 77 | 74 | 2.96 | 0.31 | MRI |
| Hertel et al.[138] | ERLS | 70 | 100 | NA | NA | Open or arthroscopic surgery |
| Calis et al.[172] | Drop-arm | 15 | 100 | NA | NA | Subacromial injection |
| Hertel et al.[138] | Drop Sign | 20 | 100 | NA | NA | Open or arthroscopic surgery |
| Calis et al.[172] | Hawkins–Kennedy | 100 | 36 | NA | NA | Subacromial injection |

## *Clinical Special Tests of Labral or Associative Tears*

The diagnostic values of most clinical special tests designed to implicate a torn labrum are poor. Only those studies that considerably biased the selection pool for the study found good diagnostic value. Subsequently, despite the high reported diagnostic values, the benefit of clinical special tests to isolate a labrum tear appears to be questionable.

### (O'Brien's) Active Compression Test—Labral Tear/AC Joint Pathology

The *Active Compression* test was described by O'Brien et al. in 1998.[142] The test is designed to detect and differentiate between a superior labral anterior-to-posterior (SLAP) tear and acromioclavicular joint abnormality. Table 9.6 outlines the diagnostic values of the *Active Compression* test.

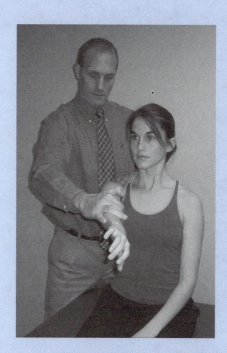

- Step One: The patient is instructed to stand with his or her involved shoulder at 90 degrees of flexion, 10 degrees of horizontal adduction, and maximum internal rotation with the elbow in full extension. The clinician stands directly behind the patient's involved shoulder.
- Step Two: The clinician applies a downward force at the wrist of the involved extremity. The patient is instructed to resist the force.
- Step Three: The patient resists the downward force and reports any pain as either "on top of the shoulder" (acromioclavicular joint) or "inside the shoulder" (SLAP lesion).
- Step Four: The patient's shoulder is then moved to a position of maximum external rotation, and the downward force is repeated.
- Step Five: A positive test is indicated by pain or painful clicking in shoulder internal rotation and less or no pain in external rotation.

**Figure 9.65**    The O'Brien's Test for Labral or AC Pathology

**TABLE 9.6**    Clinical Special Tests for Labral Pathology: Diagnostic Values

| Author (Study) | Test | Sensitivity | Specificity | +LR | −LR | Criterion Standard |
|---|---|---|---|---|---|---|
| **Superior Labral (SLAP) Tears** | | | | | | |
| Holtby & Razmjou[173] | Yergason's | 43 | 79 | 2.05 | .72 | Arthroscopy |
| Guanche & Jones[174] | Yergason's | 12 | 96 | 3.00 | .92 | Arthroscopy |
| Parentis et al.[175] | Yergason's | 13 | 93 | 1.78 | .94 | Arthroscopy |
| Holtby & Razmjou[173] | Speed's Test | 32 | 75 | 1.28 | .91 | Arthroscopy |
| Bennett[176] | Speed's Test | 90 | 14 | 1.04 | .72 | Arthroscopy |
| Guanche & Jones[174] | Speed's | 9 | 74 | .35 | 1.23 | Arthroscopy |
| Morgan et al.[177] | Speed's | 100 | 70 | 3.33 | 0 | Anterior SLAP/ Arthroscopy |
| | | 29 | 11 | .32 | 6.32 | Posterior SLAP/ Arthroscopy |
| | | 78 | 37 | 1.23 | .60 | Combined Ant and Post/Arthroscopy |

*(continued)*

| Author (Study) | Test | Sensitivity | Specificity | +LR | −LR | Criterion Standard |
|---|---|---|---|---|---|---|
| Parentis et al.[175] | Speed's | 48 | 68 | 1.49 | .77 | Arthroscopy |
| Guanche & Jones[174] | Apprehension | 30 | 63 | .81 | 1.11 | Arthroscopy |
| Guanche & Jones[174] | Jobe Relocation | 36 | 63 | .97 | 1.01 | Arthroscopy |
| Morgan et al.[177] | Jobe Relocation | 4 | 27 | .05 | 3.52 | Anterior SLAP/ Arthroscopy |
| | | 85 | 68 | 2.67 | .21 | Posterior SLAP/ Arthroscopy |
| | | 59 | 54 | 1.28 | .76 | Combined Ant and Post Arthroscopy |
| Parentis et al.[175] | Relocation | 44 | 51 | .90 | 1.10 | Arthroscopy |
| Guanche & Jones[174] | Active compression | 54 | 47 | 1.01 | .98 | Arthroscopy |
| O'Brien et al.[142] | Active compression | 100 | 99 | NA | NA | Arthroscopy but only on those suspected of having SLAP lesions |
| Morgan et al.[177] | Active compression | 88 | 42 | 1.52 | .28 | Anterior SLAP/ Arthroscopy |
| | | 32 | 13 | .37 | 5.14 | Posterior SLAP/ Arthroscopy |
| | | 85 | 41 | 1.44 | .36 | Combined Ant and Post/Arthroscopy |
| Myers et al.[145] | Active compression | 78 | 11 | .87 | 2.0 | Arthroscopy |
| McFarland et al.[178] | Active compression | 47 | 55 | 1.04 | .96 | Arthroscopy |
| Stetson & Templin[179] | Active compression | 54 | 31 | .78 | 1.48 | Arthroscopy- SLAP + Ant and Post Labral Tears |
| Parentis et al.[175] | Active compression | 65 | 49 | 1.27 | .72 | Arthroscopy |
| Guanche & Jones[174] | Crank | 39 | 67 | 1.18 | .91 | Arthroscopy |
| Myers et al.[145] | Crank | 35 | 70 | 1.16 | 0.92 | Arthroscopy |
| Stetson & Templin[179] | Crank | 46 | 56 | 1.04 | .96 | Arthroscopy- SLAP + Ant and Post Labral Tears |
| Parentis et al.[175] | Crank | 9 | 83 | .50 | 1.10 | Arthroscopy |
| Myers et al.[145] | RSERT | 83 | 82 | 4.61 | 0.20 | Arthroscopy |
| Snyder et al.[180] | Compression-rotation | ND | ND | ND | ND | Arthroscopy |
| McFarland et al.[178] | Compression-rotation | 24 | 76 | 1.0 | 1.0 | Arthroscopy |
| Kibler[146] | Anterior Slide | 78 | 92 | 9.75 | .24 | Arthroscopy |
| McFarland et al.[178] | Anterior Slide | 8 | 84 | .50 | 1.10 | Arthroscopy |
| Parentis et al.[175] | Anterior Slide | 13 | 84 | .79 | 1.04 | Arthroscopy |
| Mimori et al.[147] | Pain Provocation | 100 | 90 | NA | NA | MR Arthrography |
| Parentis et al.[175] | Pain Provocation | 17 | 90 | 1.72 | .92 | Arthroscopy |
| Kim et al.[148] | Biceps Load | 91 | 97 | 29.32 | .09 | Arthroscopy |
| Kim et al.[149] | Biceps Load II | 90 | 97 | 26.38 | .11 | Arthroscopy |
| Parentis et al.[175] | Hawkins–Kennedy | 65 | 30 | .94 | 1.15 | Arthroscopy |
| Parentis et al.[175] | Neer | 48 | 51 | .98 | 1.02 | Arthroscopy |
| **Other Labral Tears and Biceps Pathology** | | | | | | |
| Liu et al.[144] | Crank | 91 | 93 | 13 | 0.09 | Arthroscopy |
| Bennett[176] | Crank | 14 | 90 | 1.4 | 0.95 | Arthroscopy |
| Kim et al.[150] | Kim Test | 80 | 94 | 13.33 | 0.21 | Posteroinferior labral tear/Arthroscopy |
| Kim et al.[150] | Jerk Test | 73 | 98 | 36.5 | 0.27 | Posteroinferior labral tear/Arthroscopy |

## Compression–Rotation Test—SLAP Lesion

The *Compression–Rotation* test was described by Snyder et al. in 1990[143] and was designed to detect a SLAP lesion. Table 9.6 outlines the diagnostic values of the *Compression–Rotation* test.

- Step One: The patient assumes a supine position. The clinician stands to the side of the involved extremity.
- Step Two: The clinician passively places the patient's shoulder in 90 degrees of abduction and the elbow in 90 degrees of flexion.
- Step Three: The clinician first applies a compression force to the humerus and rotates the humerus back-and-forth from internal rotation to external rotation in an attempt to pinch the torn labrum.
- Step Four: A positive test is indicated by the production of a catching or snapping in the shoulder.

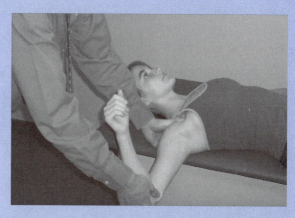

**Figure 9.66**   The Compression-Rotation Test for a SLAP Lesion

## Crank Test—Labral Tear

The *Crank test* was described by Liu et al. in 1990[144] and was designed to detect a nonspecific glenoid labrum tear. Table 9.6 outlines the diagnostic values of the Crank test.

- Step One: The patient assumes either a sitting or supine position. The clinician typically stands at the side of the involved extremity.
- Step Two: The clinician places the patient's shoulder in 160 degrees of abduction and elbow in 90 degrees of flexion.
- Step Three: The clinician first applies a compression force to the humerus and then rotates the humerus repeatedly into internal rotation and external rotation in an attempt to pinch the torn labrum.
- Step Four: A positive test is indicated by the production of pain either with or without a click in the shoulder or by reproduction of the patient's concordant complaint (usually pain or catching).

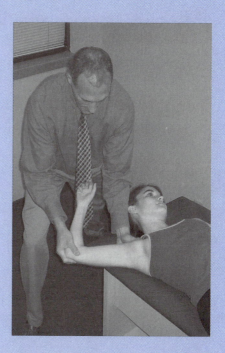

**Figure 9.67**   The Crank Test for a Labral Tear

## Resisted Supination External Rotation Test (RSERT)—SLAP Lesion

The RSERT was described by Myers et al. in 2005[145] and was designed to detect a SLAP lesion. Table 9.6 outlines the diagnostic values of the RSERT.

- Step One: The patient assumes a supine position. The clinician stands beside the patient's involved extremity.
- Step Two: The clinician grasps the patient's hand and supports the elbow. The clinician then places the patient's shoulder in 90 degrees of abduction and neutral rotation, the elbow in 65–70 degrees of flexion, and the forearm in neutral pronation/supination.
- Step Three: The clinician instructs the patient to attempt to supinate his or her arm.
- Step Four: The clinician resists supination while gradually moving the patient's shoulder to end range of external rotation.
- Step Five: A positive test is indicated by the production of pain in the anterior or deep shoulder, clicking or catching in the shoulder, or by reproduction of the patient's concordant symptoms.

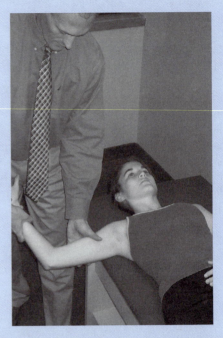

**Figure 9.68**    The RSERT Test for a SLAP Lesion

## Anterior Slide Test—SLAP Lesion

The *Anterior Slide* test was described by Kibler in 1995[146] and was designed to detect a SLAP lesion. Table 9.6 outlines the diagnostic values of the *Anterior Slide* test.

- Step One: The patient is either standing or sitting with his or her hands on his or her hips so that the thumb is positioned posteriorly. The clinician stands behind the patient.
- Step Two: The clinician places one hand superior on the shoulder to stabilize the scapula and clavicle.
- Step Three: The clinician places his or her opposite hand on the patient's elbow with the palm of the hand cupping the olecranon.
- Step Four: The clinician provides an anterior–superior force through the elbow to the glenohumeral joint while the patient resists this movement.
- Step Five: A positive test is indicated by the production of pain in the anterior shoulder, by the production of a pop or click in the shoulder, or by reproduction of the patient's concordant symptoms.

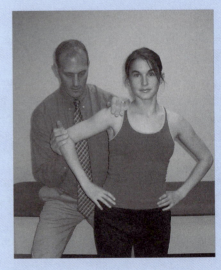

**Figure 9.69**    The Anterior Slide Test for a SLAP Lesion

## Pain Provocation Test—SLAP Lesion

The *Pain Provocation* test was described by Mimori et al. in 1999[147] and was designed to detect a SLAP lesion. Table 9.6 outlines the diagnostic values of the *Pain Provocation* test.

- Step One: The patient assumes a sitting position. The clinician stands behind the patient.
- Step Two: The clinician places the patient's shoulder in 90 degrees of abduction and toward end range external rotation. The elbow is placed at 90 degrees of flexion and the forearm in maximum supination.
- Step Three: The clinician asks the patient to rate his or her pain in this position.
- Step Four: The clinician then fully pronates the patient's forearm and asks the patient to rerate his or her pain.
- Step Five: A positive test is indicated by production of the patient's concordant pain in the forearm-pronated position or when the patient's pain is worse in pronation than in supination.

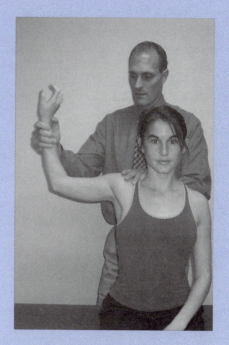

**Figure 9.70**    The Pain Provocation Test for a SLAP Lesion

## Biceps Load Test—SLAP Lesion

The *Biceps Load* test was described by Kim et al. in 1999[148] and was designed to detect a SLAP lesion. Table 9.6 outlines the diagnostic values of the *Biceps Load* test.

- Step One: The patient assumes a supine position. The clinician sits on the side of the patient's involved extremity.
- Step Two: The clinician places the patient's shoulder in 90 degrees of abduction, the elbow in 90 degrees of flexion, and the forearm in supination.
- Step Three: The clinician moves the patient's shoulder to end range external rotation (apprehension position).
- Step Four: At end range external rotation, the clinician asks the patient to flex his or her elbow while the clinician resists this movement.
- Step Five: The clinician queries the patient if and how his or her apprehension has changed after flexion of the elbow.
- Step Six: A positive test is indicated by either no change in apprehension or pain that is worsened with resisted elbow flexion.

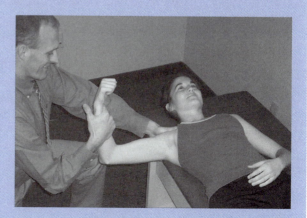

**Figure 9.71**    The Biceps Load Test for a SLAP Lesion

## Biceps Load Test II—SLAP Lesion

The *Biceps Load Test II* was described by Kim et al. in 2001[149] and was designed to detect a SLAP lesion. Table 9.6 outlines the diagnostic values of the *Biceps Load Test II.*

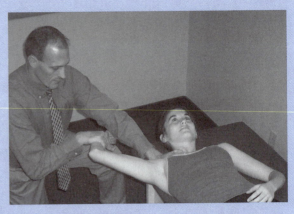

- Step One: The patient assumes a supine position.
- Step Two: The clinician sits to the side of the involved shoulder and places the patient's shoulder in 120 degrees of abduction, the elbow in 90 degrees of flexion, and the forearm in supination.
- Step Three: The clinician moves the shoulder to end range external rotation (apprehension position).
- Step Four: At end range external rotation, the clinician asks the patient to flex his or her elbow while the clinician resists this movement.
- Step Five: A positive test is indicated as a reproduction of concordant pain during resisted elbow flexion.

**Figure 9.72**    The Biceps Load Test II for a SLAP Lesion

## Kim Test—Posteroinferior Labral Lesion

The *Kim Test* was described by Kim et al. in 2005[150] and was designed to detect a posteroinferior labral lesion. Table 9.6 outlines the diagnostic values of the *Kim Test.*

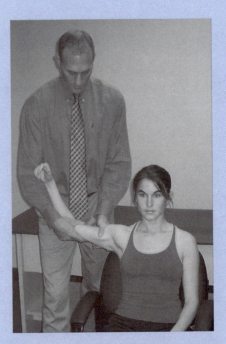

- Step One: The patient is seated in a chair with his or her back supported.
- Step Two: The clinician stands to the side of the involved shoulder and faces the patient. The clinician grasps the elbow with one hand and the mid-humeral region with the other and elevates the patient's arm to 90 degrees abduction.
- Step Three: Simultaneously the clinician provides an axial load to the humerus and a 45-degree diagonal elevation to the distal humerus concurrent with a posteroinferior glide to the proximal humerus.
- Step Four: A positive test is indicated by a sudden onset of posterior shoulder pain.

**Figure 9.73**    The Kim Test for a Posteroinferior Labral Lesion

## Jerk Test—Posteroinferior Labral Lesion

The *Jerk Test* was described by Kim et al. in 2005[150] and was designed to detect a posteroinferior labral lesion. Table 9.6 outlines the diagnostic values of the *Jerk Test*.

- Step One: The patient assumes a sitting position. The clinician stands behind the patient.
- Step Two: The clinician grasps the elbow with one hand and the scapula with the other and elevates the patient's arm to 90 degrees abduction and internal rotation.
- Step Three: The clinician provides a compression-based load to the humerus through the elbow while horizontally adducting the arm.
- Step Five: A positive test is indicated by a sharp shoulder pain with or without a clunk or click.

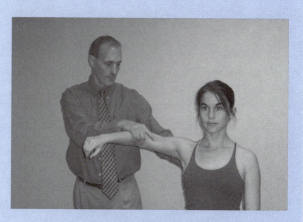

**Figure 9.74**    The Jerk Test for a Posteroinferior Labral Lesion

## *Clinical Special Tests for Joint Laxity*

Compared with other pathologies or syndromes of the shoulders, clinical special tests for joint laxity are less studied. Although several tests exist, some have yet to be examined for diagnostic value. The tests appear to demonstrate better specificity than sensitivity, indicating the ability to rule in laxity versus ruling the disorder out.

## The Sulcus Sign—Inferior Laxity

The *Sulcus Sign* is attributed to Neer and Foster[151] but was described in detail by Silliman and Hawkins in 1993[152] and was designed to detect inferior laxity. Table 9.7 outlines the diagnostic values of the *Sulcus Sign*.

- Step One: The patient assumes a sitting position. The clinician stands behind the patient.
- Step Two: The clinician grasps the elbow and pulls down, causing an inferior traction force.
- Step Three: The clinician notes, in centimeters, the distance between the inferior surface of the acromion and the superior portion of the humeral head.
- Step Four: The clinician repeats the test in supine with the shoulder in 20 degrees of abduction and in forward flexion while maintaining a neutral rotation.

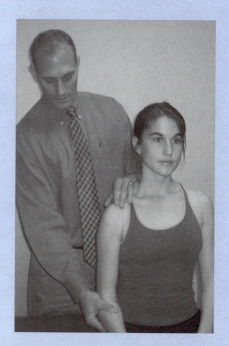

**Figure 9.75**    The Sulcus Sign for Inferior Laxity

**TABLE 9.7**    Clinical Special Tests for Joint Laxity: Diagnostic Values

| Author (Study) | Test | Sensitivity | Specificity | +LR | −LR | Criterion Standard |
|---|---|---|---|---|---|---|
| **Inferior Laxity** | | | | | | |
| Silliman & Hawkins[155] | Sulcus Sign | ND | ND | ND | ND | None |
| Gagey & Gagey[154] | Hyperabduction Test | ND | ND | ND | ND | Compared in cadavers, normal volunteers, and patients undergoing surgery for instability |
| **Anterior/Posterior Laxity** | | | | | | |
| Gerber & Ganz[153] | Anterior Drawer/ Posterior Drawer | ND | ND | ND | ND | NA |
| Silliman & Hawkins[155] | Sulcus Sign Load and Shift | ND | ND | ND | ND | NA |
| **Anterior Instability** | | | | | | |
| Lo et al.[180] | Apprehension | 53 | 99 | 53 | 0.47 | Not stated |
| Lo et al.[180] | Apprehension-relocation | 46 | 54 | 1 | 1 | Not stated |
| Gross & Distefano[158] | Anterior Release | 92 | 89 | 8.36 | 0.08 | Arthroscopy |
| Lo et al.[180] | Anterior Release | 64 | 99 | 64 | 0.36 | Not stated |

## The Hyperabduction Test—Inferior Laxity

The *Hyperabduction* test is attributed to Gagey and Gagey[154] and was designed to detect inferior instability. Table 9.7 outlines the diagnostic values of the *Hyperabduction* test.

- Step One: The patient assumes a sitting position. The clinician stands behind the patient.
- Step Two: The clinician stabilizes the scapula with a downward force on the supraclavicular region and passively places the patient's elbow in 90 degrees of flexion and the patient's forearm in pronation.
- Step Three: The clinician moves the patient's arm to maximum abduction, stabilizing the scapula to reduce rotation.
- Step Four: A positive test is indicated by passive abduction greater than 105 degrees.

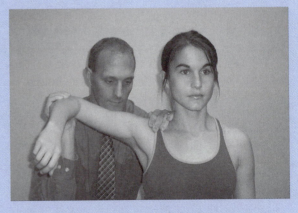

**Figure 9.76**    The Hyperabduction Test for Inferior Laxity

## The Anterior Drawer—Anterior Laxity

The *Anterior Drawer* is attributed to Gerber and Ganz[153] and was designed to detect anterior laxity. Table 9.7 outlines the diagnostic values of the *Anterior Drawer*.

- Step One: The patient assumes a supine position. The clinician stands behind the patient.
- Step Two: The clinician secures the distal arm of the patient in his or her axillary region.
- Step Three: The clinician's hands are placed so that one hand stabilizes the scapula and the other grasps the proximal humerus.
- Step Four: The clinician abducts the patient's arm to between 80 and 100 degrees, and then applies a posterior-to-anterior force (traction force) to the humerus. The clinician carefully notes the amount of translation of the glenohumeral joint compared to the uninvolved shoulder.

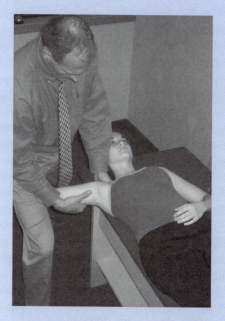

**Figure 9.77**    The Anterior Drawer Test for Anterior Laxity

## The Posterior Drawer—Posterior Laxity

The *Posterior Drawer* is attributed to Gerber and Ganz[153] and was designed to detect posterior laxity. Table 9.7 outlines the diagnostic values of the *Posterior Drawer*.

- Step One: The patient assumes a supine position. The clinician stands beside the patient to the side of the involved shoulder.
- Step Two: The clinician secures the distal arm of the patient in his or her axillary region.
- Step Three: The clinician's hands are placed so that one hand stabilizes the scapula and the other grasps the proximal humerus.
- Step Four: The clinician abducts the patient's arm to between 80 and 100 degrees then applies a posterior-to-anterior force, noting the amount of translation compared to the uninvolved shoulder.

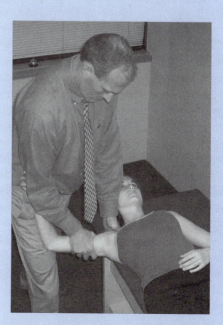

**Figure 9.78**    The Posterior Drawer Test for Posterior Laxity

## The Load and Shift Test—Anterior, Posterior, and Inferior Laxity

The *Load and Shift* test is attributed to Silliman and Hawkins in 1991[155] and was designed to detect anterior, posterior, and inferior laxity. Table 9.7 outlines the diagnostic values of the *Load and Shift* test.

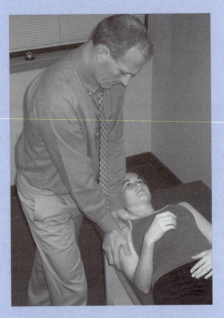

- Step One: The patient assumes a supine position. The clinician stands to the side of the patient's involved shoulder.
- Step Two: The clinician grasps the proximal humerus with one hand and stabilizes the scapula with the other hand.
- Step Three: The clinician applies an anterior-to-posterior force, noting the amount of translation as either toward the posterior rim of the glenoid or beyond the rim of the glenoid.
- Step Four: The clinician applies a posterior-to-anterior force, noting the amount of translation as either (1) to the anterior rim of the glenoid or (2) beyond the rim of the glenoid.
- Step Five: A *Sulcus Sign* (see Figure 9.79) is then performed to assess the full excursion of the humeral head in the glenoid fossa.

**Figure 9.79**    The Load and Shift Test for Anterior, Posterior, and Inferior Laxity

## The Apprehension Test—Anterior Instability

The *Apprehension* test was described by Rowe and Zarins in 1981[156] and was designed to detect anterior instability. Table 9.7 outlines the diagnostic values of the *Apprehension* test.

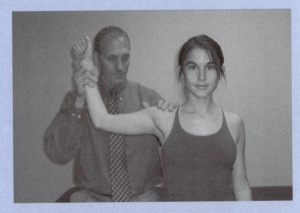

- Step One: The patient is either standing or supine. The clinician stands either behind or at the involved side of the patient.
- Step Two: The clinician grasps the wrist with one hand and maximally externally rotates the humerus with the shoulder in 90 degrees of abduction.
- Step Three: Forward pressure is then applied to the posterior aspect of the humeral head by either the clinician (if the patient is standing) or the examination table (if the patient is in supine).
- Step Four: A positive test is indicated by a show of apprehension by the patient or a report of pain.

**Figure 9.80**    The Apprehension Test for Anterior Instability

## The Apprehension-Relocation Test—Anterior Instability

The *Apprehension-Relocation* test was described by Jobe and Kvitne in 1989[157] and was designed to differentiate between anterior instability and impingement syndrome. Table 9.7 outlines the diagnostic values of the *Apprehension-Relocation* test.

- Step One: The patient assumes a supine position. The clinician stands beside the patient.
- Step Two: The clinician prepositions the shoulder at 90 degrees of abduction then grasps the patient's forearm and maximally externally rotates the humerus.
- Step Three: A posterior-to-anterior force is then applied to the posterior aspect of the humeral head by the clinician.
- Step Four: If the patient displays apprehension or reports pain, a posterior force is then applied to the proximal humerus.
- Step Five: A positive test for anterior instability is indicated by a decrease in the pain or apprehension whereas no change in pain symptoms indicates impingement.

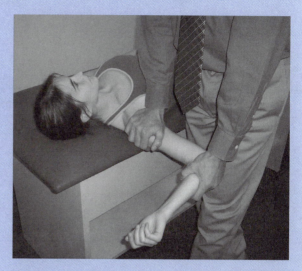

**Figure 9.81**    The Apprehension-Relocation Test for Anterior Instability

## The Anterior Release/Surprise Test—Anterior Instability

The *Anterior Release* test was described by Gross and Distefano in 1997[158] and was designed to detect anterior instability. Table 9.7 outlines the diagnostic values of the *Anterior Release* test.

- Step One: The patient assumes a supine position. The clinician stands beside the patient.
- Step Two: The clinician grasps the forearm with one hand and provides a posterior force on the humerus with the other.
- Step Three: The posterior force on the proximal humerus is maintained while the clinician moves the patient's shoulder into the apprehension position of 90 degrees abduction and end range external rotation.
- Step Four: The posterior force on the humerus is then released.
- Step Five: A positive test is indicated if the patient reports sudden pain, an increase in pain, or by reproduction of the patient's concordant symptoms.

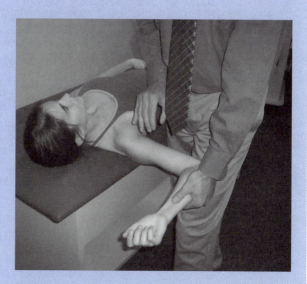

**Figure 9.82**    The Anterior Release/Surprise Test for Anterior Instability

## Clinical Special Tests for Acromioclavicular (AC) Joint Pain

Table 9.8 outlines the diagnostic value of the AC clinical special tests. The majority demonstrate good positive likelihood ratios, indicating the benefit of a positive sign.

TABLE 9.8    Clinical Special Tests for Acromioclavicular Damage: Diagnostic Values

| Author (Study) | Test | Sensitivity | Specificity | +LR | −LR | Criterion Standard |
|---|---|---|---|---|---|---|
| Walton et al.[159] | Paxino's | 79 | 50 | 1.58 | 0.42 | AC Joint injection |
| O'Brien et al.[142] | Active Compression | 100 | 97 | NA | NA | Not defined |
| Walton et al.[159] | Active Compression | 16 | 90 | 1.6 | 0.93 | AC Joint injection |
| Chronopoulos et al.[181] | AC Resisted Extension | 72 | 85 | 4.8 | 0.32 | AC Joint injection |
| Chronopoulos et al.[181] | Cross-body Adduction | 77 | 79 | 3.66 | 0.29 | AC Joint injection |
| Chronopoulos et al.[181] | Active Compression | 41 | 95 | 8.2 | 0.62 | AC Joint injection |

### Paxinos' Test—Acromioclavicular Joint Pain

*Paxinos'* test was described by Walton et al. in 2004[159] and was designed to detect AC joint pain. Table 9.8 outlines the diagnostic values of *Paxinos'* test.

- Step One: The patient is seated with the involved arm at his or her side. The clinician stands behind the patient.
- Step Two: The clinician places his or her thumb under the posterolateral aspect of the acromion and the index and middle fingers of the same hand on the distal clavicle.
- Step Three: The clinician applies an anterosuperior force with the thumb while concurrently applying an inferior force with the index and middle fingers.
- Step Four: A positive test is indicated by pain reproduction or an increase in pain at the AC joint.

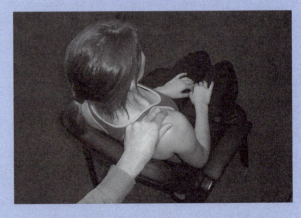

Figure 9.83    The Paxino's Test for AC Joint Pain

## AC Resisted Extension Test—Acromioclavicular (AC) Joint Abnormality

The *AC Resisted Extension* test was described by Jacob et al. in 1997[160] and was designed to detect AC joint abnormality. Table 9.8 outlines the diagnostic values of the *AC Resisted Extension* test.

- Step One: The patient is seated with his or her shoulder in 90 degrees of flexion and internal rotation, and his or her elbow in 90 degrees of flexion.
- Step Two: The clinician, standing beside the patient, asks the patient to horizontally abduct his or her arm while the clinician provides an isometric resistance to this movement.
- Step Three: A positive test is indicated by pain at the AC joint.

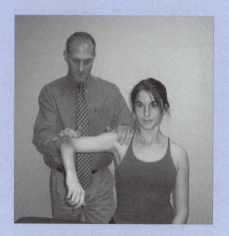

**Figure 9.84**    The AC Resisted Extension Test for AC Joint Abnormality

## Deltoid Extension Lag Sign—Axillary Nerve Palsy

The *Deltoid Extension Lag Sign* was described by Hertel et al. in 1998[161] and was designed to detect axillary nerve palsy. Table 9.8 outlines the diagnostic values of the *Deltoid Extension Lag Sign*.

- Step One: The patient assumes a seated position. The clinician stands behind the patient.
- Step Two: The clinician grasps the patient's wrist and pulls the arm into near full extension.
- Step Three: The clinician then releases the wrists.
- Step Four: A positive test is indicated by an angular drop or lag. The inability to maintain the shoulder extension is considered a positive test.
- Step Five: The clinician records any lag to the nearest 5 degrees.

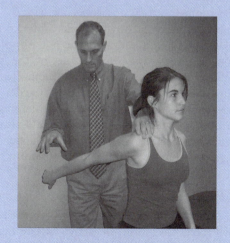

**Figure 9.85**    The Deltoid Extension Lag Sign for Axillary Nerve Palsy

## *Summary*

- Numerous clinical special tests for the shoulder have been documented, the majority demonstrating only fair diagnostic value.
- Many clinical special tests are designed to implicate impingement syndrome, but fail to isolate the structure or dysfunction associated with the impingement cause.
- Most shoulder clinical special tests are biased secondary to selection problems. For example, most labrum tests were only examined on patients with a history of instability of other predisposing factors of the shoulder.
- Clinical special tests may only offer confirmatory value in the shoulder and rarely offer definitive diagnostic value.

# TREATMENT TECHNIQUES

Recently, Winter et al.[162] outlined "shoulder pain" as synovial in origin (glenohumeral joint), shoulder girdle (may involve the cervical spine, thoracic spine, or other nonsynovial categories), and combinations (both synovial and nonsynovial). Treatment benefit depended on the classification. For example, patients without a synovial component benefited from manipulative procedures more so than those with synovial problems. Careful attention and a comprehensive examination consisting of isolation of the concordant sign are crucial to classify the origin of the pain generator.

Similar to the interventions associated with the cervical and thoracic spine and all other regions of the body, treatment selection is predicated upon the findings of the examination. However, the complexities of the shoulder require the clinician to understand the biomechanical influences of the active structures of the shoulder and the benefit associated with targeting these structures during treatment. Subsequently, the clinician should always consider the merits of a rotator cuff and upper quarter strengthening program in addition to any form of intervention.

## *Active Physiological Movements*

The majority of active physiological treatment interventions will take the form of active strengthening. A strengthening approach will depend on the form of impairment displayed by the patient and the level of recovery that patient exhibits. For example, for post-surgical patients, active physiological movements may consist of gentle, pain-free movements or subthreshold isometric exercises versus an impingement, nonsurgical patient that may receive exercises that are more aggressive.

Active physiological movements to treat the shoulder, in absence of strengthening, may be less beneficial in the shoulder. The repeated movements or sustained positions of the concordant pain that are found during the shoulder examination will rarely reduce symptoms, specifically if the patient demonstrates impingement. Nonetheless, repeated movements and sustained positions will dictate the selection of an active physiological approach, often leading the consequence of no active movements that reduce pain in the absence of a strengthening approach. The reader is suggested to explore additional textbooks or

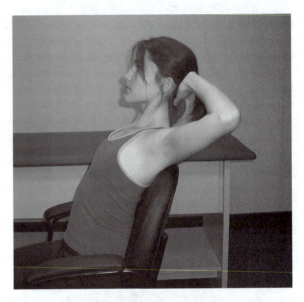

**Figure 9.86**   Upper Thoracic Extension to Improve Shoulder Range of Motion

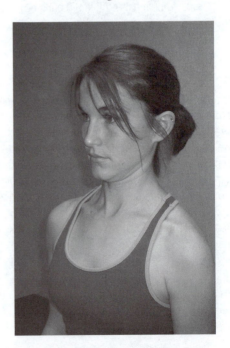

**Figure 9.87**   Repeated Neck Retraction for Improvement of Shoulder Range of Motion

manuscripts that focus on the most efficient methods of shoulder strengthening.

One non-shoulder-based program is a postural-based intervention. This treatment may consist of active exercises designed to improve the cervical and thoracic posture to improve the range of motion of the shoulder (Figures 9.86 and 9.87). Although a postural approach may not lead to reduction of pain in the shoulder, this approach has been shown to improve the overall range of motion of the shoulder or the total range available before pain is encountered.[163]

## Passive Physiological Movements

Several methods of passive physiological stretching may be beneficial for treatment of the stiff shoulder. Since the findings of the examination will drive the treatment selection, repeated or sustained movements toward end range of a restricted or painful plane-based movement will identify the correct selection of the physiological stretch. Manually assisted movements such as contract–relax or hold–relax techniques may prove beneficial and are often tolerated better during application (Figures 9.88–9.92). Because posterior capsule tightness is common in shoulder dysfunction and often corresponds with internal rotation restriction, hold–relax stretching of the internal rotators is of specific benefit.

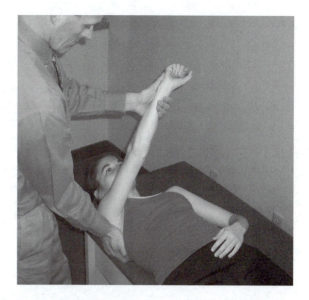

**Figure 9.90**   Hold–Relax Stretching of Horizontal Adduction

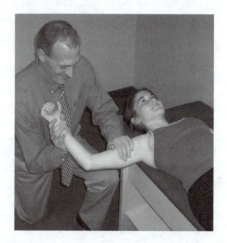

**Figure 9.91**   Hold–Relax Stretching of External Rotation

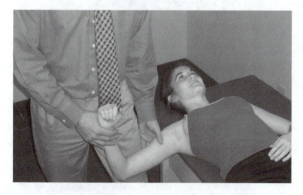

**Figure 9.88**   Hold–Relax Stretching of Shoulder Abduction

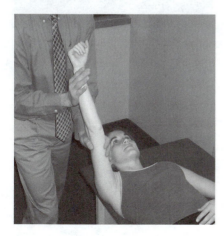

**Figure 9.89**   Hold–Relax Stretching of Shoulder Flexion

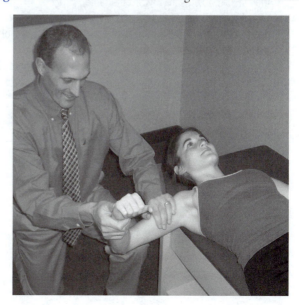

**Figure 9.92**   Hold–Relax Stretching of Internal Rotation

## Passive Accessory Movements

The capsule of the shoulder allows for a significant amount of joint play when the humerus assumes early range of motions. Because of this, mobilization procedures to increase range of motion are generally more beneficial at end ranges (at the restriction)[116] and early range of motions are more appropriately assumed for patients who exhibit pain dominance and cannot tolerate aggressive end range mobilization.

Like the active and passive physiological applications, passive accessory techniques are borne from the examination. Applications that reproduce the concordant sign and subsequent reduction of pain or increase in range during repeated movements or sustained holds are appropriate selections for treatments. Consequently, the passive accessory examination methods are all potential treatment selections for the glenohumeral, acromioclavicular, and sternoclavicular joints.

There are two instances in which subtle variations from the examination procedures are necessary and appropriate: (1) when the capsule would benefit from further tightening and (2) when the joints would benefit from a traction technique for pain control. Since these are not typically components of the examination, the procedures are described further below.

### Acromioclavicular and Sternoclavicular Traction

AC and SC traction may be beneficial when treating a pain-dominant patient or when treating conditions associated with poor posture. Both joints can be targeted during the same application if the clinician makes minor adjustments in hand position.

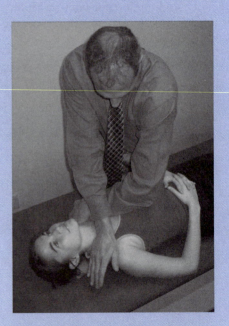

- **Step One:** The clinician places a rolled towel longitudinally on the treatment plinth. The patient assumes a supine position with the towel parallel with his or her spine.
- **Step Two:** The clinician stands to the side of the treatment plinth. The clinician stabilizes the side of the patient that is closest to him or her by placing his or her forearm on the sternum of the patient and by using his or her ulnar border to compress the clavicle downward toward the table.
- **Step Three:** To target the SC, the clinician places his or her opposite hand on the clavicle of the opposite side and places a traction force toward the shoulder.

**Figure 9.93**    Traction of the SC Joint

- Step Four: To target the AC and SC, the clinician places his or her opposite hand on the anterior head of the humerus and places a traction force toward the shoulder.
- Step Five: Treatment techniques may consist of a sustained hold or repeated movements.

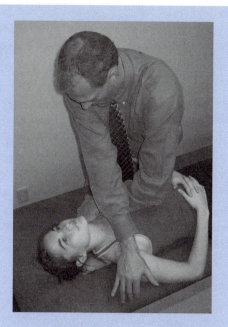

**Figure 9.94**    Traction of the AC Joint

## AC Mobilization in Preposition

The majority of the movement of the AC is required near the later ranges of glenohumeral flexion or abduction. Consequently, it is beneficial to mobilize the AC joint when the glenohumeral joint is prepositioned at near end ranges.

- Step One: The patient assumes a supine position. The clinician elevates the patient's arm into flexion or abduction then requests the patient's assistance in holding the extremity in place.
- Step Two: The clinician then applies an inferior or anterior glide (whichever is concordant) in this preposition.

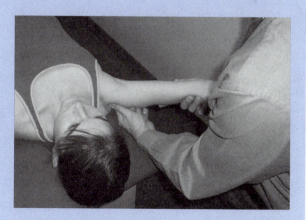

**Figure 9.95**    AC Mobilization in Preposition

## Posterior Capsule Mobilization in a Preposition of Internal Rotation and Adduction

The posterior capsule frequently contributes to range-of-motion losses and impairment at the shoulder.[34,49] Because the capsule is difficult to isolate during a planar mobilization, prepositioning of the glenohumeral joint may improve the likelihood of isolating the structure.

- Step One: The patient assumes a supine position. The clinician stabilizes the shoulder blade with his or her arm that is cephalic to the patient during standing at the side of the patient.
- Step Two: The clinician then internal rotates (to end range), adducts (just past midline), and flexes (to approximately 90 degrees) the shoulder to "wind up" the posterior capsule. The cephalic arm stabilizes the patient's shoulder blade to prevent the migration toward the patient's head.

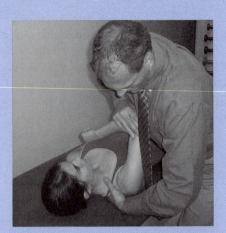

**Figure 9.96**　Preposition and Stabilization of the Shoulder

- Step Three: While maintaining the stabilization and preposition, the clinician then applies an inferior force along the shaft of the humerus. The patient should report a sharp sensation on the posterior capsule, not the medial aspect of the humerus. If pain is felt medially, structures are likely impinged and the clinician should reconsider and readjust the position.

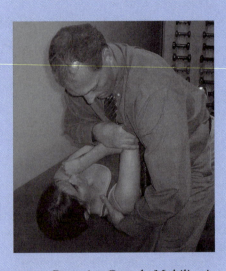

**Figure 9.97**　Posterior Capsule Mobilization

## Compression and Distraction in the Shoulder Quadrant

Maitland[164] advocates the use of compression and distraction procedures in the quadrant position to target joint and capsular structures. The quadrant position involves several combined movements of internal rotation, abduction and extension, and external rotation, flexion, and abduction. Theoretically, the movements engage the tension of the capsule throughout the available combined ranges of the glenohumeral joint and may demonstrate significant reproduction of symptoms from the patient. Clinicians may place the arm in the combined position that elicits the most significant reproduction of the concordant sign then apply either traction or compressive forces if these forces elicit further symptoms. A more detailed description of the quadrant technique and all of the facets associated with these maneuvers is available in Maitland's peripheral manipulation textbook.

- Step One: The patient assumes a supine position. To initiate the quadrant, the clinician moves the patient's shoulder toward the combined movement of internal rotation, abduction, and extension.

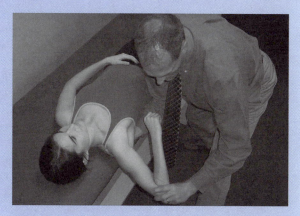

**Figure 9.98**    The Combined Movement of Internal Rotation, Abduction and Extension

- Step Two: The clinician then slowly moves the shoulder throughout the ranges of abduction by allowing external rotation to replace the preposition of internal rotation. The shoulder is slowly moved toward the patient's head, in search of a position that results in a concordant sign.
- Step Three: Once the concordant position is found, the clinician can apply a compressive or distractive force. As with all techniques, repeated movements or sustained holds should result in a reduction of symptoms for the treatment to be considered beneficial and appropriate.

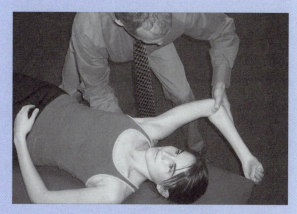

**Figure 9.99**    Compressive or Distractive Force During Preposition of External Rotation, Abduction, and Flexion

## Shoulder Manipulation

For a patient that demonstrates stiffness dominance and no signs of instability, a manipulative procedure may be beneficial.[162] Generally, the manipulative procedure involves a posterior force applied to a fixed scapula and because the procedure is very powerful, it should only be considered for a select population of patients without pain dominance. A patient who demonstrates instability, frailty, or is fearful of the technique is not a candidate for the procedure.

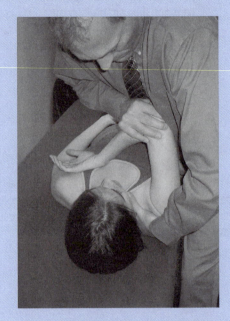

- Step One: The patient assumes a supine position. Similar to the setup and preposition of the mobilization to the posterior capsule described earlier, the clinician internally rotates, adducts, and flexes the shoulder.
- Step Two: Instead of singularly blocking the shoulder from superior migration, the clinician also elevates the scapula from the treatment table by placing his or hand under the scapula. By hooking the spine of the scapula, the clinician prevents the superior migration.
- Step Three: The clinician applies a load through the humerus to take up the capsular slack. At maximum load, the clinician applies a series of quick thrusts through the humerus. Occasionally, an audible will accompany the manipulation.

**Figure 9.100**  The Glenohumeral Manipulation

## Scapulothoracic Mobilization/Stretching

In some instances, scapulothoracic mobilization or stretching is beneficial for patient treatment. The procedure may lead to postural improvements and is generally very relaxing to a pain-dominant patient.

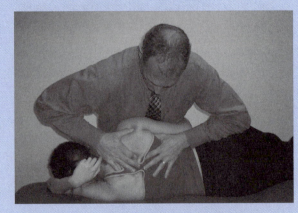

- Step One: The patient assumes a sidelying position, facing the clinician.
- Step Two: The non-plinth-sided arm of the patient is secured to the clinician by placing the thumb of the patient in a belt loop or by having the patient relax his or hand on the clinician's hip.
- Step Three: The clinician secures the inferior border of the scapula with his or her caudal-most hand and does the same for the spine of the scapula with the cephalic-most hand.
- Step Four: The clinician can apply a downward, medial, lateral, or upward force of the scapula and may combine the movements if desired. The technique selected should depend on patient tolerance and the concordant findings.

**Figure 9.101**  Multidirectional Mobilization of the Scapulothoracic Joint

## *Summary*

- Active physiological movements associated with strengthening should be a part of most manual therapy shoulder-related interventions.
- Some postural exercises may assist in improving range of motion in the shoulder, but will not likely reduce the pain associated with the shoulder impairment.
- The most effective and sensitive passive physiological movements are commonly associated with combined movements.
- Hold–relax stretching is helpful in allowing the patient to control the force of the stretch targeted at the guilty structure.
- Selection of the passive accessory mobilization method is based on the findings of the examination or careful assessment of pain versus stiffness dominance.
- Compression and distraction techniques may further improve or isolate the structure targeted during the treatment application.

## TREATMENT OUTCOMES

There appears to be strong evidence that manual therapy applied to the glenohumeral joint complex performed concurrently with strengthening exercises is more beneficial than exercises alone. Bang and Deyle[165] found significantly more reduction in pain, improved function, and increases in strength in the group that received manual therapy versus the group that received exercises alone. Conroy and Hayes[111] demonstrated that impingement syndrome patients treated with glenohumeral mobilization had decreased pain during a subacromial compression test and theorized that the decrease in pain was due to increased inferior and posterior capsule length. Their findings were only measured using short-term analyses.

There is less evidence that manual therapy is beneficial for patients with adhesive capsulitis. Mobilization has been shown to be less effective than steroid injections[166,167] and benefits may depend on the phase that the shoulder is encountered. One study, which claimed the comparison of joint mobilization with patients exhibiting adhesive capsulitis, provided very liberal inclusion criteria that most likely included patients with stiffness but not actual adhesive capsulitis.[168] The author reported significant improvement in passive shoulder abduction in patients that received various inferior, anterior, and posterior glide-based joint mobilization techniques but no reduction in pain.[168]

Mobilization and manipulation was found to be superior to modalities and/or steroid injections in the treatment of classified shoulder girdle patients.[162] The authors classified patients based on complaints that were (1) isolated to the shoulder, (2) were referred from other structures such as the cervical or thoracic spine, and (3) were a mixture of both regions. Although this finding does not profoundly implicate the use of manipulation for the shoulder, it does support the use of manipulation for pain-referring structures that mimic shoulder conditions. Patients who demonstrated "synovial pain" that was associated with the shoulder actually improved quicker using injection therapy than forms of manual therapy and modalities.

## *Summary*

- Strong evidence exists that demonstrates the benefits of mobilization for patients with impingement syndrome whereas only anecdotal evidence suggests mobilization is helpful for adhesive capsulitis.
- Patients with synovial pain may benefit from a cortisone injection versus mobilization or manipulation.

# *Chapter Questions*

1. Describe the clinical utility and validity of selected theoretical constructs such as the capsular pattern and convex–concave rule and their benefit to treatment intervention.
2. Describe the biomechanical relationship between the clavicle, the scapula, and the humerus during shoulder movements.
3. Describe how posture can affect shoulder range of motion.
4. Outline which of the concurrent movements of the spine are necessary for shoulder elevation.
5. Identify why combined movements are often beneficial and necessary to target capsuloligamentous tissues of the shoulder.
6. Outline the evidence associated with manual therapy treatment of the shoulder.

# References

1. Leclerc A, Chastang J, Niedhammer I, Landre M, Roquelaure Y. Incidence of shoulder pain in repetitive work. *Occup Environ Med.* 2004;61:39–44.

2. Bongers P. The cost of shoulder pain at work. *BMJ.* 2001;322:64–65.

3. van der Heijden GJ. Shoulder disorders: a state-of-the-art review. *Baillieres Best Pract Res Clin Rheumatol.* 1999;13(2):287–309.

4. Nygren A, Berglund A, Von Koch M. Neck and shoulder pain: an increasing problem. Strategies for using insurance material to follow trends. *Scand J Rehabil Med Suppl.* 1995;32:107–112.

5. Blasier RB, Soslowsky LJ, Malicky DM. Posterior glenohumeral subluxation: active and passive stabilization in a biomechanical model. *J Bone Joint Surg Am.* 1997;79:433–440.

6. McCluskey G, Getz B. Pathophysiology of anterior shoulder instability. *J Athletic Training.* 2000;35:268–272.

7. Rockwood C, Matsen F. *The shoulder.* Philadelphia; W.B. Saunders Publishing: 1998.

8. Renfree K, Wright T. Anatomy and biomechanics of the acromioclavicular and sternoclavicular joints. *Clin Sports Med.* 2003;22(2):219–237.

9. Urist UM. Complete dislocation of the acromioclavicular joint. *J Bone Joint Surg Am.* 1963;45:1750–1753.

10. Debski R, Parsons IM, Woo SL, Fu FH. Effect of capsular injury on acromioclavicular joint mechanics. *J Bone Joint Surg Am.* 2001;83-A(9):1344–1351.

11. Wang CH, McClure P, Pratt N, Nobilini N. Stretching and strengthening exercises: Their effect on three-dimensional scapular kinematics. *Arch Phys Med Rehabil.* 1999;80:923–929.

12. Neer CS. Anterior acromioplasty for the chronic impingement syndrome in the shoulder: a preliminary report. *J Bone Joint Surg Am.* 1972;54(1):41–50.

13. Neer CS, Craing EV, Fukuda H. Cuff-tear arthropathy. *J Bone Joint Surg Am.* 1983;65:1232–1244.

14. Bigliani LU, Kelkar R, Flatow EL, Pollock RG, Mow VC. Glenohumeral instability: Biomechanical properties of passive and active stabilizers. *Clin Orthop.* 1996;330:13–30.

15. Bigliani LU, Ticker JB, Flatow EL, Soslowsky LJ, Mow VC. The relationship of acromial architecture to rotator cuff disease. *Clin Sports Med.* 1991;10(4):823–838.

16. Kim SJ, Lee JW, Kim BS. Arthroscopic decompression for subacromial impingement syndrome. *J Korean Med Sci.* 1997;12(2):123–127.

17. Tzannes A, Murrell GA. Clinical examination of the unstable shoulder. *Sports Med.* 2002;32(7):447–457.

18. Zatsiorsky V, Aktov A. *Biomechanics of highly precise movements: Movement control: An interdisciplinary forum.* VU University Press: Amsterdam. 1991.

19. Fukuda K, Caring EV, An KN, Cofield RH, Chao EY. Biomechanical study of the ligamentous system of the acromioclavicular joint. *J Bone Joint Surg Am.* 1986;68:434–440.

20. Warwick R, Williams P. *Gray's Anatomy.* 35th ed. WB Saunders: Philadelphia. 1973.

21. Norkin CC, White JD. *Measurement of joint motion: A guide to goniometry.* 2nd ed. Philadelphia; FA Davis: 1995.

22. Sadr B, Swann M. Spontaneous dislocation of the sternoclavicular joint. *Acta Orthop Scand.* 1979;50:269.

23. Steindler A. *Kinesiology of the human body under normal and pathological conditions.* Charles C Thomas: Springfield, IL. 1955.

24. Poppen HK, Walker PS. Normal and abnormal motion of the shoulder. *J Bone Joint Surg.* 1976;58A:195–201.

25. Greenfield B, Johanson M, Donatelli R, Gonzalez Z. Treatment of instability of the shoulder with an exercise program. *J Bone Joint Surg Am.* 1993;75(2):311–312.

26. Tata GE, Ng L, Kramer JF. Shoulder antagonistic strength ratios during concentric and eccentric muscle actions in the scapular plane. *J Orthop Sports Phys Ther.* 1993;18(6):654–660.

27. Helmig P, Sojbjerg JO, Kjaersgaard-Andersen P, Nielsen S, Ovesen J. Distal humeral migration as a component of multidirectional shoulder instability. An anatomical study in autopsy specimens. *Clin Orthop Relat Res.* 1990;252:139–143.

28. Michener L, McClure P, Karduna A. Anatomical and biomechanical mechanisms of subacromial impingement syndrome. *Clin Biomech.* 2003;18:369–379.

29. MacConail M. Joint Movement. *Physiotherapy.* 1964;50:363–365.

30. McClure P, Flowers K. Treatment of limited shoulder motion: a case study based on biomechanical considerations. *Phys Ther.* 1992;72:929–936.

31. Baeyens J, Van Roy P, De Schepper A, Declercq G, Clarijs J. Glenohumeral joint kinematics related to minor anterior instability of the shoulder at the end of the later preparatory phase of throwing. *Clin Biomech.* 2001;16:752–757.

32. Baeyens J, Van Roy P, Clarijs J. Intra-articular kinematics of the normal glenohumeral joint in the late preparatory phase of throwing: Kaltenborn's rule revisited. *Ergonomics.* 2000;10:1726–1737.

33. Hsu A, Ho L, Hedman T. Joint position during anterior-posterior glide mobilization: its effect on glenohumeral abduction range of motion. *Arch Phys Med Rehabil.* 2000;81:210–214.

34. Harryman DT, Sidles JA, Harris SL, Clark JM, McQuade KJ, Gibb TD, Matsen FA. Translation of the

humeral head on the glenoid with passive glenohumeral motion. *J Bone Jnt Surg.* 1990;79A(9): 1334–1343.

35. Cyriax J. *Illustrated manual of orthopedic medicine.* 2nd ed. New York; Macmillan Publishing: 1978.

36. Mitsch J, Casey J, McKinnis R, Kegerreis S, Stikeleather J. Investigation of a consistent pattern of motion restriction in patients with adhesive capsulitis. *J Man Manipulative Ther.* 2004;12:153–159.

37. Winters JC, Groenier KH, Sobel JS, Arendzen HH, Meyboom-de Jongh B. Classification of shoulder complaints in general practice by means of cluster analysis. *Arch Phys Med Rehabil.* 1997;78: 1369–1374.

38. Rundquist P, Ludewig P. Patterns of motion loss in subjects with idiopathic loss of shoulder range of motion. *Clin Biomech.* 2004;19:810–818.

39. Rundquist PJ, Anderson DD, Guanche CA, Ludewig PM. Shoulder kinematics in subjects with frozen shoulder. *Arch Phys Med Rehabil.* 2003;84: 1473–1479.

40. Sugamoto K, Harada T, Machida A, Inui H, Miyamoto T, Takeuchi E, Yoshikawa H, Ochi T. Scapulohumeral rhythm: relationship between motion velocity and rhythm. *Clin Orthop.* 2002;401:119–124.

41. Doody SG, Feedman L, Waterland JC. Shoulder movements during abduction in the scapular plane. *Arch Phys Med Rehabil.* 1970;51(10):595–604.

42. McClure PW, Michener LA, Sennett BJ, Karduna AR. Direct 3-dimensional measurement of scapular kinematics during dynamic movements in vivo. *J Shoulder Elbow Surg.* 2001;10:269–277.

43. McQuade KJ, Wei SH, Smidt GL. Effects of local muscle fatigue on three-dimensional scapulohumeral rhythm. *Clin Biomech.* 1995;10:114–148.

44. Warner JJ, Deng XH, Warren RF, Torzilli PA. Static capsuloligamentous restraints to superior-inferior translation of the glenohumeral joint. *Am J Sports Med.* 1992;20:675–685.

45. Hebert LJ, Moffet H, McFadyen BJ, Dionne CE. Scapular behavior in shoulder impingement syndrome. *Arch Phys Med Rehabil.* 2002;83(1):60–69.

46. Abboud J, Soslowsky L. Interplay of the static and dynamic restraints in glenohumeral instability. *Clin Orthop.* 2002;400:48–57.

47. Silliman JF, Hawkins RJ. Current concepts and recent advances in the athlete's shoulder. *Clin Sports Med.* 1991;10:693–705.

48. Prescher A. Anatomical basics, variations, and degenerative changes of the shoulder joint and shoulder girdle. *Eur J Radiol.* 2000;35:88–102.

49. Brossmann J, Preidler KW, Pedowitz RA, White LM, Trudell D, Resnick D. Shoulder impingement syndrome: influence of shoulder position on rotator cuff impingement—an anatomic study. *AJR Am J Roentgenol.* 1996;167(6):1511–1515.

50. Pappas A. Overuse Syndromes of the Shoulder and Arm. *Adolesc Med.* 1991;2(1):181–212.

51. Warner JP, Boardman ND. Anatomy, biomechanics and pathophysiology of glenohumeral instability. In: Warren et al. *The unstable shoulder.* Philadelphia; Lippincott William and Wilkens: 1998.

52. Kamkar A, Irrang J, Whitney S. Nonoperative management of secondary shoulder impingement syndrome. *J Orthop Sports Phys Ther.* 1993;17:212–223.

53. Tyler TF, Nicholas SJ, Roy T, Gleim GW. Quantification of posterior capsule tightness and motion loss in patients with shoulder impingement. *Am J Sports Med.* 2000;28(5):668–673.

54. Scheib JS. Diagnosis and rehabilitation of the shoulder impingement syndrome in the overhand and throwing athlete. *Rheum Dis Clin North Am.* 1990; 16(4):971–988.

55. Hjelm R, Draper C, Spencer S. Anterior inferior capsule length insufficiency in the painful shoulder. *J Orthop Sports Phys Ther.* 1996;23:216–222.

56. Threlkeld A. The effects of manual therapy on connective tissue. *Phys Ther.* 1992;72(12):893–902.

57. Hess S. Functional stability of the glenohumeral joint. *Man Ther.* 2000;5(2):63–71.

58. Soslowsky LJ, Malicky DM, Blasier RB. Active and passive factors in inferior glenohumeral stabilization: a biomechanical model. *J Shoulder Elbow Surg.* 1997;6(4):371–379.

59. Kronberg M, Brostrom LA, Soderlund V. Retroversion of the humeral head in the normal shoulder and its relationship to the normal range of motion. *Clin Orthop Relat Res.* 1990;253:113–117.

60. Lippitt S, Matsen F. Mechanisms of glenohumeral joint stability. *Clin Orthop Relat Res.* 1993;291:20–28.

61. Wuelker N, Korell M, Thren K. Dynamic glenohumeral joint stability. *J Shoulder Elbow Surg.* 1998; 7(1):43–52.

62. Magarey ME, Jones MA. Specific evaluation of the function of force couples relevant for stabilization of the glenohumeral joint. *Man Ther.* 2003;8(4): 247–253.

63. Baquie P. Sports medicine. Dead arm. *Aust Fam Physician.* 1997;26(11):1336–1337.

64. Litaker D, Pioro M, El Bilbeisi H, Brems J. Returning to the bedside: using the history and physical examination to identify rotator cuff tears. *J Am Geriatr Soc.* 2000;48:1633–1637.

65. Manifold SG, McCann PD. Cervical radiculitis and shoulder disorders. *Clin Orthop Relat Res.* 1999;368: 105–113.

66. Miranda H, Viikari-Juntura E, Heistaro S, Heliovaara M, Riihimaki H. A population study on differences in the determinants of a specific shoulder disorder versus nonspecific shoulder pain without out clinical findings. *Am J Epidemiol.* 2005;161: 847–855.

67. Ostergren PO, Hanson BS, Balogh I, Ektor-Andersen J, Isacsson A, Orbaek P, Winkel J, Isacsson SO. Incidence of shoulder and neck pain in a working population: effect modification between mechanical and psychosocial exposures at work? Results from a one year follow up of the Malmo shoulder and neck study cohort. *J Epidemiol Community Health.* 2005;59 (9):721–728.

68. Nahit ES, Pritchard CM, Cherry NM, Silman AJ, Macfarlane GJ. The influence of work related psychosocial factors and psychological distress on regional musculoskeletal pain: a study of newly employed workers. *J Rheumatol.* 2001;28:1378–1384.

69. Vasseljen O, Holte KA, Westgaard RH. Shoulder and neck complaints in customer relations: individual risk factors and perceived exposures at work. *Ergonomics.* 2001;44(4):355–372.

70. Jull-Kristensen B, Sogaard K, Stroyer J, Jensen C. Computer users' risk factors for developing shoulder, elbow and back symptoms. *Scand J Work Environ Health.* 2004;30:390–398.

71. van der Windt DA, Thomas E, Pope DP, de Winter AF, Macfarlane GJ, Bouter LM, Silman AJ. Occupational risk factors for shoulder pain: a systematic review. *Occup Environ Med.* 2000;57:433–442.

72. MacDermid JC, Tottenham V. Responsiveness of the disability of the arm, shoulder, and hand (DASH) and patient-rated wrist/hand evaluation (PRWHE) in evaluating change after hand therapy. *J Hand Ther.* 2004;17:18–23.

73. Gummesson C, Atroshi I, Ekdahl C. The disabilities of the arm, shoulder and hand (DASH) outcome questionnaire: longitudinal construct validity and measuring self-rated health change after surgery. *BMC Musculoskelet Disord.* 2003;4:11.

74. Hudak PL, Amadio PC, Bombardier C. Development of an upper extremity outcome measure: the DASH (disabilities of the arm, shoulder and hand) [corrected]. The Upper Extremity Collaborative Group (UECG). *Am J Ind Med.* 1996;29(6):602–628.

75. Michener LA, Leggin BG. A review of self-report scales for the assessment of functional limitation and disability of the shoulder. *J Hand Ther.* 2001;14(2): 68–76.

76. Williams JW, Holleman DR, Simel DL. Measuring shoulder function with the Shoulder Pain and Disability Index. *J Rheumatol.* 1995;22(4):727–732.

77. Bot SD, Terwee CB, van der Windt DA, Bouter LM, Dekker J, de Vet HC. Clinimetric evaluation of shoulder disability questionnaires: a systematic review of the literature. *Ann Rheum Dis.* 2004;63(4): 335–341.

78. Beaton D, Richards R. Measuring function of the shoulder. A cross-sectional comparison of five questionnaires. *J Bone Joint Surg Am.* 1996;78(6): 882–990.

79. Cook KF, Gartsoman GM, Roddey TS, Olson SL. The measurement level and trait-specific reliability of 4 scales of shoulder functioning: an empiric investigation. *Arch Phys Med Rehabil.* 2001;82(11): 1558–1565.

80. Heald SL, Riddle DL, Lamb RL. The shoulder pain and disability index: the construct validity and responsiveness of a region-specific disability measure. *Phys Ther.* 1997;77(10):1079–1089.

81. Michener LA, McClure PW, Sennet BJ. American Shoulder and Elbow Surgeons Standardized Shoulder Assessment Form, patient self-report section: reliability, validity, and responsiveness. *J Shoulder Elbow Surg.* 2002;11(6):587–594.

82. Walsh RM, Sadowski GE. Systemic disease mimicking musculoskeletal dysfunction: a case report involving referred shoulder pain. *J Orthop Sports Phys Ther.* 2001;31(12):696–701.

83. Petchkrua W, Harris SA. Shoulder pain as an unusual presentation of pneumonia in a stroke patient: a case report. *Arch Phys Med Rehabil.* 2000;81(6): 827–829.

84. Khaw PY, Ball DL. Relief of non-metastatic shoulder pain with mediastinal radiotherapy in patients with lung cancer. *Lung Cancer.* 2000;28(1):51–54.

85. Gorski JM, Schwartz LH. Shoulder impingement presenting as neck pain. *J Bone Joint Surg Am.* 2003; 85-A(4):635–638.

86. Woodward T, Best T. The painful shoulder: part I. Clinical evaluation. *Am Fam Physician.* 2000;61: 3079–3088.

87. Priest J, Nagel D. Tennis shoulder. *Am J Sports Med.* 1976;4(1):28–42.

88. Bak K, Fauno P. Clinical findings in competitive swimmers with shoulder pain. *Am J Sports Med.* 1997;25(2):254–260.

89. Ludewig P, Cook T. Translations of the humerus in persons with shoulder impingement syndrome. *J Orthop Sports Phys Ther.* 2002;32(6):248–259.

90. Weiser WM, Lee TQ, McMaster WC, McMahon PJ. Effects of simulated scapular protraction on anterior glenohumeral stability. *Am J Sports Med.* 1999; 27(6):801–805.

91. Cools AM, Witvrouw EE, Danneels LA, Cambier DC. Does taping influence electromyographic muscle activity in the scapular rotators in healthy shoulders? *Man Ther.* 2002;7(3):154–162.

92. Crawford H, Jull G. The influence of thoracic posture and movement on the range of arm elevation. *Physiother Theory Pract.* 1993;9:143–148.

93. Solem-Bertoft E, Thuomas KA, Westerberg CE. The influence of scapular retraction and protraction on the width of the subacromial space. An MRI study. *Clin Orthop Relat Res.* 1993;(296):99–103.

94. Bullock MP, Foster NE, Wright CC. Shoulder impingement: the effect of sitting posture on shoulder

pain and range of motion. *Man Ther.* 2005;10(1): 28–37.

95. Culham E, Peat M. Functional anatomy of the shoulder complex. *J Orthop Sports Phys Ther.* 1993;18 (1):342–350.

96. Reeves B. The natural history of the frozen shoulder syndrome. *Scand J Rheumatol.* 1975;4(4):193–196.

97. Cyriax J. *Textbook of orthopedic medicine. Vol 1: Diagnosis of soft tissue lesions.* 7th ed. New York; Macmillan Publishing: 1978.

98. Magrarey M, Jones M. Clinical evaluation, diagnosis and passive management of the shoulder complex. *New Zealand J Physiother.* 2004;32:55–66.

99. Mulligan BR. The painful dysfunctional shoulder. A new treatment approach using 'Mobilisation with Movement'. *New Zealand J Physiother.* 2003;31: 140–142.

100. Terry GC, Hammon D, France P, Norwood LA. The stabilizing function of passive shoulder restraints. *Am J Sports Med.* 1991;19:26–34.

101. Butler D. *Mobilisation of the nervous system.* Edinburgh; Churchill Livingston: 1990.

102. Woodward T, Best T. The painful shoulder: part II. Acute and chronic disorders. *Am Fam Physician.* 2000;61(11):3291–3300.

103. de Winter A, Jans M, Scholten R, Deville W, van Schaardenburg D, Bouter L. Diagnostic classification of shoulder disorders: interobserver agreement and determinants of disagreement. *Ann Rheum Dis.* 199;58:272–277.

104. Gokeler A, Paridon-Edauw GH, DeClercq S, Matthijs O, Dijkstra PU. Quantitative analysis of traction in the glenohumeral joint. In vivo radiographic measurements. *Man Ther.* 2003;8:97–102.

105. Chesworth B, MacDermid J, Roth J, Patterson S. Movement diagram and 'end feel' reliability when measuring passive lateral rotation of the shoulder in patients with shoulder pathology. *Phys Ther.* 1998; 78:593–601.

106. Hayes K, Peterson C. Reliability of assessing end-feel and pain and resistance sequence in subjects with painful shoulders and knees. *J Orthop Sports Phys Ther.* 2001;31:432–445.

107. Peterson CM, Hayes W. Construct validity of Cyriax's selective tension examination: association of end-feels with pain at the knee and shoulder. *J Orthop Sports Phys Ther.* 2000;30:512–527.

108. Mihata T, Lee Y, McGarry MH, Abe M, Lee TQ. Excessive humeral external rotation results in increased shoulder laxity. *Am J Sports Med.* 2004;32(5): 1278–1285.

109. Johns R, Wright V. Relative importance of various tissues in joint stiffness. *J Appl Physiol.* 1962;17: 824–830.

110. Lundberg J. The frozen shoulder. Clinical and radiographical observations. The effect of manipulation under general anesthesia. Structure and glycosaminoglycan content of the joint capsule. Local bone metabolism. *Acta Orthop Scand.* 1969;Suppl 119:1–59.

111. Conroy D, Hayes K. The effect of joint mobilization as a component of comprehensive treatment for primary shoulder impingement syndrome. *J Orthop Sports Phys Ther.* 1998;28(1):3–14.

112. Warren J, Micheli L, Arslanian L, Kennedy J, Kennedy R. Scapulothoracic motion in normal shoulders and shoulders with glenohumeral instability and impingement syndrome. *Clin Orthop.* 1971; 285:191–199.

113. Edmond SL. *Manipulation and mobilization: Extremities and spinal techniques.* St Louis, MO; Mosby: 1993.

114. Wadsworth CT. Frozen shoulder. *Phys Ther.* 1986;66 (12):1878–1883.

115. Moore SM, Musahl V, McMahon PJ, Debski RE. Multidirectional kinematics of the glenohumeral joint during simulated simple translation tests: impact on clinical diagnoses. *J Orthop Res.* 2004;22(4): 889–894.

116. Hsu AT, Hedman T, Chang JH, Vo C, Ho L, Ho S, Chang GL. Changes in abduction and rotation range of motion in response to simulated dorsal and ventral translational mobilization of the glenohumeral joint. *Phys Ther.* 2002;82(6):544–556.

117. Vermeulen HM, Obermann WR, Burger BJ, Kok GJ, Rozing PM, van Den Ende CH. End range mobilization techniques in adhesive capsulitis of the shoulder joint: a multiple subject case report. *Phys Ther.* 2000;80:1204–1213.

118. Simon R, Vicenzino B, Wright A. The influence of an anteroposterior accessory glide of the glenohumeral joint on measures of peripheral sympathetic nervous system function in the upper limb. *Man Ther.* 1997;2(1):18–23.

119. O'Brien SJ, Schwartz RS, Warren RF, Torzilli PA. Capsular restraints to anterior-posterior motion of the abducted shoulder: A biomechanical study. *J Shoulder Elbow Surg.* 1995;4:298–308.

120. Brenneke SL, Reid J, Ching RP, Wheeler DL. Glenohumeral kinematics and capsulo-ligamentous strain resulting from laxity exams. *Clin Biomech.* 2000;15:735–742.

121. Wolf EM, Agrawal V. Transdeltoid palpation (the rent test) in the diagnosis of rotator cuff tears. *J Shld Elb Surg.* 2001;10(5)470–473.

122. Lyons AR, Tomlinson JE. Clinical diagnosis of tears of the rotator cuff. *J Bone Joint Surg.* 1992;74-B (3):414–415.

123. Walton J, Mahajan S, Paxinos A, Marshall J, Bryant C, Shnier R, Quinn R, Murrell GAC. Diagnostic values of tests for acromioclavicular joint pain. *J Bone Joint Surg.* 2004;86-A(4):807–812.

124. Kelly BT, Kadrmas WR, Speer KP. The manual muscle examination for rotator cuff strength. *Am J Sports Med.* 1996;24(5):581–588.

125. Park HB, Yokota A, Gill HS, El Rassi G, McFarland EG. Diagnostic accuracy of clinical tests for the different degrees of subacromial impingement syndrome. *J Bone Joint Surg.* 2005;87-A(7): 1446–1455.

126. Kendall F, McCreary EK, Provance PG. *Muscles testing and function.* Baltimore; Williams and Wilkins: 1993.

127. Wilk KE, Andrews JR, Arrigo CA, Keirns MA, Erber DJ. The strength characteristics of internal and external rotator muscles in professional baseball pitchers. *Am J Sports Med.* 1993;21(1):61–66.

128. Neer CS II. Impingement lesions. *Clin Ortho.* 1983;173:70–77.

129. Hawkins RJ and Kennedy JC. Impingement syndrome in athletes. *Am J Sports Med.* 1980;8:151–158.

130. Kessel L, Watson M. The painful arc syndrome. *J Bone Joint Surg* 1977;59:166–172.

131. McLaughlin HL. On the "frozen" shoulder. *Bull Hosp Joint Dis.* 1951;12:383–393.

132. Crenshaw AH, Kilgore WE. Surgical treatment of bicipital tenosynovitis. *J Bone Joint Surg.* 1966; 48-A:1496–1502.

133. Yergason RM. Supination sign. *J Bone Joint Surg.* 1931;13:160–165.

134. Zaslav KR. Internal rotation resistance strength test: A new diagnostic test to differentiate intra-articular pathology from outlet (Neer) impingement syndrome in the shoulder. *J Shld Elb Surg.* 2001;10: 23–27.

135. Meister K, Buckley B, Batts J. The posterior impingement sign: diagnosis of rotator cuff and posterior labral tears secondary to internal impingement in overhead athletes. *Am J Ortho.* 2004;33:412–415.

136. Gerber C, Krushell RJ. *J Bone Joint Surg.* 1991; 73-B:389–394.

137. Gerber C, Hersche O, Farron A. Isolated rupture of the subscapularis tendon. *J Bone Joint Surg.* 1996; 78-A:1015–1023.

138. Hertel R, Ballmer FT, Lambert SM, Gerber CH. Lag signs in the diagnosis of rotator cuff rupture. *J Shld Elb Surg.* 1996; 5(4):307–313.

139. Jobe FW, Jobe CM. Painful athletic injuries of the shoulder. *Clin Ortho.* 1983;173:117–124.

140. Itoi E, Kido T, Sano A, Urayama M Sato K. Which is more useful, the "full can test" or the "empty can test" in detecting the torn supraspinatus tendon. *Am J Sports Med.* 1999;27(1):65–68.

141. Moseley HF. Disorders of the shoulder. *Clin Symp.* 1959;11(3):75–102.

142. O'Brien SJ, Pagnani MJ, Fealy S, McGlynn SR, Wilson JB. The active compression test:A new and effective test for diagnosing labral tears and acromioclavicular joint abnormality. *Am J Sports Med.* 1998; 26(5):610–613.

143. Snyder SJ, Karzel RP, Del Pizzo W, Ferkel RD, Friedman, MJ. SLAP lesions of the shoulder. *Arthro* 1990;6(4):274–279.

144. Liu SH, Henry MH, Nuccion SL. A prospective evaluation of a new physical examination in predicting glenoid labrum tears. *Am J Sports Med.* 1996; 24(6):721–725.

145. Myers TH, Zemanovic JR, Andrews JR. The resisted supination test. *Am J Sports Med.* 2005;33(9):1–6.

146. Kibler BW. Specificity and sensitivity of the anterior slide test in throwing athletes with superior glenoid labral tears. *Arthro.* 1995;11(3):296–300.

147. Mimori K, Muneta T, Nakagawa T, Shinomiya K. A new pain provocation test for superior labral tears of the shoulder. *Am J Sports Med.* 1999;27(2):137–142.

148. Kim SH, Ha KI, Han KY. Biceps load test: a clinical test for superior labrum anterior and posterior lesions in shoulders with recurrent anterior dislocations. *Am J Sports Med.* 1999; 27(3):300–303.

149. Kim SH, Ha KI, Ahn JH, Kim SH, Choi HJ. Biceps load test II: a clinical test for SLAP lesions of the shoulder. *Arthro.* 2001;17(2):160–164.

150. Kim SH, Park JS, Jeong WK, Shin SK. The Kim test: a novel test for posteroinferior labral lesion of the shoulder—a comparison to the jerk test. *Am J Sports Med.* 2005;33(8):1–5.

151. Neer CS II, Foster CR. Inferior capsular shift for involuntary inferior and multidirectional instability of the shoulder: a preliminary report. *J Bone Joint Surg.* 1980;62-A:897–908.

152. Silliman JF, Hawkins RJ. Classification and physical diagnosis of instability of the shoulder. *Clin Ortho.* 1993;291:7–19.

153. Gerber C, Ganz R. Clinical assessment of instability of the shoulder with special reference to anterior and posterior drawer tests. *J Bone Joint Surg Br.* 1984;66-B:551–556.

154. Gagey OJ, Gagey N. The hyperabduction test. *J Bone Joint Surg.* 2001;83-B(1):69–74.

155. Silliman JF, Hawkins RJ. Current concepts and recent advances in the athlete's shoulder. *Clin Ortho.* 1991;10(4):693–705.

156. Rowe CR, Zarins B. Recurrent transient subluxation of the shoulder. *J Bone Joint Surg.* 1981;63-A: 863–871.

157. Jobe FW, Kvitne RS. Shoulder pain in the overhand or throwing athlete: the relationship of anterior instability and rotator cuff impingement. *Ortho Review.* 1989;18(9):963–975.

158. Gross ML, Distefano MC. Anterior release test: a new test for occult shoulder instability. *Clin Ortho.* 1997;1(339):105–108.

159. Walton J, Mahajan S, Paxinos A, Marshall J, Bryant C, Shnier R, Quinn R, Murrell GA. Diagnostic val-

ues of tests for acromioclavicular joint pain. *J Bone Joint Surg Am.* 2004;86-A(4):807–812.

160. Jacob A, Sallay P. Therapeutic efficacy of corticosteroid injections in the acromioclavicular joint. *Biomed Sci Instrum.* 1997;34:380–385.

161. Hertel R, Lambert SM, Ballmer FT. The deltoid extension lag sign for diagnosis and grading of axillary nerve palsy. *J Shld Elb Surg.* 1998;7(2):97–99.

162. Winters JC, Groenier KH, Sobel JS, Arendzen HH, Meyboom-de Jongh B. Classification of shoulder complaints in general practice by means of a cluster analysis. *Arch Phys Med Rehabil.* 1997;78: 1369–1374.

163. Lewis JS, Wright C, Green A. Subacromial impingement syndrome: the effect of changing posture on shoulder range of movement. *J Orthop Sports Phys Ther.* 2005;35(2):72–87.

164. Maitland GD. *Peripheral manipulation.* London; Butterworth Heinemann: 1986.

165. Bang M, Deyle G. Comparison of supervised exercise with and without manual physical therapy for patients with shoulder impingement syndrome. *J Orthop Sports Phys Ther.* 2000;30(3):126–137.

166. Bulgen DY, Binder AL, Hazleman BL. Frozen shoulder: a prospective clinical study with an evaluation of three treatment regimens. *Ann Rheum Dis.* 1984;43:353–360.

167. Dacre JE, Beeney N, Scott DL. Injections and physiotherapy for the painful stiff shoulder. *Ann Rheum Dis.* 1989;48(4):322–325.

168. Nicholson G. The effects of passive joint mobilization on pain and hypomobility associated with adhesive capsulitis of the shoulder. *J Orthop Sports Phys Ther.* 1985;6:238–246.

169. Turkel SJ, Panio MW, Marshall JL, Girgis FG. Stabilizing mechanisms preventing anterior dislocation of the glenohumeral joint. *J Bone Joint Surg Am.* 1981;63(8):1208–1217.

170. Ovensen J, Nielson S. Posterior instability of the shoulder: A cadaver study. *Acta Orthop Scand.* 1986; 57:436–439.

171. MacDonald PB, Clark P, Sutherland K. An analysis of the diagnostic accuracy of the Hawkins and Neer subacromial impingement tests. *J Shld Elb Surg* 2000;9(4):299–301.

172. Calis M, Akgun K, Birtane M, Karacan I, Calis H, Tuzun F. Diagnostic values of clinical diagnostic tests in subacromial impingement syndrome. *Ann of Rheum Disease* 2000; 59(1):44–47.

173. Holtby R, Razmjou H. Accuracy of the Speed's and Yergason's tests in detecting biceps pathology and SLAP lesions: comparison with arthroscopic findings. *Arthro.* 2004;20:231–236.

174. Guanche CA, Jones DC. Clinical testing for tears of the glenoid labrum. *Arthro.* 2003;19(5):517–523.

175. Parentis MA, Mohr KJ, ElAttrache NS. Disorders of the superior labrum: review and treatment guidelines. *Clin Ortho.* 2002;400:77–87.

176. Bennett WF. Specificity of Speed's test: arthroscopic technique for evaluating the biceps tendon at the level of the bicipital groove. *Arthro.* 1998;14(8): 789–796.

177. Morgan CD, Burkhart SS, Palmeri M, Gillespie M. Type II SLAP lesions: three subtypes and their relationships to superior instability and rotator cuff tears. *Arthro.* 1998;14(6):553–565.

178. McFarland EG, Kim TK, Savino RM. Clinical assessment of three common tests for superior labral anterior-posterior lesions. *Am J Sports Med.* 2002;30 (6):810–815.

179. Stetson WB, Templin K. The crank test, the O'Brien test, and routine magnetic resonance imaging scans in the diagnosis of labral tears. *Am J Sports Med.* 2002;30(6):806–809.

180. Lo IKY, Nonweiler B, Woolfrey M, Litchfield R, Kirkley A. An evaluation of the apprehension, relocation, and surprise tests for anterior shoulder instability. *Am J Sports Med.* 2004;32(2):301–307.

181. Chronopoulos E, Kim TK, Park HB, Ashenbrenner D, and McFarland EG. Diagnostic value of physical tests for isolated chronic acromioclavicular lesions. *Am J Sports Med.* 2004;32(3):655–661.

# 10

# Manual Therapy
# of the Elbow–Wrist–Hand

## Objectives

- Understand the prevalence of elbow–wrist–hand disorders and the risk factors associated with the occurrence.
- Understand the normal and pathological kinematics associated with each elbow, wrist, or hand movement.
- Recognize the patient subjective characteristics associated with elbow, wrist, or hand injuries.
- Recognize the techniques of treatment that have yielded the highest success in the literature.
- Identify the appropriate clinical special tests and the diagnostic value of these tests.

## PREVALENCE

### Occupational Injuries

Injuries to the wrist, hand, and elbow are among the most common reported dysfunctions associated with occupational medicine. The number of occupational illness cases as a result of repeated trauma increased 15-fold from 1977 to 1997.[1] Descatha et al.[2] reported an annual incidence of approximately 4–5% and a lifetime incidence of approximately 1.5%. The most common forms include lateral epicondylitis, carpal tunnel syndrome, cubital tunnel syndrome, radial tunnel syndrome, and cervicobrachial neuralgia.[3] When comparing the elbow and wrist/hand, wrist/hand injuries are more prevalent, accounting for nearly 29% of emergency room visits in the United States.[4] Selected occupations are more likely to be associated with elbow, wrist, and hand injuries, specifically those associated with heavy manual handling and repetitive work.[5] When investigated in isolation, wrist/hand injuries are more likely to occur in types of jobs that require repetitive work such as "textiles, furs & leathergoods" and "other machining occupations."[6]

Some conditions such as cubital tunnel symptoms are almost exclusively reported in occupation-related scenarios. This condition is common in occupations that require holding and using tools and in individuals that are obese. In fact, obesity, tool work, and the presence of medial epicondylitis, carpal tunnel syndrome, radial tunnel syndrome, and cervicobrachial neuralgia were the only factors associated with the likelihood of a diagnosis of cubital tunnel syndrome.[3] Other conditions such as carpal tunnel syndrome (CTS) and lateral epicondylitis are frequently reported in both occupational and nonoccupational environments and tend to be gender specific. Women are more likely to report CTS while men are more likely to acquire lateral epicondylitis.[3]

Although elbow, wrist, and hand occupation-related injuries are prevalent over nonoccupational trauma, these anatomical areas generally yield lower costs associated with disability than other regions such as the lumbar spine and shoulder. In particular, those with shoulder injuries have larger losses than those with elbow or wrist injuries, despite receiving the same disability ratings.[7] While most industry-related injuries have declined in the last 10 years[8,9] lateral epicondylar pain has increased.[10]

## Nonoccupational Injuries

The most common forms of nonoccupation-related injuries to the elbow are either fracture or overuse related.[11,12] A younger population is more apt to incur a fracture, specifically those associated with the radial head (33% of all elbow fractures) or supracondylar region (20% of all elbow fractures) of the humerus.[11,12] Older patients are more predisposed toward **tendonesis**-based injuries such as lateral epicondylitis but may also fall victim to elbow or wrist fractures, specifically olecranon fractures, which account for 20% of all elbow fractures,[13] or Colle's fractures, which are fractures of the distal radius and occasionally the ulna.

Tendonesis-based soft tissue–related conditions such as "tennis elbow" account for the majority of painful conditions in the lateral elbow, purportedly affecting 1–3% of the general population.[14,15] Tendinopathies differ from inflammatory-based problems such as tendonitis in several ways. First, tendonesis implies tendon degeneration in the absence of an active inflammatory process.[16] Second, tendonesis includes degeneration of the tendon and may or may not be symptomatic. Third, collagen fibers often lose the parallel orientation, decrease the cross-sectional fiber size, and exhibit small microtears. This results in a condition termed birefringence, which is a knotting of the tissue.[16]

Medial elbow pain is commonly referred as "little leaguer's elbow" in youths and "golfer's elbow" in older adults. The prevalence of medial elbow pain ranges from 25% of younger individuals to small percentages in older adults. Older adults are more likely to experience tendonesis-related injuries during musculoskeletal connective tissue changes associated with maturity.[17]

Lastly, degenerative conditions such as osteoarthritis may also affect the elbow, predominantly over the wrist and hand. Osteoarthritis disables about 10% of people who are older than 60 years, compromises the quality of life of more than 20 million Americans, and costs the United States economy more than $60 billion per year.[18,19] Debono et al.[20] feel the actual incidence of elbow arthritis is highly underestimated. In their clinical assessment of over 470 elbows, osteoarthritis was found in 27% of individuals.

### Summary

- Occupation-related injuries are the most common forms of elbow, wrist, and hand injuries.
- Carpal tunnel syndrome, cubital tunnel syndrome, and lateral epicondylitis are the most frequently reported elbow, wrist, and hand injuries.
- Nonoccupation-related injuries include fractures, osteoarthritis, and sports-related injuries such as golfer's elbow and little leaguer's elbow.

# Anatomy

## Osseous Structures of the Elbow

The elbow joint consists of three articulating bones: the humerus, the radius, and the ulna. The humerus is a long bone that articulates at the shoulder proximally and the elbow distally. The humerus widens significantly at the distal articulation and provides a contact point for several important muscular origins. These contact points are also common sites for fractures, although the functional recovery from fractures is generally very good.[21]

The ulna provides the distal hinge joint articulation for the humeral ulnar joint (HUJ). The ulna is a long, thin bone with a posterior and proximal protuberance called the olecranon that serves as an attachment site for the triceps and anconeus. Anteriorly, the coronoid provides stability during movement. Distally, the ulna provides a thin contact with the wrist and a shared capsular articulation with the radiocarpal joint.[22]

The radius provides the most substantial articulation with the wrist and a unique joint contact at the elbow. The concave radial head articulates with the convex capitulum forming a modified hinge joint that has a considerable amount of pivoting movement. Distally, the radius broadens and provides a wide contact surface for wrist articulation.

## Osseous Structures of the Wrist

Normally, 27 bones make up the wrist and hand complex. In some cases, sesamoid bones may increase the total of bones in the wrist. There are eight carpal bones in the normal hand (Figure 10.1). The proximal carpal row is made up of the pisiform, triquetrum, the lunate, and scaphoid. The distal row consists of hamate, the capitate, the trapezoid, and the trapezium. Of the eight carpal bones, the pisiform functions less for support and articulation and is nearly entirely embedded within the tendon of the flexor carpi ulnaris. The scaphoid is a peanut-shaped bone and is the most commonly fractured carpal bone. Approximately 65% of the fractures occur at the "waist" of the scaphoid secondary to a poor blood supply. However, pole fractures actually take longer to heal, generally taking up to 20 weeks for proper ossification and stability.[23]

## Osseous Structures of the Hand

There are five metacarpals in the hand, which are made up of 19 separate bones arranged in longitudinal order (Figure 10.2). Metacarpals are long, cylindrical bones that make up the palmar and dorsal aspect of the hand. The bones run from the carpal bones of the wrist to the articulation of metacarpal phalangeal joint. Metacarpals two and three move very little whereas metacarpal one exhibits liberal movement, allowing the thumb to oppose digits 4 and 5.[24]

There are three phalanges (proximal, middle, and distal) for each finger and two for the thumb (proximal and

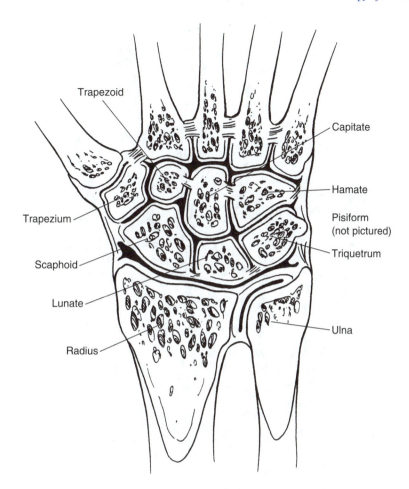

**Figure 10.1**    The Carpal Bones

distal). The phalanges are long and cylindrical with each distal joint surface exhibiting a convex presentation. Each proximal structure exhibits a concave presentation, lending to a hinge-type joint. The distal extremities are shorter and smaller than the proximal.

## Summary

- Three primary osseous structures make up the elbow joint: the humerus, the radius, and the ulna.
- The osseous structures of the wrist include the proximal structures of the ulna and radius and the carpal bones; the proximal carpal row is made up of the pisiform, triquetrum, lunate, and scaphoid. The distal row consists of hamate, capitate, trapezoid, and trapezium.
- There are five metacarpals in the hand and three phalanges for each finger and two for the thumb.

## Ligaments, Interosseous, and Capsular Structures of the Elbow

The elbow is less stable with valgus stresses than to varus stresses, although instability is not common. When instability is present, it is normally associated with valgus stress, a product of functional torque upon the joint. To counter this consequence, the medial collateral ligaments of the elbow are stronger than the lateral collateral ligaments.[25]

The medial or ulnar collateral ligaments include the anterior oblique and posterior oblique bundles and a transverse ligament (Figure 10.3).[25] The anterior oblique bundle provides medial stability throughout flexion and extension. This ligament maintains the elbow against valgus instability to a greater extent than even the bony configuration of the olecranon.[25] Morrey and Ag[26] suggested that the anterior oblique bundles provided the greatest stability to valgus forces of the ligaments of the elbow. The posterior oblique bundle provides medial stability in 60–135 degrees of flexion and extension whereas the transverse ligaments contribution is only marginal.[25]

The ulnar (medial) collateral ligament provides valgus stability (abduction) and is tightened in all positions of

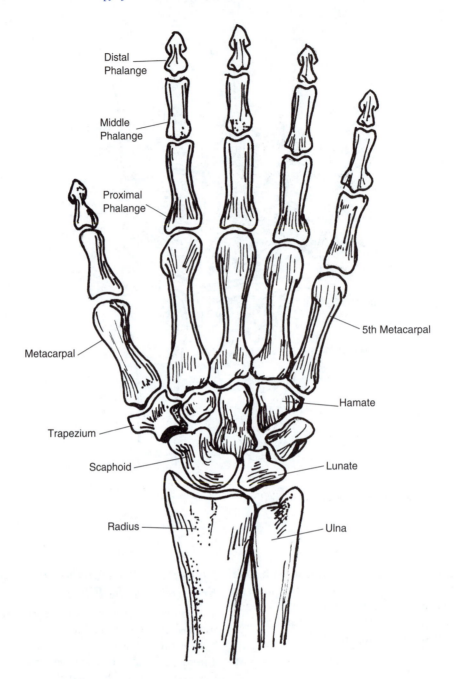

**Figure 10.2**    The Bones of the Hand

elbow because of anterior, posterior, and oblique (transverse) bands. The anterior band provides the greatest passive structure resistance to valgus force throughout the flexion and extension movements of the elbow.[22] The anterior band originates on the medial supracondylar ridge of the humerus and inserts lateral to the coronoid process of the ulna.[25] The transverse or oblique band provides medial stability at 60–135 degrees of extension to flexion movement. The transverse band originates on the distal-most aspect of the supracondylar ridge of the humerus, just distal to the humerus, and inserts on the proximal–lateral aspect of the coronoid process of the ulna.[25] The pos-

terior bundle of the medial collateral aspect of the elbow originates on the medial supracondylar ridge of the humerus and inserts just anterior to the lateral aspect of the olecranon. The ulnar ligamentous complex is most stable at 110 degrees and also most lax at this range if the ligament is disrupted.[22]

The lateral or radial collateral ligament (Figure 10.4) originates from the lateral condyle of the humerus and inserts on the annular ligament, which encircles the head of the radius. The radial collateral ligament provides varus stability (adduction) but doesn't provide the same intensity of the stabilization as does the medial collateral structures.[25]

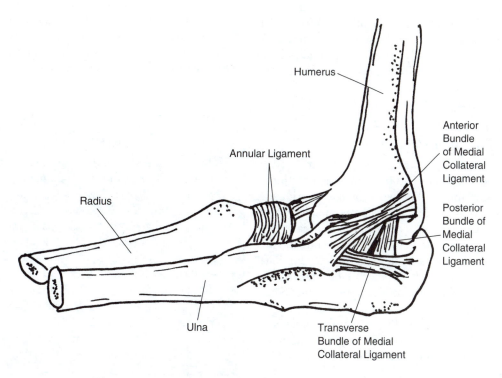

**Figure 10.3**   The Ligaments of the Medial Elbow

The annular ligament of the elbow forms a ligamentous ring that encircles the head of the radius and a ligamentous attachment to the ulna. The annular ligament allows hinge-like motion, promotes rotation of the radial head with stabilization of its position to the ulna, and contributes partially to lateral stability of the elbow. The annular ligament also prevents lateral and inferior displacement of the radial head.[25]

The capsule of the elbow (Figure 10.5) that is prepositioned in extension contributes significantly to the stability

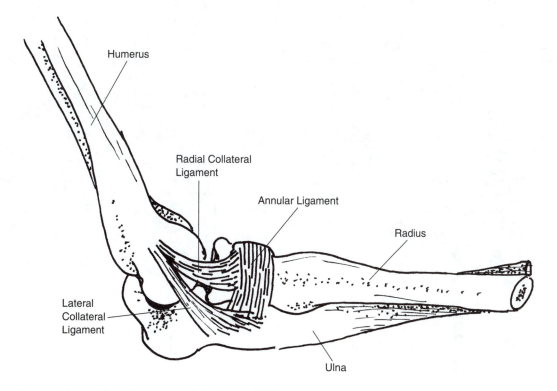

**Figure 10.4**   The Ligaments of the Lateral Elbow

of the elbow in distraction,[26] and slightly for motions of varus and valgus forces. The contribution of the capsule for stability during flexion is nearly insignificant. Studies have shown that resection of the elbow capsule does not alter valgus or varus stability; however, resection of the medial and lateral collateral ligaments certainly affects stability.[27]

### Ligaments, Interosseous, and Capsular Structures of the Wrist/Hand

The palmar ligaments (volar wrist ligaments) (Figure 10.6) are highly developed, stable, and have integrated with the volar plates in the fingers. The wrist ligaments originate from the radial styloid process and migrate in a distal and ulnar direction. These ligaments include the ulnar-sided capitohamate ligaments, the lunotriquetral ligaments, the ulnotriquetral ligament, and the ulnolunate ligament. The ulnotriquetral ligament and the ulnolunate ligament lie ulnarly whereas the radiolunate, radioscaphoid, and radioscapholunate lie radially.[28]

Like the elbow, the capsule of the wrist is synovial and contiguous. The capsule contains the joints of the wrist but does not contain the multiple tendons of the fingers, which lie outside the capsule.

The dorsal surface of the hand also demonstrates excellent stability. The superficial layers include the dorsal oblique radiotriquetral ligaments, the dorsal transverse intercarpal (trapezoid-triquetral ligament), while the deep

## Summary

- The ligaments of the elbow include the medial structures, the anterior oblique and posterior oblique bundles, a transverse ligament, the lateral collateral ligament, and the annular ligament.
- The capsule within the elbow is contiguous.
- The wrist consists of both medial and lateral ligaments as well as multiple interosseous ligaments between each carpal bone.
- The hand also consists of numerous ligaments that guide motion and provide structure to the hand and fingers.
- The capsule of the wrist is contiguous but does not contain the tendons of the wrist.

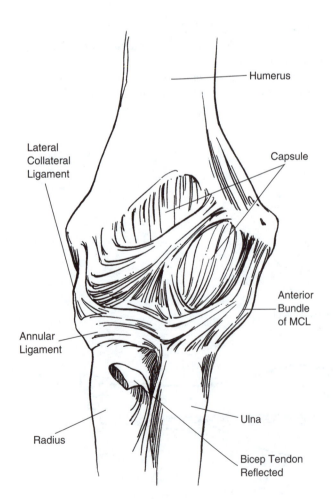

**Figure 10.5**   The Contiguous Capsule of the Elbow

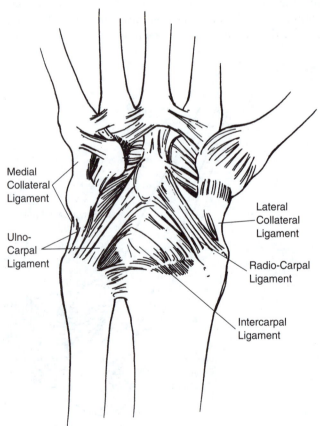

**Figure 10.6**   The Palmar Ligaments of the Wrist

layers include the scapholunate interosseous ligament and the unotriquetral interosseous ligament. Each of the deep and superficial ligaments plays an important role during stabilization of the wrist.[28]

# Biomechanics

## The Elbow

The center of rotation for sagittal movement of the elbow moves very little throughout flexion and extension physiological movements.[29] This suggests that the humeroulnar joint (HUJ) is a simple hinge joint with only slight alterations of variability. Others have found up to 8 degrees of variability[30] with concurrent varus and valgus movements of 4–8 degrees in the coronal plane. This movement is associated with the contribution of the capitellum and the freedom of varus and valgus translation during this motion.

Individually, the radial head can turn clockwise and counterclockwise. The axis of rotation for pronation and supination lies in an oblique plane between the ulna and the radius and passes through the interosseous membrane at the distal fourth of the ulna.[29] During pronation, the radius moves both proximally and laterally whereas the ulna concurrently internally rotates. During supination the ulna exhibits external rotation while the radius moves distally and medially. Prepositioning of the elbow in pronation or supination alters the axis of the HUJ and humeroradial joint (HRJ), creating differences in the amount of force that is translated through the joint.[29]

## Joints of the Elbow

The two most proximal joints of the elbow, the HUJ and the HRJ, have two degrees of freedom: (1) flexion–extension at the HUJ and (2) pronation–supination at the HRJ. The third joint, the proximal radio-ulnar joint (PRUJ), is enveloped within the same capsule as the HUJ and the HRJ.

### Humeroulnar Joint (HUJ)

The HUJ is a hinge joint, demonstrating the primary movements of flexion and extension (Figure 10.7). The complete range of motion of the joint varies but generally exhibits 0–5 degrees of hyperextension to 135–150 degrees of flexion. The 5 degrees of hyperextension is considered normal and functional.

Extension is limited either by the olecranon process of the posterior articulation or by the anterior ligaments of the elbow. Occasionally, tightness in the origin and insertions of the anterior muscles may limit extension as well. Flexion is limited by the coronoid process of the elbow, soft tissue of the anterior forearm and biceps, and posterior and anterior ligaments.

When the elbow is fully extended and supinated, the forearm is angled slightly away from the long axis of the humerus. This angle is called the "carrying angle" and is a product of function and the fulcruming action of the bi-

ceps tuberosity. The head of the radius will translate medially during supination and laterally during pronation as a result of the fulcruming action of the biceps tuberosity of the radius.[29]

### Humeroradial Joint (HRJ)

The articulation between the humerus and the radius is the HRJ (see Figure 10.7). The articulation is hallmarked by the smooth junction of the convex capitulum of the humerus as the structure articulates with the top of the concave radial head. This biomechanical relationship allows for a spinning movement around the capitulum by the radial head during flexion, which contributes to flexion and extension and pronation and supination of the joint.[29]

### Proximal Radial Ulnar Joint (PRUJ)

The PRUJ is a pivot joint and consists of the articulations of the proximal one-third of the ulna and radius. The radius is attached to the ulna by the annular ligament, which assists in guiding the movement of pronation and supination. Normal pronation values are approximately 70 degrees of range of motion whereas supination is approximately 85 degrees of range. During supination and extension, the radial head is displaced medially, allowing for an increased carrying angle. During pronation, the radial head translates laterally, promoted by the biceps tubercle as a pivot point and fulcrum.

The complex movements associated with elbow and wrist motion are manufactured by the collective movements of numerous muscles (Figures 10.8 and 10.9). The biceps, brachioradialis, and the brachialis provide the majority of torque for flexion. The anconeus and the triceps provide extension torque. Pronation is produced primarily from the pronator teres whereas supination is produced by the supinator and the biceps. Damage to the muscle may lead to movement dysfunction and subsequent restrictions and impairments (Table 10.1).

## Summary

- The two most proximal joints of the elbow, the ulnohumeral and the radiohumeral, have two degrees of freedom allowing flexion and extension as well as pronation and supination.
- The elbow also exhibits a small degree of varus and valgus motion during flexion and extension.
- Pronation requires the lateral translation of the radial head while supination requires a medial translation of the radial head.
- Multiple muscles produce the complex active movements of the elbow, some contributing to movements in more than one plane.

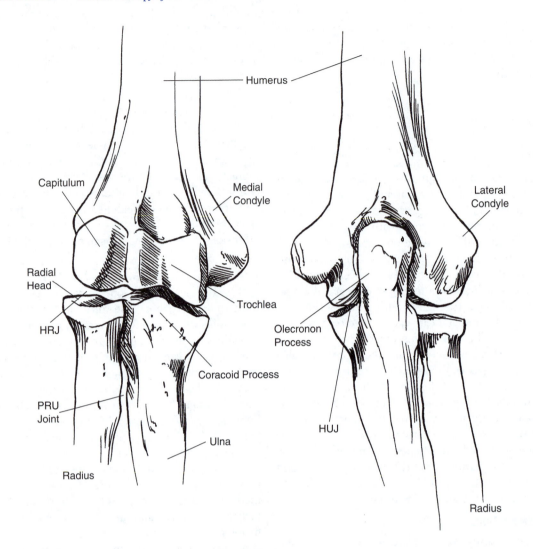

**Figure 10.7**    The Joints of the Elbow Complex

## The Wrist

Wrist motion is the summated movements of the collective joints of the wrist and is infinitely complex. This motion includes the intricate motions of the carpal bones and the movements with the distal aspect of the radius. Individual ranges of motion between the distal carpal bones range from as little as 6 degrees of flexion–extension, or radial–ulna deviation to as great as 12 degrees.[31] The carpal bones in the distal row generally move in concert more often than the carpal bones in the proximal row, but do exhibit isolated movements. The reason the proximal row demonstrates greater isolated movements is that the carpal bones are less tightly bound to one another through ligamentous and capsular connections.[32,33] In general, carpal bones within the distal row synergistically move with flexion and ulnar deviation during flexion and conversely, with extension, extension and radial deviation.

The proximal carpal bones that exhibit the greatest amount of movement are the scaphoid, which moves up to 80 degrees with respect to the radius,[33] and the lunate and triquetrum, which move only slightly less.[34] It is imperative to acknowledge that movement occurs in multiple planes, with respect to the radius and with respect to other carpal bones. For example, the scaphoid not only moves toward extension during wrist extension but also supinates and deviates into a radial direction.[31] Wrist flexion promotes the combined movements of flexion, ulnar deviation, and pronation of the scaphoid. In contrast, during extension, the lunate extends, pronates, and ulnarly deviates.

Range of motion is also dependent on the laxity of the intercarpal joints, the shape of the distal radius, the function of the **triangular fibrocartilagenous complex (TFCC)**, and the ulnocarpal joint. Movements are always combined, are very complex, and are dependent on a myriad of structures.

In summary, motion of the wrist is coupled and multiplanar. Movements such as flexion and ulnar deviation and extension and radial deviation occur concurrently and have a linear relationship. As much as 75% of ulnar and

**TABLE 10.1   Muscles and Function of the Elbow and Forearm**

| Muscle | Movement and Function | Joint Motion | Spinal Segment |
|---|---|---|---|
| Biceps Brachii | Flexion and supination | Flexes arm and forearm | C5-C6 |
| • Long Head | | | |
| • Short Head | | Supinates hand | |
| Brachialis | Flexion | Flexes forearm | C5-C6 |
| Triceps | Extension | Extends arm and forearm | C7-C8 |
| • Long Head | | | |
| • Lateral Head | | | |
| • Medial Head | | | |
| Pronator Teres | Pronation and flexion | Pronates hand, flexes forearm | C6-C7 |
| Supinator | Supination | Following pronation, the supinator supinates the radius | C6 |
| Flexor Carpi Radialis | Flexion, pronation, and radial deviation | Flex forearm and hand aid in pronation and abduction of hand | C6-C7 |
| Palmaris Longus | Flexion | Flexes hand and wrinkles skin of palm of hand | C6-C7 |
| Flexor Digitorum Superficialis | Flexion | Flexes phalanges, wrist, and forearm | C6,C7,T1 |
| Flexor Carpi Ulnaris | Flexion and ulnar deviation | Flexes forearm and hand, adducts hand | C8-T1 |
| Flexor Pollicis Longus | Flexion | Flexes thumb | C8-T1 |
| Flexor Digitorum Profundus | Flexion | Flexes phalanges | C8-T1 |
| Pronator Quadratus | Pronation | Pronates hand | C8-T1 |
| Extensor Carpi Radialis Longus | Extension and radial deviation | Extends and abducts the wrist | C6-C7 |
| Extensor Carpi Radialis Brevis | Extension and radial deviation | Extends and abducts the wrist | C6-C7 |
| Extensor Carpi Ulnaris | Extension and ulnar deviation | Extends and adducts the hand | C6,C7,C8 |
| Anconeus | Extension | Extends forearm | C7-C8 |

radial deviation is associated with flexion and extension movements.[35] Additionally, pronation and supination of the elbow require pronation and supination contributions from the wrist.[36] The mean degree of movement of pronation and supination that originates at the wrist is 17 degrees, respectively, for both.[36]

## Joints of the Wrist Hand

The global movements of the wrist hand include flexion and extension with normative values of 80–90 degrees of flexion and 75–80 degrees of extension. Thirty-five de-

grees of ulnar deviation and 20 degrees of radial deviation are considered normal, as is metacarpal phalangeal flexion and extension of 135 and 25 degrees, respectively. Adduction and abduction values are 20–25 degrees, respectively, and proximal interphalangeal flexion and extension values are 115 and 0 degrees, respectively. Finally, distal interphalangeal extension and flexion demonstrate 0–90 degrees of movement.

Although there are numerous joints of the wrist hand, each joint is synovial and contributes to the astonishing functional movements of the wrist hand. For order, the

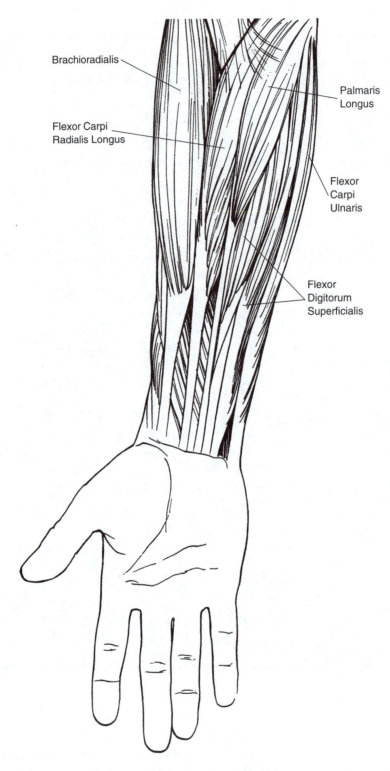

Brachioradialis

Flexor Carpi
Radialis Longus

Palmaris
Longus

Flexor
Carpi
Ulnaris

Flexor
Digitorum
Superficialis

**Figure 10.8**   Forearm Muscles-Anterior View

joints will be discussed primarily by row; however, in real- ity, movement may occur between carpal bones, in multiple axes, and through highly complicated mechanisms.[37,38]

### Proximal Carpal Row

The proximal carpal row (Figure 10.10) consists of the lateral articulations of the lunate and scaphoid with the ra-

dius (radiolunate and radioscaphoid) and the medial articu- lation of the ulna, TFCC, and the lunate (ulnolunate), and TFCC and triquetrum. The radiocarpal joints (radiolunate and radioscaphoid) include a biconvex carpal segment and the biconcave radial aspect. The ulnocarpal joint is further complicated by the presence of the TFCC that merges with the volar edge of the ulnocarpal ligaments and, at its

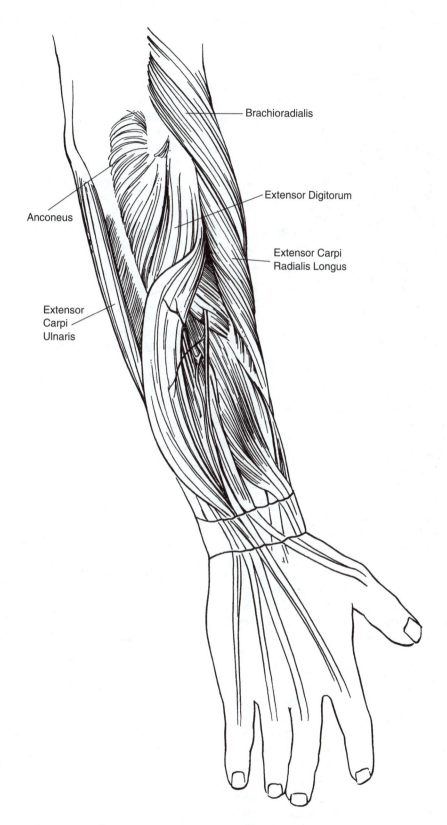

**Figure 10.9**   Forearm Muscles-Posterior View

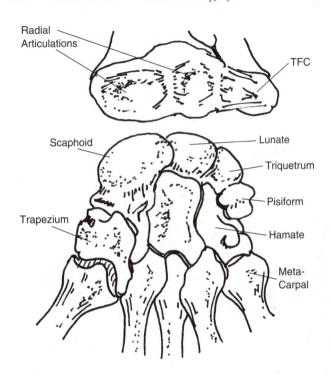

**Figure 10.10**    The Proximal Carpal Row

dorsal edge, with the floors of the extensor carpi ulnaris and extensor digiti minimi and separates the ulna and the proximal carpal row.[39] The TFCC has numerous functions at the proximal carpal row. First, the disc provides a smooth and conformed gliding surface across the entire distal face of the ulna and proximal carpal row. Second, the disc allows flexion, extension, rotation, and translational movements. Third, the disc cushions forces that are transmitted through this region, thus reducing the risk of fracture.[39] Lastly, the disc connects the two boney regions together in an otherwise poorly congruent region.

### Mid-Carpal Row

The mid-carpal row (Figure 10.11) consists of the articulations of the triquetrum, lunate, and scaphoid (proximal row) with the hamate, capitate, trapezoid, and trapezium (distal row). The distal surfaces of the triquetrium, lunate, and scaphoid are biconcave whereas the distal surfaces of most of the scaphoid is either convex or planar. The proximal surfaces of the capitate and hamate are convex, and the proximal surface of the trapezoid and trapezium are concave or planar.

Under normal situations movements of the mid-carpal joint are disparate from the movements of the pisotrique-tral, radiocarpal, and first carpometacarpal joints.[22] This complex joint provides numerous interosseous articulations, providing movement that is much more complex than simple extension/flexion or radial and ulnar deviation. Because the large capitate crosses the axis of the mid-carpal row and encroaches into the proximal carpal joint, the mid-carpal joint will always demonstrate lower values of motion as compared to the proximal row.

### Intercarpal Joints

Multiple intercarpal joints are present throughout the two rows of carpal bones. The joints are stabilized by ligamentous and capsular components but do allow movements such as shear, rotation, flexion, and extension relative to one another. Range-of-motion values differ among joints yet each intercarpal structure can be a pain generator. Instability may occur in many forms; the most common are identified as a **volar intercalated segmental instability** (VISI) and a DISI, a **dorsal intercalated segmental instability.** A VISI results from a disruption between the triquetrum and lunate, allowing volar drift of the lunate and problems during physiological flexion of the wrist.[40] A VISI pattern is usually associated with triquetrolunate dissociation or triquetral–hamate instability. A DISI results from a disruption between the scaphoid and the lunate, allowing the scaphoid to float into volar flexion.[40] A patient with a DISI (scapho-ligamentous disruption) exhibits problems with physiological dorsiflexion and is diagnosed by the presence of a scapholunate angle greater than 70 degrees.

### Carpometacarpal Joints

The carpometacarpal joints are the articulations of the distal carpal row and the metacarpals of all five digits. The first carpometacarpal joint (Figure 10.12) lies laterally to the rest of the palm, which promotes oppositional movements of the thumb. The joint is a sellar, saddle joint with

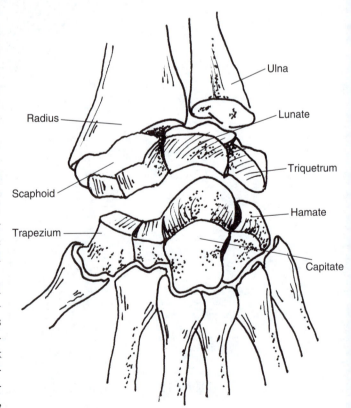

**Figure 10.11**    The Articulation of the Mid-Carpal Row

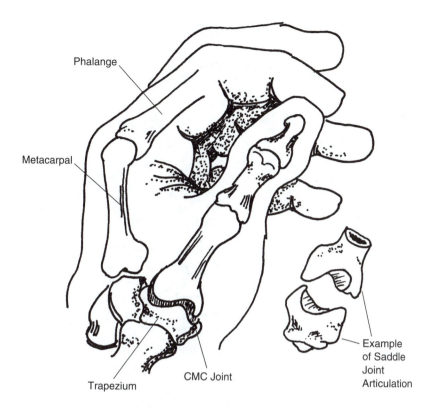

**Figure 10.12**    The First Carpometacarpal Joint

two main axes (a radiolulnar axis for flexion and extension and a dorsopalmar axis for abduction and adduction). Some rotation is possible at this joint when the thumb is adducted or placed in slight flexion.[41] The closed packed position of the thumb occurs during full abduction. Normally, the capsule of the carpometacarpal joint is lax, which allows opposition.

## Joints of the Hand

There are numerous movements within the hand. Structurally, the hand exhibits three primary arches to promote stabile grasps and gripping functions.[41] The proximal transverse arch forms at the posterior border of the carpal tunnel and is rigid and stable. The distal transverse arch is formed by the metacarpal heads and is maintained by the intrinsic muscles of the hand. The longitudinal arch allows the fourth and fifth metacarpals to oppose the palm longitudinally.

### Intermetacarpal Joints

The intermetacarpal joints allow movements within the distal transverse axis of the hand. The intermetacarpal joints help create an arch in the palm, an arch that is progressively more angular near the ulnar aspect of the hand. By far, the majority of transverse movement occurs at metacarpals 4 and 5, allowing further opponens movements toward the thumb of the hand.[41] Overall, the amount of movement available at these joints is minimal,

but is necessary for appropriate fist making and hand manipulation.

### Metacarpophalangeal Joints

The metacarpophalangeal joint (Figure 10.13) is a condyloid classification that allows flexion, extension, abduction, rotation, and circumduction. The joint is well stabilized anteriorly, medially, and laterally. The joints are most stable in flexion and allow the greatest amount of mobility in extension.[41]

### Proximal and Distal Phalangeal Joints

The phalangeal joints include the proximal interphalangeal joint (PIP) and the distal interphalangeal joints (DIP). Both joints have a fibrous capsule, collateral ligaments that stabilize lateral displacement, volar plates that stabilize against hyperextension forces, and additional soft tissue stabilization from muscle and fascia. Both joints are considered hinge joints and are important in manipulation of objects.

Numerous muscles in the hand are responsible for the complex and delicate movements required for grasp and manipulation of objects. Table 10.2 outlines the muscles and movements associated with the fingers and the distal hand.

The extensor mechanism of the hand is a complex mechanism of passive and active tension. Prime movement occurs through the insertion of the extensor

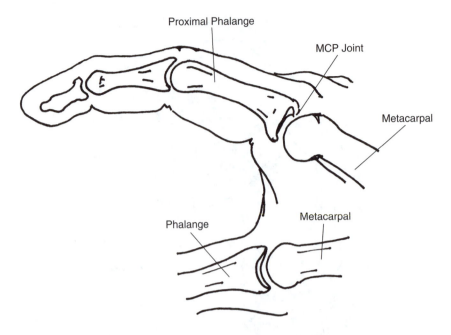

**Figure 10.13**    The Metacarpophalangeal Joints-Side View

**TABLE 10.2    Finger Motion**

| Muscle | Movement and Function | Joint Motion | Spinal Segment |
|---|---|---|---|
| Abductor digiti minimi | Abduction | Abduction of the 5th digit | C8-T1 |
| Dorsal interossei | Abduction, flex proximal, extend middle and distal phalanges | Extension of the PIP and DIP and abduction of the MCP | C8-T1 |
| Extensor digiti minimi | Extension | Isolated extension of the 5th digit | C6-C8 |
| Extensor digitorum | Extension | Extension of digits 2 to 5 | C6-C8 |
| Extensor indicis | Extension | Extension of the 2nd digit | C7-C8 |
| Flexor digiti minimi | Flex metacarpo-phalangeal joint | Isolated flexion of the 5th digit | C8-T1 |
| Flexor digiti profundus | Flex metacarpo-phalangeal, proximal, and distal interphalangeal joints | Flexion of the 2nd through 5th digits to the DIP | C8-T1 |
| Flexor digiti superficialis | Flex metacarpo-phalangeal and proximal interphalangeal joints | Flexion of the 2nd through the 5th digits to the PIP | C7-T1 |
| Lumbricals | Flex metacarpo-phalangeal joints, extend middle and distal phalanges | Flexion of the 2nd through 5th MCP and extension (in concert with other muscles) of the PIP and DIP of the 2nd through 5th digits | C7-C8 |
| Volar interossei | Adduction, flex proximal, extend middle and distal phalanges | Extension of the PIP and DIP and adduction of the MCP | C8-T1 |

**TABLE 10.3**    Thumb Muscles and Movements

| Muscle | Movement and Function | Joint Motion | Spinal Segment |
|---|---|---|---|
| Flexor pollicis brevis | Thumb flexion | 1st digits metacarpo-phalangeal flexion | C6-C7 |
| Flexor pollicis longus | Thumb flexion and some adduction | 1st digit interphalangeal flexion and slight adduction | C8-T1 |
| Extensor pollicis brevis | Thumb extension | 1st digit metacarpo-phalangeal extension | C6-C7 |
| Extensor pollicis longus | Thumb extension | 1st digit interphalangeal extension | C6-C7 |
| Adductor pollicis | Thumb adduction | CMC and PIP adduction | C8-T1 |
| Abductor pollicis brevis Abductor pollicis longus | Thumb abduction | CMC and PIP abduction | C8-T1 |
| Opponens pollicis Opponens digiti minimi | Thumb opposition | CMC and PIP opposition | C6-C7 |

digitorum comunis (and the extensor indicis and extensor digiti minimi at the second and fifth digits, respectively) in the dorsum of each phalanx just distal to the metacarpal–phalangeal (MCP) joint. This connection is responsible for extension of the MCP and contributes to the elaborate further extension of the proximal interphalangeal (PIP) and distal interphalangeal (DIP).[42] A central tendon proceeds from the extensor insertion to the base of the middle phalanx (just distal to the PIP) and contributes to extend the PIP. Structures called "lateral bands" receive tendinous attachments from the lumbricals and the interossei and create tension (during contraction) of the DIP. The oblique retinacular ligament creates passive tension on the DIP during PIP extension and subsequently extends the DIP.[43] Dysfunctions such as mallet finger (central insertion rupture at the DIP) and Boutonniere deformity (rupture of the central slip of the extensor tendon at the level of the proximal interphalangeal joint) can lead to the inability to straighten the finger at the middle joint or distal joint and subsequent contractures.

### The First Carpometacarpal Joint (The Thumb)

The articular surface of the thumb involves the contact of the trapezium and the first metacarpal. The first metacarpal conforms to the biplanar articular surface of the trapezium, creating a saddle joint with six degrees of freedom. This degree of freedom allows a great range of mobility in all directions so that the pad of the thumb can oppose any finger pad. Individually, the metacarpal-phalangeal joint of the thumb is capable of the movements of metacarpophalangeal flexion and extension, and interphalangeal flexion and extension. Conversely, the additional movements of abduction and adduction occur at the carpometacarpal joint through the interplay of numerous muscles (Table 10.3) such as the abductor pollicis brevis and longus, adductor and flexor pollicis, and extensor pollicis muscles (Figure 10.14).

## Summary

- There are numerous joints of the wrist/hand, too numerous to note.
- Joints at the wrist are typically described by location and are generally divided into the proximal carpal row, the mid-carpal row, and the distal carpal row.
- The joints of the hand are typically described by location and include the carpometacarpal, the metacarpal phalangeal, the proximal interphalangeal, and the distal interphalangeal joints.
- Movement at the wrist is coupled and depends on the complex interplay between the carpal bones.
- The carpometacarpal joint of the thumb has a biplanar articular surface of the trapezium, creating a saddle joint with six degrees of freedom.

# ASSESSMENT AND DIAGNOSIS

## Subjective Considerations

### Elbow Symptoms

A number of elbow-related symptoms may assist in identifying selected elbow impairments. To improve the ability of isolation of the disorder, it is best to categorize elbow impairments by location. Lateral elbow pain is commonly associated with lateral epicondalgia but requires differentiation from less common disorders such as radial tunnel syndrome or posterolateral rotary instability.[44] Additionally, patients who report a history of trauma require a diagnostic work-up to determine the presence of a radial head fracture, an injury that typically occurs during a fall on an outstretched forearm. Medial impairments of the

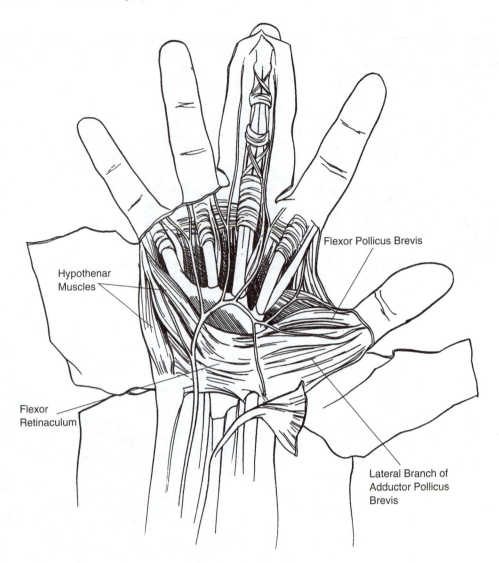

**Figure 10.14**    Hand and Thumb Muscles-Reflected

elbow include golfer's elbow, little leaguer's elbow, and cubital tunnel syndrome. Anterior problems at the elbow may include biceps bursitis or tumor. Lastly, posterior elbow pain may include olecranon bursitis, an olecranon fracture, or triceps tendonitis.

It is critical that a thorough patient history is performed to outline the potential causes and contributions to the elbow-related pain.[45] Cervical radiculopathy can masquerade as an impairment of the elbow. Selected elbow conditions can refer pain to the forearm and wrist/hand. Lateral epicondylitis may refer pain to the proximal forearm extensor muscle mass.[17] Additionally, in some fractures such as a humerus fracture, it is common to see radial and medial nerve trauma in adults more so than in children.[21]

## *Wrist/Hand Symptoms*

Patient report of wrist and hand symptoms provides the examiner with useful information, specifically in the capacity to differentiate selected forms of wrist/hand dys-function. Wrist fractures are relatively common and are generally associated with trauma. The most common fracture of the wrist is a scaphoid fracture, which involves an injury either by a fall on an outstretched hand or by a direct blow to the palm. A lunate fracture is relatively uncommon, is often reported as weakness of the wrist, and generally involves hyperextension of the wrist or impact to the heel of the hand during a fall. A triquetrum fracture is also injured during forced hyperextension but generally the wrist is placed in ulnar deviation versus the injury associated with radial deviation (scaphoid). A capitate fracture may occur during a fall on an outstretched hand with forced dorsiflexion and a degree of radial deviation of the wrist or during direct impact or a crush injury to the dorsum of the wrist.[46] Because of the difficulty with identifying the number of possible wrist-related fractures the use of a radiograph is essential when a traumatic history is present with poor improvement or reduction of symptoms over time.[47]

Inflammatory processes are common in patients with osteoarthritis or rheumatoid arthritis. Patients with these conditions often exhibit morning stiffness, disuse pain, and pain with extreme overuse.[40] Commonly, patients may complain of heat with erythema of selected joints. Complaints of pain with passive movement may be present during a number of dysfunctions including tenosynovitis, wrist instability, and arthritic conditions. Motor weakness is generally associated with muscular atrophy (if chronic) and may be a consequence of an upper motor neuron dysfunction or carpal tunnel syndrome.[40]

Symptoms associated with carpal tunnel syndrome (CTS) and other focal peripheral neuropathy include pain, numbness, and tingling in the distribution of the median nerve in at least two of the digits 1, 2, or 3, and the palm or dorsum of the hand.[48,49] These symptoms generally are present with or without pain and may radiate to the forearm, elbow, and shoulder.[49] CTS symptoms are usually worse at night and can awaken patients from sleep.[49–51]

Instability is associated with pain during or shortly after a recent injury to the wrist. Pain is frequently present during grasping wide objects, shaking hands, handling work tools, and other activities that require a power grip.[40] Often, the wrist will exhibit popping and cracking noises during movements.

## Psychosocial Factors

Psychosocial factors such as work stress, poor locus of control, poor social support, and elevated perceptions of work-related stress have been associated with increased subjective complaints of the upper extremity.[52] Henderson et al.[53] identified the prevalence of high pain intensity scores, depression, and helplessness covariates with the likelihood of reported carpal tunnel syndrome. Several studies have found common covariate traits among occupationally-related elbow, wrist, and hand injuries; the most significant were as follows. Individuals who indicated they had poor social support and limited peer contact were more likely to report elbow, wrist, and hand pain.[54–57] Job situations in which perceived high work demand was prevalent were also linked to report of wrist and hand symptoms.[55–57] Lastly, some report of lack of control, specifically during work-related demands, was also related to an increased risk of reporting hand-, elbow-, and wrist-related symptoms.[56]

## Functional Assessment Tools

The *Disability of the Arm, Shoulder and Hand Instrument* (DASH) is a relative region-specific outcome instrument that measures self-rated upper-extremity disability and symptoms. The questionnaire was designed to measure a number of conditions associated with activities of daily living that affect the shoulder, elbow, wrist, and hand.[58] The DASH has been validated on populations of shoulder-, elbow-, and wrist/hand-related dysfunction.[59] The DASH consists of a 30-item disability/symptom scale, scored 0 (no disability) to 100, and was originally introduced by the American Academy of Orthopedic Surgeons in collaboration with a number of other organizations.[60]

The *American Shoulder and Elbow Surgeons* (ASES) elbow form is designed to measure pain, disability, and patient satisfaction with the treatment associated with the patient's elbow pathology. The format includes a patient rating scale for pain (0–10), a Likert-type scale to measure function, and a 0–10 scale for measuring patient satisfaction. The scale has demonstrated good reliability, the responsiveness is unknown, and the measure appears to correlate well with physician-identified factors of physical examination.[61,62]

The *Boston Questionnaire* (BQ) is a self-administered, multidimensional[63] outcome instrument specific for use in carpal tunnel syndrome. The BQ has two sections, one that assesses symptoms such as pain and paraesthesia and the second that analyzes function associated with activities of daily living. The symptom severity scale consists of 11 questions whereas the functional status scale consists of eight questions. Each question has a 1–5 Likert-type scale, in which 1 indicates no symptom and 5 indicates severe symptoms.[64] The symptom severity scale assesses the symptoms with respect to severity, frequency, time, and type. The functional status scale assesses the effect of carpal tunnel syndrome on daily living. This questionnaire has been compared with many different outcome measures[65–67] and has been validated in other languages.[63,64,67] The Boston questionnaire is scored using a mean score for both symptom severity and functional status.

## *Summary*

- Conditions at the elbows are frequently described via location. Lateral elbow pain is commonly associated with lateral epicondalgia, radial tunnel syndrome, or posterolateral rotary instability. Medial impairments of the elbow include golfer's elbow, little leaguer's elbow, and cubital tunnel syndrome. Anterior problems at the elbow may include biceps bursitis or tumor. Lastly, posterior elbow pain may include olecranon bursitis, an olecranon fracture, or triceps tendonitis.
- Conditions at the wrist may include fractures (most common), instability, or inflammatory responses.
- Covariate psychosocial conditions have been associated with lateral elbow pain and carpal tunnel syndrome.
- The functional assessment tool known as the DASH (Disability of the Arm, Shoulder and Hand Instrument) is a valid measure of function for the regions of the shoulder, elbow, and wrist.

## Objective/Physical Examination

### *Observation*

The use of location of pain for differential diagnosis also does exhibit some merit. Conditions such as lateral epicondylitis use location of pain for two of the three diagnostic criteria: pain over the lateral epicondyle, tenderness over the same area, and exacerbation of pain by resisted wrist extension.[68,69] Medial epicondylitis is less investigated, but for diagnosis, also requires pain exhibition over the medial elbow (which may radiate distally or proximally), local tenderness, as well as pain aggravated by resisted wrist flexion with the forearm extended.[70]

A **hand diagram** has been frequently used for the diagnosis of carpal tunnel syndrome. Typically, this method of assessment demonstrates good sensitivity and very good specificity.[71–74] Symptom patterns from a hand diagram identified preoperatively are effective in predicting the outcome of carpal tunnel release and are independent of psychosocial covariates that may influence outcome.[75,76] Tenosynovitis of the first dorsal compartment is characterized by pain on the radial side of the wrist, impairment of thumb function, and thickening of the ligamentous structure covering the tendons in the first dorsal compartment of the wrist.[70]

Individuals with significant elbow effusion often hold his or her arm in a position of 70–80 degrees of flexion.[77] Additionally, swelling often increases joint fullness just distally to the lateral epicondyle of the humerus. Dislocations of the elbow present with prominence of the olecranon of the ulna or radial head since most elbow dislocations are posterior or posterior-lateral.[77] Olecranon bursitis is visible during extreme swelling and should be noted.

Observation may be useful in identifying hand dysfunction associated with resting position.[78] The resting attitude of the normal quiescent hand may identify an underlying pathology.[40] At rest, the hand demonstrates approximately 20–30 degrees of extension and 10–15 degrees of ulnar deviation.[79] The fingers and the thumb are slightly flexed and the palm demonstrates an arch that is progressively more flexed from radial to ulnar. Additionally, the fingers are more flexed as the digits progress ulnarly. Ulnar palsy is occasionally termed "bishop's hand" because the second and third digits maintain an extended posture whereas digits four and five are significantly flexed secondary to lack of intrinsic muscle innervation.[80] Flexor or extensor tendon ruptures generally result in a resting position of extension or flexion, respectively.[78] Radial nerve palsy results in the inability to actively extend the rest and a resting position of slight wrist flexion.[80] Medial nerve palsy results in weakness of the flexor pollicus longus and flexor digitorum profundus. During pinch tests the patient will exhibit pad-to-pad pinching and an inability to distally flex the interphalangeal joint.

Hand texture including color, moisture, edema, and atrophy require careful assessment. Absence of moisture on the distal phalanx may indicate a digital nerve injury.[78] Additionally, differences in skin color (blanched or hyperemic) or the inability to appropriately sweat at a localized region may also be related to a digital nerve dysfunction.[78] Edema may be associated with soft tissue–related injuries or a fracture and significant atrophy may be associated with an upper motor neuron lesion.[81,82]

### *Introspection*

It is intuitive to assume that most elbow, wrist, and hand injuries are associated with some form of trauma or overuse. Subsequently, careful attention to the lifestyle, occupation, and activities of the patient is required in order to fully comprehend the likely outcome for the patient. Effective orthopedic manual therapy may require strengthening, modification, and bracing as well as diligent assessment of potential proximal contributors such as the shoulder and cervical and thoracic spine.

## *Summary*

- The use of a pain diagram to outline the location of symptoms may be more useful for the hand than for the elbow.
- When examining a patient with elbow–wrist–hand injuries, it is imperative to evaluate the work performance requirements of the patient.
- Hand texture may assist in diagnosis of nerve-related impairments or fractures.

# Clinical Examination

## Active Physiological Movements

Active movements at the elbow may be limited by a number of pathological structures. Full ranges of extension are often limited either by the abnormalities in the olecranon process after a fracture, loose bodies associated with degeneration or trauma, edema, or by damage or compensatory changes in the anterior ligaments of the elbow. Full ranges of flexion can be limited by the damage to the coronoid process of the elbow, edema, excessive soft tissue of the anterior forearm and biceps, and specifically selected damage to the posterior and anterior ligaments.

The active movements at the wrist and hand are extremely complex and rarely involve isolated planar movements. It is necessary to watch for deviations during movements, substitution patterns, and recruitment of the elbow joint during limitations in active motion. It is also important to address wrist motions in patients with elbow pain since both joints house two joint muscle systems that can influence symptom reproduction.

Several nonmechanical pathologies can cause wrist and hand pain and must be differentiated during the clinical examination process. Pain may be associated with disease processes that affect the bone, cartilage, synovium, nerves, blood vessels, muscle, or connective tissue.[40] Neoplasms in the hand may arise insidiously, causing local swelling, pain, and dysfunction. A rare disorder, Reiter's syndrome, may cause symptoms associated with arthritis acutely, and can progress to fever, weight loss, and anorexia.[40] Lupis is more common than Reiter's syndrome and may cause swan neck deformities and ulnar deviation similar to rheumatoid arthritis. Scleroderma, a connective tissue dis-

order, may exhibit skin thickening or symptoms similar to arthritis. Disorders such as vasculitis, polychondritis, and septic infections can be differentiated with careful history and clinical examinations.

Goniometric range-of-motion values are important to consider at the elbow and the wrist/hand and have demonstrated reliability.[83–85] These measures generally involve single planar movements that are not necessarily the functional ranges of the elbow, wrist, and hand; however, loss of these movements has been associated with decline in perceived function.[86]

It is useful to perform the elbow wrist/hand examination at the same time because many structures contribute concurrently to elbow and wrist/hand pain. Throughout this chapter, elbow wrist/hand examination is performed concurrently, although there is a strong chance that structures may be isolated for pain.

## Active Elbow and Wrist Flexion

Normal values for active range of elbow flexion arc range from 0 degrees of extension to 140 degrees of flexion.[87–89] The carrying angle changes from valgus to varus, substantially altering the ability to assess resting carrying angle in patients with significant swelling.[90]

Active wrist flexion allows assessment of the proximal, mid-, and distal carpal joints, although it is hypothesized that the radiocarpal joint moves more substantially than the others.[91] Active restriction with pain may be associated with capsular restriction, a volar intercalated segmental instability or pain in the extensor structures of the forearm.

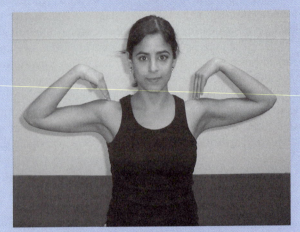

- Step One: The patient sits or stands. Resting symptoms are assessed.
- Step Two: It is beneficial to perform the movements bilaterally for observational assessment.
- Step Three: The patient is instructed to abduct his or her shoulder to approximately 90 degrees bilaterally.
- Step Four: The patient is instructed to flex his or her elbow and wrist to the first point of pain. Pain is assessed for the concordant sign.
- Step Five: The patient is instructed to move beyond the first point of pain toward end range. Pain is assessed to determine the effect on the concordant sign.

**Figure 10.15**   Elbow and Wrist Flexion

## Active Elbow and Wrist Extension

Active extension normally allows full extension or functional hyperextension.[87] The presence of heterotrophic ossification, osteophytes, or medial elbow tightness may limit the ability to move into full extension, as does joint edema. Nearly 50% of baseball players exhibit limitations in the ability to achieve full extension secondary to hypertrophy of the medial structures of the elbow.[87]

Active wrist extension also involves assessment of the proximal, mid-, and distal carpal joints and again it is hypothesized that the radiocarpal joint substantially moves more than the others.[91] This emphasis of movement is most likely associated with the biomechanical variability and complexity of the mid-carpal joint and the relative stability of the carpo–metacarpal complex.

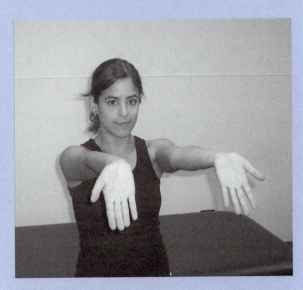

- Step One: The patient sits or stands. Resting symptoms are assessed.
- Step Two: It is beneficial to perform the movements bilaterally for observational assessment.
- Step Three: The patient is instructed to extend his or her elbow and wrist to the first point of pain. Pain is assessed for the concordant sign.
- Step Four: The patient is instructed to move beyond the first point of pain toward end range. Pain is assessed to determine the effect on the concordant sign.

**Figure 10.16**   Elbow, Wrist and Hand Extension

## Active Elbow and Wrist Supination and Pronation

Normal values of supination and pronation are 80–90 degrees when the elbow is held at 90 degrees of flexion.[87–89] Variations will occur with significant swelling at the elbow secondary to the shared capsule. Additionally, the inability to achieve 90 degrees of flexion may reduce the capacity to fully translate the radius with respect to the ulna, further altering movement.

Some degree of radial–ulnar supination is a product of wrist movement. Noticeable reductions of movement are associated with individual carpal bone fractures or dysfunction associated with carpal-to-carpal ligamentous groups. McGee[92] suggests that up to 20 degrees of the available supination range of motion is associated with wrist movement.

Since pronation requires lateral translation of the radius with respect to the ulna, a fair degree of mobility is required within the shared capsule and within the radial head. Like supination, some degree of radial–ulnar pronation is a product of wrist movement. McGee[92] suggests that up to 15 degrees of the available pronation range of motion is associated with wrist movement.

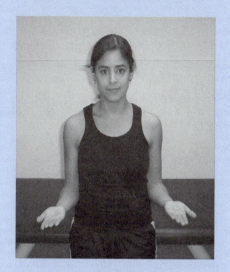

- Step One: The patient sits or stands. Resting symptoms are assessed.
- Step Two: It is beneficial to perform the movements bilaterally for observational assessment.
- Step Three: The patient is instructed to first flex the elbow to 90 degrees or the maximum available range of motion up to 90 degrees.
- Step Four: The patient is then instructed to supinate his or her elbow to the first point of pain. Pain is assessed for the concordant sign.
- Step Five: The patient is instructed to move beyond the first point of pain toward end range. Pain is assessed to determine the effect on the concordant sign.

**Figure 10.17**    Elbow and Wrist Supination

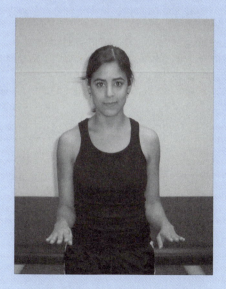

- Step Six: The patient is then instructed to pronate his or her elbow to the first point of pain. Pain is assessed for the concordant sign.
- Step Seven: The patient is instructed to move beyond the first point of pain toward end range. Pain is assessed to determine the effect on the concordant sign.

**Figure 10.18**    Elbow and Wrist Pronation

## Active Wrist Radial and Ulnar Deviation

Wrist radial and ulnar deviation is in some fashion a product of concurrent flexion and extension of the wrist. Radial deviation tends to couple with wrist extension and the end feel is generally restricted by the osseoligamentous structures of the carpal bones. Ulnar deviation tends to couple with wrist flexion. Like radial deviation the end feel associated with wrist ulnar deviation is generally restricted by the osseoligamentous structures of the carpal bones.

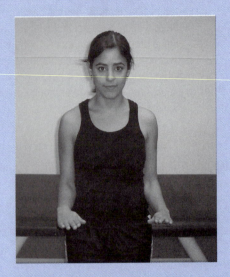

- Step One: The patient sits or stands. Resting symptoms are assessed.
- Step Two: The patient is instructed to flex elbow for prepositioning.
- Step Three: The patient is instructed to move in radial deviation to the first point of pain. The pain is assessed to determine if concordant.
- Step Four: The patient is then instructed to move beyond the first point of pain toward end range. Pain is assessed to determine the effect on the concordant sign.

**Figure 10.19**    Wrist Radial Deviation

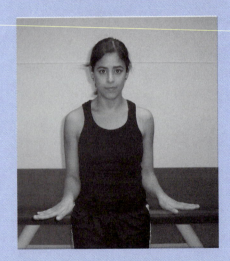

- Step Five: The patient is then instructed to move in ulnar deviation to the first point of pain. The pain is assessed to determine if concordant.
- Step Six: The patient is then instructed to move beyond the first point of pain toward end range. Pain is assessed to determine the effect on the concordant sign.
- Step Seven: It is beneficial to perform these motions bilaterally.

**Figure 10.20**    Wrist Ulnar Deviation

## Active Group Finger Flexion and Extension

Finger flexion requires the passive engagement of the finger extensors and the active engagement of the finger flexors (primarily the superficialis and profundus). Finger flexion should be symmetric and pain free in the undamaged hand.

The extensor mechanism of the fingers is a complex system of intercrossed fibers from the extensor digitorum communis, the extensor indicis, the lumbricals, and the first volar interosseous muscles. The fibers work in concert to create a hood structure over the dorsum of the finger that collectively extends the middle and distal interphalangeal joints.[93] Failure of the extensor mechanism may be the result of tightness in ligaments, disruption of the extensor tendon, or other phenomena.

- Step One: The patient sits or stands. Resting symptoms are assessed.
- Step Two: The patient is instructed to extend the wrist to neutral and elbow for prepositioning.
- Step Three: For finger flexion, the patient is instructed to concurrently flex his or her fingers to the first point of pain. The pain is assessed to determine if concordant.
- Step Four: The patient is then instructed to move beyond the first point of pain toward end range. Pain is assessed to determine the effect on the concordant sign.
- Step Five: For finger extension, the patient is instructed to concurrently extend his or her fingers to the first point of pain. The pain is assessed to determine if concordant.
- Step Six: The patient is then instructed to move beyond the first point of pain toward end range. Pain is assessed to determine the effect on the concordant sign.
- Step Seven: It is beneficial to perform these motions bilaterally.

## Active Group Finger Adduction and Abduction

Abduction at the thumb is produced by the abductor pollicis longus and abductor pollicis brevis. Finger abduction is produced by the dorsal interossei and the abductor digiti minimi. Thumb adduction is provided by the adductor pollicis whereas finger adduction is a product of palmar interossei contraction.

- Step One: The patient sits or stands. Resting symptoms are assessed.
- Step Two: The patient is instructed to extend the wrist to neutral for prepositioning.
- Step Three: For finger adduction, the patient is instructed to concurrently adduct his or her fingers against the adjacent fingers to the first point of pain. The pain is assessed to determine if concordant.
- Step Four: The patient is then instructed to move into further adduction beyond the first point of pain toward end range. Pain is assessed to determine the effect on the concordant sign.
- Step Five: The patient is instructed to extend the wrist to neutral for prepositioning.
- Step Six: For finger abduction, the patient is instructed to concurrently abduct his or her fingers to the first point of pain. The pain is assessed to determine if concordant.
- Step Seven: The patient is then instructed to move into further abduction beyond the first point of pain toward end range. Pain is assessed to determine the effect on the concordant sign.
- Step Eight: It is beneficial to perform these motions bilaterally.

## Functional Active Movements

Conventional wrist and hand assessment evaluates movements in single planes in isolated directions.[35] Actual movement of the wrist/hand involves coupled movements in multiple planes (Figures 10.21 and 10.22). These movements are generally considered more functional than single plane excursions.

Several studies have evaluated and proposed range-of-motion parameters for "functional" range at the wrist. Range-of-motion parameters are important measurement features of the wrist and have been associated with disability both functionally and through patient perception.[86] Generally, functional range-of-motion values of the wrist include 5–10 degrees of flexion, 15–30 degrees of extension,[94,95] 10 degrees of radial deviation, and 15 degrees of ulnar deviation.[94]

Hand movements involve a complex set of functional patterns to accomplish tasks such as grip and manipulation, and tasks that require dexterity. For the manual clinician, the inability to accomplish the following functional tasks, if associated with joint or soft tissue restrictions, may be an indication for range-of-motion gains. The clinician is encouraged to evaluate tip-to-tip and pad-to-pad movements as well as two different forms of gripping methods: power grip and narrow grip (Figures 10.23 and 10.24).

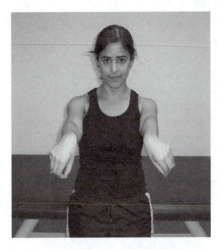

Figure 10.21    Coupled Flexion and Ulnar Deviation

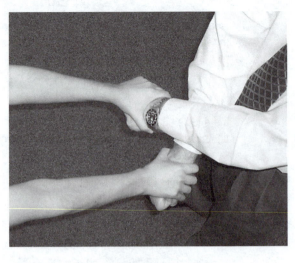

Figure 10.23    Power Grip Shake

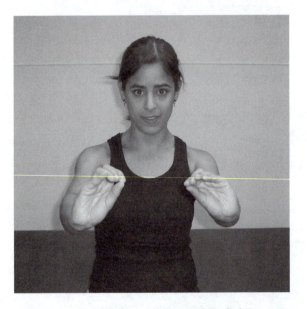

Figure 10.22    Coupled Extension and Radial Deviation

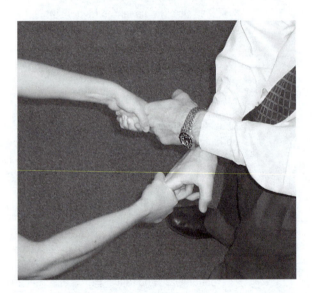

Figure 10.24    Narrow Grip Shake

## Summary

- Because of the multiple planes of movement associated with the elbow–wrist–hand, a general screen that examines general planar active movement is a quick method to identify movement dysfunction.
- Most wrist motion is coupled as is the elbow to a minor degree. When a movement is isolated as pathological to a specific joint, the coupled movements may benefit from assessment.
- Functional movements such as finite finger motions and power movements such as a grip or handshake provide the examiner with additional active assessment features.

## Passive Movements

### Passive and Combined Physiological Movements of the Elbow

Because combined movements are such a critical aspect of the elbow,[30] the passive examination procedures are presented in concert. The concerted presentation allows for a smoother examination and the ability to compare similar movements that may demonstrate concordant findings.

There are myriad potential causal structures for an elbow–wrist–hand dysfunction. Consequently, it is imperative that the clinician isolate the findings to a selected region, in order to more comprehensively passively examine the region. The most effective method of selection involves the judicious use of overpressure and the results of the overpressure in identifying the concordant pain.

## Passive Elbow Flexion

A significant amount of valgus to varus conversion occurs during extension to flexion movement. Additionally, it is likely that changes in pronation and supination will coexist with movements into flexion.

- Step One: The patient is placed in a supine position. The forearm is prepositioned in a supinated posture. Resting symptoms are assessed.
- Step Two: The clinician stabilizes the humerus of the patient by cupping the posterior aspect of the upper arm in his or her hand and supporting the upper arm on the plinth.
- Step Three: The clinician passively flexes the elbow to the first point of pain. The pain is assessed to determine if concordant.
- Step Four: The clinician passively flexes the elbow past the first point of pain. The pain is reassessed to determine if worse, better, or the same.

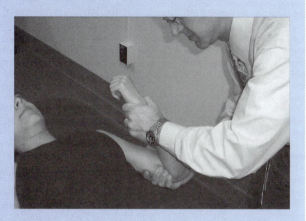

**Figure 10.25**    Passive Elbow Flexion

## Passive Elbow Flexion with Overpressure

Overpressure into flexion is necessary to truly isolate a flexion-based assessment. End feel in terminal flexion is generally soft associated with compression of soft tissues.

- Step One: At the limit of active elbow flexion, the clinician passively supplies an end range movement.
- Step Two: At the passive end range, a quick overpressure of sustained and/or repeated movements is supplied. Adjustments of force are appropriate specifically if prepositioning of valgus or varus is desired. Pain is assessed to determine the effect on the concordant sign.
- Step Three: Compression through the long axis of the lower arm is another potential tool used to sensitize the overpressure procedure.

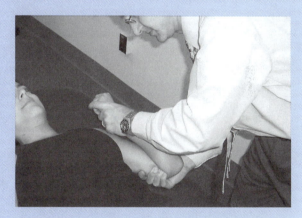

**Figure 10.26**    Elbow Flexion with Overpressure

## Passive Elbow Flexion with Varus and Valgus Force

A significant amount of valgus to varus conversion occurs during extension to flexion movement.[30] Passive elbow flexion with varus is the motion required during the combined movements of flexion and supination of the wrist. Passive elbow flexion with a valgus force is the motion required during the combined movements of extension and pronation of the wrist.

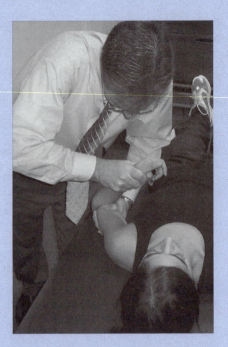

- Step One: The patient is placed in a supine position. The forearm is prepositioned in a supinated posture. Resting symptoms are assessed.
- Step Two: The clinician stabilizes the humerus of the patient by cupping the posterior aspect of the upper arm in his or her hand and supporting the upper arm on the plinth. To reduce potential internal rotation at the shoulder, the arm is prepositioned in slight external rotation.
- Step Three: The clinician passively and concurrently flexes and places a varus force at the elbow to the first point of pain. The pain is assessed to determine if concordant.
- Step Four: The clinician passively and concurrently flexes and places a varus force at the elbow past the first point of pain. The pain is reassessed to determine if worse, better, or the same.

**Figure 10.27**    Passive Elbow Flexion with a Varus Force

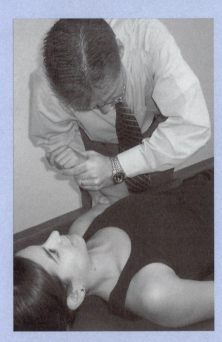

- Step Five: To reduce potential external rotation at the shoulder during flexion and a valgus force, the arm is prepositioned in slight internal rotation.
- Step Six: The clinician passively and concurrently flexes and places a valgus force at the elbow to the first point of pain. The pain is assessed to determine if concordant.
- Step Seven: The clinician passively and concurrently flexes and places a valgus force at the elbow past the first point of pain. The pain is reassessed to determine if worse, better, or the same.

**Figure 10.28**    Passive Elbow Flexion with a Valgus Force

## Passive Elbow Extension

Passive elbow extension may be limited by the presence of heterotrophic ossification, edema, osteophytes, or medial elbow tightness.

- Step One: The patient is positioned in supine. Resting symptoms are assessed.
- Step Two: The clinician places his or her forearm over the anterior aspect of the shoulder and loops his or her wrist around the posterior aspect of the distal humerus. This creates a stable support at the elbow joint and reduces the tendency of the shoulder to rise during elbow extension.
- Step Three: The clinician then passively moves the elbow into extension to the first point of pain. The pain is assessed to determine if concordant.
- Step Four: The clinician then passively moves the elbow beyond the first point of pain to determine the effect of further range of motion on the symptoms.

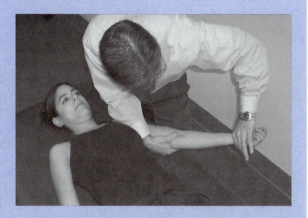

**Figure 10.29**    Passive Elbow Extension

## Passive Elbow Extension with Overpressure

Overpressure is necessary to rule out the presence of pain during extension. A bony end feel is associated with the olecranon block; a softer end feel generally means a ligamentous block. An empty end feel may be associated with pain, fear, or significant swelling.

- Step One: At the limit of passive physiological elbow extension, the clinician passively supplies an end range movement.
- Step Two: At the passive end range, a quick overpressure of sustained and/or repeated movements is supplied. Adjustments of force are appropriate specifically if prepositioning of valgus or varus is desired. Pain is assessed to determine the effect on the concordant sign.
- Step Three: Compression through the long axis of the lower arm is another potential tool used to sensitize the overpressure procedure.

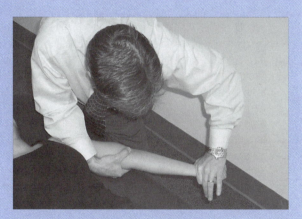

**Figure 10.30**    Elbow Extension with Overpressure

## Passive Elbow Extension with a Varus and Valgus Force

Passive elbow extension with a varus force is the motion required for the combined movements of extension and pronation.[30] Passive elbow extension with a valgus force is the motion required for the combined movements of extension and supination.

- Step One: The patient is positioned in supine. Resting symptoms are assessed.
- Step Two: The clinician places his or her forearm over the anterior aspect of the shoulder and loops his or her wrist around the posterior aspect of the distal humerus. This creates a stable support at the elbow joint and reduces the tendency of the shoulder to rise during elbow extension. To reduce the tendency of shoulder internal rotation, the upper arm is prepositioned into slight external rotation.
- Step Three: The clinician then passively moves the elbow into extension and a varus force to the first point of pain. The pain is assessed to determine if concordant.
- Step Four: The clinician then passively moves the elbow beyond the first point of pain to determine the effect of further range of motion on the symptoms.

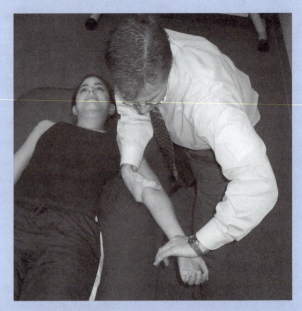

**Figure 10.31**    Elbow Extension with Varus

- Step Five: For assessment of elbow extension with a valgus force, the clinician places his or her forearm over the anterior aspect of the shoulder and loops his or her wrist around the posterior upper arm of the patient. This creates a stable support at the elbow joint and reduces the tendency of the shoulder to rise during elbow extension. To reduce the tendency of shoulder external rotation, the upper arm is prepositioned into slight internal rotation.
- Step Six: The clinician then passively moves the elbow into extension and a valgus force to the first point of pain. The pain is assessed to determine if concordant.
- Step Seven: The clinician then passively moves the elbow beyond the first point of pain to determine the effect of further range of motion on the symptoms.

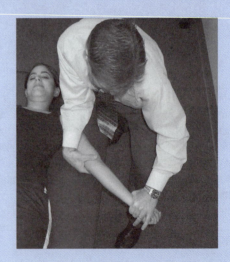

**Figure 10.32**    Elbow Extension with Valgus

## Passive Physiological Supination

Both supination and pronation involve movement at the proximal and distal radioulnar joint and movement within the wrist carpals. To ensure specific assessment of the proximal and distal radioulnar joint, the contact point for the clinician should be proximal to the radiocarpal row.

- Step One: The patient is positioned in supine. Resting symptoms are assessed.
- Step Two: The clinician flexes the elbow to 90 degrees and stabilizes the distal wrist using an adduction grasp between the thumb and index finger.
- Step Three: The clinician then slowly rotates the radioulnar joint into supination to the first point of pain. Pain is assessed to determine if concordant.
- Step Four: The clinician then slowly rotates past the first point of pain into further supination. If painful, the clinician may provide repeated motions or sustained holds to determine the outcome.

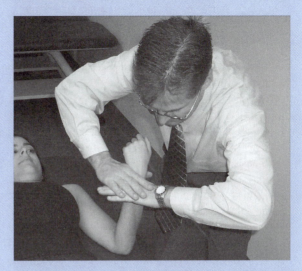

**Figure 10.33** Proximal and Distal Radioulnar Supination

### Passive Wrist Supination

Up to 20–30% of forearm supination is a product of carpal joint movements. The movements may occur at the proximal row (predominantly), mid-carpal row (less predominant), or carpo-metacarpal junctions (even less pre-dominant). To differentiate between carpal contributions it is essential to assess each row individually if supination was concordant during active movements.

## Proximal Row Supination

Supination of the proximal row requires the stabilization of the radius and ulna while performing supination of the proximal carpal row.

- Step One: The patient is positioned in supine. Resting symptoms are assessed.
- Step Two: The clinician flexes the elbow to 90 degrees and stabilizes the radius and ulnar using an adduction grasp between the thumb and index finger of one hand and places the other hand around the proximal carpal row of the wrist.
- Step Three: The clinician passively moves the proximal carpal row into supination while stabilizing the radius and the ulna. Movement is stopped at the first point of pain and pain is assessed to determine if concordant.
- Step Four: The clinician then passively moves the proximal row further into supination to determine the effect on pain. The clinician may apply repeated movements or a sustained hold to determine the effect.
- Step Five: If the passive movement is not painful, overpressure is applied to the movement.

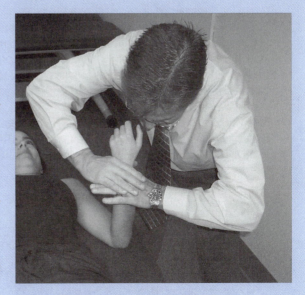

**Figure 10.34** Proximal Row Supination

## Mid-Carpal Joint Supination

Assessment of the mid-carpal row requires the stabilization of the proximal row during subsequent movement of the distal row into supination.

- Step One: The patient is positioned in supine. Resting symptoms are assessed.
- Step Two: The clinician flexes the elbow to 90 degrees and stabilizes the proximal carpal bones using an adduction grasp between the thumb and index finger of one hand and places the other hand around the distal carpal row of the wrist.
- Step Three: The clinician passively moves the distal carpal row into supination while stabilizing the proximal carpal row. Movement is stopped at the first point of pain and pain is assessed to determine if concordant.
- Step Four: The clinician then passively moves the distal row further into supination to determine the effect on pain. The clinician may apply repeated movements or a sustained hold to determine the effect.
- Step Five: If the passive movement is not painful, overpressure is applied to the movement.

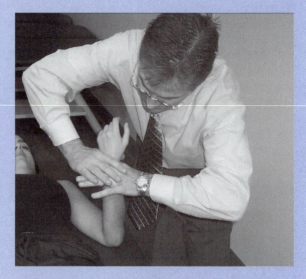

**Figure 10.35**   Mid-carpal Row Supination

## Passive Carpo-metacarpals Wrist Supination

The carpo-metaphalangeal joint, which also contributes to supination, must be isolated for appropriate assessment.

- Step One: The patient is positioned in supine. Resting symptoms are assessed.
- Step Two: The clinician flexes the elbow to 90 degrees and stabilizes the proximal and distal carpal bones using an adduction grasp between the thumb and index finger of one hand and places the other hand around the metacarpals of the hand.
- Step Three: The clinician passively moves the metacarpals of the hand into supination while stabilizing the proximal and distal carpals. Movement is stopped at the first point of pain and pain is assessed to determine if concordant.
- Step Four: The clinician then passively moves the metacarpals further into supination to determine the effect on pain. The clinician may apply repeated movements or a sustained hold to determine the effect.
- Step Five: If the passive movement is not painful, overpressure is applied to the movement.

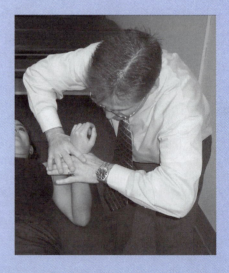

**Figure 10.36**   Carpo-metacarpals Wrist Supination

Overpressure is necessary to isolate supinatory motion. Careful attention must be made to apply the overpressure to end range since myriad structures contribute to guiding and stabilizing the motion of supination and resistance is often encountered early during active movement. The overpressure movements are similar to those that distinguish general supination, radiocarpal, mid-carpal, and CMC movements as previously described.

## Passive Physiological Elbow Pronation

To ensure specific assessment of the proximal and distal radioulnar joint, the contact point for the clinician should be proximal to the radiocarpal row.

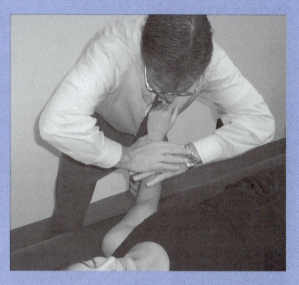

- Step One: The patient is positioned in supine. Resting symptoms are assessed.
- Step Two: The clinician flexes the elbow to 90 degrees and stabilizes the distal wrist at the radius and the ulna using an adduction grasp between the thumb and index finger.
- Step Three: The clinician then slowly rotates the radioulnar joints into pronation to the first point of pain. Pain is assessed to determine if concordant.
- Step Four: The clinician then slowly rotates past the first point of pain into further pronation. If painful, the clinician may provide repeated motions or sustained holds to determine the outcome.
- Step Five: If the passive movement is not painful, overpressure is applied to the movement.

**Figure 10.37**    Proximal and Distal Radioulnar Pronation

## Passive Proximal Row Pronation

Isolated pronation of the proximal row requires the stabilization of the radius and ulna while performing pronation of the proximal carpal row.

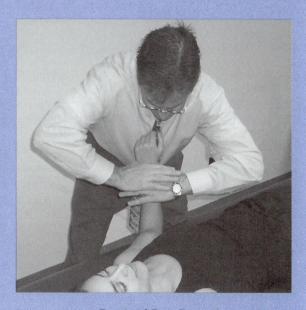

- Step One: The patient is positioned in supine. Resting symptoms are assessed.
- Step Two: The clinician flexes the elbow to 90 degrees and stabilizes the distal wrist using an adduction grasp between the thumb and index finger of one hand and places the other hand around the proximal carpal row of the wrist.
- Step Three: The clinician passively moves the proximal carpal row into pronation while stabilizing the radius. Movement is stopped at the first point of pain and pain is assessed to determine if concordant.
- Step Four: The clinician then passively moves the proximal row further into pronation on the radius to determine the effect on pain. The clinician may apply repeated movements or a sustained hold to determine the effect.
- Step Five: If the passive movement is not painful, overpressure is applied to the movement.

**Figure 10.38**    Proximal Row Pronation

## Passive Mid-Carpal Wrist Pronation

Assessment of the mid-carpal row requires the stabilization of the proximal row during subsequent movement of the distal row into pronation.

- Step One: The patient is positioned in supine. Resting symptoms are assessed.
- Step Two: The clinician flexes the elbow to 90 degrees and stabilizes the proximal carpal bones using an adduction grasp between the thumb and index finger of one hand and places the other hand around the distal carpal row of the wrist.
- Step Three: The clinician passively moves the distal carpal row into pronation while stabilizing the proximal carpal row. Movement is stopped at the first point of pain and pain is assessed to determine if concordant.
- Step Four: The clinician then passively moves the distal row further into pronation to determine the effect on pain. The clinician may apply repeated movements or a sustained hold to determine the effect.
- Step Five: If the passive movement is not painful, overpressure is applied to the movement.

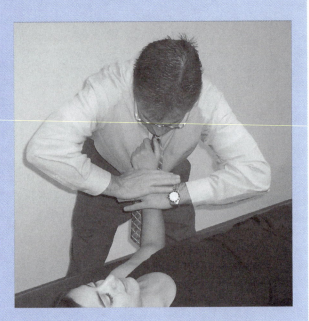

**Figure 10.39**    Mid-Carpal Row Pronation

## Passive Carpo-metacarpals Wrist Pronation

Lastly, the carpo-metaphalangeal joint, which also contributes to pronation, must be isolated for appropriate assessment.

- Step One: The patient is positioned in supine. Resting symptoms are assessed.
- Step Two: The clinician flexes the elbow to 90 degrees and stabilizes the proximal and distal carpal bones using an adduction grasp between the thumb and index finger of one hand and places the other hand around the metacarpals of the hand.
- Step Three: The clinician passively moves the metacarpals of the hand into supination while stabilizing the proximal and distal carpals. Movement is stopped at the first point of pain and pain is assessed to determine if concordant.
- Step Four: The clinician then passively moves the metacarpals further into pronation to determine the effect on pain. The clinician may apply repeated movements or a sustained hold to determine the effect.
- Step Five: If the passive movement is not painful, overpressure is applied to the movement.

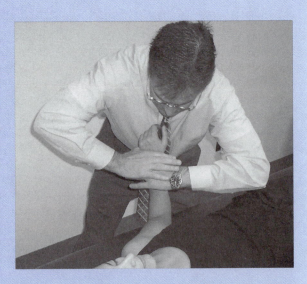

**Figure 10.40**    Carpo-metacarpals Wrist Pronation

## *Passive and Combined Physiological Movements of the Wrist and Hand*

Because combined movements are such a critical aspect of the wrist and hand, the passive examination procedures are presented in concert. The concerted presentation allows for a smoother examination and the ability to compare similar movements that may demonstrate concordant findings.

---

### Passive Physiological Wrist Flexion

Pain associated with wrist instability such as a VISI is typically reproduced during passive flexion or extension of the wrist during focused movements of the metacarpals.[40] Wrist flexion often involves the combined movements of flexion, ulnar deviation, and supination. Single plane movements such as isolated flexion, extension, and ulnar and radial deviation may require advanced assessment of combined movements if the single movements are concordant.

 Because of the elasticity of the forearm extensor muscles and the contribution of these muscles to the mobility of wrist flexion, significant diligence should be used to ensure end range overpressure assessment. Resistance is encountered early in wrist flexion and overpressure at midranges may fail to implicate actual pathology isolated at this junction.

- Step One: The patient is positioned in supine. Resting symptoms are assessed.
- Step Two: The clinician flexes the elbow to 90 degrees and stabilizes the radius on the palmar aspect of the wrist with one hand while the other secures the dorsal aspect of the wrist.
- Step Three: The clinician passively moves the wrist into flexion. Movement is stopped at the first point of pain and pain is assessed to determine if concordant.
- Step Four: The clinician then passively moves the wrist further into flexion to determine the effect on pain. The clinician may apply repeated movements or a sustained hold to determine the effect.
- Step Five: At the limit of active wrist flexion, the clinician passively supplies an end range movement of overpressure into further flexion.

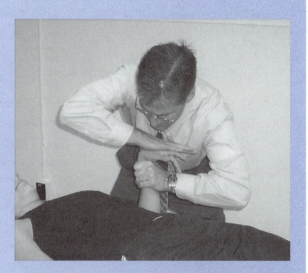

**Figure 10.41**    Passive Physiological Wrist Flexion

## Passive Wrist Extension

Pain associated with wrist instability such as a DISI is typically reproduced during passive flexion or extension of the wrist during focused movements of the metacarpals.[40] Wrist extension promotes the combined movements of extension, pronation, and radial deviation. Painful single plane movements of extension may require advanced assessment of combined movements if concordant. As with wrist flexion overpressure assessment, the end range of wrist extension encounters significant resistance providing false suggestions of actual end feel.

- Step One: The patient is positioned in supine. Resting symptoms are assessed.
- Step Two: The clinician flexes the elbow to 90 degrees and stabilizes the radius on the dorsal aspect of the wrist with one hand while the other secures the palmar aspect of the wrist.
- Step Three: The clinician passively moves the wrist into extension. Movement is stopped at the first point of pain and pain is assessed to determine if concordant.
- Step Four: The clinician then passively moves the wrist further into extension to determine the effect on pain. The clinician may apply repeated movements or a sustained hold to determine the effect.
- Step Five: At the limit of active wrist extension, the clinician passively supplies an end range movement of overpressure into further extension.

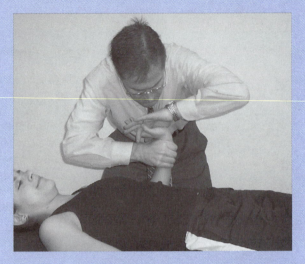

**Figure 10.42** Passive Physiological Wrist Extension

## Passive Ulnar and Radial Deviation

Limitation of ulnar and radial deviation is commonly associated with intercarpal restrictions, fractures, or other capsular injuries. Overpressure into ulnar deviation is required to clear this planar movement and because ulnar movement is frequently coupled with flexion, it is common to see some concurrent discomfort with flexion and ulnar deviation. Because radial movement is frequently coupled with extension, it is common to see some concurrent discomfort with extension and radial deviation.

- Step One: The patient is positioned in supine. Resting symptoms are assessed.
- Step Two: The clinician flexes the elbow to 90 degrees and stabilizes the wrist on the ulnar aspect with one hand while the other secures the radial aspect of the wrist and hand.
- Step Three: The clinician passively moves the wrist into ulnar deviation. Movement is stopped at the first point of pain and pain is assessed to determine if concordant.
- Step Four: The clinician then passively moves the wrist further into ulnar deviation to determine the effect on pain. The clinician may apply repeated movements or a sustained hold to determine the effect.
- Step Five: At the limit of active wrist ulnar deviation and if the passive movement does not produce pain, the clinician passively supplies an end range movement of overpressure.

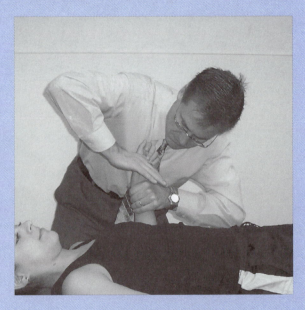

**Figure 10.43** Passive Physiological Ulnar Deviation of the Wrist

328

- Step Six: For radial deviation, the clinician flexes the elbow to 90 degrees and stabilizes the wrist on the radial aspect with one hand while the other secures the ulnar aspect of the wrist and hand.
- Step Seven: The clinician passively moves the wrist into radial deviation. Movement is stopped at the first point of pain and pain is assessed to determine if concordant.
- Step Eight: The clinician then passively moves the wrist further into radial deviation to determine the effect on pain. The clinician may apply repeated movements or a sustained hold to determine the effect.
- Step Nine: At the limit of active wrist radial deviation and if the passive movement does not produce pain, the clinician passively supplies an end range movement of overpressure.

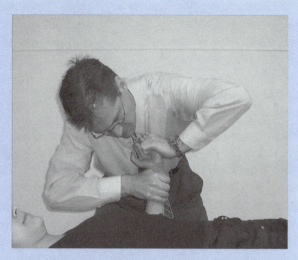

**Figure 10.44**    Passive Physiological Radial Deviation of the Wrist

## Passive Movements of the Carpo-metacarpal Extension and Flexion

The movements associated with the carpometacarpal joints of the second through fifth digits are minimal but necessary. Along with the previous assessments of pronation and supination of this region, flexion and extension may provide further isolation of the concordant impairment of the wrist/hand.

Because the joint is inherently stable and is difficult to isolate, a counter point procedure is necessary for passive physiological assessment.

- Step One: The patient is positioned in supine. Resting symptoms are assessed.
- Step Two: The clinician flexes the elbow to 90 degrees and stabilizes the wrist in neutral at the proximal and mid-carpal joints.
- Step Three: Using the other hand the clinician applies a counter point procedure by applying an extension movement at the carpo-metacarpal (CMC) joint. For CMC extension, the clinician's thumb applies a palmar movement just distal to the CMC while the hand applies a dorsal movement at the distal aspect of the metacarpal.
- Step Four: The procedure is repeated at the second through fifth digits using appropriate repeated motions and overpressure if warranted.

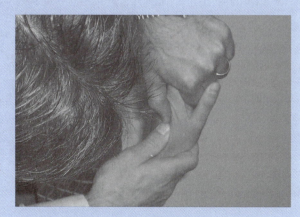

**Figure 10.45**    CMC Extension of the Second through Fifth Digits

*(continued)*

- Step Five: For CMC flexion, the clinician's thumbs apply a dorsal movement just distal to the CMC while the hand applies a palmar movement at the distal aspect of the metacarpal.
- Step Six: The procedure is repeated at the second through fifth digits using appropriate repeated motions and overpressure if warranted.

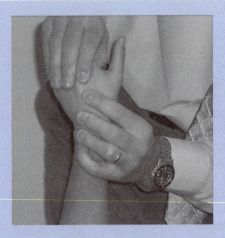

**Figure 10.46**    CMC Flexion of the Second through Fifth Digits

## Passive Physiological Flexion and Adduction of the Thumb

The articular complex of the first CMC joint (the thumb) allows multiple variations of physiological movements. The movements of flexion and adduction, although different, share a common end point just adjacent and flush to the second metacarpal. It is uncommon to see physiological restrictions of these movements.

- Step One: The patient is positioned in supine. Resting symptoms are assessed.
- Step Two: Using one hand, the clinician can stabilize the trapezium of the wrist to isolate movement to the CMC and distal joints of the thumb. If physiological movement without stabilization is solicited, no stabilization of the trapezium is necessary.
- Step Three: From a starting point of thumb extension or abduction, the thumb is passively moved medially toward the second metacarpal. Movement is stopped at the first point of pain. The pain is assessed to determine if concordant.
- Step Four: As with the previous assessments, repeated movements or end range movements are used to determine if movement is a helpful treatment option.

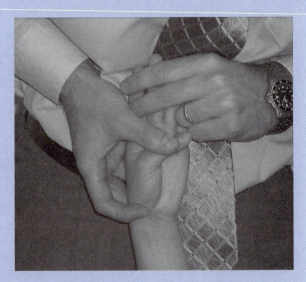

**Figure 10.47**    Passive Physiological Flexion/ Adduction of the Thumb

## Passive Physiological Extension and Abduction of the Thumb

Passive extension of the thumb is limited by the volar and radial structures of the hand. Passive extension occurs in the coronal plane while passive abduction occurs in the sagittal plane. PIP extension and abduction may be limited during disease processes such as arthritis or sepsis.

- Step One: The patient is positioned in supine. Resting symptoms are assessed.
- Step Two: Using one hand, the clinician stabilizes the trapezium (if desired) of the wrist to isolate movement to the CMC and distal joints of the thumb. If movement specific to the distal segments is desired the stabilization force should move proximal to the proximal aspects of the PIP and the DIP.
- Step Three: For thumb extension the starting point should be thumb flexion. The thumb is passively moved within the coronal plane toward extension. Movement is stopped at the first complaint of pain. If painful the complaint is assessed to determine if concordant.
- Step Four: As with the previous assessments, repeated movements or end range movements are used to determine if this movement is a helpful treatment option. Overpressures are required to rule out the joints of the thumb and the opposite side should be tested if appropriate.

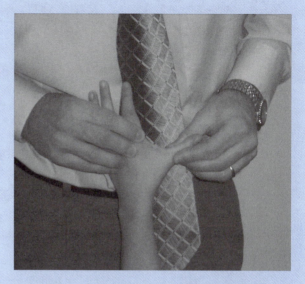

**Figure 10.48**  Passive Physiological Extension and Abduction of the Thumb

## Passive Physiological Abduction of the Thumb

- Step One: For thumb abduction the starting point for motion should be thumb adduction.
- Step Two: Using one hand, the clinician stabilizes the trapezium (if desired) of the wrist to isolated movement to the CMC and distal joints of the thumb. If movement specific to the distal segments is desired the stabilization force should move proximal to the proximal aspects of the PIP and the DIP.
- Step Three: From a starting point of thumb flexion, the thumb is passively moved within the sagittal plane toward abduction. Movement is stopped at the first complaint of pain. If painful the complaint is assessed to determine if concordant.
- Step Four: As with the previous assessments, repeated movements or end range movements are used to determine if this movement is a helpful treatment option. Overpressures are required to rule out the joints of the thumb and the opposite side should be tested if appropriate.

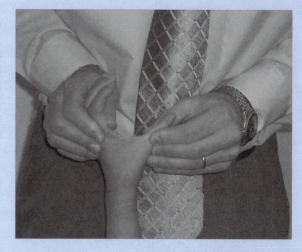

**Figure 10.49**  Passive Physiological Abduction of the Thumb

## Passive Physiological MCP Flexion and Extension

Manipulation of small objects requires the coupled movements of MCP flexion/extension, rotation, and abduction/adduction. Rotation occurs primarily in extension but assessment in selected degrees of flexion may also be beneficial.

Flexion of the MCP joints of digits 2 through 5 reduces the simultaneous movements of abduction/ adduction and rotation of the same joint. "Joint play," subsequently, is greater during MCP extension, introducing an increased frequency of MCP flexion restrictions versus extension restrictions.

### Passive Physiological Flexion of the MCP

- Step One: The patient is positioned in supine. Resting symptoms are assessed.
- Step Two: Using one hand, the clinician individually grasps the distal aspect of the metacarpal of digits 2 through 5 depending on where the desired movement is required.
- Step Three: rom a starting point of extension, the proximal phalange (and subsequent middle and distal phalange) is moved into flexion while concurrently stabilizing the articulating metacarpal. Movement is stopped upon the first point of pain. Any pain is assessed to determine if concordant.
- Step Four: As with the previous assessments, repeated movements or end range movements are used to determine if this movement is a helpful treatment option. Overpressures are required to rule out the movement.

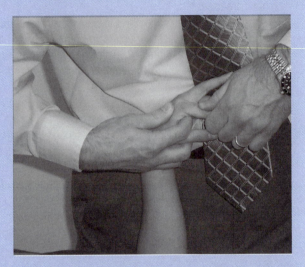

**Figure 10.50**    Passive Physiological Flexion of the MCP

- Step Five: For MCP extension the MCP is prepositioned into flexion. From a starting point of flexion, the proximal phalange (and subsequent middle and distal phalange) is moved into extension while concurrently stabilizing the distal metacarpal. Movement is stopped upon the first point of pain. Any pain is assessed to determine if concordant.
- Step Six: As with the previous assessments, repeated movements or end range movements are used to determine if this movement is a helpful treatment option. Overpressures are required to rule out the guilt of the movement.

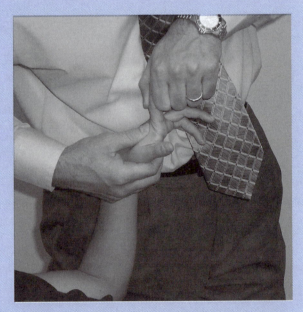

**Figure 10.51**    Passive Physiological Extension of the MCP

**MCP Rotation (in extension)**

- Step One: The patient is positioned in supine. Resting symptoms are assessed.
- Step Two: Using one hand, the clinician individually grasps the distal aspect of the metacarpal of digits 2 through 5 depending on where the desired movement is required. The metacarpal is stabilized distally.
- Step Three: The PIP is prepositioned into flexion allowing a sturdy structure for grasp by the clinician.
- Step Four: Rotation into both directions is applied to the first point of pain. Pain is assessed to determine if concordant.

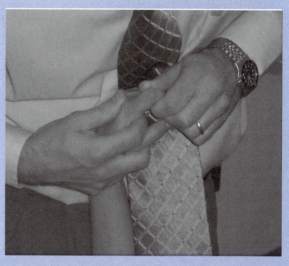

**Figure 10.52**     Passive Physiological Rotation of the MCP

**MCP Abduction and Adduction**

- Step One: Using one hand, the clinician individually grasps the distal aspect of the metacarpal of digits 2 through 5 depending on where the desired movement is required.
- Step Two: The PIP may be prepositioned into flexion allowing a sturdy structure for grasp by the clinician, although maintaining extension will not affect the abduction or adduction.
- Step Three: Abduction and subsequent adduction is applied to the first point of pain. Pain is assessed to determine if concordant.
- Step Four: Repeated movements, end range holds, and overpressures may be necessary to further distal information regarding the joint.

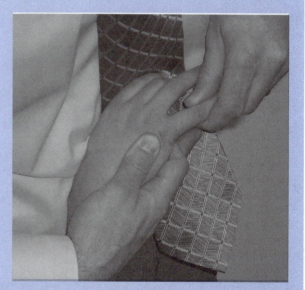

**Figure 10.53**     Passive Physiological Abduction and Adduction of the MCP

## PIP and DIP Flexion and Extension

Restriction into PIP flexion may occur secondary to tightness in the lateral and dorsal structures of the second through fifth digits. Restrictions of extension may be associated with tightness of the volar plate of the finger or tightness in the oblique lateral ligaments of the finger.

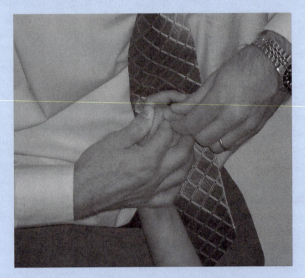

**Figure 10.54**    Passive Physiological PIP Flexion and Extension

- Step One: The patient is positioned in supine. Resting symptoms are assessed.
- Step Two: Using one hand, the clinician individually grasps the distal aspect of the proximal phalange, just proximal to the PIP. Using the opposite hand, the clinician grasps the middle phalange. For the DIP, the clinician individually grasps distal aspect of the middle phalange, just proximal to the DIP. Using the opposite hand, the clinician grasps the distal phalange just distal to the DIP.

- Step Three: Flexion and subsequent extension are performed to the PIP and DIP. Movement is restricted to the first point of pain. Pain is assessed to determine if concordant.
- Step Four: Repeated movements, end range holds, and overpressures may be necessary to further distal information regarding the joint.

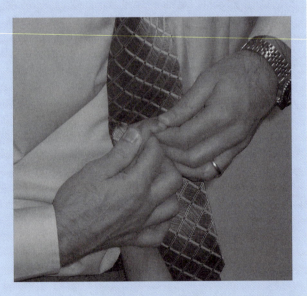

**Figure 10.55**    Passive Physiological DIP Flexion and Extension

## *Passive Accessory Movements of the Elbow*

### Posterior Anterior (PA) of the Humeroulnar Joint

A PA of the humeroulnar joint most likely is a combination of physiological and slight accessory movement. The congruence of the humeroulnar joint reduces the plausibility of a direct PA motion because the olecranon will compress against the humerus.

- Step One: The patient is positioned in prone. The arm is placed in a preposition of extension at the side of the patient. Baseline symptoms are assessed.
- Step Two: The anterior aspect of the arm is cradled by the fingers of the clinician. The thumbs are placed on the posterior aspect of the olecranon using a pad-to-pad placement.
- Step Three: The clinician applies a combined movement of lifting the anterior aspect of the arm while applying a posterior–anterior force to the olecranon of the elbow. The clinician pushes to the first point of pain. Pain is assessed to determine if concordant.
- Step Four: The clinician then applies a PA force beyond the first point of pain toward end range. Sustained holds or repeated movements are performed to determine the effect on the patient's condition.

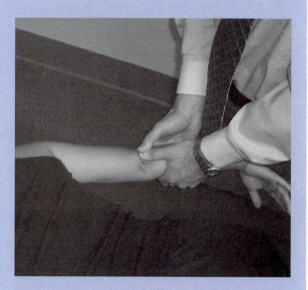

**Figure 10.56**    Posterior Anterior of the Humeroulnar Joint

### Posterior Anterior (PA) of the Humeroradial Joint

Though less common, an isolated impairment to the humeroradial joint can restrict full extension. Additionally, a PA to the humeroradial joint may be beneficial if the patient exhibits complaints during the combined movements of extension and supination.

- Step One: The anterior aspect of the arm is cradled by the fingers of the clinician. The thumbs are placed on the posterior–lateral aspect of the radial head using a pad-to-pad placement.
- Step Two: The clinician applies a combined movement of lifting the anterior aspect of the arm while applying a posterior–anterior force to the elbow. The clinician pushes to the first point of pain. Pain is assessed to determine if concordant.
- Step Three: The clinician then applies a PA force beyond the first point of pain toward end range. Sustained holds or repeated movements are performed to determine the effect on the patient's condition.
- Step Four: The opposite side is assessed if appropriate.

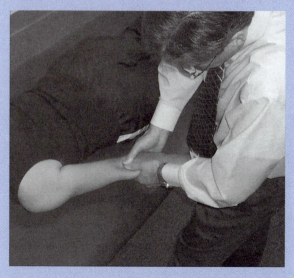

**Figure 10.57**    Posterior Anterior of the Humeroradial Joint

## Anterior Posterior (AP) of the Humeroulnar Joint

The congruent articular arrangement of the humeroulnar joint reduces the amount of passive joint play. Essentially, the majority of the movement at this joint is a traction-based movement where the ulna is distracted from the convex humerus.

- Step One: The patient is positioned in supine. The arm is placed in a preposition of flexion at the side of the patient. Baseline symptoms are assessed.
- Step Two: The posterior aspect of the arm is cradled by the fingers of the clinician. The thumbs are placed on the anterior aspect of the ulna through the soft tissue of the brachium.
- Step Three: The clinician applies a combined movement of lifting the posterior aspect of the forearm while applying an anterior-to-posterior force to the anterior aspect of the ulna. The clinician pushes to the first point of pain. Pain is assessed to determine if concordant.
- Step Four: The clinician then applies an AP force beyond the first point of pain toward end range. Sustained holds or repeated movements are performed to determine the effect on the patient's condition.

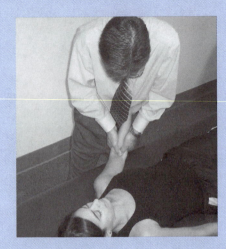

**Figure 10.58**    Anterior Posterior of the Humeroulnar Joint

## Anterior Posterior (AP) of the Humeroradial Joint

An AP of the humeroradial joint may be effective if the patient exhibits restrictions in the combined movements of flexion and pronation.

- Step One: The posterior aspect of the arm is cradled by the fingers of the clinician. The thumbs are placed on the anterior aspect of the radial head through the soft tissue of the anterior aspect of the extensor group.
- Step Two: The clinician applies a combined movement of lifting the posterior aspect of the arm while applying an anterior-to-posterior force to the elbow. The clinician pushes to the first point of pain. Pain is assessed to determine if concordant.
- Step Three: The clinician then applies an AP force beyond the first point of pain toward end range. Sustained holds or repeated movements are performed to determine the effect on the patient's condition.
- Step Four: The opposite side is assessed if appropriate.

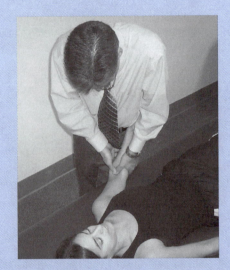

**Figure 10.59**    Anterior Posterior of the Humeroradial Joint

## PA of the Radioulnar Joint (Medial Glide of the Radial Head)

During supination the ulna exhibits external rotation while the radius moves distally and medially. Prepositioning of the elbow in supination alters the axis of the PRUJ, which increases the intensity of force that is translated through the joint.[29]

- Step One: The patient assumes a sitting position. Resting symptoms are assessed.
- Step Two: The patient assists in stabilizing the distal wrist using his or her opposite hand.
- Step Three: The clinician applies a posterior-to-anterior force to the first point of pain to the posterior–lateral aspect of the radial head. The pain is assessed to determine if concordant.
- Step Four: The movement is repeated, pushing beyond the first point of pain toward end range. Repeated movements or sustained holds may be helpful to determine the effect of movement on the joint.
- Step Five: The patient may enhance the intensity of the movement by passively supinating the wrist.
- Step Six: If required, the same procedure can be applied to the opposite extremity.

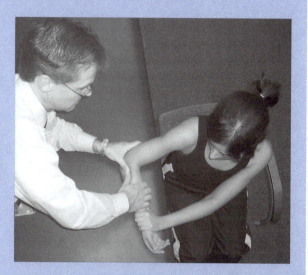

**Figure 10.60**    Posterior Anterior (PA) of the Radioulnar Joint

## AP of the Radioulnar Joint (Lateral Glide of the Radial Head)

During pronation, the radius moves both proximally and laterally while the ulna concurrently internally rotates. By altering the preposition of pronation or supination the clinician can adjust the intensity of force and implicate different aspects of the capsule and ligaments.[29]

- Step One: The patient assumes a sitting position. Resting symptoms are assessed.
- Step Two: The patient assists in stabilizing the distal wrist using his or her opposite hand.
- Step Three: The clinician applies an anterior-to-posterior force to the first point of pain to the anterior–medial aspect of the radial head. The pain is assessed to determine if concordant.
- Step Four: The movement is repeated, pushing beyond the first point of pain toward end range. Repeated movements or sustained holds may be helpful to determine the effect of movement on the joint.
- Step Five: The patient may enhance the intensity of the movement by passively pronating the wrist.
- Step Six: If required, the same procedure can be applied to the opposite extremity.

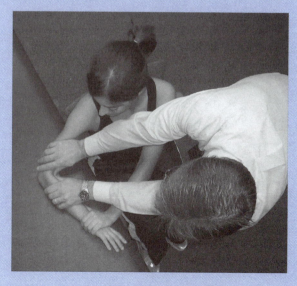

**Figure 10.61**    Anterior Posterior (AP) of the Radioulnar Joint

## *Passive Accessory Movements of the Wrist*

### PA and AP Glide of the Proximal Carpal Row

PA and AP glide of the proximal carpal row may benefit movement such as extension and flexion and may indirectly improve restrictions in pronation and supination.

- Step One: The patient assumes a sitting position. Resting symptoms are assessed. For a PA glide the patient's forearm is pronated. For an AP glide the patient's forearm is supinated.
- Step Two: The clinician stabilizes the proximal wrist by firmly grasping the radius and ulna. With the other hand the clinician grasps the patient's carpal bones just distal to the proximal carpal row.
- Step Three: The clinician applies an anterior-to-posterior force to the first point of pain to the proximal carpal row. The pain is assessed to determine if concordant.
- Step Four: The movement is repeated, pushing beyond the first point of pain toward end range. Repeated movements or sustained holds may be helpful to determine the effect of movement on the joint.

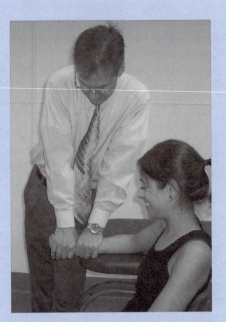

**Figure 10.62**    AP Glide of the Proximal Carpal Row

- Step Five: The patient's wrist is pronated for the PA glide. The clinician applies a posterior-to-anterior force to the first point of pain to the proximal carpal row. The pain is assessed to determine if concordant.
- Step Six: The movement is repeated, pushing beyond the first point of pain toward end range. Repeated movements or sustained holds may be helpful to determine the effect of movement on the joint.

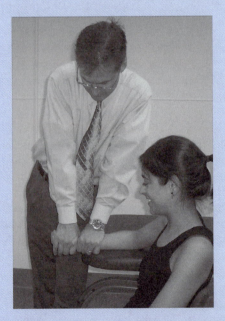

**Figure 10.63**    PA Glide of the Proximal Carpal Row

## PA and AP Glide of the Mid-Carpal Row

Although less mobile than the proximal row, PA and AP of the mid-carpal row may also improve movements such as flexion and extension as well as indirectly improving the movements of pronation and supination.

- Step One: The patient assumes a sitting position. Resting symptoms are assessed. The positioning and set-up is identical to the proximal carpal row.
- Step Two: The clinician stabilizes the proximal carpal row by firmly grasping the proximal carpal bones. With the other hand the clinician grasps the carpal bones just distal to the proximal carpals or mid-carpal joint.
- Step Three: The clinician applies an anterior-to-posterior force to the first point of pain to the mid-carpal row. The pain is assessed to determine if concordant.
- Step Four: The movement is repeated, pushing beyond the first point of pain toward end range. Repeated movements or sustained holds may be helpful to determine the effect of movement on the joint.
- Step Five: The patient's wrist is pronated for the PA glide. The clinician applies a posterior-to-anterior force to the first point of pain to the mid-carpal row. The pain is assessed to determine if concordant.
- Step Six: The movement is repeated, pushing beyond the first point of pain toward end range. Repeated movements or sustained holds may be helpful to determine the effect of movement on the joint.
- Step Seven: To isolate the carpo-metacarpal joint the clinician follows the same procedures outlined for the proximal and mid-carpal rows but stabilizes the distal carpal bones and moves the metacarpals in an AP or PA fashion.

## Radial and Ulnar Glide of the Wrist

In theory, radial and ulnar glide should improve the movements of ulnar and radial deviation.

- Step One: The patient assumes a sitting position. Resting symptoms are assessed. It is essential that the patient assume a slightly pronated posture for these mobilizations (palm down) for the proper direction of glide.
- Step Two: The clinician stabilizes the proximal wrist by firmly grasping the radius and ulna. With the other hand the clinician grasps the carpal bones just distal to the proximal carpal row.
- Step Three: The clinician applies an ulnar glide to the first point of pain to the proximal carpal row. The pain is assessed to determine if concordant.
- Step Four: The movement is repeated, pushing beyond the first point of pain toward end range. Repeated movements or sustained holds may be helpful to determine the effect of movement on the joint.

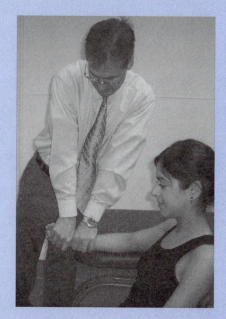

**Figure 10.64**    Ulnar Glide of the Proximal Carpal Row

*(continued)*

- Step Five: The clinician alters his or her position to apply a radial glide. The clinician applies a radial glide to the first point of pain to the proximal carpal row. The pain is assessed to determine if concordant.
- Step Six: The movement is repeated, pushing beyond the first point of pain toward end range. Repeated movements or sustained holds may be helpful to determine the effect of movement on the joint.
- Step Seven: The ulnar and medial glide can be repeated using the same landmarks as the AP and PA glide to target the midcarpal and carpo-metacarpal rows.

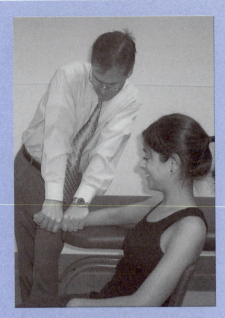

**Figure 10.65**    Radial Glide of the Proximal Carpal Row

## Medial Glide (Extension and Abduction) of the First CMC Joint

Injury to the thumb often leads to a reduction of abduction and extension at the CMC and MCP. Tightness in the medial structures and stretching of the lateral structures results in an imbalance in tissues. The medial glide technique is designed to improve the mobility of the soft tissue structures, thus normalizing motion.

- Step One: The patient assumes a sitting position. Resting symptoms are assessed. The thumb is prepositioned into slight extension or abduction, whichever the focus of motion that is desired.
- Step Two: The clinician places one thumb distal to the CMC (or MCP) and the other proximal. The fingers of the clinician are laced around the medial aspect of the thumb and hand as a counterforce.
- Step Three: The clinician applies medial glide to the first point of pain. The pain is assessed to determine if concordant.
- Step Four: The movement is repeated, pushing beyond the first point of pain toward end range. Repeated movements or sustained holds may be helpful to determine the effect of movement on the joint.

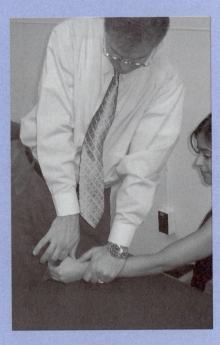

**Figure 10.66**    CMC Medial Glide

## AP and PA Glides of the MCP, PIP, and DIP

AP and PA glides of the MCP, PIP, and DIP are designed to improve the range of motion of flexion and extension of the fingers.

- Step One: The patient assumes a sitting position. Resting symptoms are assessed. For a PA glide the patient's forearm is pronated. For an AP glide the patient's forearm is supinated.
- Step Two: Using a pincer grasp the clinician stabilizes the joint (MCP, PIP, or DIP) just proximal to the joint line and grasps the joint with the other hand just distal to the joint line.
- Step Three: The clinician applies an AP or PA glide to the first point of pain. The pain is assessed to determine if concordant.
- Step Four: The movement is repeated, pushing beyond the first point of pain toward end range. Repeated movements or sustained holds may be helpful to determine the effect of movement on the joint.

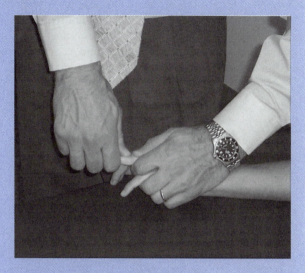

**Figure 10.67**    PA Glide of the PIP

## Summary

- Because of the multiple planes of movement associated with the elbow–wrist–hand, a general screen that examines general planar passive movement is a quick method to identify movement dysfunction.
- Most wrist motion is coupled. When a passive or an accessory movement is isolated as pathological to a specific joint, assessment of the coupled movements may be beneficial.
- The primary purpose of assessment of passive motion is to determine whether the passive movement may be beneficial as a treatment mechanism. Subsequently, it is imperative to determine the effect of sustained holds or repeated movements during a passive or accessory movement.

## Clinical Special Tests

### Palpation

Palpation at the elbow includes both bony and soft tissue palpation. Bony palpation should include the medial and lateral epicondyles of the humerus, the olecranon process of the humerus, and the radial head of the radius specifically at the contact point of the capitulum.

Soft tissue palpation should include the lateral, posterior, and medial musculature, the biceps tendon anteriorly, the ulnar nerve medially, and the ulnar collateral ligament medially. The medial collateral ligaments are easier to expose and palpate when the arm is suppinated and flexed to approximately 90 degrees.

Sucher[96] advocates the benefit of palpation for carpal tunnel syndrome of the hand. Others have reported that isolated tenderness to the snuff-box may be indicative of a scaphoid fracture, pain directly on the scaphoid tubercle may indicate instability, and tenderness to the hook of the hamate may indicate a hamate fracture.[78] Isolated tenderness to the pisiform may also implicate a fracture of the pisiform.[78]

### Muscle Testing

Manual muscle testing at the elbow using a dynamometer has been shown to demonstrate comparable validity to pain report in patients with medial elbow pain.[97] It has been suggested that isolating the middle finger of the extensor digitorum communis is beneficial in isolating pain associated with lateral epicondylitis.[98] This suggestion lacks investigation and may yield imprecise findings. Nonetheless, this method, identified as the Maudsley test, is described further in the clinical special tests section. Additional forms of manual muscle testing of the wrist and hand are less discriminative and therefore should be used in concert with other examination methods.[99]

## Clinical Special Tests for the Elbow

### Cozen's Test

Cozen's test (Figure 10.68) is best described as resisted simultaneous wrist extension and supination[100] and is considered a clinical test for the detection of lateral epicondylitis. Despite the prevalence of use, no studies have examined this test for diagnostic value. Consequently, the discriminatory nature of this clinical examination is unknown. Performance requires a simultaneous resisted contraction of supination and extension at the wrist.

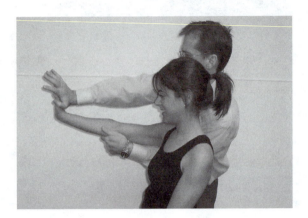

**Figure 10.68**    Cozen's Test

### Maudsley's Test

Maudsley's test (Figure 10.69), also referred to as the middle finger test, is a purported test for radial tunnel syndrome.[101] The test is considered positive when pain is encountered during resisted extension of the middle finger.[98] This action purportedly tests the contribution of the origin of the extensor digitorum communis to compression of the radial nerve. Although there is controversy regarding the actual occurrence of radial tunnel syndrome, both radial tunnel syndrome and posterior interosseous nerve (PIN) compression syndrome can be caused by compression of the posterior interosseous nerve.[102,103] True neurogenic radial tunnel syndrome is an uncommon condition caused by entrapment of the radial or posterior interosseous nerve in the radial tunnel and is usually easily identifiable by focal motor weakness in the distribution of the posterior interosseous nerve.[104] Patients who lack motor weakness are most appropriately diagnosed with lateral tendonesis, thus Maudsley's test most likely contributes to many findings of false positives.[104] To date, no tests have measured the diagnostic value of this study.

### Valgus and Varus Stress Test

Varus (Figure 10.70) and valgus (Figure 10.71) tests are useful in determining the integrity of the medial and lateral collateral ligaments of the elbow. Although commonly used, the tests lack diagnostic assessment for the presence of a specific pathology but should yield additional findings for the potential of instability.

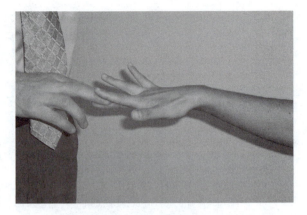

**Figure 10.69**    Maudsley's Test

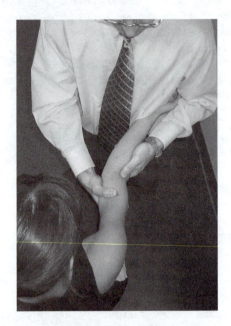

**Figure 10.70**    The Valgus Stress Test

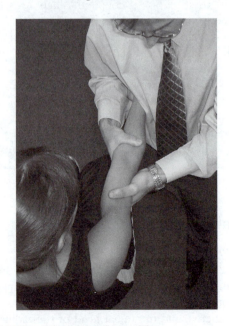

**Figure 10.71**    The Varus Stress Test

### Fat Pad Sign for Fractures

The Fat Pad Sign is a radiographic measure for the presence of an elbow fracture. The test is considered positive when the evidence of joint distention is prevalent on an x-ray. Most notably, the diagnosis is made when the anterior fat pad is displaced further anteriorly and superiorly, and the posterior fat pad is displaced posteriorly and superiorly.[105] In addition to fractures, conditions such as joint effusion from trauma, infection, or inflammation can distend the joint capsule and displace the fat pads and provide a false positive.[105] De Maeseneer et al.[106] found moderate kappa agreement among radiologists (Anterior Fat Pad, 0.6; Posterior Fat Pad, 0.49). Irshad et al.[107] reported that the test did provide poor to fair diagnostic value, identifying a sensitivity of 85.4 and a specificity of 50.1 (+LR = 1.71) on a sample of 193 patients with elbow injuries associated with trauma (Table 10.4).

### Tinel's Sign at the Elbow

Tinel's (Figure 10.72) at the elbow purportedly measures the propensity of cubital tunnel syndrome. Cubital tunnel syndrome is a clinical condition associated with ulnar nerve compression at the medial collateral ligament (MCL) and the overlying retinaculum during physiological flexion.[108] Typically, a prepositioning of end range flexion to the elbow is used to increase the sensitivity of the test.

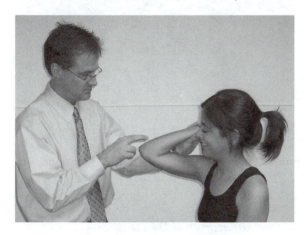

**Figure 10.72**    Tinel's Sign at the Elbow

## Clinical Special Tests for the Wrist/Hand

### Phalen's Test

Phalen's test (Figure 10.73) is a purported test for carpal tunnel syndrome. Phalen's test supposedly increases the pressure within the carpal canal through the action of prolonged flexion. Phalen's test involves the patient placing the dorsums of both hands together then forcing the wrists into flexion. The test should be held for a full minute for complete reproduction of symptoms.[109–117] Generally, the reliability of the test is considered fair to moderate as is the diagnostic power of the test.[76]

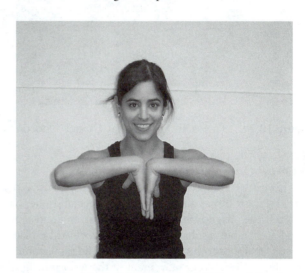

**Figure 10.73**    Phalen's Test for Carpal Tunnel Syndrome

### Tinel's Sign

Tinel's sign (Figure 10.74) at the wrist is a purported test for carpal tunnel syndrome. Tinel's test is designed to determine if an abnormal amount of pressure is present over the medial nerve. The wrist is prepositioned in an extended position and the clinician taps on the median nerve directly over the carpal tunnel.[48] Positive findings are a reproduction of neurological symptoms.[118] The reliability of Tinel's test is considered comparable to Phalen's test,[76] although some authors feel it is less diagnostic than Phalen's test (see Table 10.5).[119–121]

**TABLE 10.4**    Diagnostic Values of Elbow Special Tests

| Study | Sensitivity | Specificity | +LR | −LR | Criterion Standard |
|---|---|---|---|---|---|
| **Fat Pad Sign** | | | | | |
| Irshad et al.[107] | 85.4 | 50.1 | 1.71 | 0.29 | Radiograph |
| **Tinel Sign for Cubital Compression** | | | | | |
| Novak et al.[108] | 70 | 97 | 23.3 | 0.31 | Electrodiagnostic evaluation |
| **Flexion and Compression Test** | | | | | |
| Novak et al.[108] | 91 | 97 | 30.3 | 0.09 | Electrodiagnostic evaluation |

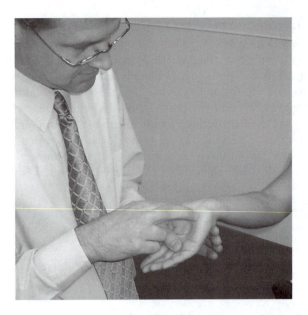

**Figure 10.74**   Tinel's Test for Carpal Tunnel Syndrome

### Carpal Compression Test

The carpal compression test (Figure 10.75) is a purported test for carpal tunnel syndrome. Several studies have analyzed the diagnostic value of this test and most have found acceptable results. The test is performed by placing direct pressure over the median nerve in the retinaculum of the palm.[48] Concurrent movement of the wrist into flexion increases the sensitivity of the test (see Table 10.5).

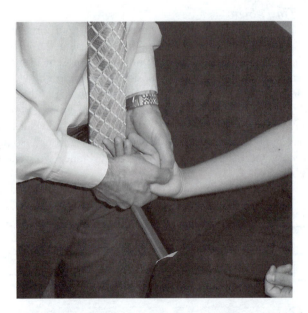

**Figure 10.75**   The Carpal Compression Test for Carpal Tunnel Syndrome

### Flick Test

The flick test is a purported test for carpal tunnel syndrome. The flick sign occurs when a patient shakes his or her hand to reduce symptoms associated with carpal tun-

nel syndrome.[48] The flick sign is often described as similar to shaking down a thermometer. Table 10.5 outlines the diagnostic accuracy.

### Finkelstein's Test

Finkelstein's test (Figure 10.76) is a purported clinical test for De Quervain's tenosynovitis.[122] The test involves a passive combined ulnar and flexion deviation while maintaining thumb opposition within a "grip" of the fingers. A recent biomechanical analysis suggests that the Finkelstein's test is more appropriately isolated to the extensor pollicis brevis versus the abductor pollicis longus.[123] This finding and the relative provocative nature of the test leads to numerous false positive findings,[124] and, unfortunately, there are no tests that have examined the diagnostic value of this particular clinical test.

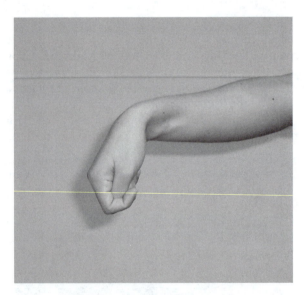

**Figure 10.76**   Finkelstein's Test for De Quevain's Tenosynovitis

### Ulnomeniscotriquetral Dorsal Glide

The ulnomeniscotriquetral glide test (Figure 10.77) is designed to place distraction on the structures of the distal ulna, TFCC, and the triquetrum.[125] The test can be used to determine the integrity of the triangular ligament of the distal ulna. Table 10.5 outlines the diagnostic accuracy of the test.

1. The patient assumes a supine or seated position.
2. With one hand, the clinician stabilizes the thumb and gently moves the wrist into slight ulnar deviation. The clinician blocks the distal ulna with the thumb by placing the contact point on the dorsum of the ulna.
3. The index finger of the clinician contacts the palmar aspect of the pisiform.
4. The clinician then pinches the index and thumb toward one another, creating a dorsal glide of the pisiform and triquetrum.

5. Reproduction of symptoms and/or excessive laxity (clicking) is considered a positive test for ulnomeniscotriquetral laxity.

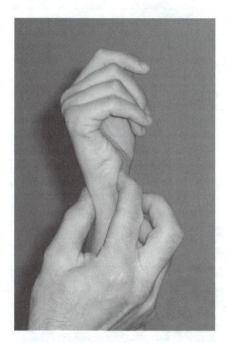

**Figure 10.77**   The Ulnomeniscotriquetral Dorsal Glide Test

### Ballottement Test

The ballottement test (Figure 10.78), which is intermittently and inconsistently called the shuck test, is a purported test for triquetrolunate strain and instability.[126] Lunotriquetral instability may appear after a hyperpronation injury,[126,127] but more often after a hyperextension injury with an impact on the ulnar side.[128] The test is performed by applying a shear force to the triquetrolunate joint while stabilizing lunate dorsally and pisotriquetral plane volarly. A positive test is crepitus and notable swelling (excursion) of the pisotriquetral (Table 10.5).[129]

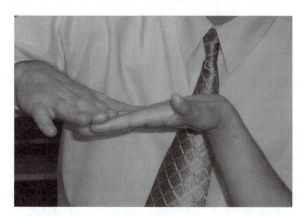

**Figure 10.78**   The Ballottement Test (Alternative Method)

An alternative method requires no stabilization of the carpal bones. The clinician provides a posterior-to-anterior force to the fingers as the patient resists and holds his or her hand in wrist flexion and finger and MCP extension. The same findings are indicative of a positive test.

### Scaphoid Shift Test

The scaphoid shift test (Figure 10.79) is designed to test the stability of the scaphoid bone, specifically with respect to adjacent structures. Normally, the scaphoid translates volarly and in a rotational motion when moving toward a radial direction.[129] To accurately perform the test, the clinician blocks the proximal movement of the scaphoid tubercle during passive radial deviation of the wrist. A positive test results in pain and instability during the movement. A normal finding is a stable block during radial glide (see Table 10.5).

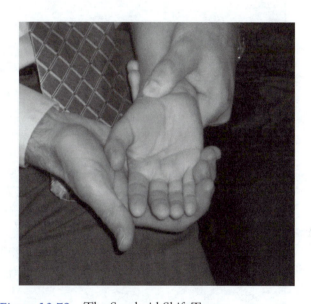

**Figure 10.79**   The Scaphoid Shift Test

## Summary

- The use of palpation may be helpful to localize symptoms in the elbow–wrist–hand.
- Manual muscle testing of the elbow may be a valid method of determining strength loss.
- Most elbow clinical special tests have not undergone conclusive diagnostic accuracy assessment and have unknown benefit.
- The majority of carpal tunnel clinical special tests have been measured for diagnostic accuracy and a number of the tests appear valid and reliable.
- Other forms of tests for the wrist/hand have not been tested as extensively for diagnostic accuracy and may present with limited benefit.

**TABLE 10.5** Diagnostic Value of Wrist/Hand Special Tests

| Study | Sensitivity | Specificity | +LR | −LR | Criterion Standard |
|---|---|---|---|---|---|
| **Scaphoid Shift Test** | | | | | |
| LaStayo and Howell[129] | 69 | 66 | 2.02 | 0.47 | Arthroscopic findings |
| **Ballottement Test** | | | | | |
| LaStayo and Howell[129] | 64 | 44 | 1.14 | 0.82 | Arthroscopic findings |
| **Ulnomeniscotriquetral Dorsal Glide** | | | | | |
| LaStayo and Howell[129] | 66 | 64 | 1.83 | 0.53 | Arthroscopic findings |
| **Phalen's Test** | | | | | |
| Ahn[164] | 67.5 | 91 | 7.5 | 0.36 | Electrodiagnostic evaluation |
| Heller et al.[115] | 60 | 59 | 1.46 | 0.68 | Electrodiagnostic testing |
| Hansen et al.[165] | 34 | 74 | 1.31 | 0.89 | Electrodiagnostic testing |
| Tetro et al.[166] | 61 | 83 | 3.58 | 0.47 | Electrodiagnostic testing |
| Szabo et al.[167] | 75 | 95 | 15 | 0.26 | Nerve condition velocity tests |
| **Tinel's Sign** | | | | | |
| Ahn[164] | 67.5 | 90 | 6.75 | 0.36 | Electrodiagnostic evaluation |
| Heller et al.[115] | 67 | 77 | 2.91 | 0.43 | Electrodiagnostic testing |
| Hansen et al.[165] | 27 | 100 | NA | NA | Electrodiagnostic testing |
| Tetro et al.[166] | 74 | 91 | 8.22 | 0.29 | Electrodiagnostic testing |
| Szabo et al.[167] | 64 | 99 | 64 | 0.36 | Nerve condition velocity tests |
| **Flick Sign** | | | | | |
| Hansen et al.[165] | 37 | 92 | 4.6 | 0.68 | Electrodiagnostic testing |
| **Carpal Compression Test** | | | | | |
| Kaul et al.[168] | 52.5 | 61.8 | 1.37 | 0.77 | Electrodiagnostic testing |
| Wainner et al.[169] | 36 | 57 | 0.83 | 1.12 | Nerve conduction velocity |
| Tetro et al.[166] | 75 | 93 | 10.7 | 0.27 | Electrodiagnostic testing |
| Szabo et al.[167] | 89 | 91 | 9.88 | 0.12 | Nerve condition velocity tests |

# TREATMENT TECHNIQUES

## Soft Tissue Techniques—Friction Massage

Deep friction massage has been used frequently as a treatment method for various elbow- and wrist-related pain. The technique can be applied either perpendicular to the direction of the fibers of the muscle or parallel with the fibers of the muscle.

## Active Physiological Movements

The propensity for elbow stiffness following a trauma is very high.[130,131] Large amounts of range-of-motion loss are common, often in the extensors greater than the flexors.[130] Both intrinsic and extrinsic factors are related to range-of-motion losses[132] and both may benefit from active plane-based movements.

## Passive Physiological Movements

Many of the same passive physiological assessment movements and hand holds used within the examination process are plausible treatment techniques, specifically if sustained holds or repeated movements lead to a reduction of pain. For the elbow, it is useful to incorporate the coupled movements of elbow extension and flexion with varus and valgus forces.

## Passive Accessory Movements

Like passive physiological techniques, the crux behind patient-based indices of assessment suggests that treatment methods are selected based on concordant examination findings. Subsequently, many of the passive accessory treatments reflect the same position and stabilization demonstrated during the examination section of this chapter. However, some alterations are plausible during passive accessory treatment that may improve the outcome of the intervention.

### Cervical Mobilization or Manipulation for Elbow Pain

There is also moderate evidence to support that manual therapy provides an excitatory effect on sympathetic nervous system activity.[133–136] Specially, the manual therapy mobilization techniques associated with anteroposterior and lateral glides have been well documented (Figures 10.80–10.82).[137] An excitatory effect on the sympathetic nervous system occurs concurrently with a reduction of hypoanalgesia and may parallel the effects of stimulation of the dorsal periaqueductal gray area of the midbrain, a process that has occurred in animal research.[138] Documented evidence supports the benefit of modulation of pain and remarkably has a nonlocalized effect. Stimulation of the cervical spine has demonstrated upper extremity changes in pain response (pressure-pain) and a measurable sympathoexcitatory effect.[139,140]

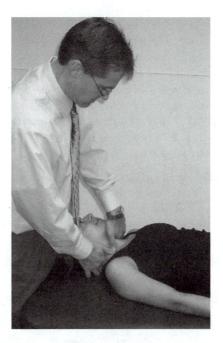

**Figure 10.82**    Anterior Posterior Glide of the Cervical Spine

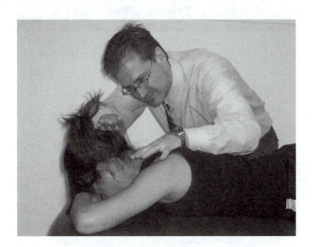

**Figure 10.80**    Lateral Glide of the Cervical Spine

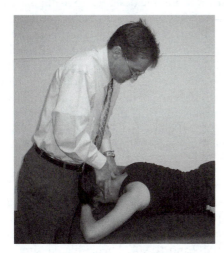

**Figure 10.81**    Posterior Anterior Glide of the Cervical Spine

### The Use of a Belt during Elbow Distraction

Stabilization during elbow distraction (Figure 10.83) can be challenging, specifically during prepositioning of elbow flexion. The judicious use of a mobilization belt can improve the stabilization of the humerus to allow a more vigorous mobilization of the humeroulnar or humeroradial joint.[141] When using a belt, careful attention must be placed on the friction and pressure the belt places on human tissue.

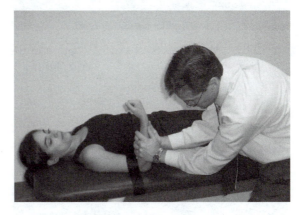

**Figure 10.83**    Mobilization of the Elbow Using the Belt to Brace the Humerus

## Manually Assisted Movements

### Manually Assisted Movements of the Elbow

Paungmali et al.[142] and Vicenzino[141] describe a mobilization technique for lateral epicondylalgia in which a lateral glide is performed at the elbow. This technique is performed by stabilizing the internally rotated shoulder at the distal humerus, while concurrently performing a lateral glide at the ulna by contact on the medial side. The patient performs a gripping procedure during the mobilization in order to reproduce the patient's pain, albeit only to threshold levels. Their findings suggest that the mobilization with movement technique yielded physiological effects similar to those produced with spinal manipulation. Abbott[143] and Abbott et al.[144] describe a similar technique that involves repeated wrist extension by the patient versus gripping an object.

### Manually Assisted Movements of the Wrist

In a single case study, Backstrom[145] describes a manually assisted mobilization to the wrist (Figure 10.84) for the treatment of De Quervain's tenosynovitis. This technique uses pain-free radial glides from the clinician during concurrent thumb extension by the patient.

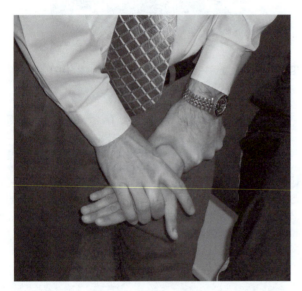

**Figure 10.84**    Manually Assisted Mobilization of the Proximal Row of the Wrist; Radial Glide

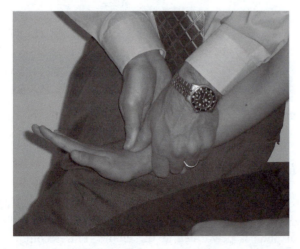

**Figure 10.85**    Manually Assisted Mobilization PA of the Columns

Maitland[38] promoted the use of passive physiological movement of the wrist during concurrent passive accessory motion at the carpal bones. These column mobilizations are designed to improve the AP or PA movement of the carpal bones during physiological flexion and extension at the wrist (Figures 10.85 and 10.86). If the wrist is divided into three theoretical columns (medial, middle, and lateral), the pressure from the thumb can promote an AP or PA movement on the adjacent columns.

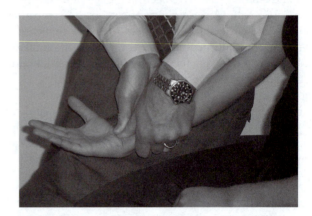

**Figure 10.86**    Manually Assisted Mobilization AP of the Columns

## Manipulation

### Manipulation of the Elbow

Kaufman[146] described the use of manipulation method in the treatment of lateral epicondylitis of the elbow (Figure 10.87). The technique is performed by rapidly driving the elbow into extension after a prepositioning of pronation and wrist flexion. This positive finding was with a single case and as of yet no single protocol that demonstrates beneficial outcome for manipulative therapy of the elbow exists.

### Watson's Manipulation

Recently a technique designed to manipulate the carpal bones was used as a treatment technique for lateral epicondylitis. The technique involves a prepositioning of the patient with his or her forearm of the affected side on a table with the palmar side of the hand facing down. The clinician grasps the patient's scaphoid bone between the clinician's thumb and index finger and extends the wrist dorsally at the same time the scaphoid bone was manipulated ventrally (Figure 10.88). The authors repeated this procedure 20 times and alternated by either forced passive extension of the wrist or extension against resistance.

### Manipulation of the Carpal Joints

Kaufman and Bird[147] describe a series of radiocarpal wrist manipulations used in the treatment of a patient with chronic dysfunction associated with a Colles' fracture (Figures 10.89 and 10.90). Their isolated, single case findings advocate the use of manipulation for increase in range of motion and grip strength.

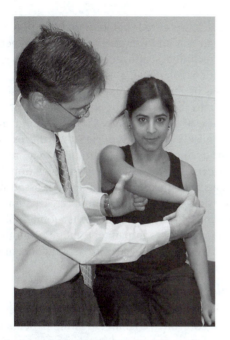

**Figure 10.87**    Manipulation of the Elbow

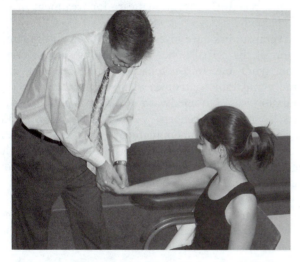

**Figure 10.88**    The End Position of the Manipulation Technique

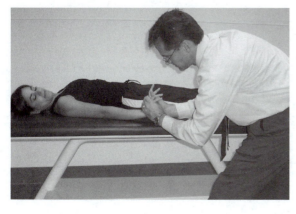

**Figure 10.89**    Longitudinal Distraction Manipulation-Preposition of Extension

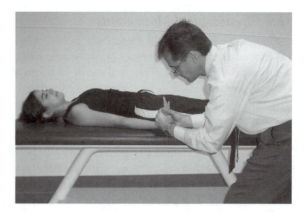

**Figure 10.90**    Longitudinal Distraction Manipulation-Preposition of Flexion.

## Summary

- The majority of the treatment techniques used for the elbow–wrist–hand is borne from the examination methods.
- Selected treatment methods may be enhanced by using the coupled movements of the elbow and wrist and by incorporating patient assistance during movements.

# TREATMENT OUTCOMES

## Soft Tissue Techniques—Friction Massage

Although deep friction massage has been used frequently as a treatment method for various elbow- and wrist-related pain, no studies have demonstrated benefit when compared with pragmatic control.[148] Although the technique may be helpful when combined with other methods of treatment, used alone the procedure has limited value.

## Active Range-of-Motion Exercises

Early elbow movement may help reduce the range-of-motion losses; however, it is common to see degenerative changes, fibrous tissue adhesions, musculotendinous structures, ectopic ossification, loose bodies, and/or osteophytes.[131,132] Lastly, age (> 70 years) is a more significant factor in active and passive range of motion loss versus gender,[149] most likely associated with the biomechanical changes of degeneration.

Active movement for the treatment of the wrist/hand has a well-documented benefit. Early movement, focusing on separate exercises of the wrist and hand, after surgical treatment of carpal tunnel syndrome has been associated with better outcomes versus immobilization.[150] Others have reported the benefit of an active range-of-motion treatment in the intervention of uncomplicated distal radius fractures.[151]

## Passive Physiological Movements

Few studies have examined the benefits of passive physiological movements of the elbow or wrist. Coyle et al.[152] reported improvement in radiocarpal range of motion in a small trial of patients who had encountered a distal radius fracture, although oscillations resulted in a better overall outcome and were more effective in reducing pain.

Clinically, elbow extension is generally the most different range of motion to improve with treatment. Although Cyriax[153] reported that the capsular pattern of the elbow is flexion loss greater than extension, there has been no studies that have substantiated or refuted this finding.

The movements associated with passive physiological stretching and oscillatory glides may be beneficial in the treatment of elbow, wrist, and hand pain. As with the patient response-based guidelines, treatment methods are selected based on concordant examination findings are warranted. Treatments such as passive elbow flexion with and without varus and valgus forces, passive elbow extension with and without varus and valgus forces may improve the outcome of a manual therapy intervention. By using the stabilization methods discussed earlier, the clinician improves the dosage of the force applied through the elbow, wrist, and hand.

## Nerve Glides

Radial nerve glides and radial head mobilization for elbow pain has demonstrated better outcomes than a standard approach that included ultrasound, strengthening, and friction massage.[154] Case studies have reported the benefit of nerve gliding exercises in patients with cubital tunnel syndrome.[155] More studies have investigated the benefit in wrist- and hand-related regions. Median nerve gliding exercise relieved pain and improved range of motion more than patients who received no treatment but demonstrated comparable outcomes to joint mobilization in patients with carpal tunnel syndrome (CTS).[156] In another population of CTS, splinting performed with nerve glides demonstrated a reduction of pain and an improvement in grip strength; however, the effect was not significantly better than splinting alone.[157]

## Passive Accessory Mobilizations

A significant amount of literature has been dedicated to the outcome associated with passive accessory movements. Coyle and Robertson[152] demonstrated improvements in pain and function using a treatment approach of passive accessory glides in patients' status post Colles' fracture. Their findings suggested that oscillatory mobilization was more effective (specifically on pain) than static stretching.

Randall et al.[158] reported that joint mobilization was more effective than a home exercise program of general exercises. The techniques utilized were standard carpal joint glides to patient tolerance.

Variations in application have included the use of compression versus distraction, prepositioning in a restriction versus the use of a "loose-packed" mobilization and other nuances. Ishikawa et al.[24] reported that the use of wrist distraction during carpal mobilization may reduce the amount of carpal excursion during mobilization. The authors suggest that the nonuse of traction is associated with greater physiological, coupled, and intercarpal movement. Tal-Akabi and Rushton[156] report that joint mobilization leads to improvements in pain and range of motion more so than no treatment and lead to a reduction in surgical intervention.[156]

## Manipulation Procedures

Manipulation of the carpal bones has shown benefit in a randomized controlled trial investigating patients with lateral epicondylitis. Those who received "conventional" care and wrist manipulation performed better than those who just received conventional care for treatment of lateral epicondylitis.[15]

Several studies have investigated the benefit of manipulation of the carpal bones in conditions such as carpal tunnel syndrome. In a comparative trial, Davis et al.[159] found comparable outcomes to medical care when manipulation was combined with ultrasound and wrist supports. In two case reports, Valente and Gibson[160] and Russell[161] advocated manipulation to the neck, wrist, and elbow in the treatment of two 40+-year-old females with conditions of CTS and cubital tunnel syndrome (respectively). Hafner et al.[162] reported comparable outcomes of medical and chiropractic intervention of manipulation of the wrist. Despite the purported benefits, Ernst[163] acknowledged that no hard evidence exists to support "chiropractic" manipulation for the care of CTS.

## Summary

- Significant evidence exists to support early controlled active movement for healing of fractures and ligamentous injuries of the elbow–wrist–hand.
- Evidence exists of the benefit of cervical mobilization for reduction of elbow pain in lateral epicondylitis.
- Some evidence exists to support the use of manipulation of the wrist for both elbow and wrist pain.

# Chapter Questions

1. Describe the overlap in contribution of potential concordant pain between the elbow, wrist, and hand.
2. Briefly outline the biomechanical characteristics of the elbow. Identify how the degrees of freedom are passively assessed. Repeat this process for the wrist and hand.
3. Identify the benefits and disadvantages of using a single scale for the elbow, wrist, and hand.
4. Suggest the potential manual therapy treatments used in conditions associated with stiffness, laxity, and pain for the elbow, wrist, and hand.

# References

1. National Institute for Occupational Safety and Health. Musculoskeletal disorders and workplace factors. A critical review of epidemiologic evidence for work-related musculoskeletal disorders of the neck, upper extremity, and low back. 1997; DHHS no. 97–141.
2. Descatha A, Leclerc A, Chastang JF, Roquelaure Y; the Study Group on Repetitive Work. Medial epicondylitis in occupational settings: prevalence, incidence and associated risk factors. *J Occup Environ Med.* 2003;45(9):993–1001.
3. Descatha A, Leclerc A, Chastang JF, Roquelaure Y; Study Group on Repetitive Work. (abstract). Incidence of ulnar nerve entrapment at the elbow in repetitive work. *Scand J Work Environ Health.* 2004;30(3):234–240.
4. Bauer W. Occupational finger injuries. *Morbidity and Mortality Weekly Reports.* 1983;32:589–591.
5. Walker-Bone K, Palmer KT, Reading I, Coggon D, Cooper C. Prevalence and impact of musculoskeletal disorders of the upper limb in the general population. *Arthritis Rheum.* 2004;51(4):642–651.
6. Zakaria D. Rates of carpal tunnel syndrome, epicondylitis, and rotator cuff claims in Ontario workers during 1997. *Chronic Dis Can.* 2004;25(2):32–39.
7. Reville RT, Neuhauser FW, Bhattacharya J, Martin C. Comparing severity of impairment for different permanent upper extremity musculoskeletal injuries. *J Occup Rehabil.* 2002;12(3):205–221.
8. Sizer P, Brismée JM, Cook C, Dedrick L, Phelps V. Ergonomic pain, part 1: Etiology, epidemiology & prevention. *Pain Prac.* 2004;4:41–52.
9. Sizer P, Phelps V, Brismée J, Cook C, Dedrick L. Ergonomic pain part 2: Differential diagnosis and management considerations. *Pain Prac.* 2004;4:136–162.
10. Silverstein B, Viikari-Juntura E, Kalat J. Use of a prevention index to identify industries at high risk for work-related musculoskeletal disorders of the neck, back, and upper extremity in Washington State, 1990–1998. *Am J Ind Med.* 2002;41(3):149–169.
11. Liow RY, Cregan A, Nanda R, Montgomery RJ. Early mobilization for minimally displaced radial head fractures is desirable. *Injury.* 2002;33:801–806.
12. Hildebrand KA, Patterson SD, King GJ. Acute elbow dislocations: simple and complex. *Orthop Clinics North Am.* 1999;20:63–79.
13. Kim DH, Kam AC, Chandika P, Tiel RL, Kline DG. Surgical management and outcome in patients with radial nerve lesions. *J Neurosurg.* 2001;95(4):573–583.
14. Nirschl R. Elbow tendinosis/tennis elbow. *Clin Sports Med.* 1992;11:851–870.
15. Struijs PA, Kerkhoffs GM, Assendleft WJ, Van Dijk CN. Conservative treatment of lateral epicondylitis. *AM J Sports Med.* 2004:32:462–469.
16. Maffulli N, Wong J, Almekinders LC. Types and epidemiology of tendinopathy. *Clin Sports Med.* 2003;22(4):675–692.
17. Sanders M. *Management of cumulative trauma disorders.* Boston; Butterworth-Heinemann: 1997.
18. Buckwalter JA, Saltzman C, Brown T. The impact of osteoarthritis: implications for research. *Clin Orthop Relat Res.* 2004;(427 Suppl):S6–15.
19. McAuliffe J, Miller R. Osteoarthritis and traumatic arthritis of the elbow. *J Hand Ther.* 2000;13(2):136–147.
20. Debono L, Mafart B, Jeusel E, Guipert G. Is the incidence of elbow osteoarthritis underestimated? Insights from paleopathology. *Joint Bone Spine.* 2004;71(5):397–400.
21. Kim DH, Kam AC, Chandika P, Tiel RL, Kline DG. Surgical management and outcome in patients with radial nerve lesions. *J Neurosurg.* 2001;95(4):573–583.
22. Van de Graaff. *Human anatomy.* 6th edition. St. Louis, MO; McGraw Hill: 2002.
23. Short WH, Werner FW, Green JK, Masaoka S. Biomechanical evaluation of the ligamentous stabilizers of the scaphoid and lunate: Part II. *J Hand Surg [Am].* 2005;30(1):24–34.
24. Ishikawa J, Cooney W, Niebur G, Kai-Nan A, Minami A, Kaneda K. The effects of wrist distraction on carpal kinematics. *J Hand Surg.* 1999;24A:113–120.
25. Safran M. Soft-tissue stabilizers of the elbow. *J Shoulder and Elbow Surgery.* 2005;14:S179–S185.

26. Morrey BF, An KN. Articular and ligamentous contributions to the stability of the elbow joint. *Am J Sports Med.* 1983;11(5):315–319.

27. Nielsen KK, Olsen BS. No stabilizing effect of the elbow joint capsule. A kinematic study. *Acta Orthop Scand.* 1999;70(1):6–8.

28. Mayfield JK, Johnson RP, Kilcoyne RK. Carpal dislocations: pathomechanics and progressive perilunar instability. *J Hand Surg [Am].* 1980;5(3):226–241.

29. An N-K, Morrey B. Biomechanics of the elbow. In Morrey B. *The elbow and its disorders.* 3rd ed. Philadelphia; Saunders: 1993.

30. Von Lanz T, Wachsmuth W. *Praktische anatomie.* Berlin; Springer-Verlag: 1959.

31. Garcias Elias M, Horii E, Berger R. Individual carpal bone motion. In An K-N, Berger R, Cooney W. (ed), *Biomechanics of the wrist joint.* New York; Springer-Verlag: 1991.

32. de Lange A, Krauer J, Hiskes R. Kinematic behavior of the human wrist joint: a roentgen-stereophotogrammetric analysis. *J Orthop Res.* 1985;3: 56–64.

33. Ruby L, Cooney W, An K-N. Relative motion of selected carpal bones: a kinematic analysis of the normal wrist. *J Hand Surg (AM).* 1988;13:1–10.

34. Horii E, Garcia-Elias M, An KN, Bishop AT, Cooney WP, Linscheid RL, Chao EY. A kinematic study of luno-triquetral dissociations. *J Hand Surg [Am].* 1991;16(2):355–362.

35. Li ZM, Kuxhaus L, Fisk JA, Christophel TH. Coupling between wrist flexion-extension and radial-ulnar deviation. *Clin Biomech.* 2005;20(2):177–183.

36. Gupta A, Moosawi NA. How much can carpus rotate axially? An in vivo study. *Clin Biomech.* 2005; 20(2):172–176.

37. Walker M. Manual physical therapy examination and intervention of a patient with radial wrist pain: a case report. *J Orthop Sports Phys Ther.* 2004;34: 716–769.

38. Maitland GD. *Peripheral manipulation.* 3rd ed. ed. London; Butterworth-Heinemann, 1986.

39. Munk B, Jensen SL, Olsen BS, Kroener K, Ersboell BK. Wrist stability after experimental traumatic triangular fibrocartilage complex lesions. *J Hand Surg [Am].* 2005;30(1):43–49.

40. Haque M, Adams J, Borenstein D, Wiesel S. *Hand and wrist pain.* 2nd ed. Danvers MA. Lexis Publishing. 2000.

41. Cooney W, Linscheid R, Dobyns J. *The wrist; diagnosis and operative treatment.* Vol 1. St. Louis MO; Mosby. 1998.

42. Rodriguez-Niedenfuhr M, Vazquez T, Golano P, Parkin I, Sanudo JR. Extensor digitorum brevis manus: anatomical, radiological and clinical relevance. A review. *Clin Anat.* 2002;15(4):286–292.

43. Schweitzer TP, Rayan GM. The terminal tendon of the digital extensor mechanism: Part I, anatomic study. *J Hand Surg [Am].* 2004;29(5):898–902.

44. Mehta JA, Bain GI. Posterolateral rotatory instability of the elbow. *J Am Acad Orthop Surg.* 2004;12 (6):405–415.

45. Higgs PE, Young VL. Cumulative trauma disorders. *Clin Plast Surg.* 1996;23(3):421–433.

46. Kiuru MJ, Haapamaki VV, Koivikko MP, Koskinen SK. Wrist injuries; diagnosis with multidetector CT. *Emerg Radiol.* 2004;10(4):182–185.

47. Pao VS, Chang J. Scaphoid nonunion: diagnosis and treatment. *Plast Reconstr Surg.* 2003;112(6): 1666–1676.

48. Macdermid JC, Wessel J. Clinical diagnosis of carpal tunnel syndrome: A systematic review. *J Hand Ther.* 2004;17(2):309–319.

49. Gupta K, Benstead T. Symptoms experienced by patient with carpal tunnel syndrome. *J Canadian Neuro Sci.* 1997;24(4):338–342.

50. Viera A. Management of Carpal Tunnel Syndrome. *Am Fam Physic.* 2003;68(2);265–273.

51. Lehtinen I, Kirjavainen T, Hurme M, Lauerma H, Martikainen K, Rauhala E. Sleep-related disorder in carpal tunnel syndrome. *Acta Neuro Scand.* 1996; 93:360–365.

52. Bongers P, Kremer A, ter Laak J. Are psychosocial factors, risk factors for symptoms and signs of the shoulder, elbow or wrist/hand?: A review of the epidemiological literature. *Am J Ind Med.* 2002;41: 315–342.

53. Henderson M, Kidd BL, Pearson RM, White PD. Chronic upper limb pain: an exploration of the biopsychosocial model. *J Rheumatol.* 2005;32(1): 118–122.

54. Bergqvist U, Wolgast E, Nilsson B, Voss M. Musculoskeletal disorders among visual display terminal workers: individual, ergonomic, and work organizational factors. *Ergonomics.* 1995;38(4):763–776.

55. Bernard B, Sauter S, Fine L, Petersen M, Hales T. Job task and psychosocial risk factors for work-related musculoskeletal disorders among newspaper employees. *Scand J Work Environ Health.* 1994; 20(6):417–426.

56. Engstrom T, Hanse JJ, Kadefors R. Musculoskeletal symptoms due to technical preconditions in long cycle time work in an automobile assembly plant: a study of prevalence and relation to psychosocial factors and physical exposure. *Appl Ergon.* 1999;30(5): 443–453.

57. Lagerstrom M, Wenemark M, Hagberg M, Hjelm EW. Occupational and individual factors related to musculoskeletal symptoms in five body regions among Swedish nursing personnel. *Int Arch Occup Environ Health.* 1995;68(1):27–35.

58. MacDermid J, Tottenham V. Responsiveness of the Disability of the Arm, Shoulder, and Hand (DASH) and Patient-Rated Wrist/Hand Evaluation (PRWHE) in evaluating change after hand therapy. *J Hand Ther.* 2004;17(1):18–23.

59. Gummesson C, Atroshi I, Ekdahl C. The disabilities of the arm, shoulder and hand (DASH) outcome questionnaire: longitudinal construct validity and measuring self-rated health change after surgery. *BMC Musculoskelet Disord.* 2003;4(1):11.

60. Hudak P, Amadio P, Bombardier C. Development of an upper extremity outcome measure: the DASH (disabilities of the arm, shoulder, and hand). *Am J Ind Med.* 1996;29:602–608.

61. King GJ, Richards RR, Zuckerman JD, Blasier R, Dillman C, Friedman RJ, Gartsman GM, Iannotti JP, Murnahan JP, Mow VC, Woo SL. A standardized method for assessment of elbow function. Research Committee, American Shoulder and Elbow Surgeons. *J Shoulder Elbow Surg.* 1999;8(4):351–354.

62. MacDermid JC. Outcome evaluation in patients with elbow pathology: issues in instrument development and evaluation. *J Hand Ther.* 2001;14(2):105–114.

63. Levine DW, Simmons BP, Koris MJ, Daltroy LH, Hohl GG, Fossel AH, Katz JN. A self-administered questionnaire for the assessment of severity of symptoms and functional status in carpal tunnel syndrome. *J Bone Jnt Surg.* 1993;75A:1585–1592.

64. Heybeli N, Kutluhan S, Demirci S, Kerman M, Mumcu EF. Assessment of outcome of carpal tunnel syndrome: a comparison of electrophysiological findings and a self-administered Boston questionnaire. *J Hand Surg [Br].* 2002;27(3):259–264.

65. Amadio P, Silverstein M, Ilstrup D, Schleck C, Jensen L. Outcome assessment for carpal tunnel surgery: The relative responsiveness of generic, arthritis-specific, disease-specific and physical examination measures. *J Hand Surg.* 1996;21A:338–346.

66. Atroshi I, Gummesson C, Johnsson R, Sprinchorn A. Symptoms, disability and quality of life in patients with carpal tunnel syndrome. *J Hand Surg.* 1999;24A:398–404.

67. Atroshi I, Johnsson R, Sprinchorn A. Self-administered outcome instrument in carpal tunnel syndrome. *Acta Orthopaedica Scandinavia.* 1998;69:82–88.

68. Bystrom S, Hall C, Welander T, Kilbom A. Clinical disorders and pressure-pain threshold of the forearm and hand among automobile assembly line workers. *J Hand Surg.* 1995;20B:782–790.

69. Ono Y, Nakamura R, Shimaoka M, Hiruta S, Hattori Y, Ichihara G. Epicondylitis among cooks in nursery schools. *Occup Environ Med.* 1998;55:172–179.

70. Walker-Bone KE, Palmer KT, Reading I, Cooper C. Criteria for assessing pain and nonarticular soft-tissue rheumatic disorders of the neck and upper limb. *Semin Arthritis Rheum.* 2003;33(3):168–184.

71. Katz JN, Larson MG, Sabra A, Krarup C, Stirrat CR, Sethi R, Eaton HM, Fossel AH, Liang MH. The carpal tunnel syndrome: diagnostic utility of the history and physical examination findings. *Ann Intern Med.* 1999;112:321–327.

72. Atroshi I, Breidenbach W, McCabe S. Assessment of the carpal tunnel outcome instrument in patients with nerve-compression symptoms. *J Hand Surg.* 1997;22:222–227.

73. Gunnarsson L, Amilon A, Hllestrand P, Leissner P, Philipson L. The diagnosis of carpal tunnel syndrome. Sensitivity and specificity of some clinical and electrophysiological tests. *J Hand Surg.* 1997;22:34–27.

74. O'Gradiagh D, Merry P. A diagnostic algorithm for carpal tunnel syndrome based on Bayes's theorem. *Rheumatology.* 2000;39:1040–1041.

75. Bessette L, Keller RB, Lew RA, Simmons BP, Fossel AH, Mooney N, Katz JN. Prognostic value of a hand symptom diagram in surgery for carpal tunnel syndrome. *J Rheumatol.* 1997;24(4):726–734.

76. Priganc V, Henry S. The relationship among five common carpal tunnel syndrome tests and the severity of carpal tunnel syndrome. *J Hand Ther.* 2003;16:225–236.

77. Dugas J, Andrews J. In Altchek D, Andrews J. *The athlete's elbow.* Philadelphia; Lippincott Williams and Wilkins: 2001.

78. Daniels J, Zook E, Lynch J. Hand and wrist injuries. Part 1: Non-emergent evaluation. *Am Family Phys.* 2004;69:1941–1948.

79. Kapandji I. *The physiology of the joint: The elbow. Flexion and extension.* 2nd ed. Vol 1. London; Livingstone: 1970.

80. Chaparro A, Rogers M, Fernandez J, Bohan M, Choi SD, Stumpfhauser L. Range of motion of the wrist: implications for designing computer input devices for the elderly. *Disabil Rehabil.* 2000;22(13–14):633–637.

81. Ebara S, Yonenobu K, Fujinara K, Yamashita K, Ono K. Myelopathic hand characterized by muscle wasting. A different type of myelopathic hand in patients with cervical spondylosis. *Spine.* 1988;13:785–791.

82. Colebatch J, Gandevia S. The distribution of muscular weakness in upper motor neuron lesions affecting the arm. *Brain.* 1989;112:749–763.

83. LaStayo PC, Wheeler DL. Reliability of passive wrist flexion and extension goniometric measurements: a multicenter study. *Phys Ther.* 1994;74(2):162–174.

84. Horger MM. The reliability of goniometric measurements of active and passive wrist motions. *Am J Occup Ther*. 1990;44(4):342–348.

85. Mayerson NH, Milano RA. Goniometric measurement reliability in physical medicine. *Arch Phys Med Rehabil*. 1984;65(2):92–94.

86. Adams BD, Grosland NM, Murphy DM, McCullough M. Impact of impaired wrist motion on hand and upper-extremity performance(1). *J Hand Surg [Am]*. 2003;28(6):898–903.

87. Morrey BF, Chao EY. Passive motion of the elbow joint. *J Bone Joint Surg Am*. 1976;58(4):501–508.

88. Youm Y, Dryer RF, Thambyrajah K, Flatt AE, Sprague BL. Biomechanical analyses of forearm pronation-supination and elbow flexion-extension. *J Biomech*. 1979;12(4):245–255.

89. Morrey BF, Askew LJ, Chao EY. A biomechanical study of normal functional elbow motion. *J Bone Joint Surg Am*. 1981;63(6):872–877.

90. Wagner C. Determination of the rotary flexibility of the elbow joint. *Eur J Appl Physiol Occup Physiol*. 1977;37(1):47–59.

91. Sarrafian S, Melamed J, Goshgarian G. Study of wrist motion in flexion and extension. *Clin Orthop*. 1977;126:153–159.

92. McGee D. *Orthopedic physical assessment*. 4th ed. Philiadelphia; Saunders. 2002.

93. Garcia-Elias M, An KN, Berglund L, Linscheid RL, Cooney WP, Chao EY. Extensor mechanism of the fingers. I. A quantitative geometric study. *J Hand Surgery*. 1991;16A:1130–1136.

94. Palmer AK, Skahen JR, Werner FW, Glisson RR. The extensor retinaculum of the wrist: an anatomical and biomechanical study. *J Hand Surg [Br]*. 1985;10(1):11–16.

95. Brumfield RH, Champoux JA. A biomechanical study of normal functional wrist motion. *Clin Orthop Relat Res*. 1984;(187):23–25.

96. Sucher B. Palpatory diagnosis and manipulative management of carpal tunnel syndrome. *J Am Osteopathic Assoc*. 1994;94:647–663.

97. Rosenberg D, Conolley J, Dellon AL. Thenar eminence quantitative sensory testing in the diagnosis of proximal median nerve compression. *J Hand Ther*. 2001;14(4):258–265.

98. Fairbank SR, Corelett RJ. The role of the extensor digitorum communis muscle in lateral epicondylitis. *J Hand Surg [Br]*. 2002;27(5):405–409.

99. Szabo RM, Slater RR Jr, Farver TB, Stanton DB, Sharman WK. The value of diagnostic testing in carpal tunnel syndrome. *J Hand Surg [Am]*. 1999;24(4):704–714.

100. Cozen L. The painful elbow. *Ind Med Surg*. 1962;31:369–71.

101. Maudsley RH, Roles NC. Trapped nerves. *Br Med J*. 1972;3;2(813):593–594.

102. Kalb K, Gruber P, Landsleitner B. (abstract). Compression syndrome of the radial nerve in the area of the supinator groove. Experiences with 110 patients. *Handchir Mikrochir Plast Chir*. 1999;31(5):303–310.

103. Lister GD, Belsole RB, Kleinert HE. The radial tunnel syndrome. *J Hand Surg [Am]*. 1979;4(1):52–59.

104. Rosenbaum R. Disputed radial tunnel syndrome. *Muscle Nerve*. 1999;22(7):960–967.

105. Goswami GK. The fat pad sign. *Radiology*. 2002;222 (2):419–420.

106. De Maeseneer M, Jacobson JA, Jaovisidha S, Lenchik L, Ryu KN, Trudell DR, Resnick D. Elbow effusions: Distribution of joint fluid with flexion and extension and imaging implications. *Invest Radiol*. 1998;33(2):117–125.

107. Irshad F, Shaw N, Gregory R. Reliability of fat-pad sign in radial head/neck fractures of the elbow. *Injury*. 1997;28:433–435.

108. Novak et al. Provocative testing for cubital tunnel syndrome. *J Hand Surg Am*. 1994;19:817–820.

109. Phalen G. The carpal tunnel syndrome. Seventeen years experience in diagnosis and treatment of six hundred fifty four hands. *J Bone Jnt Surg Am*. 1966;48:211–228.

110. Phalen G. The birth of a syndrome, or carpal tunnel revisited. *Am J Hand Surg*. 1981;6:109–110.

111. Kuhlman KA, Hennessey WJ. Sensitivity and specificity of carpal tunnel syndrome signs. *Am J Phys Med Rehabil*. 1997;76(6):451–457.

112. Fertl E, Wober C, Zeitlhofer J. The serial use of two provocative tests in the clinical diagnosis of carpal tunnel syndrome. *Acta Neurol Scand*. 1998;98(5):328–332.

113. Gunnarsson LG, Amilon A, Hellstrand P, Leissner P, Philipson L. The diagnosis of carpal tunnel syndrome. Sensitivity and specificity of some clinical and electrophysiological tests. *J Hand Surg [Br]*. 1997;22(1):34–37.

114. Gellman H, Gelberman RH, Tan AM, Botte MJ. Carpal tunnel syndrome. An evaluation of the provocative diagnostic tests. *J Bone Joint Surg Am*. 1986;68(5):735–737.

115. Heller L, Ring H, Costeff H, Solzi P. Evaluation of Tinel's and Phalen's signs in diagnosis of the carpal tunnel syndrome. *Eur Neurol*. 1986;25(1):40–42.

116. Katz JN, Stirrat CR, Larson MG, Fossel AH, Eaton HM, Liang MH. A self-administered hand symptom diagram for the diagnosis and epidemiologic study of carpal tunnel syndrome. *J Rheumatol*. 1990;17 (11):1495–1498.

117. Katz JN, Stirrat CR. A self-administered hand diagram for the diagnosis of carpal tunnel syndrome. *J Hand Surg [Am]*. 1990;15(2):360–363.

118. Spicher C, Kohut G, Miauton J. At which stage of sensory recovery can a tingling sign be expected? A

review and proposal for standardization and grading. *J Hand Ther.* 1999;12(4):298–308.

119. Kuschner S, Ebramzadeh E, Johnson D, Brien W, Sherman R. Tinel's sign and Phalen's test in carpal tunnel syndrome. *Orthopedics.* 1992;15:1297–1302.

120. Walters C, Rice V. An evaluation of provocative testing in the diagnosis of carpal tunnel syndrome. *Mil Med.* 2002;167(8):647–652.

121. De Krom M, Knipschild P, Kester A, Spaans F. Efficacy of provocative tests for diagnosis of carpal tunnel syndrome. *Lancet.* 1990;335:393–395.

122. Murtagh J. De Quervain's tenosynovitis and Finkelstein's test. *Aust Fam Physician.* 1989;18(12):1552.

123. Kutsumi K, Amadio PC, Zhao C, Zobitz ME, Tanaka T, An KN. Finkelstein's test: a biomechanical analysis. *J Hand Surg [Am].* 2005;30(1):130–135.

124. Elliott BG. Finkelstein's test: a descriptive error that can produce a false positive. *J Hand Surg [Br].* 1992; 17(4):481–482.

125. Hertling S, Kessler R. *Management of common musculoskeletal disorders: Physical therapy principles and methods.* Philadelphia; Lippincott: 1990.

126. Taleisnik J: Current concepts review. Carpal instability. *J Bone Joint Surg Am.* 1988;70:1262–1268.

127. Lichtman DM, Noble WH, Alexander CE: Dynamic triquetrolunate instability: case report. *J Hand Surg Am.* 1984;9:185–188.

128. Pin PG, Young VL, Gilula LA, Weeks PM: Management of chronic lunotriquetral ligament tears. *J Hand Surg Am.* 1989;14:77–83.

129. LaStayo P, Howell J. Clinical provocative tests used in evaluating wrist pain: a descriptive study. *J Hand Ther.* 1995;8(1):10–17.

130. Morrey B. The posttraumatic stiff elbow. *Clin Orthop.* 2005;431:26–35.

131. Kim S, Shin S. Arthroscopic treatment for limitation of motion of the elbow. *Clin Orthop.* 2000;375: 1401–1448.

132. Chinchalker S, Szekeres M. Rehabilitation of elbow trauma. *Hand Clinic.* 2004;20:363–374.

133. Vicenzino B, Collins D, Wright A. Sudomotor changes induced by neural mobilization techniques in asymptomatic subjects. *J Manual Manipulative Therapy.* 1994;2:66–74.

134. Chiu T, Wright A. To compare the effects of different rates of application of a cervical mobilization technique on sympathetic outflow to the upper limb in normal subjects. *Man Ther.* 1996;1:198–203.

135. Vicenzino B, Collins D, Wright A. An investigation of the interrelationship between manipulative therapy-induced hypoalgesia and sympathoexcitation. *J Manipulative Physiol Ther.* 1998;21:448–453.

136. Sterling M, Jull G, Wright A. Cervical mobilization: concurrent effects on pain, sympathetic nervous system activity and motor activity. *Man Ther.* 2001;6: 72–81.

137. Wright A. Pain-relieving effects of cervical manual therapy. In Grant R. *Physical therapy of the cervical and thoracic spine.* 3rd ed. New York; Churchill Livingston: 2002.

138. Brosseau L, Casimiro L, Milne S, Robinson V, Shea B, Tugwell P, Wells G. Deep transverse friction massage for treating tendonitis. *Cochrane Database Syst Rev.* 2002;(4):CD003528.

139. Lovick T. Interactions between descending pathways from the dorsal and ventrolateral periaqueductal gray matter in the rat. In: Depaulis A, Bandler R. (eds) *The midbrain periaqueductal gray matter.* New York; Plenum Press: 1991.

140. Vicenzino B, Paungmali A, Buratowski S, Wright A. Specific manipulative therapy treatment for chronic lateral epicondylalgia produces uniquely characteristic hypoalgesia. *Man Ther.* 2001;6:205–212.

141. Simon R, Vicenzino B, Wright A. The influence of an anteroposterior accessory glide of the glenohumeral joint on measures of peripheral sympathetic nervous system function in the upper limb. *Man Ther.* 1997;2(1):18–23.

142. Vincenzion B. Lateral epicondylalgia: a musculoskeletal physiotherapy perspective. *Man Ther.* 2003;8:66–79.

143. Paungmali A, O'Leary S, Souvlis T, Vincenzino B. Naloxone fails to antagonize initial hypoalgesic effect of a manual therapy treatment for lateral epicondylalgia. *J Manipulative Physiol Ther.* 2004;27: 180–185.

144. Abbott J. Mobilization with movement applied to the elbow affects shoulder range of movement in subjects with lateral epicondylagia. *Man Ther.* 2001; 6:170–177.

145. Abbott J, Patla C, Jensen P. The initial effects of an elbow mobilization with movement technique on grip strength in subjects with lateral epicondylagia. *Man Ther.* 2001;6:163–169.

146. Backstrom K. Mobilization with movement as an adjunct intervention in a patient with complicated de Quervain's tenosynovitis: a case report. *J Orthop Sports Phys Ther.* 2002;32:86–97.

147. Kaufman RL. Conservative chiropractic care of lateral epicondylitis. *J Manipulative Physiol Ther.* 2000;23(9):619–622.

148. Kaufman RL, Bird J. Manipulative management of post-Colles' fracture weakness and diminished active range of motion. *J Manipulative Physiol Ther.* 1999;22(2):105–107.

149. Lin C, Ju M, Huang H. Gender and age effects on elbow joint stiffness in healthy subjects. *Arch Phys Med Rehabil.* 2005;86:82–85.

150. Cook A, Szabo R, Birkholz S, King E. Early mobilization following carpal tunnel release. A prospective randomized study. *J Hand Surg (Br).* 1995;20: 228–230.

151. Kay S, Haensel N, Stiller K. The effect of passive mobilization following fractures involving the distal radius: a randomized study. *Aust J Physiother.* 2000; 46:93–101.

152. Coyle J, Robertson V. Comparison of two passive mobilizing techniques following Colles' fracture: a multi-element design. *Man Ther.* 1998;3(1):34–41.

153. Cyriax J, Cyriax P. *Cyriax's illustrated manual of orthopaedic medicine.* Oxford; Boston; Butterworth-Heineman. 1993.

154. Trudel D, Duley J, Zastrow I, Kerr EW, Davidson R, MacDermid JC. Rehabilitation for patients with lateral epicondylitis: a systematic review. *J Hand Ther.* 2004;17(2):243–266.

155. Coppieters MW, Bartholomeeusen KE, Stappaerts KH. Incorporating nerve-gliding techniques in the conservative treatment of cubital tunnel syndrome. *J Manipulative Physiol Ther.* 2004;27(9):560–568.

156. Tal-Akabi A, Rushton A. An investigation to compare the effectiveness of carpal bone mobilization and neurodynamic mobilization as methods of treatment for carpal tunnel syndrome. *Man Ther.* 2000;5:214–222.

157. Akalin E, El O, Peker O, Senocak O, Tamci S, Gulbahar S, Cakmur R, Oncel S. Treatment of carpal tunnel syndrome with nerve and tendon gliding exercises. *Arch Phys Med Rehab.* 2002;81(2):108–113.

158. Randall T, Portney L, Harris B. Effects of joint mobilization on joint stiffness and active motion of the metacarpal-phalangeal joint. *J Orthop Sports Phys Ther.* 1985;6:30–36.

159. Davis P, Hulbert J, Kassak K, Meyer J. Comparative efficacy of conservative medical and chiropractic treatments for carpal tunnel syndrome: a randomized controlled trial. *J Manipulative Physiol Ther.* 1998;21:317–326.

160. Valente R, Gibson H. Chiropractic manipulation in carpal tunnel syndrome. *J Manipulative Physiol Ther.* 1994;17:246–249.

161. Russell B, A suspected case of ulnar tunnel syndrome relieved by chiropractic extremity adjustment methods. *J Manipulative Physiol Ther.* 2003;26:602–627.

162. Hafner E, Kendall J, Kendall P. Comparative efficacy of conservative medical and chiropractic treatments for carpal tunnel syndrome: a randomized clinical trial. *J Manipulative Physiol Ther.* 1999;22(5):348–349.

163. Ernst E. Chiropractic manipulation for non-spinal pain: a systematic review. *N Z Med J.* 2003;116(1179):539.

164. Ahn D. Hand elevation: A new test for carpal tunnel syndrome. *Ann Plast Surg.* 2001;46:120–124.

165. Hansen P, Mickelsen P, Robinson L. Clinical utility of the flick maneuver in diagnosing carpal tunnel syndrome. *Am J Phys Med Rehabil.* 2004;83:363–367.

166. Tetro AM, Evanoff BA, Hollstien SB, Gelberman RH. A new provocative test for carpal tunnel syndrome. Assessment of wrist flexion and nerve compression. *J Bone Joint Surg Br.* 1998;80(3):493–498.

167. Szabo RM, Slater RR. Diagnostic testing in carpal tunnel syndrome. *J Hand Surg [Am].* 2000;25(1):184.

168. Kaul M, Pagel K, Wheatley M, Dryden J. Carpal compression test and pressure provocative test in veterans with median-distribution paresthesias. *Muscle Nerve.* 2001;24:107–111.

169. Wainner RS, Boninger ML, Balu G, Burdett R, Helkowski W. Durkan gauge and carpal compression test: accuracy and diagnostic test properties. *J Orthop Sports Phys Ther.* 2000;30(11):676–682.

# 11

# Manual Therapy of the Lumbar Spine

## Objectives

- Understand the basic aspects of lumbar spine biomechanics and anatomy
- Identify the prevalence and etiology of low back pain
- Identify the role of physical and psychosocial factors and low back pain
- Identify the common classification systems for low back pain
- Demonstrate the active physiological assessment components for low back pain
- Demonstrate the passive physiological assessment components for low back pain
- Demonstrate the passive accessory components for low back pain
- Identify common lumbar spine special tests and their respective diagnostic values
- Identify the pertinent treatment methods for lumbar spine impairment classifications

## PREVALENCE

Low back pain (LBP) is a major health burden in the United States, affecting 60–80% of Americans within their lifetime.[1,2] Low back pain is the leading cause of injury and disability for those under the age of 45, and the third most prevalent impairment for those 45 and older.[2] Americans are projected to report 16 million new low back pain impairments and 8 million LBP disabilities for 2004.[2]

Low back pain also leads to major costs associated with work loss. This disorder is the second leading cause of illness or missed work in the United States, annually affecting 15–20% of the workforce.[3,4] Annual costs associated with worker's compensation claims equate to millions of dollars, with low back pain accounting for 40% of worker's compensation physical therapy treatments.[5,6] In 1997, over 1 million worker's compensation claims were filed,[7] leading to 2–5% of the annual workforce mired in work loss and rehabilitation programs.[8] Nearly seven million visits to physical therapists occurred under worker's compensation in 1990.[8]

Typically, low back pain is a self-limiting disorder. Up to 90% of patients recover in 3–4 months, 70% recover in 1 month, and 50% in 2 weeks with no formal treatment. Five percent (5%) of the remaining 10% will not respond to conservative care such as physical therapy or care from other rehabilitation professionals.[5,9] For this 5%, removal from work has a negative effect on recovery. If an individual is out of work for 6 months, they have less than a 40% chance of returning to their occupation. If the time away from work extends to 1 year, the number decreases to less than 20%. If the impairment is severe enough to cause 2 years of work loss, the chance of returning is nearly nonexistent.[9]

### Summary

- Low back pain is a huge financial burden in the United States.
- Low back pain is generally self-limiting, but may progress to a disability in 5% of patients.
- Much of low back treatment is untested, is potentially ineffective, and may offer little toward the recovery process of low back pain.

At present, a standardized approach that is responsible for the recovery of the 5% is undetermined.[5] Ninety-five percent (95%) of patients may improve with little or no treatment, or may be treated by a method that has little or no scientific basis for effectiveness. Techniques that have been investigated and show significant benefit in clinical trials are the focus of this chapter. When uninvestigated, techniques that are patient response-based are demonstrated.

# ANATOMY

## Lumbar Vertebra

The lumbar spine consists of five lumbar vertebrae, five corresponding intervertebral discs, 12 **zygopophyseal joints** (T12-L1 to L5-S1), and multiple ligaments, muscular, and neurological contributions. The design of the lumbar spine allows viscoelastic motion, absorbs energy, moves with six degrees of freedom, and has limited fatigue tolerance. These functions depend on muscular, bone, and ligamentous components for mechanical tasks.[10]

The typical lumbar vertebrae display dramatic height increase when compared to the thoracic spine. The lower vertebrae and discs are wedge shaped, lending to the natural postural lordosis. The anterior aspect of the vertebra is generally concave and the posterior aspects are flattened and stable.[10]

Lumbar vertebrae can be divided into three sections from anterior to posterior (Figure 11.1). The anterior portion in the vertebral body is essentially flat on the superior

and inferior surfaces and provides contact points for the intervertebral disc.[10] The middle section in the lumbar spine includes the pedicles, which are strong posterior projections. The posterior portion of the vertebral body includes the inferior and superior articular processes, the spinous process, and the transverse processes. The spinous processes are heavy and rectangular.

## The Vertebral and Intervertebral Foramen

The anterior wall of the vertebral canal is flattened and the discs demonstrate no propensity of bulging into the spinal canal. The anterior wall of the vertebral canal is

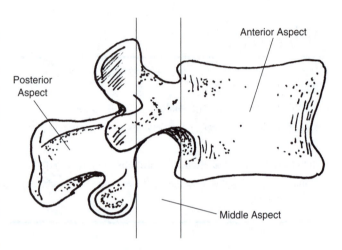

**Figure 11.1**    The Three Divisions of a Typical Lumbar Vertebral Body

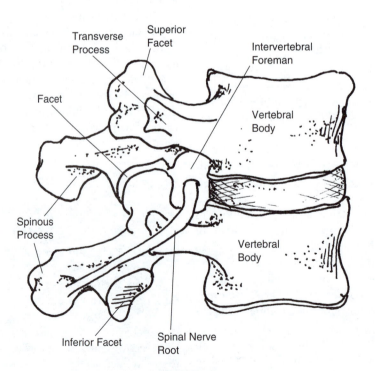

**Figure 11.2**    The Intervertebral Foramen

formed by the posterior surfaces of the lumbar vertebra and the posterior wall is formed by the lamina and ligamentum flava of the same vertebra.[10] The disc surrounds the intervertebral foramen anteriorly, the pedicle inferiorly and superiorly, and by the zygopophyseal joints posteriorly (Figure 11.2).[10]

## Joints of the Lumbar Spine

### The Zygopophyseal Joints

The zygopophyseal joints (Figure 11.3), also known as facets or apophysial joints, are enclosed in a fibrous capsule that contains menisci. The menisci are invaginations of the joint capsule and may occasionally project into joint space.[11] Facets do not have "free" motion as does the disc and are limited both structurally and by the capsule. Movement is generally restricted to large sagittal motions guided by the shape of the zygopophyseal joints.

The facets flatten anteroposterior and run slightly dorsally and upward.[10] The zygopophyseal joints and the surrounding structure represent attachment sites for several intertransverse ligaments and muscles. The intertransverse ligaments attach to each transverse process and limit side flexion to the opposite side. The transverse process of L5 attaches to the medial portion of the iliac crest by several strong strands of the iliolumbar ligament, which tends to ossify at older ages. The anterior portions of the lumbar facets oriented coronally (promote side bend forces). The posterior facets face sagittal and resist rotational and side bend forces.[11]

### The Intervertebral Disc (Interbody Joints)

The intervertebral disc (Figure 11.4) functions as a shock absorber, a deformable space, and resists compressive forces of the spine.[8] There are three major components of the disc: (1) the annulus fibrosis, (2) the nucleus pulposis, and (3) the cartilaginous end plate. The nucleus pulposis accounts for up to 50% of the disc area and includes collagen fibers without specific orientation. The major constituents include proteoglycans, collagen, and water.

The nucleus is responsible for nutrient transport via osmosis of the middle cartilaginous end plate and articulation with the disc. The actual compression tolerance is derived from the properties in the water (at lower levels) through proteoglycans imbibitions of joint fluid. The nucleus transfers much of the weight to the annulus when loads are high or when damage has occurred to the intervertebral segment.

The annulus gradually blends into the nucleus in a gradual transition rather than an abrupt transition between two separate structures.[12] The annulus consists of multiple concentric rings called lamella, which provide tension in all directions when force is encountered. The lamella consists of concentric-oriented rings, lying at a 30-degree plane from the horizon.[13] Lamellae are designed to counter compression, side bending, shear, and distraction forces. Nerve endings in the outer border of the annulus are responsible for pain generation and somatic referral of symptoms.

The disc integrates with the vertebrae at the cartilaginous end plate. The inner two-thirds of the disc attach to the cartilaginous end plate while the outer two-thirds attach to the intervertebral body. The cartilaginous end plate is responsible for nutrient transfer to the disc from the vertebral body and becomes thicker and less permeable with increasing age. This structure is composed of hyaline cartilage and is thicker and more calcified at the periphery.[14] The vertebral end plate also contributes in confining the annulus and nucleus.[15]

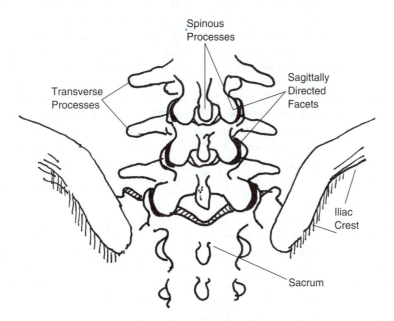

**Figure 11.3** Zygopophyseal Joints of the Lumbar Spine

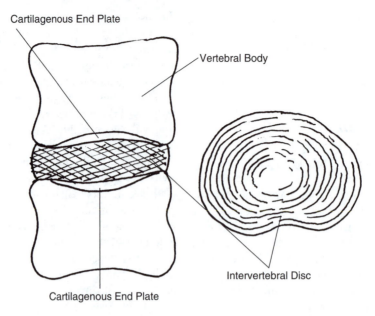

**Figure 11.4**    The Three Major Components of the Intervertebral Disc

The intervertebral disc is the major load bearing and motion control element in lateral and anterior shear, axial compression, flexion, and side flexion. The intervertebral disc guides the motion of rotation whereas the facet restricts motion beyond disc boundaries.[16,17] This is in contrast to the facet, which contributes to motion control during posterior shear, extension, and axial torsion. During lateral and anterior shear with high external forces, the facets may transmit a portion of the load.[17]

In a healthy lumbar spine, the disc transfers the forces evenly and transmits forces to the ligaments of the back (specifically the anterior longitudinal ligament and the posterior longitudinal ligament), through an interplay of the thoracolumbar fascia and abdominal musculature.[17,18] In the nondamaged disc up to 85% of the movement is controlled through the interplay of disc dispensation. A damaged disc will encounter a different percentage, typically dispensing force to the facets and other supportive structures, including the vertebral endplate. The vertebral endplate is the most significant potential point of weakness and is the quickest healing area of the lumbar disc segment.[10] Unfortunately, no known clinical examination features outline vertebral end plate damage, thus these impairments may remain undetected.

### Nerves of the Lumbar Spine

The spinal nerves of the lumbar spine subdivide into ventral and dorsal rami. Each spinal nerve lies within the intervertebral foramen and are numbered according to the vertebra above the nerve. Subsequently the L4 nerve root runs below the L4 vertebra, in between L4 and L5. Each spinal nerve arises from a ventral and a dorsal nerve root, which meet to form the spinal nerve in the intervertebral foramen.[10] Each dorsal root communicates to a dorsal root ganglion that

contains the cell bodies of the sensory fibers of the dorsal roots. The dorsal root transmits sensory fibers whereas the ventral root primarily transmits motor fibers.[19] Each spinal nerve exits the intervertebral foramen with dural structures, an extension of the dura mater and arachnoid mater, commonly referred to as the dural sleeve.[19] In the intervertebral foramen, the amount of space is extremely limited, thus the structures in this region are predisposed to problems associated with space occupying lesions.

Branching from each ventral rami are sinuvertebral nerves that are considered mixed (motor and sensory) nerves. The sinuvertebral nerve complex innervates the outer border of the annulus, posterior longitudinal ligament, and contributes fibers to the joint capsule and articular facet. Posteriorly, the lumbar spine is innervated by branches of the dorsal rami that run to the zygopophyseal joints and muscles. Anterior and posterior plexuses innervate the anterior longitudinal ligament (ALL) and posterior longitudinal ligament (PLL), additionally supplying innervation to the intervertebral disc and periosteum of the vertebral bodies.[10,19] This complex innervation pattern reduces the likelihood of unambiguous pain referral patterns from one specific structure.

### Ligaments of the Lumbar Spine

Numerous ligaments restrain free motion. The anterior longitudinal ligament (ALL) and posterior longitudinal ligament (PLL) interconnect the vertebral bodies and are deeply associated with the annulus fibrosis of the discs. The ALL serves primarily to resist vertical separation of the anterior ends of the vertebral bodies and resists anterior bowing during extension movements.[10] The PLL also resists separation of vertebra and aids in posterior support with the intimate connection with the annulus fibrosis.[10]

Posterior ligaments include the ligamentum flavum, the interspinous ligaments, and the supraspinous ligament. The ligamentum flavum is a short, thick ligament that joins each lamina of consecutive vertebrae. This ligament also resists separation of vertebrae, although the exact mechanics of the ligament are unknown.[10,14] The interspinous ligaments connect adjacent spinous processes and most likely resist separation of the spinous processes. The supraspinous ligament attaches to the posterior ends of the spinous processes and are likely heavily embedded with proprioceptive nerve endings.[20] In general, the posterior spinous ligaments are slack in upright standing but will tighten during forward flexion and rotation.

The iliolumbar ligaments are well-developed ligaments, are anterior, superior, and vertical in nature, and are one of few structures that actually cross the sacroiliac joint.[21] Bodguk and Twomey[22] outlined five separate bands of the iliolumbar ligament, which traverse from the transverse process of L5 to the quadratus lumborum, the iliac crest, and the posterior aspect of the iliac tuberosity. The iliolumbar ligament ossifies by the fifth decade and is demarcated from the quadratus lumborum muscle.[22] The iliolumbar ligament appears to restrict sagittal nutation and counternutation of the SIJ.[21,23]

## *Muscular Stabilization of the Spine*

Stability of the lumbar spine is a joint responsibility of the passive and active structures of the lumbar spine. Studies have suggested that the multifidi are responsible for postural, multidirectional, and individual segmental control.[24–26] The multifidi are the largest and most medial of the lumbar paraspinal muscles, originating from a spinous process and spreading caudo-laterally from the midline, inserting into the mamillary processes of the facet joint, the iliac crest, and the sacrum. The multifidi maintain lumbar lordosis by acting like a bowstring transmitting some of the axial compression force to the ALL. These muscles protect discs by preventing unwanted wobbling movements associated with torsion and flexion.

The transverse abdominus plays an important role in dynamic isometric stabilization during twisting and rotation motions.[27–30] Selected authors have suggested that for individuals with passive spine instability, sagittal torsion or rotation strains are more responsible for damaging structures than linear forces.[31] The hypothesized contribution occurs through increasing the stiffness of the lumbar spine (i.e., increasing intra-abdominal pressure and tensioning the thoracolumbar fascia resisting torsion). The transverse abdominus increases in stiffness in anticipation of limb movement and limits intersegmental translation and rotational forces. This action may provide a more stable lever with the other trunk muscles.[30]

Other contributors to spine movement and stability include the erector spinae, external and internal obliques, and the thoracolumbar fascia. The thoracolumbar fascia that inserts on the gluteus maximus and latissimus dorsi

and integrates with the deep lamina of the inferior aspect of the lumbar pedicle works in concert with the lumbar musculature to stabilize during dynamic movement. The internal and external obliques work in concert with the thoracolumbar fascia to stabilize the core pressure but are primarily prime movers of diagonal rotational motions and poor stabilizers of the lumbar spine. The erector spinae consist of the longissimus thoracic and iliocostalis lumborum groups.[32] Van Dieën et al.[33] reported that subjects with low back pain demonstrated a higher recruitment of the lumbar erector spinae in an effort to increase stability.

The psoas major is not a significant contributor to spine stability and is primarily a hip flexor.[32] The psoas fibers originate near the anterior spine (T12 through L4-5) and transverse process and inserts on the hip. This lever mechanism is too inefficient to produce lumbar movement.[32] Many clinicians misperceive the role of the psoas as a significant contributor to low back pain. Bogduk states, "The isometric morphology of the psoas indicates that the muscle is designed exclusively to act on the hip".[32] Although a maximum contraction can increase intradiscal loads,[32] this muscle may not contribute to stabilize the spine.

## *Summary*

- Much of low back movement is controlled and guided by the intervertebral disc.
- The shape of the lumbar vertebral body and disc promotes a natural lordosis.
- The orientation of the facets limits lumbar rotation and aids in stability during rotation.
- Several muscles of the lumbar spine are the primary source of dynamic stability functioning as prime movers and stabilizers.

# BIOMECHANICS

Many manual therapy disciplines base specific mobilization and manipulation techniques on selected theories of lumbar coupling direction, theories that are often inconsistently reported.[34] Biomechanical analysis, including investigation of **coupled motion,** is often reported as an essential concept to low back evaluation.[35–39] The two principle components of lumbar coupling are quantity of motion, used in detection of hypo- and hypermobility, and direction of coupling behavior. The most controversial of the two assessment methods is the theory of directional lumbar coupling, a theory based on the invalidated premise that a "normal" lumbar coupling pattern exists in nonpathological individuals.[40–42] It has been suggested that the link between pathology of the lumbar spine may be best represented by addressing the pattern or direction of coupling behavior.[39,43–48]

Coupled motion is the rotation or translation of a vertebral body about or along one axis that is consistently associated with the main rotation or translation about another axis.[48] During movement, translation occurs when movement is such that all particles in the body at a given time have the same direction of motion relative to a fixed coordinate system.[48] With movement, rotation occurs as a spinning or angular displacement of the vertebral body around some axis.

Historic, foundational works on coupling mechanics used observation or controversial two-dimensional (2-D) radiographic imagery.[39] Past 2-D studies involved cadaveric tissue, X-rays of live subjects, or single X-rays of segments, and used a small sample of subjects.[39,49] Prior to 1969, only 2-D studies were executed for spinal coupling, signifying that any study performed prior to 1969 encompassed these errant methods.[39] 2-D imagery leads to magnification errors, projection of translations as rotations, and misleading results.[39,50] Theories such as Fryettes Laws I and II of the lumbar spine have not held up well to modern science and are generally recognized by researchers as incorrect.[34,39]

Contemporary studies use three-dimensional (3-D) assessment, which more accurately measures the six degrees of freedom associated with coupling motion.[34] All of the studies reported no coupling present in at least some of the specimens/subjects at L1-2, with two reporting opposite results.[34] Inconsistency is also present at L2-3 and L3-4 where results are split between no report of coupling, opposite rotational coupling with side bending, and both.[34]

The spinal levels of L4-5 and L5-S1 exhibited the greatest degree of variability. Two studies reported that no coupling was present at L4-L5, three others recognized opposite rotational coupling with side bending, and one indicated same side, rotational coupling with side bending.[34] The same two studies that found no coupling at previous segments found no coupling at L5-S1, three others found opposite rotational coupling to side bending, and one found both opposite and no coupling.[34]

Recent *in vivo* and *in vitro* studies find coupling pattern disparities specifically when dealing with symptomatic patients with low back pain.[36,43,51–59] According to Panjabi et al.,[60] "diseases and degeneration affect the physical properties of the spinal components (ligaments, discs, facet joints, and vertebral bodies) which, in turn, alter the overall spinal behavior." Current research addresses the contribution of coupling motion from the disc and the facets.[34] An *in vivo* study[61] found that a narrowed intervertebral disc led to increased lateral bending, increased disc shear at the level of abnormality, and asymmetric coupling patterns throughout adjacent functional spine units. Lower lumbar levels (L3-4, L4-5) increased their coupling behavior and range while decreasing at higher levels

(L1-2, L2-3). Surgical fusion created increased mobility immediately above the fused site.[62] The coupling movement was abnormal and relied heavily on increased motion in the posterior facet joints and shear of the intervertebral discs. Posterior–lateral disc removal *in vitro* does significantly affect normal spinal kinematics. The alteration is not only present in the single functional spinal unit but also the neighboring joints.[47] **Chronic back pain** diagnoses such as post-laminectomy, post-discectomy, and disc degeneration leads to variability in *in vivo* coupling at lower levels of the lumbar spine.[46]

There seems to be little evidence to support that knowledge of lumbar spine coupling characteristics are important in understanding and treating patients with low back pain.[38] Many manual therapy techniques use coupling-based mobilizations and the validity of this approach is questionable. Several authors have suggested that the use of symptom reproduction to identify the level of pathology is the only accurate assessment method.[63–69] Because no pathological coupling pattern has shown to be consistent, an assessment method in absence of symptom reproduction may yield inaccurate results. Therefore, biomechanical coupling theory may only be useful if assessed with symptom reproduction within a clinical examination.[70] There is little evidence to support a limited focus on biomechanical coupling patterns, therefore techniques that are based on this "theory" is excluded from this textbook.

## Range of Motion

Troke et al.[71] report global flexion and extension range-of-motion values of 72 degrees to 40 degrees of flexion and 29 degrees to 6 degrees of extension. Their findings suggest that range of motion declines with age changes from 16 to 90 years. These findings are in accordance with others who have reported similar numbers and similar declines with advancing age.[72,73] Rotation and side flexion have also been studied extensively. The motions are reported in Tables 11.1 and 11.2 and represent individual segmental movements in rotation and side flexion.

## Summary

- Little to no evidence exists to support the use of directional lumbar coupling biomechanics for manual therapy techniques.
- The use of coupling assessment as a basis for treatment is not scientific, not evidence based, and therefore may be inappropriate for certain patients.
- The majority of segmental range of the motion in the lumbar spine occurs within a sagittal plane, followed by coronal, and lastly transverse.

**TABLE 11.1    Mean Range of Motion for Physiological Side Bending**

| Author | L-2 | L2-3 | L3-4 | L4-5 | L5-S1 |
|---|---|---|---|---|---|
| White & Panjabi[256] | 6 | 6 | 8 | 6 | 8 |
| Pearcy & Tibrewal[257] | 10 | 11 | 10 | 6 | 8 |
| Panjabi et al.[38] | 4.2 | 5.8 | 5.3 | 5.1 | 4.3 |
| Panjabi et al.[47] | 4 | 6.2 | 6 | 5.7 | 5.5 |
| Goel[258] | 2.5 | 2.5 | 2.5 | 2.5 | 2.5 |
| Soni[259] | 4.2 | 5.7 | 4.8 | 6 | Not reported |

# ASSESSMENT AND DIAGNOSIS

## Differential Diagnosis

Differential diagnosis of low back disorders into subcategories should result in more effective treatment.[74–77] Subcategorization into diagnostic classifications is also beneficial for improvements in research, consistency in terminology, development of pertinent treatment algorithms, and optimization of surgical selection. McCarthy et al.[78] outline three categorization processes during the initial diagnostic triage: (1) identification of nerve root–related problems, (2) identification of disorders that represent serious pathology, and (3) identification of patients who fall under the classification heading of nonspecific low back pain. This process allows the clinician to differentiate those subjects that are appropriate for care and to categorize further patients into homogenized groups for optimal treatment.

### Step One: Nerve Root Assessment

The first step, identification of patients who exhibit nerve root–related problems, is discussed in detail in Chapter Five. Essentially, three forms of referred pain to the lower extremities may originate from structures of the lumbar spine: (1) myelopathy, (2) radiculopathy, and (3) somatic referred pain. Presence of myelopathy is generally outlined by upper motor neuron signs and symptoms, and requires further medical intervention outside a traditional rehabilitative approach. Selected conditions of radiculopathy require careful, specific intervention and may involve a variety of different conditions. Somatic referred pain that involves referred pain originating from a structure outside of a nerve root is generally treated differently than radiculopathic pain.

### Step Two: Red Flag Assessment

A concurrent second step involves the differentiation of patients that are appropriate for conservative care. Within this step, it is imperative to isolate **sinister disorders** and red flags as well as other factors that may retard outcome or foster progression of chronicity. The majority of low back impairments are generally benign self-limiting disorders;[79–83] nonetheless, in approximately 5% or less of cases, patients may present with a serious, specific disease process that requires emergency intervention.[79] Lurie[79] outlines three major categories of serious, specific disease processes that may not recover well during conventional care. In addition, the reader is recommended to refer to Chapter Five to assist in understanding the selected "red flags" associated with differential diagnosis. The three major categories include: (1) nonmechanical spine disorders, (2) visceral disease, and (3) miscellaneous. Table 11.3 outlines the selected disorders under each specific category and the estimated prevalence of the dysfunction.

Patient history is more useful than a clinical examination in detecting malignancy, which is rare, accounting for less than 1% of low back pain.[79] Jarvik and Deyo[84]

**TABLE 11.2    Physiological Range of Rotational Motion**

| Author | L-2 | L2-3 | L3-4 | L4-5 | L5-S1 |
|---|---|---|---|---|---|
| White & Panjabi[256] | 2 | 2 | 2 | 2 | 1 |
| Pearcy & Tibrewal[257] | 2 | 2 | 3 | 3 | 2 |
| Panjabi et al.[38] | 1.75 | 2.2 | 2.2 | 2.2 | 1.05 |
| Panjabi et al.[47] | 1 | 2 | 1.5 | 1.5 | 1 |
| Goel[258] | 1 | 1 | 1 | 1 | 1 |
| Tencer et al.[116] | 1 | 2 | 2 | 2 | Not reported |
| Pearcy et al.[35] | 1 | 1 | 1.5 | 1.5 | .5 |

**TABLE 11.3** Serious, Specific Low Back Diseases[79]

| Category | Specific Disorders | Examples of Disorders |
|---|---|---|
| 1) Nonmechanical spine disorders (± 1%) | Neoplasia | Metastases, lymphoid tumor, spinal cord tumor |
| | Infection | Infective spondylitis, epidural abscess, endocarditis, herpes zoster, Lyme disease |
| | Seronegative spondyloarthritides | Ankylosing spondylitis, psoriatic arthritis, reactive arthritis, Reiter's syndrome, inflammatory bowel disease |
| 2) Visceral disease (1–2%) | Pelvic | Prostatitis, endometriosis, pelvic inflammatory disease |
| | Renal | Nephrolithiasis, pyelonephritis, renal papillary necrosis |
| | Aortic aneurysm | Aortic aneurysm |
| | Gastrointestinal | Pancreatitis, cholecystitis, peptic ulcer disease |
| 3) Miscellaneous | Paget's disease | Paget's disease |
| | Parathyroid disease | Parathyroid disease |
| | Hemoglobinopathies | Hemoglobinopathies |

reported that the most diagnostic combination of red flags used to identify malignancy were age >50, history of cancer, unexplained weight loss, and failure of conservative care. The cluster of these variables demonstrated a sensitivity of 100% and a specificity of 60%. Another nonmechanical condition, infective spondylitis, is generally associated with a fever (sensitivity of 98%), although this finding is not specific to this disorder (specificity of 50%).[79] Ankylosing spondylitis is often associated (specificity of 82%) with early or slow onset, age <40, long-term discomfort (>3 months), morning stiffness, and improvement of discomfort with exercise, although a combination of these factors results in low sensitivity (23%). Lurie[79] suggests including historical factors such as family history, thoracic stiffness, thoracic pain, and heel pain to improve the specificity. The detection of cauda equina problems are most accurately identified by urinary retention (sensitivity of 90%, specificity of 95%).[85] In addition, red flags are potentially significant physiological risk factors for developing chronic low back pain if not appropriately assessed. These physical factors include evidence of radicular symptoms into the lower extremity, peripheralization of symptoms during treatment or movements, and narrowing of the intervertebral space upon radiological examination. Others have warned that no hard evidence exists that allows identification of the presence of specific physical factors that may lead to negative outcomes.[86–90]

### Step Three: Diagnostic Classification

The third and final phase of diagnostic classification involves categorizing patients into homogenized groups for better treatment. Low back classification models categorize homogeneous conditions by using one of three classification index strategies: (1) status index, (2) prognostic index, and (3) the patient-response model. Status index models such as those created by Bernard and Kirkaldy-Willis[91] and Moffroid et al.[92] involve the use of physical impairment classifications (diagnoses) designed to discriminate among faulty pathological tissue. Groups are subdivided into homogenous categories based on suspected pain generators. Prognostic index models such as pain-related fear, coping behavior, and so on are primarily used to predict the future outcome of the patient and to target prospectively those with potentially poor progression.[93] Prognostic index models are typically obtained from statistical analysis of preexisting data and may involve subclassifications based on like type outcomes. Prognostic index models are retrospective in nature but have been suggested for use prospectively.[94]

Patient-response models provide clinicians with potential exercise and treatment selections based on the patient's response to movements during an examination. Classification using the patient-response method addresses symptom elicitation (using pain provocation or reduction methods) with various movements for diagnostic assessment. This classification model (provocation, reproduction, and reduction) assesses the response of singular or repeated movements and/or positions on the patient's concordant complaint of pain or abnormality of movement. Treatment techniques are often similar to the direction and form of the assessment method. The particular treatment technique is based on the movement method that reproduces the patient's pain in a way designed to yield a result that either reduces pain or increases range of motion. The direction, amplitude, forces, and speed of the treatment depends on the patient response during and after the application. This method consists of within-treatment and between-treatment patient response parameters of provocation, reproduction, and reduction that have shown to predict good outcomes overall.[94–97] Within the literature, this process of classification has further been subdivided into two primary forms: (1) diagnostic classification based on signs and symptoms and (2) classification based on expectations of treatment outcomes. It is arguable whether classification based on treatment outcomes is not considered diagnostic.

Diagnostic classification based on signs and symptoms is the hallmark of most low back classification systems. Physicians have developed many classification techniques that place diagnostic labels to implicate the "guilty structure." The usefulness of these diagnostic labels seldom guide rehabilitation clinicians' decisions related to the prognosis or treatment of patients with low back pain.[93] Numerous ICD-9 codes outline specific back impairments, each with subtle differences in characteristics. In many cases, diagnostic equipment that is frequently used to classify low back pain is not discriminatory enough to specify a disorder. Lastly, some physicians do not agree on the occurrence of certain impairments, which may lead to over- or underreporting of the prevalence. These "labels" offer little or no confirmation of the nature, severity, irritability, or stage of the back impairment.

The patient response-based classification is a mechanism commonly referred to throughout this textbook. This classification occurs after results from assessment are analyzed.[93] An example, such as the *McKenzie method*, allows for modification of classification based on follow-up findings.[94] Each classification is dependent upon each patient response to the assessment methods and the corresponding change in treatment approach. This approach does not rely on specific paradigms because each patient may exhibit unique symptoms, which do not lend to one dogmatic approach. However, these methods also have weaknesses as well as strengths. The McKenzie classification does not recognize spine instability or categories consisting of sinister pathologies such as tumors or fractures.[93]

A recent classification system by Peterson et al.[99,100] involves the merger of diagnostic and patient-response indices into a single diagnostic classification. The purpose of this system is to identify clinically homogenous subgroups of patients with nonspecific low back pain that are outlined specifically with the symptomatic causal structures.[99] The process involves three steps in classifying a patient's condition, much of which is based on McKenzie's classification system. However, the system is designed to strengthen some of the areas in which McKenzie fails to cover, such as subclassification for the categories of zygopophyseal joint syndrome, sacroiliac joint syndrome, myofascial pain, adverse neural tension, and abnormal pain syndromes.[100]

Perhaps the most common low back impairment classification system is the *Quebec Task Force* (QTF) classification model. This model consists of 12 categories of impairments, often based on location of symptoms, imaging results, and chronicity of pain. One challenge to this model is that rehabilitation clinicians often do not have access to imaging and occasionally the imaging results are flawed. In addition, the intertester reliability between the QTF is unknown.[93] All categories are not mutually exclusive, leading to the chance of classification into more than one group.[93] The QTF model does not associate treatment with diagnosis.[101] Lastly, like the treatment response-based classification, not all impairment categories are represented (i.e., spine instability, fracture).

One reason the task of classification is difficult is that there is sparse evidence to support the relationship between specific physical factors and the ability to predict the severity of a lumbar pathology.[102,103] Similarly, there is little evidence to support that specific physical factors are accurate predictors of disability.[104,105] Essentially, low back recovery is poorly related to the severity of impairment, the type of treatment received, and/or the surgical procedure.

At present, no single diagnostic classification system has demonstrated superiority over another.[99,100] There are numerous pain generators of the lumbar spine, many that are clinically difficult to isolate secondary to convergence.[32] Sources can include the bone, which is innervated by the sympathetic trunk, gray rami communicantes, and the plexuses of the anterior and posterior longitudinal ligament. Additionally, muscles, thoraco-lumbar fascia (which contains nociceptive nerve endings), dura mater (which is innervated by an extensive plexus of the lumbar sinuvertebral nerve complex), the epidural plexus, ligaments, zygopophyseal joints that are innervated by the medial branches of the lumbar dorsal rami, and frequently, the intervertebral discs all share common nerve attachments.[106–108]

Spitzer et al. reports that most incidences of low back pain do not have a readily demonstrable and identifiable pathologic basis.[103] Often the selected pathological process is generally not the established cause of the pain[109] or may not occur in isolation. Despite these challenges, selected authors have suggested prevalence of "at-fault" structures that may be the pain generators of low back impairment. Bogduk[109] reported the most common site is typically discogenic (39%), followed by the zygopophyseal joints (15%), the sacroiliac joint (13%), and undefined (33%). Laslett et al. report estimates of 15–40% of low back pain originating in the zygopophyseal joints.[110]

## *Summary*

- Even with clinical and diagnostic tests, the cause of most low back impairments is unknown.
- The lumbar intervertebral disc is the primary pain generator in the lumbar spine, accounting for the majority of impairments.
- Physical factors offer little predictive evidence for low back pain recovery.
- A lumbar spine classification system may yield homogeneous outcomes for research, treatment, and assessment.
- The treatment response-based classification system may offer the most clinician-friendly classification model and typically does not suffer from many of the validity challenges of other classification models.
- At present, no classification system has been proven more valid than another has, but for manual therapy clinicians, the treatment response-based classification may allow adaptability to each individual patient.

# CLINICAL EXAMINATION

## *Observation*

For individuals with **postural syndromes**, observation and the symptoms associated with long-term positioning is a prime assessment tool. Recently, O'Sullivan[18] used observations to determine positional preferences of spine instability patients. His classifications were based on position intolerance and theoretical instabilities on these positions. Additionally, Cook, Sizer, and Brismee[111] reported that certain postural intolerances were characteristic to patients with clinical lumbar spine instability. Granata and Wilson have associated the maintenance of selected trunk postures with the propensity for spine instability.[112]

A decreased **willingness to move** is also an observational method worth addressing and has been related to poor treatment outcomes.[113,114] Avoidance of certain movements because of fear of reinjury or increased pain is common in patients with chronic low back impairment.[115] This reluctance may be associated with fear of movement–related pain that may lead to a cascade of further problems. **Catastrophising behavior,** a symptom frequently associated with decreased willingness to move, is also common in those with poor low back–related outcomes.[115]

Although not conclusively definitive, physiometric findings may assist the clinician in categorizing patient presentations. Physiometric findings are poorly reliable and not always associated with patient outcomes but when combined with other indicators are useful in patient as-

**TABLE 11.4** Objective Observational Findings of Low Back Pain

| Structure | Observational Finding |
| --- | --- |
| Herniated disc | Flattened back |
| Radiographic instability | Excessive lordosis |
| Sacroiliac dysfunction | Flattened back |
| Degenerative disc disease | Hypertrophic supraspinous ligament |
| Spine stenosis | Flattened back |
| Facet impingement | Flexed back, usually unilateral |
| Nerve root adhesion | Bad posture, avoids forward flexion |

sessment. Abnormal side-to-side weight-bearing asymmetry has been recognized in patients with low back pain versus controls.[116] Other nonempirical-based findings such as flattened posture, excessive lordosis, or generalized poor posture may be associated with selected pathologies (Table 11.4).

Riddle and Rothstein[117] found that detection of a lateral shift (Figure 11.5) demonstrated poor interrater reliability during an examination. Kilpikoski et al.[118] also found poor reliability for visual detection of lateral shift

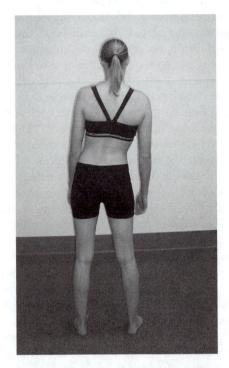

**Figure 11.5** Patient with a right lateral shift. Shift detection is determined by analyzing the position of the trunk over the pelvis. In this example, the patient's trunk is shifted right over the pelvis.

but did agree on the directional preference of each centralizing patient. The directional preference corresponds to a movement that decreases pain symptoms, a movement that may include any active range of motion in the sagittal or coronal plane. Clare, Adams, and Maher[119] found moderate reliability (0.48–0.64) in the detection of a lateral shift and proposed the use of a photograph to dissect the sagittal plane to improve results. Tenhula et al.[120] suggested that response to a shift correction demonstrated useful clinical information during an examination, confirming the presence of a lateral shift in patients with low back pain. The authors advocated the use of repeated side glides for analysis of centralization or peripheralization of symptoms, a finding supported by Young et al.[121] in association with repeated movement testing. Centralization of symptoms is associated with positive outcomes and a reduced tendency for disability.[104]

Patients may exhibit a lateral shift toward or away from his or her report of pain. If the shift is toward the pain, the shift is described as an ipsilateral shift and may be associated with a central disc herniation. If the shift is away from the report of pain, the shift is described as a contralateral shift and may be associated with a posterolateral disc herniation.

## Subjective History

Vroomen et al.[122] found that consistency in history taking varied among clinicians and was strongest in the areas of muscle strength and sensory losses, intermediate for reflex changes, and poor in the areas of a specific spine examination. Most significantly, the authors suggested that the clinicians should concentrate further on history taking to extract useful components for clarification. This suggestion is supported by other studies that found that gender differences,[123] occupations that require vigorous activity, occupations that expose the individual to vibration, the report of an unpleasant work environment,[123–126] prior history of back problems,[127] and a sedentary lifestyle[125,127] all correspond to certain classifications of low back pain. A standardized approach to the subjective evaluation provides a useful format for the clinician and reduces the potential of errors of omission.

Young et al.[128] reported the link between patient history and physical examination factors in order to associate common subjective complaints with specific impairments. Their findings suggested that pain while rising from sitting was positively associated with both sacroiliac pain and discogenic pain, but negatively associated with zygopophyseal pain. O'Sullivan et al.[129] reported correlations between complaint of back pain and time spent sitting. Relief during immediate sitting is strongly suggestive of spinal stenosis,[86] demonstrating a sensitivity of 0.46 and a specificity of 0.93. Difficulty with toileting and the Valsalva maneuver during sitting is not specific to a particular disorder but is recognized as a common complaint of

low back pain.[81] Wide-based gait or abnormalities of gait are commonly associated with stenosis; however, these symptoms are not specific to stenosis and may involve any lower back–related pathology.[79]

Deyo et al.[85] suggests that when attempting to ascertain information that may be helpful to determine outcome based on history, the most useful items are failed previous treatments, substance abuse history, and disability compensation. Additionally, reviewing for the presence of depression may be helpful in determining whether this potential covariate will reduce the chance of successful recovery. Since no single scale exists that succinctly identifies all of these psychosocial characteristics, a careful and judicious history may be the only mechanisms for evaluation.

## Area of the Symptoms

Although radicular and referred pain is caused by many structures, isolation of pain origination will help identify the "guilty" structure or movement impairment. Discounting myelopathy, essentially two types of referred pain can arise from the lumbar spine: (1) somatic referred pain, which is caused by noxious stimulation of structures or tissue intrinsic to the lumbar spine and (2) radicular pain, which is caused by irritation of the lumbar or sacral nerve roots that pass through the lumbar vertebral canal or foramina.[130] Somatic referred pain may arise from nearly any source of local lumbar or lumbosacral pain secondary to convergence.[10] Clinically, the characteristics of the pain are often described as deeply perceived, diffuse, and hard to localize.[10] Causal structures may include ligaments, the surrounding musculature, zygopophyseal joints, and/or the intervertebral discs, each of which can refer pain to the lower extremities.[10,130]

Several studies have suggested that pain originating from the zygopophyseal joints can refer pain to the greater trochanter, posterior lateral thigh, buttock, groin, and below the knee.[131,132] Pain originating in the dura may cause back or leg pain. Smyth and Wright[133] found that dural-pain is typically isolated with traction stimulus. Kuslich et al.[134] found that dural-pain may be referred to the back, buttock, and the upper and lower leg. Typically, zygopophyseal, disc, and dural-pain have no predictable pain patterns but it is common to see symptoms below the knee for all three conditions.[130] Robinson[130] reported that common somatic referred pain descriptors are characterized by predictable identifiers. Pain is typically in the back or lower extremities, characterized as deep, achy, diffuse, poorly localized, dull, and cramp-like.

Radicular pain indicates that the origin of the pain generator is in the nerve root and may be associated with chemical or mechanical trauma. Radicular pain typically displays "hard" nerve findings that may include motor losses, sensory deficits, or pain in a dermatome distribution.[135] Like somatic referred pain, radicular symptoms tend to correspond to the level of dysfunction. L4 will radiate to the hip and anterolateral aspect of thigh (never to foot). L5 will radiate to the posterior side of leg into great toe, S1 to the posterior leg, distal-lateral to foot and little toe, and S2 to the posterior side of thigh, down to the bend of the knee, but never into the foot. McCullough and Waddell[136] and Smyth and Wright[133] differentiated L5 and S1 by the location of the symptoms; L5 is located at the dorsum of the foot and S1 is located at the lateral aspect of the foot. However, studies acknowledged that L5-S1 pain does not always cause pain that refers to the foot or toe.

In general, radicular pain is characterized by the identifiers of intense, radiating, severe, sharp, darting, lancinating, and well localized in comparison to somatic referred pain.[130] Caution should be used in diagnosing based on complaint of radiculopathy since description of the pain yields low diagnostic value.[137] To summarize, the area of the symptoms for low back pain may be associated with numerous structures including ligaments, dura, vertebrae, musculature, zygopophyseal, and intervertebral discs. Anterior thigh pain can be L2-3 dermatome or somatic pain from multiple structures. Groin pain can be somatic pain from local structures, somatic pain from the back, or L1-2 dermatomes. Posterior thigh pain can be somatic referred pain from many structures, S1-2 dermatomes, and L5-S1 disc or joint structures. Lastly, foot pain can be L5-S1 radiculopathy, somatic referred pain from disc (more rare), sacroiliac (rare), dura (rare), or zygopophyseal (rare).[130]

## Functional Scales

The relationship of lumbar disability, pain, and quality of life scores is tenuous at best. Concepts such as pain, psychosocial factors, and biomechanical covariates often correlate poorly, and rarely determine the extent of disability.[138] Because these disparate concepts have demonstrably variable relationships with disability and quality of life measures, these constructs are best investigated separately using disparate forms.[138,139]

Two commonly used outcome instrument scales are the *Roland Morris Disability Questionnaire* (RMQ) and the *Oswestry Disability Index* (ODI). Both have been well documented in the literature and both are recognized as reliable instruments for low back pain assessment. The ODI is a multidimensional scale and has been used to document changes in muscle activity, pain, psychological factors, and work status.[140] The ODI has been used to evaluate pre- and post-surgical outcomes, as well as a benchmark for determination of treatment effectiveness. Four versions of the ODI are available in English and in nine other languages. The data for the ODI provide both validation and standards for other users and indicate the power of the instrument for detecting change in sample populations.[141]

The RMQ is a unidimensional scale and is an excellent short functional disability questionnaire that focuses on activity intolerances related to the low back impairment. The RMQ was originally developed from the *Sickness Impact Profile* (SIP), although the RMQ is simpler, quicker, and easier to use.[140] Like the ODI, the RMQ has been used in all forms of outcome investigation including research. Like most valuable outcome instruments, it is particularly responsive to change in acute back pain populations.[142]

Waddell suggests that when compared to the ODI, the RMQ is simpler, faster, and more acceptable to patients.[143] He implies that it is a more sensitive measure of activity intolerances in acute and subacute patients but the ODI is more sensitive for identifying activity intolerances in chronic patients. Rasch analysis of the RMQ questionnaire confirms the unidimensionality of the instrument.[144] Rasch analysis of the ODI suggests that reorganization may improve the instrument, providing more appropriate findings.[141]

The *Tampa Scale for Kinesiophobia* (TSK) is designed to measure whether a patient has an irrational, excessive, and debilitating fear of physical movement and activity secondary to fear of pain and resultant reinjury.[145] The TSK, first presented in 1991, is a 17-item, 4-point Likert-type scale in which the total score varies from 17 to 68. The scale has demonstrated reliability (0.91; CI 0.85–0.94) and validity obtained through factor analysis.[146] Like the *Fear Avoidance Beliefs Questionnaire*, the TSK was developed primarily for musculoskeletal pain syndromes.[147]

## Summary

- The subjective may be the most important process of the low back examination.
- The clinician should target the patient's concordant sign during each examination.
- A measurable baseline is imperative for comparative analysis before, during, and after each intervention and treatment technique.
- The use of validated outcome measures such as the ODI and RMQ may improve data gathering and measurement of treatment progression.

# Active Physiological Movements

## Centralization Phenomenon

The **centralization phenomenon,** a hallmark of many manual therapy classification programs, was initially recognized by McKenzie in the 1950s and documented in the 1980s.[147] Centralization is liberally defined as a movement, mobilization, or manipulation technique targeted to pain radiating or referring from the spine, which when applied abolishes or reduces the pain distally to proximally in a controlled, predictable pattern.[148] This procedure has been well documented as a predictor of patient care outcomes, specifically suggesting that noncentralizers (those in which peripheral pain does not centralize with movements, mobilization, or manipulation) have poorer outcomes than those who do.[101,104] Others have used the centralization phenomenon to subclassify patients for research study.[149–152] Werneke and Hart[104] found patients' failure to centralize (noncentralizers) were at greater odds for higher pain intensity, failure to return to work, for interference with daily outcomes, and had a higher likelihood of further healthcare costs. Additionally, centralizing behavior is 95% sensitive and 52% specific for the presence of disc syndrome.[149] Without question, the evidence suggesting the inclusion of the centralization phenomenon in a spinal evaluation is quite compelling.

## Available Range of Motion

While useful in detecting asymmetries in available range of spinal motion, there is little evidence to support the singular use of "total available range of motion" as a predictor for low back impairment. Poor range of spinal motion is a common finding among asymptomatic spines as is "normal" total range of motion in symptomatic spines. Parks et al. found a very poor correlation between total range of motion and functional assessment scores[153] and

Haswelll et al.[154] reported poor to moderate Kappa values for reproduction of active physiological movements within an examination session.

## The Use of Repeated Movements

Young et al.[128] suggested that repeated movements are essential in detection of discogenic pain symptoms. Repeated motions are useful to determine the irritability of a patient and the directional preference of their movements. If a patient's condition is easily exacerbated with minimal repeated motions, then further care should advance cautiously. The term "directional preference" reflects the preference of repeated movement in one direction that will improve pain and the limitation of range, whereas movement in the opposite direction causes signs and symptoms to worsen.[155]

## The Use of Sustained Movements or Postures

Sustained movements or postures also are essential to detect the pain behavior of the patient. Patients may exhibit preferences in directions of sustained holds or may demonstrate reduction of pain once a segment is stretched or tension is released.

## Active Physiological Flexion

The purpose of active physiological flexion is to examine the effect of the movement on the patient's concordant sign and to determine the effect of repeated or sustained movements and whether this response centralizes the patient's concordant pain.

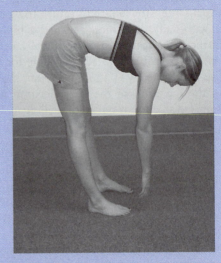

- Step One: The patient is first positioned in a neutral standing position. Baseline pain and radicular/referred symptoms are requested.
- Step Two: The patient is instructed to flex forward to his or her first point of pain. The pain is queried to determine if concordant.
- Step Three: The patient is then instructed to progress past the first point of pain. Symptoms are again queried.
- Step Four: The patient is then instructed to perform repeated movements past and/or near the end range of the motion. During the movement the patient is instructed to report whether his or her symptoms are worsening, improving, or staying the same and/or centralizing, peripheralizing, or neither.
- Step Five: It is imperative that the clinician also identify whether range of motion increases or decreases during movement.

**Figure 11.6**     Flexion of the Lumbar Spine

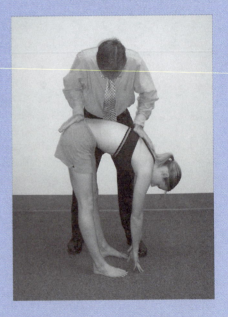

- Step Six: If repeated flexion to end range was pain-free, gently "take up the slack" and apply firm pressure to engage the end feel.
- Step Seven: At the end feel position, if pain-free, apply small, repeated oscillations to rule out this motion. If pain is engaged at any movement, the overpressure is unnecessary.

**Figure 11.7**     Flexion with Overpressure

If the repeated or sustained movements and overpressure are pain-free, the movement can be identified as discordant or nonprovocative. Maitland[156] stated that a joint (or movement) couldn't be classified as normal unless the range is pain-free during movement and passively with the inclusion of overpressure. He suggests placing firm pressure at the end of the available range, then applying small oscillatory movements at that end range. Only one study has investigated this phenomenon in rehabilitation assessment. Peterson and Hayes[157] reported that abnormal-pathologic end feels are associated with more pain than normal end feels during passive physiologic motion testing at the knee or shoulder. They suggested that the presence of this finding may indicate dysfunction and thus should be assessed during the clinical examination.

## Active Extension-Repeated Movements

The purpose of active physiological extension is to examine the effect of the movement on the patient's concordant sign and to determine the effect of repeated or sustained movements and whether this response centralizes the patient's concordant pain.

- Step One: The patient is first positioned in a neutral standing position. The hands of the patient are placed on each side of his or her hips. Baseline pain and radicular/referred symptoms are requested.
- Step Two: The patient is instructed to extend backward to his or her first point of pain. The pain is queried to determine if concordant.
- Step Three: The patient is then instructed to progress past the first point of pain. Symptoms are again queried.
- Step Four: The patient is then instructed to perform repeated movements past and/or near the end range of the motion. During the movement the patient is instructed to report whether his or her symptoms are worsening, improving, or staying the same and/or centralizing, peripheralizing, or neither.
- Step Five: It is imperative that the clinician also identify whether range of motion increases or decreases during movement.

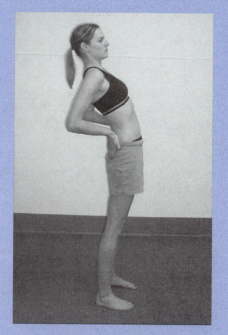

**Figure 11.8**    Repeated Extension of the Lumbar Spine

- Step Six: If end range repeated extension was pain-free, gently "take up the slack" and apply firm pressure to engage the end feel.
- Step Seven: At the end feel position, if pain-free, apply small, repeated oscillations to rule out this motion. If pain is engaged at any movement, the overpressure is unnecessary.

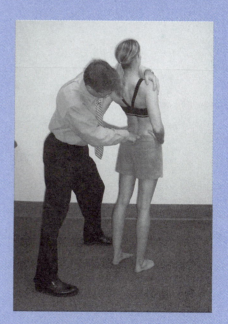

**Figure 11.9**    Extension with Overpressure

In the event that a patient does not demonstrate centralization with standing repeated movements, it may be relevant to assess the movements in a prone or supine position. Patients who demonstrate a high degree of irritability may require off-loading of the spine in order to centralize with repeated movements or sustained postures. The clinician may adopt this examination position if they suspect a high degree of irritability and an increased likelihood of centralization with prone or supine movements.

## Active Side Flexion with Repeated Motions

Past studies have suggested that a reduction or asymmetry of side-bending range of motion is a good predictor of disability[158] and is associated with severity of low back pain symptoms.[159] Causes of range-of-motion loss may include posterolateral disc irritation on one side versus the other, nerve root irritation with traction, and/or disc-degenerative height changes that affect the axis of motion.

- Step One: The patient is first positioned in a neutral standing position. The hands of the patient are placed on each side of his or her hips. Baseline pain and radicular/referred symptoms are queried.
- Step Two: The patient is instructed to bend to the right side to his or her first point of pain. The pain is queried to determine if concordant.
- Step Three: The patient is then instructed to progress past the first point of pain. Symptoms are again queried.
- Step Four: The patient is then instructed to perform repeated movements past and/or near the end range of the motion. During the movement the patient is instructed to report whether his or her symptoms are worsening, improving, or staying the same and/or centralizing, peripheralizing, or neither.
- Step Five: It is imperative that the clinician also identify whether range of motion increases or decreases during movement.

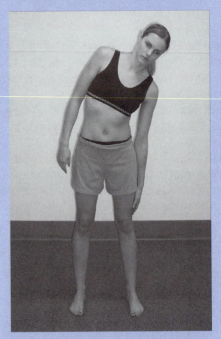

**Figure 11.10**     Repeated Side Flexion of the Lumbar Spine

- Step Six: If end range repeated side flexion was pain-free, gently "take up the slack" and apply firm pressure to engage the end feel.
- Step Seven: At the end feel position, if pain-free, apply small, repeated oscillations to rule out this motion. If pain is engaged at any movement, the overpressure is unnecessary.
- Step Eight: The movement is repeated on the opposite side.

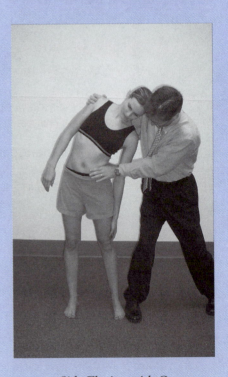

**Figure 11.11**     Side Flexion with Overpressure

## Active Rotation (Sitting) No-Repeated Motions

Very little axial rotation of the lumbar spine exists in normal subjects. Previous studies (outlined in Table 11.2) suggest that normal rotation range of motion varies from a high of 3 degrees at L3-4 to a low of .5 degrees at L5-S1.

- Step One: The patient is instructed to cross (tightly) his or her arms on his or her chest and sit straddling the treatment table, to stabilize the pelvis.
- Step Two: Further instructions and emphasis on proper posture will ensure the lumbar spine is isolated.
- Step Three: The patient is instructed to rotate as far as possible to the left side. Pain is queried. If painful, it is imperative to determine if the pain is concordant.

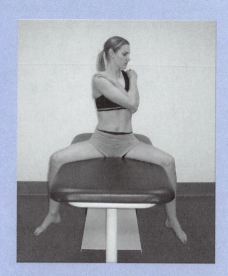

**Figure 11.12**    Active Rotation to the Left

- Step Four: If pain-free, gently "take up the slack" and apply firm pressure to engage the end feel.
- Step Five: At the end feel position, if pain-free, apply small, repeated oscillations to rule out this motion. If pain is engaged at any movement, the overpressure is unnecessary.
- Step Six: Repeat on the opposite side.

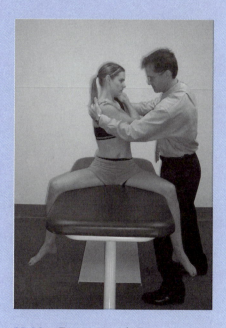

**Figure 11.13**    Rotation with Overpressure

## Combined Active Physiological Movements

Combining physiological movements allows movement to occur in a number of planes and may improve the ability to implicate a specific structure. Sizer et al.[160] reports the significance of sagittal-versus rotational-based motions in detection of discogenic symptoms. Pain, reproduced during sagittal repeated motions, is typically indicative of a dysfunction of discogenic origin, while pain during rotation may indicate facet joint pathology.

Combined movements or "quadrant" movements may be useful in ruling out pain origination from the lumbar spine. The motions are considered very provocative (sensitive) but do not have the capacity to define the origin or specific structure at fault. A negative finding during the combined tests may be more useful than a positive finding.

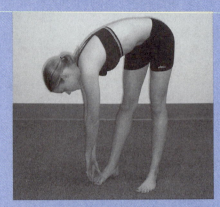

- Step One: The patient is first positioned in a neutral standing position. The patient is instructed to reach downward with both hands toward the left ankle.
- Step Two: The patient is queried for reproduction of symptoms.
- Step Three: The patient is instructed to reach down with both hands toward the right ankle. Again, the patient is queried for reproduction of symptoms.

**Figure 11.14**    Combined Flexion, Side Flexion, and Rotation

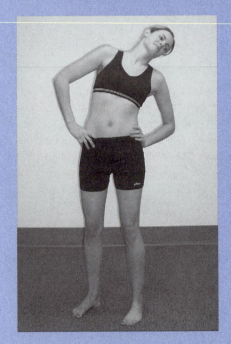

- Step Four: The patient is instructed to extend, rotate, and side flex toward the left side. Symptoms are assessed.
- Step Five: The patient is instructed to extend, rotate, and side flex toward the right side.

**Figure 11.15**    Combined Extension, Side Flexion, and Rotation

## *Summary*

- Active range of motion is necessary to elicit the concordant sign of the patient.
- Repeated motions will dictate whether the patient is a centralizer versus a peripheralizer, whether they exhibit a directional preference, and will contribute to predicting the likelihood of a positive long-term outcome.
- Detection of total range-of-motion value is less beneficial for the clinician than asymmetrical findings during bilateral movements.

## Passive Movements

### *Passive Physiological Movements*

The primary benefit of passive physiological assessment is to determine if the response associated with passive movements is the same as the requested active movements. Passive physiological coupling assessment of the spine does not provide useful information because there is no specific "normal" coupling pattern.[34]

Strender et al.[161] demonstrated good reliability among experienced manual therapists for detection of passive physiological movements in a side lying position. Others[162] have found relatively poor percent agreement between two manual therapists using a similar method of assessment. Most authors have debated the clinical utility, reliability, and validity of passive physiological findings, suggesting that passive physiological assessment of segmental motion may be too discrete, too minute, and thus too unreliable to yield beneficial information.[66–68]

Essentially, the most useful benefit to passive physiological assessment may be the comparison of active to passive movement. More passive range of motion may suggest a decreased willingness to move when requested actively or pain that is present during weight bearing. Although the usefulness of this assessment section is debated, some clinicians would argue that their palpation capabilities provide helpful information for treatment selection.

### Physiological Flexion and Extension

Physiological flexion and extension may provide the clinician with an understanding of the available sagittal movements of the lumbar spine.

- Step One: Patient is asked to lay on his or her side with his or her hips bent to 45 degrees and his or her knees to 60 degrees.
- Step Two: The clinician places the knees of the patient against his or her anterior superior iliac spine. This allows the clinician to move the patient into flexion and extension using his or her trunk to support the lower extremities. It may require the clinician to lift up the knees of the patient (into slight side flexion) in order to reduce the drag on the plinth.
- Step Three: During the movements of flexion and extension, the clinician palpates the spinous processes to determine available movement.

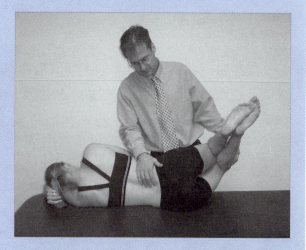

**Figure 11.16**    Passive Physiological Flexion and Extension

## Physiological Side Bending

During passive physiological side flexion, the clinician is concerned with determining the level of motion for each selected spinal segment in comparison to adjacent segments.

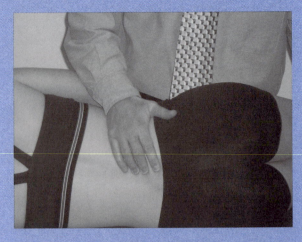

- Step One: Patient is asked to lay on his or her side with his or her hips bent to 45 degrees and his or her knees to 60 degrees.
- Step Two: The clinician then wraps the ankles of the patient in order to lift both legs as one. If the patient is large, the clinician can substitute by using one leg.
- Step Three: The clinician palpates the interspinous spaces using a "piano" grip.

**Figure 11.17**    The Piano Grip for Intersegmental Palpation

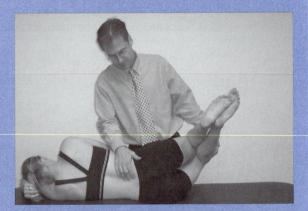

- Step Four: The clinician gently lifts the legs, feeling for separation and movement between the spinous processes (with caudal lifting at the legs, expect movement distal to proximal).
- Step Five: The clinician then compares the available passive range to the active range.
- Step Six: The method is repeated for the opposite side.

**Figure 11.18**    Passive Physiological Side Flexion

## Physiological Rotations

Physiological rotations involve isolated rotation of a single passive segment of the lumbar spine.

- Step One: Patient is asked to lie on his or her side and is positioned at 45 degrees of hip flexion and approximately 60 degrees of knee flexion.
- Step Two: The clinician uses his or her forearm to take up the slack in the hip and his or her finger to loop underneath the spinous process of S1.
- Step Three: Using a force of his or her forearm placed on the side of the rib cage and by gently applying a force on L5 toward the treatment table with his or her thumb, the clinician applies a distraction moment at the L5-S1 facet.
- Step Four: The force is in a diagonal to emphasize the direction of the facets. Excessive movement, pain, or gapping should be noted since ideally, rotation is minimal in nature.
- Step Five: Progress cephalically and perform the same procedure for L4-L5 and the corresponding cephalic segments.
- Step Six: Turn the patient onto the opposite side and repeat.

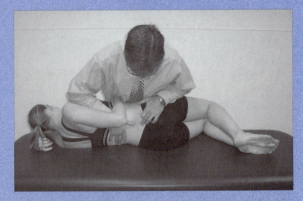

**Figure 11.19**    Physiological Rotation, Passive Assessment

## Summary

- Passive physiological range-of-motion assessment is marred by poor reliability of motion detection.
- The most useful information collected during passive physiological assessment is the comparison between active physiological motions.

## Passive Accessories

Passive accessory assessment is designed to address the relationship of pain intensity with pathological movement or the level of stiffness, information that must be confirmable from patient to therapist.[163] Most authors use the terms "joint stiffness" and "motion detection" interchangeably, hypothesizing that stiffness is the detection of motion available within the examined joint,[164–170] although this concept is not always synonymously agreed upon by all clinicians.[170] The behavior and location of movement stiffness may dictate the level of pathology and theoretically may qualify a determinable level of motion loss.

Physiological accessory motions may include many of the traditional principles of arthrokinematic motion, including a central posterior–anterior (PA), anterior–posterior (AP), arthrokinematic glide, and joint compression. The posterior–anterior accessory motion is a commonly used therapeutic assessment tool for the low back and is a fundamental assessment tool in clinical judgment of both pain provocation and motion assessment.[171,172]

While detecting spinal accessory stiffness alone has not been shown to be consistently reliable,[170–173] several authors have suggested that palpating for pain accompanying stiffness or movement dysfunction is both reliable and valid.[163,164,174] Phillips and Twomey[174] examined 32 subjects with a format of both verbal and nonverbal responses accompanied with passive intervertebral and passive accessory intervertebral movements. In both a prospective and retrospective study, they too found that the manual clinicians displayed a higher level of sensitivity with verbal versus nonverbal manual diagnosis.

Dickey et al.[175] reported a strong relationship between reported pain and the measured amount of vertebral accessory motion during physiologic movement. They reported that both intervertebral motions (translations and rotations) and deformations (compression and distraction movements) have a high degree of interaction with pain (as one increases so does the other). Jull et al.[164] used passive articular intervertebral movements (PAIVMs) to identify proven symptomatic zygopophyseal levels with very high levels of sensitivity. A similar study found reliability of motion detection to vary widely (kappa .00 to .23) compared to verbal response (kappa .22 to .65).[65] Others[176] found similar findings but to a lesser degree. Pain during these studies was reported during active physiological movements (flexion extension, right to left side bending, and vice versa) but does suggest the importance of intersegmental motion assessment and accessory joint play.

Posterior–anterior (PA) mobilization has been used as a component of a clinical prediction rule for manipulation of the spine in two studies.[177,178] Both studies indicated that detectable PA stiffness in combination with other factors found during the examination was related to a higher likelihood that the patient would benefit with manipulation. This suggests that detection of stiffness by the clinician, when used in concert with other findings, may be beneficial for treatment outcomes. Fritz and colleagues[179] has correlated the treatment outcome with the assessment of posterior–anterior stiffness in a clinical population. The authors found that patients who displayed hypomobility during the clinician's assessment in the examination were more likely to improve with manipulation and patients who displayed hypermobility were more likely to improve with stabilization. Conversely, Hicks et al.[180] has identified that the presence of hypermobility (along with other variables) found during the examination (using a PA) is a predictor of success for patients undergoing a stabilization approach.

## Central Posterior Anterior (CPA)

Maitland suggests the application of a CPA when report of midline or bilateral symptoms is present.[156] The process involves a three-point movement targeted to the spinous process of the patient. Under force application, all lumbar segments translate and rotate in a three-point fashion, although the segment that receives the direct force application moves greater than the surrounding segments.[181]

- Step One: Using a thumb pad to thumb pad grip, apply gentle force perpendicular to the spinous process of the lumbar spine. The force should be about 4 kg or thumbnail blanching at first followed by progressing intensities.
- Step Two: The clinician starts proximal and moves distal on the patient's spine, asking for the reproduction of the concordant sign of the patient.
- Step Three: A joint can only be cleared if a significant amount of PA force is applied.
- Step Four: A guilty joint will elicit the concordant sign during the mobilization, and may reproduce radicular or referred symptoms. Repeated movement or sustained holds help determine the appropriateness of the technique.

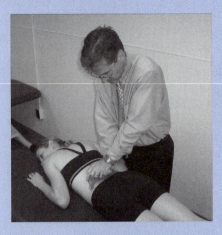

**Figure 11.20**    Central Posterior Anterior Intervertebral Assessment

## Unilateral Posterior Anterior (UPA)

A UPA also involves a three-point movement targeted to the facet, lamina, or transverse process of the guilty segment.[181]

- Step One: Using a thumb pad to thumb pad grip, the clinician applies a gentle force perpendicular to the targeted transverse process of the lumbar spine (right or left). The force should be about 4kg or thumbnail blanching at first.
- Step Two: By placing the PA force laterally on the transverse process, more rotation is elicited.
- Step Three: The UPAs are preformed proximal with a proximal-to-distal progression.
- Step Four: The clinician should ask for the reproduction of the concordant sign of the patient. Repeated movement or sustained holds help determine the appropriateness of the technique.
- Step Five: A joint can only be cleared if a significant amount of PA force is applied.

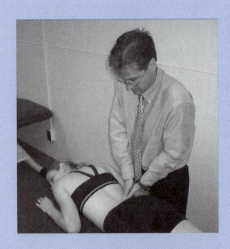

**Figure 11.21**    Unilateral Posterior Anterior Intervertebral Assessment

## L5-S1 Differentiation

The proximity of the L5-S1 facet to the sacroiliac joint may lead to confusion during differential assessment. The L5-S1 facet lies midway between the L5 spinous process and the deep-set sacroiliac joint. In most patients, the joints are less than one inch from one another. Correct palpation can effectively target each segment and allow the clinician to perform a UPA pain provocation maneuver.

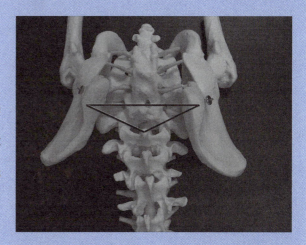

- Step One: The clinician palpates the sacral base by first identifying the superior border of the posterior superior iliac spine (PSIS).
- Step Two: The fifth lumbar vertebra is then palpated as the first prominent spinous process superior to the sacral base.
- Step Three: The clinician then, visually or with a pen, outlines the theoretical triangle where the L5-S1 segment exists.

**Figure 11.22**    The Theoretical Triangle of L5-S1 and the Sacroiliac Joint

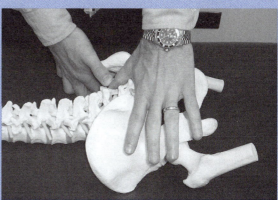

- Step Four: The clinician applies a UPA force midway between the spinous process of L5 and the PSIS (sacroiliac joint). This force should identify the L5-S1 facet.

**Figure 11.23**    UPA Force to L5-S1 Facet

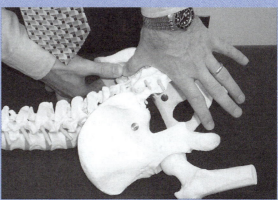
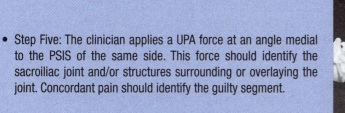

- Step Five: The clinician applies a UPA force at an angle medial to the PSIS of the same side. This force should identify the sacroiliac joint and/or structures surrounding or overlaying the joint. Concordant pain should identify the guilty segment.

**Figure 11.24**    UPA Force (at Angle) to Sacroiliac Joint

## Transverse Glide

The transverse glide is a combined translation and rotation assessment method used to target guilty segments. In most cases, the transverse glide is identified by the patient as a greater provocateur than a UPA or CPA. This assessment method should be used with caution since it may lead to soreness and easier reproduction of symptoms.

- Step One: Using a thumb pad, hook the spinous process, the clinician takes up the slack of motion.
- Step Two: If the lesion is reported by the patient to be on the right, the clinician should move to the left side of the patient and push the spinous process to the right. By placing the lateral force on the spinous process, rotation is elicited.
- Step Three: The lateral glides are initiated proximal with a proximal-to-distal progression.
- Step Four: The clinician should ask for the reproduction of the concordant sign of the patient.
- Step Five: A guilty joint will elicit the concordant sign of the patient during the mobilization, and may reproduce radicular or referred symptoms. Repeated movement or sustained holds help determine the appropriateness of the technique.

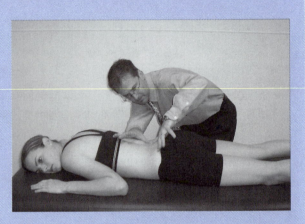

**Figure 11.25**    Transverse Glide of the Lumbar Spine

## Summary

- Passive accessory assessment may yield useful information in the detection of lumbar pathology.
- Passive accessory assessment is useful in isolating the guilty segment of dysfunction.
- Passive accessory assessment may be unreliable when assessment of stiffness is the only goal.
- Passive accessory assessment is beneficial when pain provocation is the purpose of the segmental examination.

## Clinical Special Tests

### Palpation

Generally, palpation of the lumbar spine may not be useful in implicating selected tissue because of the problems with convergence. However, palpation is useful in order to identify specific structures during mobilization or manipulation. Billis et al.[182] reported poor reproducibility among clinicians for identifying the L5 spinous process. Clinicians and manual therapists demonstrated more reproducibility than students did, but all subjects were seemingly inaccurate. French et al.[183] reported similar findings for palpatory mechanisms used prior to the administration of chiropractic techniques. Subsequently, palpation-based treatments in the absence of patient report of concordant pain may yield variable findings among clinicians.

### Manual Muscle Testing

The use of manual muscle testing of the lumbar musculature is controversial. The construct of a manual muscle test for lumbar impairment assumes the resisted weakness, implicating weakness and subsequent impairment. However, because the lumbar spine's musculature is complex, the global musculature (prime movers) may exhibit no strength losses whereas the local musculature may be both weak and may demonstrate motor control problems. Local musculature weakness (multifidi and transverses abdominus) and motor loss commonly demonstrates subtle quantifiable clinical features[184] with negative or inconsistent findings during manual muscle testing. In essence, gross manual muscle testing of the trunk does not yield very useful information. Finite muscle testing using a stabilizer or blood pressure cuff may yield information that is more useful.

### Special Tests for Discogenic Pathologies

There are several special tests for the presence of discogenic pathology. Most clinical tests operate on the assumption that additional nerve tension placed on an abnormally preactivated nerve root will lead to reproduction of symptoms.

## The Slump Sit Test (SS)

The SS is typically positive when tension on a nerve root is painful, specifically during the onset of discogenic pain. Findings may implicate a primary disc herniation or a chronic nerve root adhesion. Lew and Briggs[185] reported that regardless of hamstring tension, the sensitization methods of the SS do not affect any hamstring-related symptoms. The test can specifically distill out hamstring tightness versus neurogenic origins.

To distill a positive test, the SS must be sequentially performed. Butler[186] explains that the SS is positive only upon the inclusion of three criteria. First, the findings must be asymmetrical from the concordant sign to the normal side. Second, the pain produced during the examination should be the same radicular pain reported by the patient. Lastly, the pain should have a sensitization quality, thus movement from a distal or proximal area that engages the tension of the nerve root should increase the symptoms. Johnson and Chiarello[187] demonstrated that in healthy males, false positives for range-of-motion restriction in the knee are common. Table 11.5 provides the diagnostic value of the SS test.

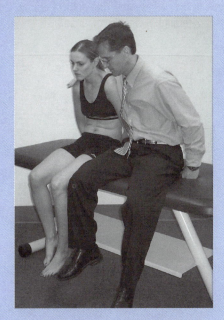

- Step One: The subject sits straight with the arms behind the back, the legs together, and the posterior aspect of the knees against the edge of the treatment table.
- Step Two: The subject slumps so that the sacrum is vertical to the sitting structure, producing trunk flexion. The examiner applies firm overpressure to bow the subject's back, being careful to keep the sacrum vertical.

**Figure 11.26**  Step Two: Trunk Is Loaded (Compressed)

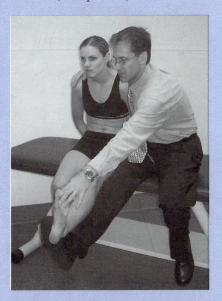

- Step Three: The subject is asked to flex his or her head, and overpressure is then added to the neck flexion.
- Step Four: While maintaining full spinal and neck flexion with overpressure, the examiner asks the subject to extend the knee.
- Step Five: The clinician then moves the foot into dorsiflexion while maintaining knee extension.

**Figure 11.27**  Step Five: Dorsiflexion Is Added to Sensitize the Maneuver

*(continued)*

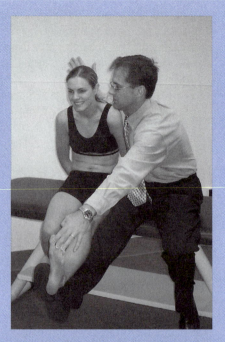

- Step Six: Neck flexion is then released, and the subject is asked to further extend the knee.
- Step Seven: Dorsiflexion and knee extension are released and neck flexion is resumed. The subject is then asked to perform steps 3 through 6 with the other leg.

**Figure 11.28**    Neck Flexion Is Released and Symptoms Are Reassessed

## Straight Leg Raise

The straight leg raise test (SLR) was first described by Forst in 1880.[188] Presently, several iterations of the passive straight leg exist with little agreement.[188] Like the slump test, the SLR is best performed sequentially and requires three criteria to avoid false positives. First, the findings must be asymmetrical from the concordant sign to the normal side. Second, the pain produced during the examination should be the same radicular pain reported by the patient. Lastly, the pain should have a sensitization quality, thus movement from a distal or proximal area that engages the tension of the nerve root should increase the symptoms. Breig and Troup[189] suggested the following standardization of the straight leg raise assessment. Table 11.5 provides the diagnostic value of the SLR.

- Step One: The patient should lie on a firm but comfortable surface, the neck and head in the neutral position.
- Step Two: The patient's trunk and hips should remain neutral; avoid internal or external rotation, lacking adduction or abduction.
- Step Three: The clinician then supports the patient's leg at the heel, maintaining knee extension and neutral dorsiflexion at the ankle. The leg should be raised to the point of symptom reproduction.

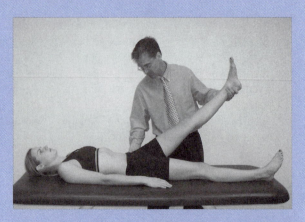

**Figure 11.29**    The Leg Is Passively Raised to the Point of Symptoms

- Step Four: If the passive straight leg raise is unilaterally positive for reproduction, or bilaterally positive at 50 degrees or less, raise to the onset of pain, lower a few degrees to reduce symptoms, then successively dorsiflex the ankle, medially rotate the hip, and flex the neck. If symptom reproduction occurs, then the test may be interpreted as a positive finding.

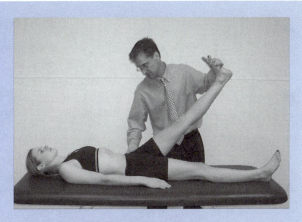

**Figure 11.30**    Dorsiflexion Is Added to the Passive Leg Raise

- Step Five: To further sensitize the test, the patient is instructed to lift his or her head into flexion. Further increase in symptoms is indicative of a positive test.

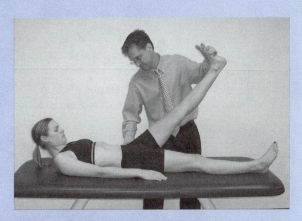

**Figure 11.31**    Neck Flexion Is Added to the DR and Passive Leg Raise

The clinical utility of the SLR may be hampered by the physiological process that occurs during the provocation procedure. Investigators have documented as much as 5 millimeters of linear excursion and 2–4% strain of the lumbosacral nerve roots and associated dura in fresh cadavers during a straight leg raise maneuver[190,191], excursion that is increased with the addition of ankle dorsiflexion and hip internal rotation. A SLR procedure increases the segmental flexion at the lower lumbar levels, which can place tension on the ventral nerve root.[192] Root tension increases transverse compression of the ventral root against a disc, an anatomical consequence of proximal and distal root anchoring by the ligaments of Hoffman[193,194] and interforaminal ligaments.[195] Any disorder or movement such as head and neck flexion that produces pretensioning of the lumbosacral plexus[185] can increase the sensitivity of the test and subsequently may reduce the specificity.

## Well Leg Raise—1° Disc

A positive well leg raise (also known as the crossed leg raise) is typically indicative of a disc derangement or serious pathology. This test generally exhibits low sensitivity but high specificity. When used in combination with the SLR, which is more sensitive than specific, the crossed SLR may be a useful instrument. The well leg raise is performed using the same procedure as the straight leg raise but with the opposite, nonsymptomatic limb. Table 11.5 provides the diagnostic value of the well leg raise.

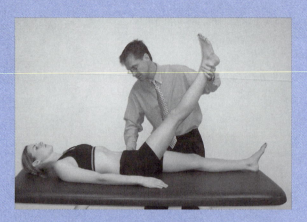

**Figure 11.32**    The Well Leg Raise

## Femoral Nerve Tension Test

Wasserman first described the Femoral Nerve Tension test for patients who demonstrated anterior thigh symptoms that were intermittently positive or absent with a straight leg raise.[196] This test is designed to implicate the femoral nerve in thoracic or upper lumbar discogenic pain[197] and has been shown to implicate extreme lateral disc herniations with a fair degree of sensitivity.[196,198] By adding sensitization methods such as plantarflexion and neck side flexion or extension, enhancement of the stress to the nerve roots is facilitated.

Variations exist, including the use of the "cross femoral nerve test" in which the opposite limb is tested to elicit symptoms on the contralateral or affected side.[199,200] The test is known to demonstrate a fair amount of false positives, having demonstrated like findings in patients with ruptured aortic aneurysms, retroperitoneal hemorrhages,[197] and tightness in the iliopsoas.[197] Clinicians should expect these patients to demonstrate motor weaknesses greater than sensory losses with positive findings.[196,197] Geraci and Alleva[201] suggest improving sensitivity by using extension of the hip in combination with knee flexion.

- Step One: The patient lies prone in a symmetric pain-free posture.
- Step Two: The clinician places one hand on the PSIS, the same side of the knee that the clinician will bend into flexion.
- Step Three: The clinician then gently moves the lower extremity into knee flexion, bending the knee until the onset of symptoms.

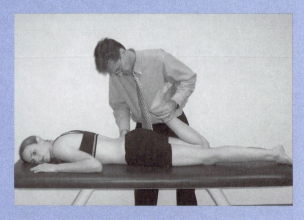

**Figure 11.33**    Step Three: Knee Flexion to the Point of Symptoms

- Step Four: Once symptoms are engaged, the clinician slightly backs out of the painful position.
- Step Five: At this point, the clinician may use plantarflexion, dorsiflexion, or head movements to sensitize the findings.
- Step Six: Further sensitization can be elicited by implementing hip extension. The clinician can repeat on the opposite side if desired.

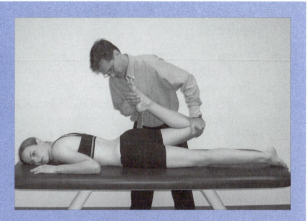

**Figure 11.34**   Step Five: Sensitizing the Movements with Plantarflexion

**TABLE 11.5**   Diagnostic Value of Special Tests for Discogenic Pain

| Study | Sensitivity | Specificity | +LR | −LR | Criterion Standard |
|---|---|---|---|---|---|
| **Slump Sit Test** | | | | | |
| Stankovic et al.[202] | 82.6 | 54.7 | 1.82 | 0.32 | Surgery |
| **Straight Leg Raise** | | | | | |
| Charnley[203] | 78 | 64 | 2.16 | 0.34 | Surgery |
| Knuttson[204]* | 96 | 10 | 1.06 | 0.40 | Surgery |
| Hakelius & Hindmarsh[205] | 96 | 17 | 1.15 | 0.24 | Surgery |
| Spangfort[206] | 97 | 11 | 1.08 | 0.27 | Surgery |
| Kosteljanetz et al.[207] | 76 | 45 | 1.38 | 0.53 | Surgery |
| Kosteljanetz et al.[208] | 89 | 14 | 1.03 | 0.78 | Surgery |
| Kerr et al.[209] | 98 | 44 | 1.75 | 0.05 | Surgery |
| Lauder et al.[210]* | 21 | 87 | 1.61 | 0.90 | Electrodiagnosis |
| Albeck[211] | 82 | 21 | 1.03 | 0.86 | Surgery |
| Gurdjian et al.[212] | 81 | 52 | 1.68 | 0.36 | Surgery |
| **Well Leg Raise** | | | | | |
| Knuttson[204]* | 25 | 95 | 5 | 0.79 | Surgery |
| Hakelius & Hindmarsh[205] | 28 | 88 | 2.33 | 0.82 | Surgery |
| Spangfort[206] | 23 | 88 | 1.91 | 0.86 | Surgery |
| Kosteljanetz et al.[208] | 24 | 100 | NA | NA | Surgery |
| Kerr et al.[209] | 43 | 97 | 14.3 | 0.59 | Surgery |

*Authors did not isolate HNP but tested vs. nerve root compression.*

## *Special Tests for Segmental Mobility or Provocation*

Manual therapists commonly use clinical special tests or other manual techniques for the assessment of spine stiffness. Previously, Paris[213] and Kirkaldy-Willis and Farfan[214] suggested that manual palpation is effective in detection of instability, simply by determining if motion is greater than that found with conditions of hypermobility, and some evidence exists that supports the reliability of palpation mechanisms for spinal instability assessment.[215] Nonetheless, numerous clinical instability tests exist with varied reported levels of reliability that have never been tested for validity.[216,217] A majority of spine instability

clinical special tests are designed to measure pain, displacement, or degree of stiffness.[218]

In 2003, Hicks et al.[176] studied the interrater reliability of several clinical special tests and identifiers for lumbar spine instability. The authors selected the clinical special tests of "Posterior shear test," "Prone instability test," and "Posterior–anterior" segmental mobility test. The authors did find reliability in selected tests, specifically those associated with pain provocation. A 2005 study by Fritz et al.[215] found that a lack of hypomobility during intervertebral motion testing (PA Spring test) provided 95% sensitivity and 9% specificity for detection of radiographic instability. Furthermore, findings such as hypermobility demonstrated 81% sensitivity and 2.4% specificity during the examination.[218]

---

### Intervertebral Motion Testing

Intervertebral motion testing, as described by Fritz et al.[215] and Hicks et al.,[180] is identical to the posterior–anterior procedure described during the passive accessory examination. Although the test is generally described to provoke pain in a patient, the test does appear to have diagnostic value in detecting radiographic instability of the spine in absence of report of pain[215] and in identifying subjects that may response to manipulative treatment (if stiffness is detected). Table 11.6 provides the diagnostic value of intervertebral spring testing.

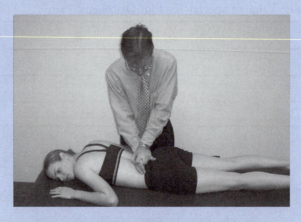

**Figure 11.35**    Prone Intervertebral Motion Testing

---

**TABLE 11.6**    Diagnostic Value of Spine Instability Testing

| Study | Sensitivity | Specificity | +LR | −LR | Criterion Standard |
|---|---|---|---|---|---|
| Fritz et al.[215] Lack of hypomobility present | 95 | 9 | 1.04 | 0.56 | Radiographic findings |
| Fritz et al.[215] Any hypermobility present during testing | 81 | 2.4 | 2.4 | 7.91 | Radiographic findings |

## Sidelying PA Glide

The sidelying PA glide is designed to measure the quantity of translation from posterior to anterior.

- Step One: The patient is placed in a sidelying position. The patient's arms are locked in extension and his or her hands are placed on the ASIS of the assessing clinician.
- Step Two: The clinician applies a posterior-to-anterior (PA) force at the caudal level (i.e., at L5 when assessing L4-L5 mobility).

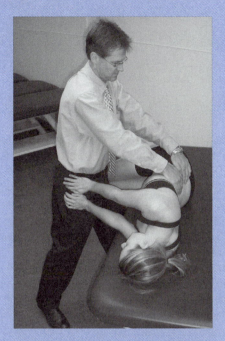

**Figure 11.36**    The Sidelying PA Segmental Assessment

- Step Three: The cephalic segment is palpated just inferior at the interspinous space (i.e., during L4-L5 assessment, the interspinous space is palpated to assess movement). One may repeat on the other side though most likely results are similar.

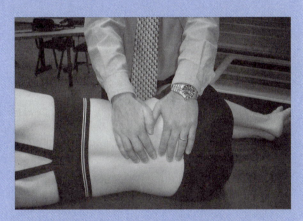

**Figure 11.37**    Hand Position for the Sidelying PA Assessment

## Sidelying AP Glide

Like the sidelying PA glide, no studies exist that examine the reliability or radiographic verification of this test, and none exist that measure the sensitivity or specificity of this test motion. This clinical test has been used widely to assess the anterior-to-posterior translation of specific spinal segments. While some clinicians report the use to detect "stiffness," others use this method to detect clinical instability.

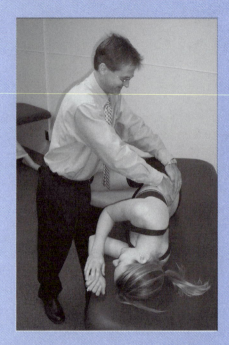

- Step One: The patient is placed in a sidelying position. The hips of the patient are flexed to 90 degrees and the patient's knees are placed against the ASIS of the clinician.
- Step Two: The clinician stabilizes the superior segments by pulling posterior to anterior on the patient's spine. The clinician applies an anterior-to-posterior force at the caudal level (i.e., at L5 when assessing L4-L5 mobility) by applying force through the flexed femurs.
- Step Three: The cephalic segment is palpated just inferior at the interspinous space (i.e., during L4-L5 assessment, the interspinous space is palpated to assess movement.
- Step Four: One may repeat on the other side, though most likely results are similar.

**Figure 11.38**    The Sidelying AP Glide

## Specific Lumbar Spine Torsion Test

Transverse torsion testing may be the most effective tool for detecting facet instability.[30] However, there are no studies that have examined the reliability, sensitivity, or specificity of this procedure. One possible mechanism to improve the validity of this test is to examine whether pain and hypermobility are present. Since torsion theoretically compromises facet instability more so than linear methods, pain should accompany hypermobility.

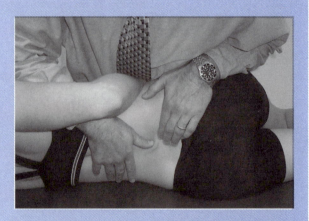

- Step One: Patient is asked to lie down on his or her side and is positioned at 60 degrees of hip flexion and approximately 45 degrees of knee flexion.
- Step Two: The clinician uses his or her forearm to take up the slack in the hip and his or her finger to loop underneath the spinous process of S1.

**Figure 11.39**    Hand Position for the Specific Lumbar Spine Torsion Test

- Step Three: Using a force of their forearm placed on the side of the rib cage and by gently applying a force on L5 toward the treatment table with their thumb, the clinician applies a distraction moment at the L5-S1 facet.
- Step Four: The force is in a diagonal to emphasize the direction of the facets.
- Step Five: Excessive movement, pain, or gapping should be noted since ideally, rotation is minimal in nature.
- Step Six: Progress cephalically and perform the same procedure for L4-L5.

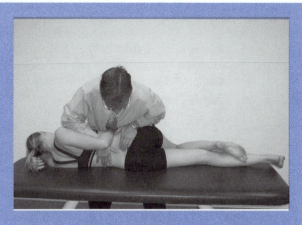

**Figure 11.40**    The Specific Lumbar Spine Torsion Test

## Prone Spine Torsion Test

No studies examine the reliability or radiographic verification of this test. In theory, maximum rotation is less than 1–2 mm and we should feel no motion at any segment. If the clinician "feels" movement of more than 1–2 mm, it may implicate rotational hypermobility or passive instability of that segment. As with most special tests, adding provocation to the finding should improve the integrity of the test.

- Step One: The patient lies in prone. The therapist applies a transverse directed force medially on the level above and the level below the suspected lesion. The force is concentrated on the lateral aspect of the spinous processes.
- Step Two: The therapist feels for excessive gapping while questioning the patient regarding recreation of painful symptoms.
- Step Three: Repeat by applying the same medially directed force but switching contact points from caudal (right) to cephalic (left) to cephalic (right) to caudal (left).

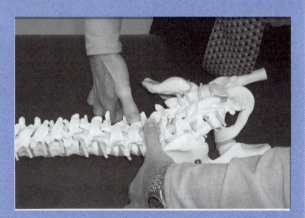

**Figure 11.41**    Skeletal View of the Prone Spine Torsion Test

### Prone Instability Test

Hicks et al.[176,180] and Fritz et al.[215] found good reliability with the prone instability test. A positive prone instability test occurs when pain is provoked during the PA but disappears when the test is repeated with the legs off the floor.[176] Hicks et al.[180] included this finding in a clinical prediction rule for spine stabilization. This and other factors were associated with an increased chance of benefiting from a lumbar stabilization intervention program.

- Step One: The patient is prone with the torso on the examining table and the legs over the edge of the plinth and the feet resting on the floor.
- Step Two: The clinician performs a PA spring on the low back to elicit back pain using the pisiform grip.

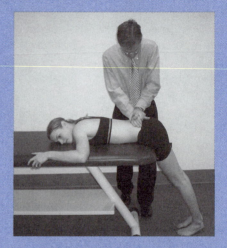

**Figure 11.42**   The Spring Test during the Prone Spine Instability Test

- Step Three: The patient is requested to lift his or her legs off the floor by using a back contraction.
- Step Four: The clinician maintains the PA force to the low back. A positive test is a reduction of symptoms while lifting the legs off the ground.

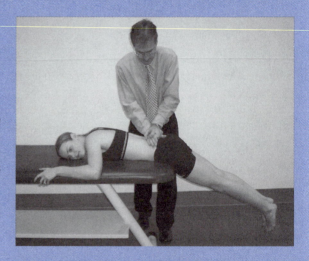

**Figure 11.43**   End Step of the Prone Spine Stability Test

## Summary

- Several studies have demonstrated that the SLR is a sensitive instrument, beneficial in ruling out disorders, but lacks specificity.
- Few studies have investigated the manual therapist's ability to differentiate lumbar instability.
- Selected spine instability tests are useful in detecting which patients may benefit from manipulation and stabilization.

# TREATMENT TECHNIQUES

## Targeted Outcome

The purpose of each treatment technique selected should have a singular focus toward improving the outcome of the patient. Treatment should directly affect the concordant sign of the patient. Therefore, active, positional, and passive techniques should directly stimulate the concordant sign during the application of the technique. Treatment techniques that initially cause an increase in symptoms or peripheralizing pain (temporary) may be appropriate techniques. These techniques are inappropriate to use if the patient exhibits worsening symptoms, particularly peripheralization during continued application and at the end of treatment.

Understanding when to use a specific technique was outlined in the examination section. The patient's response to repeated movements and/or sustained stretches are indicators of whether a specific treatment choice is appropriate or not for continuation. The selections can provide one of three potential positive outcomes: (1) reduction of pain, (2) normalization of range, and (3) centralization or abolishment of symptoms. The obtainment of any of these three outcomes will validate the treatment method used in the previous treatment. A treatment selection that provides no change in the patient, or results in negative consequences, is either an inappropriate treatment selection or is designed to provide benefits in due time (e.g., lumbar stabilization exercises). The nexus of the patient-response method requires that the clinician identify the effectiveness of the specific manual therapy approach within and between each patient session.[97]

## Treatment-Based Classification

Delitto and colleagues have advocated the use of a treatment-based classification (TBC) model.[151,219] They based their classification partly on the response of a patient to treatment constructed from key history and examination findings. Like the McKenzie classification, the TBC placed patients into homogenous groups purportedly to allow more specific treatment intervention, yet, unlike the McKenzie classification, the TBC provided a classification for groups unrepresented such as instability.

The focus of the TBC model is less on diagnosis and more on improvement of treatment[219] and has recently been reduced to four specific classifications that involve categorization based on key history and clinical findings. These categories include (1) specific exercise, (2) mobilization, (3) immobilization, and (4) traction.[222] The specific exercise category involves patients who may demonstrate postural preferences, may exhibit centralization behavior with selected movements, or may demonstrate reduction of pain during active and passive techniques. The mobilization group generally demonstrates local, unilateral low back pain, or SIJ-related pain. The immobilization group may exhibit frequent bouts of similar back pain and could be associated with instability. Lastly, the traction group exhibits signs and symptoms of nerve root compression, no improvement with lumbar movements, and a potential lateral shift that is unimproved with lateral translations. Although this model has demonstrated poor reliability,[220] there is evidence of construct validity.[219]

The benefit of using the TBC classification is that the examination distills out which categories of the TBC in which the patient falls (Figure 11.44). For example, if a patient exhibits centralization behavior, they would fall into the specific exercise group. If a patient exhibits radiculopathy, they fall into the traction group. If a patient centralizes during active movements and improves with mobilization, they could qualify in both categories. Each category is not considered mutually exclusive.

### Specific Exercise Classification

Within the TBC model, the specific exercise classification involves directional preferences of patients and improvements with specific directionally based exercises. The hallmark of this approach is associated with the centralization phenomenon. As mentioned, the centralization phenomenon is a useful tool in identifying the presence of a discogenic pain[149] and whether the patient will exhibit a positive outcome versus a concordant group that does not demonstrate centralization behavior.[104] Centralization is defined as "a situation in which pain arising from the spine and felt laterally from the midline or distally is reduced and transferred to a more central or near midline position when certain movements are performed".[147,148] Examination techniques that lead to centralization behavior during the examination are carried over to treatment. In some cases, it may take several treatment visits to ascertain the result of repeated motions and to determine if the patient is a centralizer.

This text adopts a very liberal definition for the term centralization. Active or passive techniques that centralize, reduce, or *abolish* symptoms during application are considered plausible techniques of choice. Unlike the definitions supported by other authors, a centralization response may occur from a number of structures, which are nondiscogenic, that originate from radiculopathic or somatic referred pain.

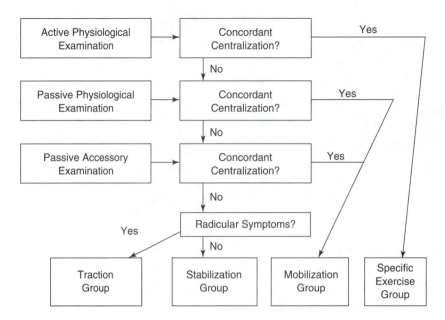

**Figure 11.44**    Algorithm for the Treatment Based Classification

## Active Treatment Techniques—Repeated Motions

Treatment involving repeated motions should directly relate to the findings of the examination. If the patient exhibited decreases or centralization of symptoms during repeated extension, the repeated extension is advocated. The same process occurs if the patient demonstrates improvement with another direction of movement such as flexion or side flexion. Repeated movements in prone are advocated if the patient is irritable and does not demonstrate centralization in a loaded position. Repeated movements such as extension are performed in standing or prone.

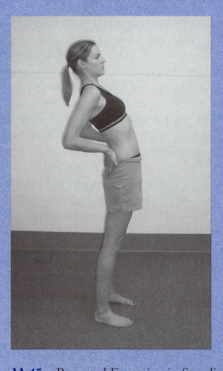

**Figure 11.45**    Repeated Extension in Standing

## Active Physiological Sustained Postural Holds

Treatment involving a postural hold is also distilled out of the examination. In some cases, the postural hold may serve as prepositioning for a mobilization procedure.

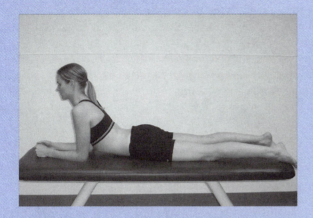

**Figure 11.46**   Static Hold for Low Back Extension

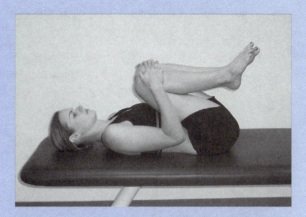

**Figure 11.47**   Static Hold for Low Back Flexion

## Treatment Techniques—Side Glides

Side glides are a positional or movement-based technique designed to correct a positional shift. Typically, patients exhibit a lateral shift described by analyzing the position of the thoracic trunk over the pelvis. In Figure 11.48, the patient exhibits a left lateral shift as the thoracic spine is shifted over the pelvis. Correcting the shift would require a pull to the patient's trunk in the opposite direction as the shift, or a technique described as a "right" side glide. This technique is appropriate to use if the symptoms centralize upon completion of a bout of therapy.

- Step One: The patient stands with shifted side facing the clinician.
- Step Two: After instructing the patient regarding the procedure at hand, the clinician places one shoulder compressed to the trunk of the patient while wrapping his or her arms around the pelvis of the patient.
- Step Three: Using sequential movements, the clinician glides the pelvis in the opposite direction as he or she pulls the pelvis.
- Step Four: Treatment is based on a positive response during repeated trials for the patient. If the patient exhibits centralization, the process is repeated several bouts. If the patient peripheralizes during the procedure, the patient is a candidate for traction under the TBC criteria.

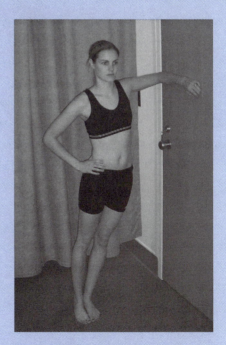

**Figure 11.48**   Side Glide for Lateral Shift Correction

## Combined Movements—Passive Accessory Mobilization in Prepositioning

This textbook adopts a liberal definition of the specific exercise classification of the TBC.[219] The use of passive procedures to enhance the movement in a specific direction is plausible if this movement positively affects the concordant sign of the patient. For example, with the exception of an isolated L5-S1 dysfunction, if a patient benefits from repeated end range extension the patient may benefit from repeated passive accessory mobilization to the spine at a preposition of end range extension because both actions create a three-point movement of the spine.[181] Subsequently, prepositions such as side flexion, extension, or a nerve tension–related position may be useful prior to the application of a CPA or UPA technique. Each technique is only performed if the effects are similar to what occurs during the specific active physiological movement and if the concordant sign is improved.

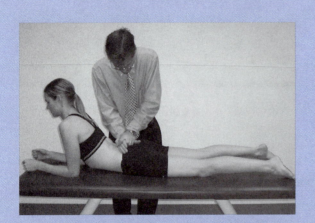

**Figure 11.49**    Passive Accessory CPA during Prone on Elbows Extension

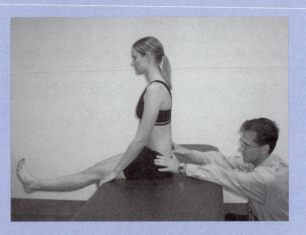

**Figure 11.51**    UPA during Sitting with SLR

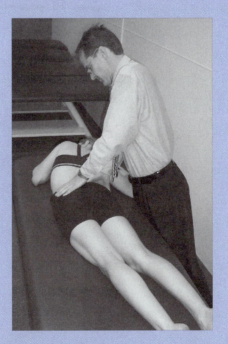

**Figure 11.50**    Passive Accessory UPA during Side Flexion

## *Mobilization Classification*

Patients that fall within the mobilization classification may benefit from mobilization or manipulation. This text adopts the likelihood that a considerable amount of overlap exists between the specific exercise and mobilization classifications.

---

### Manipulation Clinical Prediction Rule

Flynn et al.[177] developed a clinical prediction rule for determining if patients are appropriate for manipulation early within the care cycle. The authors outlined duration of symptoms, (1) < 16 days, (2) hip internal rotation of at least 35 degrees, (3) lumbar segmental hypomobility tested with a spring test (a version of a central posterior–anterior mobilization), (4) no symptoms distal to the knee, and (5) a score of < 19 on the work subscale of the *Fear-Avoidance Beliefs Questionnaire,* as the five mechanisms of the clinical prediction rule. Four of 5 of these findings increased the odds of a short-term positive response from manipulation by 25-fold and demonstrated better outcomes than exercises.[178]

   The manipulation procedure performed to the experimental group is a technique commonly associated with SIJ manipulation.

- Step One: The patient lies in a supine position and is requested to lace both hands behind the neck.
- Step Two: The clinician places his or her arm through the arms of the patient's and grasps the arm of the patient closest to the table. An alternative method involves the clinician reaching posteriorly and contacting the scapula of the patient.
- Step Three: The clinician side bends the patient away and rotates/flexes the patient toward them while applying pressure to the distal ASIS.
- Step Four: The clinician continues to apply rotation toward him- or herself until the ASIS begins to rise from the table
- Step Five: Once resistance is encountered, the clinician applies an AP force through the ASIS.

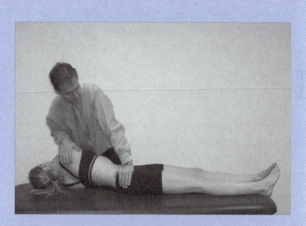

**Figure 11.52**    Grade V of Ileum on Sacrum

---

### Sidelying Rotational Mobilization (Grade III or Grade IV)

A common mobilization procedure used to gap the zygopophyseal joints superiorly from the table or "close" the segment inferiorly on the table is a sidelying rotational mobilization.

- Step One: The patient lays sidelying depending on the intent of the procedure. If the clinician desires to "open" a facet, the patient lies with the painful side up. If the clinician plans to "close" the segment, the clinician lies with the painful side down. The decision of which side to place the patient is based on the examination results.
- Step Two: The patient's lower leg is straightened and the upper leg is slightly flexed (the knee does not rest on the table).
- Step Three: The clinician grasps the upper arm and gently flexes and rotates the patient cephalically. By using a "piano grip" hand placement within the spinous processes, the clinician palpates to feel the level of movement.

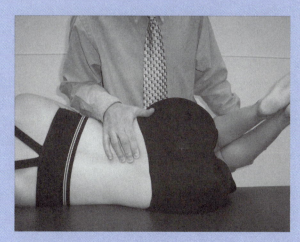

**Figure 11.53**    Hand Position for the Mobilization

*(continued)*

- Step Four: The clinician only rotates to the point they feel movement at the segment superior to his or her targeted joint. Once found, the clinician places the hand of the patient underneath the side of his or her head.
- Step Five: The clinician places his or her ASIS just cephalic to the patient's ASIS. His or her forearm then pulls the patient's pelvis snuggly to the clinician's thigh and hip.
- Step Six: The clinician then places his or her forearm posteriorly on the rib cage (interlocked through the arm of the patient). The patient is rotated slightly to further stabilize or "lock" the position.
- Step Seven: For additional isolation, the clinician loads the patient through his or her body and can shift the emphasis of the procedure toward the upper, middle, and lower segments by weight shifting cephalically to caudally (cephalic shift emphasizes upper segments, caudal shift lower segments).
- Step Eight: The clinician pulls upward caudally on the lateral aspect of the spinous process of the caudal segment by pulling up away from the table. Conversely, the clinician uses his or her thumb to push downward toward the table on the lateral aspect of the cephalic spinous process.
- Step Nine: Mobilization is performed based on patient response. The technique is applied as a gentle oscillation by loading the patient and by pushing down toward the table with the cephalic hand and pulling upward away from the table with the caudal hand.

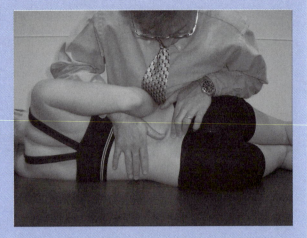

**Figure 11.54**   Opening Procedure Causing Gapping of Superior Zygopophyseal Joints

## Sidelying Rotational Manipulation

The rotational manipulation is useful for patients with chronic stiffness of the lower back. The technique may be indicated if UPAs or transverse glides do not provide enough vigor to relieve (completely) the patient's symptoms. Prime patient candidates include those that report difficulty moving into rotation or another direction due to a limitation or block.

- Step One: The same placement principles used in the sidelying mobilization procedure are used in the setup for the manipulation.
- Step Two: The thrust is performed by taking up the slack and prepositioning the patient at the limit. Since the limit is a combined movement of side flexion and rotation, the technique is not performed at end range rotation.

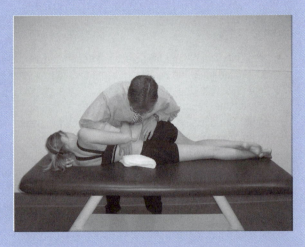

**Figure 11.55**   Preposition Prior to Manipulative Thrust

- Step Three: The final procedure involves a quick thrust performed by loading downward (toward the table) on the patient. A common mistake involves pulling and pushing too vividly with the fingers. The technique involves more loading through the body of the patient than forceful hand movements.

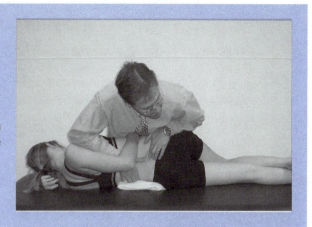

**Figure 11.56** Thrust Procedure

## Mobilization Procedures from the Examination

Mobilization methods selected based on the response of the patient's examination may also be plausible treatment options. Generally, the methods are selected based on the desired response of the patient once the techniques were applied during the examination. Chiradejnant et al.[221] reported that the direction of the technique made little difference in the outcome of the patient. Randomly selected spine mobilization techniques performed at the *targeted* level demonstrated no difference when compared to therapist-selected techniques. Nevertheless, the technique does result in the best outcome when applied directly to the desired concordant segment.[222]

## *Immobilization Group*

Individuals that fall within the immobilization group may exhibit a long-term history of trauma, generalized laxity, an instability catch, and frequent episodes of low back pain. These individuals may demonstrate radiographic instability or clinical instability. Radiologic appreciable instability reflects marked disruption of passive osseoligamentous anatomical constraints[223] and is typically diagnosed by appropriate radiographic measurements.[218] Clinical instability is more challenging to diagnose and may involve discrepancies in radiographic findings.[218] Theoretically, clinical dynamic stabilizers include the neural feedback systems and the muscles and tendons of the spinal column and comprise force or motion transducers that include muscle spindles and Golgi tendon organs that exhibit proprioceptive and kinesthetic neural properties. Clinical instability commonly demonstrates subtle quantifiable clinical features[184] with negative or inconsistent findings during traditional radiographic analysis.[224] Studies by Cook et al. have outlined the multiple facets of clinical instability. In their studies, the authors outlined proposed patient history and clinical examination findings of instability as advocated by consensus from expert clinical practitioners.[111,225–226] Hicks et al.[180] have developed a clinical prediction rule to identify those patients who may benefit from a stabilization intervention program. Three of four clinical findings of (1) age < 40, (2) SLR > 91 degrees, (3) aberrant movements during the examination, and (4) positive prone instability test during the examination are identifiers that may warrant stabilization.

## Transverse Abdominus Contraction

Isolating a transverse abdominus contraction is challenging for both the patient and the clinician. The ability to isolate this muscle from the surrounding muscle requires a contraction that is much lesser in intensity than one may expect. A subthreshold contraction is required and endurance training versus resistance training should be the focus. The reader is suggested to read further elsewhere for more information regarding stabilization training.

- Step One: The patient assumes a supine hooklying position.
- Step Two: The clinician places his or her fingers just medial and just inferior to the ASIS of the patient.
- Step Three: The patient is instructed to tighten his or her pelvic floor muscles. Usually, this process firms the transverse abdominus and solicits the warranted contraction of the TA.
- Step Four: If no contraction of the TA is palpated, the patient is instructed to "draw in" his or her abdomen just inferior to his or her "belly button." The patient should be instructed not to tighten the obliques.
- Step Five: A correct contraction allows the TA to hollow out. An incorrect contraction pushes upward against the clinician's fingers or a pelvic tilt is performed by the patient.

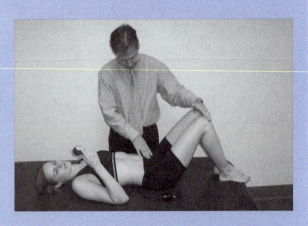

**Figure 11.57**    Transverse Abdominus Contraction

## Multifidi Progression

Several exercises trigger the multifidi muscles. The easiest to perform is in a four-point stance. The patient must be instructed to contract at subthreshold. The reader is suggested to read further elsewhere for more information regarding stabilization training.

- Step One: The patient assumes a four-point position. The clinician places his or her hands just cephalic to the sacral base pre-contract the TA.
- Step Two: Initially, the patient is instructed to "gently swell" his or her multifidi into the fingers of the therapist. Because this commonly leads to the inability to contract the multifidi or substitutions, the clinician may have to adopt an alternative method to isolate the contraction. The patient is instructed to "telescope" his or her leg up manually on one side. He or she should be instructed to only lift the leg approximately 1 inch.
- Step Three: The patient is then instructed to extend the hip approximately 10 degrees. This action should lift the leg approximately 1–3 inches posteriorly to the earlier placement in four-point.
- Step Four: An individual can progress performing similar exercises with greater weights, time of holds, and different positions.

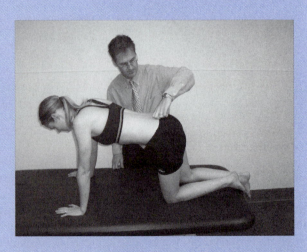

**Figure 11.58**    Multifidi Exercises

## *Traction Group*

Many clinicians use motorized traction to treat lumbar disc–related problems. This textbook advocates the use of manual traction to more appropriately isolate the force and direction of treatment to the targeted regions. Essentially, any activity that decompresses the intervertebral foreman is considered a plausible traction-related technique because there is little evidence to support a "reduction" of the disc with traction.

### Hooklying Traction

For irritable patients, lumbar traction may provide enough relief to advance to techniques that are more vigorous. Although the benefit of distraction for the disc is disputed, the benefit of gentle traction techniques for pain relief is substantiated.

- Step One: The patient assumes a hooklying position in supine.
- Step Two: The clinician hooks the distal aspect of his or her thigh with the elbows or hands and gently pulls caudally.
- Step Three: The intent of the treatment is to reduce symptoms

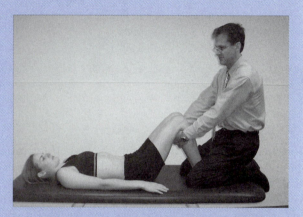

**Figure 11.59**    Hooklying Lumbar Traction

### Sidelying Traction

- Step One: The patient assumes a sidelying position, with the painful disc up.
- Step Two: The clinician promotes side bending, either through a caudal pressure placed on the patient's iliac crest or through prepositioning.
- Step Three: The clinician then applies a PA force, maintaining the pressure placed caudally.
- Step Four: The intent of the treatment is to reduce and centralize symptoms.

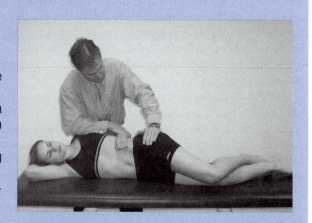

**Figure 11.60**    Side Lying Traction Technique: Incorporation of Anterior Rotation

## Leg Pull Procedure

Another traction technique involves a single distraction of the lumbar spine with the hip in internal rotation. The procedure allows the lumbar spine to side flexion away and open the symptomatic side.

- Step One: The patient assumes a supine position.
- Step Two: The clinician lifts the patient's leg approximately 2 feet from the table.
- Step Three: The clinician pulls the leg while monitoring the symptoms of the patient.

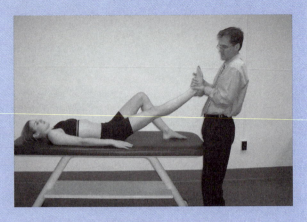

**Figure 11.61**  Leg Pull Traction

### Psychosocial Factors

It is important to note that despite the best efforts toward clinical treatment, some patients exhibit factors that retard their progress toward recovery. Past authors have suggested the existence of blue, yellow, and black flags that may hamper recovery during low back treatment. Both blue and black flags are occupationally related. **Blue flags** include perceived occupational factors believed by patients to impede their recovery. These factors include litigation, long-term worker's compensation, and a negative relationship with their supervisor.[90] **Black flags** include objective occupational or workplace factors that may initially lead to the onset of low back pain, and may promote disability once the acute episode has occurred. These factors include low job grade, low job salary, newness at position, low rating by supervisor, and low job satisfaction.[5] Lastly, **yellow flags** are potentially significant psychosocial risk factors for developing chronic low back pain. These include sociodemographic, abnormal pain behavioral responses, compensation-related responses, and psychological elements.[227,228]

Ironically, nonphysical items such as psychosocial factors are the best predictors of return to work, recovery from acute low back pain,[1,113,114] advancement of chronicity,[5,229–233] and recovery from surgical intervention.[234] These psychosocial factors include abnormalities in pain perception, job-related intricacies, psychological dysfunction, social support challenges, and disability perceptions. There are mixed findings whether the demographic and attribute variables of age, gender, smoking, and education are associated with low back pain disability and chronicity.

### Summary

- The clinician must first identify the concordant sign of the patient and treatment should be directed toward this finding.
- The TBC is a classification method that allows categorizing of patient treatment approaches.
- The four divisions of the TBC include a stabilization group, mobilization group, specific exercise group, and a traction group.
- Psychosocial factors provide greater predictive evidence for negative outcomes.
- For unknown reasons, conditions with the same diagnosis may lead to dissimilar outcomes.
- Numerous "flags" exist that may alter the outcome of the rehabilitation treatment.
- Failure to acknowledge and investigate each of the "flags" may yield inappropriate and ineffective treatment.

## TREATMENT OUTCOMES

It is imperative to note that factors that increase one's risk for injury are not necessarily the same factors that increase one's risk for poor prognosis.[235] A challenge to the rehabilitation clinician is that injuries, which are intrinsically similar and involve similar treatment methods, often result in a wide range of outcomes.[235]

Up to 85% of low back pain does not have a readably demonstrable pathological basis,[80–82] nor does an identified pathologic process automatically establish the cause of the pain. No one treatment approach has excelled over another. Frankly stated, we are still uncertain what truly works superiorly over other interventions.

## Treatment Based on Classification

This textbook advocates a patient response-based treatment homogenized into a classification model. At present, only a few studies have investigated this form of analysis but have yielded positive results. One study established criterion validity[219] whereas another found better outcomes when compared against a control group that received exercises based on standardized suggested guidelines.[236]

Recently, Cook et al.[94] reported the outcomes of exercise programs based on the patient-response method of classification. In their study, the authors limited study selection to those that compared the classified approach to a pragmatic or true control. Only five studies were included, four of which demonstrated evidence of improvement over pragmatic controls.

## Active Physiological Exercise

The majority of active physiological exercise approaches were performed on patients with nonhomogeneous low back pain. A recent study and subsequent update by van Tulder and colleagues of the *Cochrane Collaboration Back Review Group* suggests that evidence to support one specific exercise approach for low back pain has yet to be demonstrated beyond doubt.[139] There are several points of concern regarding soundness of the van Tulder et al. findings. First, the review included studies with all forms of exercise interventions failing to specify in the inclusion criteria if the approach necessitated the clinical application by a physical therapist. Second, the majority of studies included heterogeneous classifications of patients treated homogeneously and lumped into time-based categories of "acute," "subacute," or "chronic" low back pain. Third, to select the "high-quality trials" van Tulder used, a modified scale was originally developed for pharmacological intervention trials.[237] This scale included criteria such as blinding of the patient and therapist, two components that have a low likelihood of occurring in a physical therapy–associated clinical trial. The scale did not include assessment criteria for the timeframe and quality of the exercises.[238] There was no criterion designed to measure the consistency in timing of the outcome assessment of one intervention versus another.[239]

## Manipulation/Mobilization

Most studies have not compared outcomes of treatment-based classifications. In a meta-analysis of 39 articles, two reviewers from the *Cochrane Back Review Group*[240] reported that for patients with acute low back pain compared with preselected, possibly harmful, ineffective modalities, spinal manipulation was not significantly bet-

ter when combined in analysis. They also reported that compared with sham spinal manipulation, manipulation was better (but not significantly) in pain reduction. For patients with chronic back pain, when the subjects were compared with preselected, possibly harmful, ineffective modalities, spinal manipulation was not significantly better, and when compared with sham, spinal manipulation was better (but not significantly) in pain reduction. Lastly, when compared with sham manipulation, spinal manipulation was better but not significantly.

Oddly, the authors found no significant difference when subjects had chronic or acute pain, or patients with any form of sciatica, no significant difference, even when the highest rated studies were selected, and no evidence to support that manipulation/mobilization can help this impairment classification.[240] The authors stated, "For patients, clinicians, and policymakers, our findings that spinal manipulation therapy is substantially less effective than previously estimated should temper enthusiasm for this treatment as "the recommended therapy for patients with low back pain." Additionally, "We found no evidence that spinal manipulative therapy is superior to other advocated therapies including analgesics, exercises, physical therapy, and back schools."

Two recent reviews found similar information,[241,242] indicating there is no compelling evidence for the use of manipulative therapy for the lumbar spine specifically by chiropractors. Since this condemnation, several smaller, less comprehensive studies have been published that suggest the benefit of manual therapy (including mobilization and manipulation) for low back impairment. Future studies involving larger clinical trials may improve the conclusiveness of this approach and improve our ability to ascribe manual therapy to the lumbar spine (Table 11.7).

## Traction

At present, there is poor evidence to include or exclude the use of lumbar traction during treatment of low back pain.[252,253] The primary problem associated with determining the effectiveness of traction is the failure of appropriate design and study control.[254] A preponderance of studies included subjects that would have fallen into a different classification advocated by this textbook and would

## Summary

- Few clinical trials have examined the benefit of mobilization and manipulation of the lumbar spine.
- Most positive results have occurred in small, poorly designed studies.
- Future studies are needed to examine the benefit of mobilization and manipulation of the lumbar spine.

**TABLE 11.7**   Outcomes Associated with Mobilization and/or Manipulation

| Author | Type of Study | Subjects | Findings | Clinician |
|---|---|---|---|---|
| Childs et al.[178] | RPT | 131 patients with LBP | When patients were categorized into the clinical prediction rule, manip group demonstrated better outcomes than exercise-only group. | PT |
| Hurwitz et al.[243] | RPT | N = 681, LBP patients | Chiro manip group, medical supervision only, and PT intervention group were compared. Chiro and medical group were similar at 6 months; the PT group was superior significantly over the medical only but not significantly over the Chiro group. | PT, MD, DC |
| Burton et al.[244] | Retro | N = 252, LBP | 78% of patients reported reoccurrence of symptoms within 1 year after receiving manip only care. Over ½ opted for additional Rx as well. At 4 years out, depressive symptoms appeared to be more related to reoccurrence than anything. | DC, PT |
| Haas et al.[245] | RPT | N = 72 | Two-group comparison between SMT and modalities. At 4 weeks, SMT proved to be better than modalities. No differences at 12 weeks. | DC |
| Hoiriis et al.[246] | RPT | N = 192, LBP | Three-group comparison of SMT, sham adjustments and muscle relaxants, and Sham and sham medicine. SMT was better (significantly) than both groups for pain and disability. | DC, MD |
| Haas et al.[247] | RPT | N = 2870 | A cohort of Chiro patients were compared against medical intervention only in a 1-year trial. Chiro patients demonstrated better benefit in acute and chronic patients, as well as those with leg pain. | DC, MD |
| UK BEAM Trial Team[248] | RPT | N = 1334 LBP | Manipulation was most cost-effective, followed by manipulation and exercise, then exercise alone. No modalities. | PT, DO, DC |
| Niemisto et al.[249] | RPT | N = 204, Chronic LBP | Manipulation lead to decreased pain when compared to stabilization exercises. Stab exercises were taught by physician. No modalities. | PT, MD |
| Wand et al.[250] | RCT | N = 102, Acute LBP | Two-group comparison between a group who received Rx of manual therapy, exercise, and biopsychosocial education, vs. a group who received advice and no treatment. Significant improvement in 6 weeks for Rx group. No modalities. | PT |
| Niemisto et al.[251] | RPT | N = 102, Chronic LBP | Severe affective distress, over 25 days of sick leave, poor life control, and generalized somatic symptoms were associated with poor response to manipulation. No modalities. | PT |

*RPT, Randomized Pragmatic Trial*
*RCT, Randomized Controlled Trial*

inherently not be good candidates for traction. Because motorized traction is the only form of traction that is adequately standardized for research comparisons, this area is the only iteration studied. Krause et al.[255] suggested that traction is most likely to benefit patients with acute (> 6 weeks' duration) radicular pain with concomitant neurological deficit but agree that little support exists to substantiate these suggestions. Subsequently, results to support the use of manual traction are significantly lacking.

# Chapter Questions

1. Which factors have a higher degree of association to impairment or disability: physical or psychosocial?
2. What role do the multifidi and transverse abdominus play in the stability of the lumbar spine?
3. Which movement-based phenomenon has been shown to relate to positive outcomes?
4. How does the physiological anatomy of the facet joint limit rotation?
5. Which physiological motion allows more degrees of movement in the lumbar spine: flexion-extension, rotation, or side flexion?
6. Which special tests of discogenic-related symptoms have the highest sensitivity and specificity?
7. Why do tests that require manual assessment of minute movements have poor reliability?
8. At present, is the literature definitive in its exploration of the benefits of manual therapy for the lumbar spine?
9. Which method of assessment, pain provocation or movement assessment, has the highest degree of reliability?
10. What procedure is suggested initially for patients who exhibit centralization behavior of the lumbar spine?

# References

1. Burton A, Tillotson K, Main C, Hollis S. Psychosocial predictors of outcome in acute and subchronic low back trouble. *Spine.* 1995;20:722–728.
2. Truchon M. Determinants of chronic disability related to low back pain: towards an integrative biopsychosocial model. *Disabil Rehabil.* 2001;23: 758–767.
3. Andersson GB. Low back pain. *J Rehabil Res Dev.* 1997;34(4):ix–x.
4. Peate WF. Occupational musculoskeletal disorders. *Prim Care.* 1994;21(2):313–327.
5. Gatchel R, Polatin P, Mayer T. The dominant role of psychosocial risk factors in the development of chronic low back pain disability. *Spine.* 1995;20: 2702–2709.
6. Gomez T. Symmetry of lumbar rotation and lateral flexion range of motion and isometric strength in subjects with and without back pain. *J Orthop Sports Phys Ther.* 1994;19:42–48.
7. Frymoyer JW, Durett CL. The economics of spinal disorders. In *The adult spine: Principles and practice,* eds. J.W. Frymoyer. Philadelphia; Lippincott-Raven: 1997.
8. Frymoyer J, Cats-Baril W. Predictors of low back pain disability. *Clin Orthop.* 1987;221:89–98.
9. DeBerard M, Masters K, Colledge A, Schieusener R, Schlegel J. Outcomes of posterolateral lumbar fusion in Utah patients receiving worker's compensation: A retrospective cohort study. *Spine.* 2001;26: 738–746.
10. Bogduk N. *Clinical anatomy of the lumbar spine and sacrum.* 3rd ed. New York; Churchill Livingstone: 1997.
11. Little JS, Khalsa PS. Material properties of the human lumbar facet joint capsule. *J Biomech Eng.* 2005;127(1):15–24.
12. Pope MH, Panjabi M. Biomechanical definitions of spinal instability. *Spine.* 1985;10(3):255–256.
13. Peng B, Wu W, Hou S, Li P, Zhang C, Yang Y. The pathogenesis of discogenic low back pain. *J Bone Joint Surg Br.* 2005;87(1):62–67.
14. Eyre DR. Biochemistry of the intervertebral disc. *Int Rev Connect Tissue Res.* 1979;8:227–291.
15. Humzah MD, Soames RW. Human intervertebral disc: structure and function. *Anat Rec.* 1988;220(4): 337–356.
16. Tencer A, Ahmed A, Burke D. Some static mechanical properties of the lumbar intervertebral joint, intact and injured. *J Biomech Eng.* 1982;104:193–201.
17. Gracovetsky S, Farfan H, Helleur C. The abdominal mechanism. *Spine.* 1985;10(4):317–324.
18. O'Sullivan P. Lumbar segmental instability: clinical presentation and specific stabilizing exercise management. *Man Ther.* 2000;5(1):2–12.
19. Bogduk N: The Innervation of the Lumbar Spine. *Spine.* 1983;6:286–293.
20. Cavanaugh JM, el-Bohy A, Hardy WN, Getchell TV, Getchell ML, King AI. Sensory innervation of soft tissues of the lumbar spine in the rat. *J Orthop Res.* 1989;7(3):378–388.

21. Bogduk N, Twomey L. *Clinical anatomy of the lumbar spine*. Melbourne; Churchill Livingstone: 1987.

22. Luk K, Ho H, Leong J. The iliolumbar ligament: a study of its anatomy, development and clinical significance. *J Bone Jnt Surg*. 1986;68:197–200.

23. Pool-Goudzwaard A, van Dijke G, Mulder P, Spoor C, Snijders C, Stoeckart R. The iliolumbar ligament: its influence on stability of the sacroiliac joint. *Clin Biomech*. 2003;18:99–105.

24. Panjabi M. The stabilizing system of the spine: Part I. Function, dysfunction, adaptation, and enhancement. *J Spinal Disord*. 1992;5:383–389.

25. Hides J, Richardson C, Jull G. Multifidus recovery is not automatic after resolution of acute, first-episode low back pain. *Spine*. 1996;21(23):2763–2769.

26. Cresswell A, Thortensson A. Changes in intra-articular pressure, trunk muscle activation and force during isokinetic lifting and lowering. *Eur J Appl Physiol*. 1994;68:315–321.

27. Juker D, McGill S, Kropf P, Steffen T. Quantitative intramuscular myoelectric activity of lumbar portions of psoas and the abdominal wall during a wide variety of tasks. *Med Sci Sports Exerc*. 1998;30: 301–310.

28. Cresswell A. Responses of intra-abdominal pressure and abdominal muscle activity during dynamic loading in man. *Eur J Appl Physiol* 1993;66:315–320.

29. Hodges P, Richardson C. Inefficient muscular stabilization of the lumbar spine associated with low back pain: a motor control evaluation of transverse abdominis. *Spine*. 1996;21(22):2640–2650.

30. Taylor J, O'Sullivan P. Lumbar segmental instability: Pathology, diagnosis, and conservative management. In: Twomey L, Taylor J, eds. *Physical Therapy of the low back. 3rd ed.* Philadelphia: Churchill Livingstone; 2000.

31. Farfan H. *Mechanical disorders of the low back*. Philadelphia: Lea & Febiger, 1973.

32. Bogduk N, Macintosh JE, Pearcy MJ. A universal model of the lumbar back muscles in the upright position. *Spine*. 1992;17(8):897–913.

33. van Dieen JH, Selen LP, Cholewicki J. Trunk muscle activation in low-back pain patients, an analysis of the literature. *J Electromyogr Kinesiol*. 2003;13(4): 333–351.

34. Cook C. Lumbar Coupling biomechanics—A literature review. *J Man Manipulative Ther*. 2003;11(3): 137–145.

35. Pearcy M, Portek I, Shepherd J. The effect of low back pain on lumbar spine movements measured by three-dimensional x-ray analysis. *Spine*. 1985;10: 150–153.

36. Mellin G, Harkapaa K, Hurri H. Asymmetry of lumbar lateral flexion and treatment outcome in chronic low back pain patients. *J Spinal Disorders*. 1995;8:15–19.

37. Winkel D, Aufdemkampe G, Matthijs O, Phelps V. *Diagnosis and treatment of the spine*. Gaithersburg, MD; Aspen: 1996.

38. Panjabi M, Oxland T, Yamamoto I, Crisco J. Mechanical behavior of the human lumbar and lumbosacral spine as shown by three-dimensional load-displacement curves. *Am J Bone Joint Surgery*. 1994; 76:413–424.

39. Harrison D, Harrison D, Troyanovich S. Three-dimensional spinal coupling mechanics: Part one. *J Manipulative Physiol Ther*. 1998;21(2):101–113.

40. Gibbons P, Tehan P. Spinal manipulation: indications, risks and benefits. *J Bodywork Movement Therapies* 2001;5(2):110–119.

41. Fryette H. *The Principles of Osteopathic Technique*. Carmel, CA; Academy of Applied Osteopathy: 1954.

42. Faye LJ. *Motion palpation of the spine*. Huntington Beach, CA; Motion Palpation Institute: 1984.

43. Gertzbein S, Seligman J, Holtby R. Centrode patterns and segmental instability in degenerative disc disease. *Spine*. 1986;14:594–601.

44. Plaugher G. *Textbook of clinical chiropractic: A specific biomechanical approach*. Baltimore; Williams & Wilkins: 1993.

45. Gracovetsky S, Newman N, Pawlowsky M, Lanzo V, Davey B, Robinson L. A database for estimating normal spinal motion derived from noninvasive measurements. *Spine*. 1995;20(9):1036–1046.

46. Lund T, Nydegger T, Schlenzka D, Oxland T. Three-dimensional motion patterns during active bending in patients with chronic low back pain. *Spine*. 2002;27(17):1865–1874.

47. Panjabi M, Hult J, Crisco J, White A. Biomechanical studies in cadaveric spines. In Jayson M., ed. *The Lumbar Spine and Back Pain*. 4th ed. London; Churchill Livingstone: 1992.

48. Evans F, Lissner H. Biomechanical studies on the lumbar spine and pelvis. *J Bone Joint Surg Am*. 1959; 41:278–290.

49. Harrison D, Harrison D, Troyanovich S, Hansen D. The anterior-posterior full-spine view: the worst radiographic view for determination of mechanics of the spine. *Chiropractic Technique*. 1996;8:163–170.

50. Rab G, Chao E. Verification of roentgenographic landmarks in the lumbar spine. *Spine*. 1977;2:287–293.

51. Grice A. Radiographic, biomechanical and clinical factors in lumbar lateral flexion: Part 1. *J Manipulative Physiol Ther*. 1979;2:26–34.

52. Gomez T. Symmetry of lumbar rotation and lateral flexion range of motion and isometric strength in subjects with and without back pain. *J Orthop Sports Phys Ther*. 1994;19:42–48.

53. Gertzbein S, Seligman J, Holtby R. Centrode patterns and segmental instability in degenerative disc disease. *Spine*. 1986;14:594–601.

54. Kaigle A, Holm S, Hansson T. Experimental instability in the lumbar spine. *Spine.* 1995;20:421–430.

55. Kaigle A, Wessberg P, Hansson T. Muscular and kinematic behavior of the lumbar spine during flexion-extension. *J Spinal Disord.* 1998;11:163–174.

56. Panjabi M, Krag M, Chung T. Effects of disc injury on mechanical behavior of the human spine. *Spine.* 1984;9(7):707–713.

57. Seligman J, Gertzbein S, Tile M, Kapasouri A. Computer analysis of spinal segment motion in degenerative disc disease with and without axial loading. *Spine.* 1984;9:566–573.

58. Weitz E. The lateral bending sign. *Spine.* 1981;6: 388–397.

59. Parnianpour M, Nordin M, Frankel V, Kahanovitz N. Trunk triaxial coupling of torque generation of trunk muscles during isometric exertions and the effect of fatiguing isoinertial movements on the motor output and movement patterns. *Spine.* 1988;13: 982–992.

60. Panjabi M, Hult E, Crisco J, White A. Biomechanical studies in cadaveric spines. In: White A, & Panjabi M. *Clinical biomechanics of the spine.* Philadelphia; Lippincott: 1978.

61. Lai PL, Chen LH, Niu C, Fu T, Chen WJ. Relation between laminectomy and development of adjacent segment instability after lumbar fusion with pedicle fixation. *Spine.* 2004;29(22):2527–2532.

62. Panjabi M, Krag M, Chung T. Effects of disc injury on mechanical behavior of the human spine. *Spine.* 1984;9(7):707–713.

63. Keating J, Bergman T, Jacobs G, Finer B, Larson K. The objectivity of a multi-dimensional index of lumbar segmental abnormality. *J Manipulative Physiol Ther.* 1990;13:463–471.

64. Hardy G, Napier J. Inter- and intra-therapist reliability of passive accessory movement technique. *New Zealand J Physio.* 1991;22–24.

65. Vilkari-Juntura E. Inter-examiner reliability of observations in physical examinations of the neck. *Phys Ther.* 1987;67(10):1526–1532.

66. Lee M, Latimer J, Maher C. Manipulation: investigation of a proposed mechanism. *Clin Biomech.* 1993; 8:302–306.

67. Maher C, Adams R. Reliability of pain and stiffness assessments in clinical manual lumbar spine examinations. *Phys Ther.* 1994;74(9):801–811.

68. Maher C, Latimer J. Pain or resistance: the manual therapists' dilemma. *Aust J Physiother.* 1992;38(4): 257–260.

69. Boline P, Haas M, Meyer J, Kassak K, Nelson C, Keating J. Interexaminer reliability of eight evaluative dimensions of lumbar segmental abnormality: Part II. *J Manipulative Physiol Ther.* 1992;16(6): 363–373.

70. Li Y, He X. Finite element analysis of spine biomechanics. *J Biomech Engineering.* 2001;18(2)288–289, 319.

71. Troke M, Moore AP, Maillardet FJ, Hough A, Cheek E. A new, comprehensive normative database of lumbar spine ranges of motion. *Clin Rehabil.* 2001;15:371–379.

72. Dvorak J, Vajda EF, Grob D, Panjabi MM. Normal motion of the lumbar spine as related to age and gender. *Eur Spine J.* 1995;20:2421–2428.

73. Van Herp G, Rowe PJ, Salter PM. Range of motion in the lumbar spine and the effects of age and gender. *Physiotherapy.* 2000;86:42.

74. Borkan JM, Koes B, Reis S, Cherkin DC. A report from the second international forum for primary care research on low back pain. Re-examining priorities. *Spine.* 1998;23:1992–1996.

75. Bouter LM, van Tulder MW, Koes BW. Methodologic issues in low back pain research in primary care. *Spine.* 1998;23:2014–2020.

76. Leboeuf-Yde C, Lauritsen JM, Lauritsen T. Why has the search for causes of low back pain largely been nonconclusive? *Spine.* 1997;22:877–881.

77. Spitzer WO. Scientific approach to the assessment and management of activity related spinal disorders. A monograph form clinicians. Report of the Quebec Task Force on Spinal Disorders. *Spine.* 1987;Suppl. S1–59.

78. McCarthy C, Arnall F, Strimpakos N, Freemont A, Oldham J. The biopsychosocial classification of nonspecific low back pain: a systematic review. *Physical Therapy Reviews.* 2004;9:17–30.

79. Lurie JD. What diagnostic tests are useful for low back pain? *Best Pract Res Clin Rheumatol.* 2005;19(4): 557–575.

80. Deyo R, Phillips W. Low back pain. A primary care challenge. *Spine.* 1996;21(24):2826–2832.

81. Deyo RA. Nonsurgical care of low back pain. *Neurosurg Clin N Am.* 1991;2(4):851–862.

82. Hart LG, Deyo RA, Cherkin DC. Physician office visits for low back pain. Frequency, clinical evaluation, and treatment patterns from a U.S. national survey. *Spine.* 1995;20(1):11–19.

83. Frymoyer JW. Back pain and sciatica. *N Engl J Med.* 1988;318(5):291–300.

84. Jarvik JG, Deyo RA. Imaging of lumbar intervertebral disk degeneration and aging, excluding disk herniations. *Radiol Clin North Am.* 2000;38(6):1255–1266.

85. Deyo RA, Rainville J, Kent DL. What can the history and physical examination tell us about low back pain? *JAMA.* 1992;268(6):760–765.

86. McIntosh G, Frank J, Hogg-Johnson S. Prognostic factors for time receiving workers' compensation benefits in a cohort of patient with low back pain. *Spine.* 2000;26:758–765.

87. Hadijistavropoulos H, Craig K. Acute and chronic low back pain: cognitive, affective, and behavioral dimensions. *J Consult Clin Psychol.* 1994;62:341–349.

88. Hunter S, Shaha S, Flint D, Tracy D. Predicting return to work. A long-term follow-up study of railroad workers after low back injuries. *Spine.* 1998;23:2319–2328.

89. Frymoyer J. Predicting disability from low back pain. *Clin Orthop.* 1992;(279):101–109.

90. Schultz et al. Biophysical multivariate predictive model of occupational low back disability. *Spine.* 2001;27(23):2720–2728.

91. Bernard T, Kirkaldy-Willis W. Recognizing specific characteristics of nonspecific low back pain. *Clin Orthop.* 1987;217:266–280.

92. Moffroid M, Haugh L, Henry S, Short B. Distinguishable groups of musculoskeletal low back pain patients and asymptomatic control subjects based on physical measures of the NIOSH Low Back Atlas. *Spine.* 1994;19:1350–1358.

93. Riddle DL. Classification and low back pain: a review of the literature and critical analysis of selected systems. *Phys Ther.* 1998;78:708–737.

94. Cook C, Hegedus E, Ramey K. Physical therapy exercise intervention based on classification using the patient response method: a systematic review of the literature. *J Manual Manipulative Ther.* 2005;13:158–168.

95. Aina A, May S, Clare H. The centralization phenomenon of spinal symptoms—a systematic review. *Man Ther.* 2004;9:134–143.

96. Tuttle N. Do changes within a manual therapy treatment session predict between-session changes for patients with cervical spine pain? *Aust J Physiother.* 2005;51:43–48.

97. Hahne AJ, Keating JL, Wilson SC. Do within-session changes in pain intensity and range of motion predict between-session changes in patients with low back pain? *Aust J Physiother.* 2004;50(1):17–23.

98. Delitto A, Cibulka MT, Erhard RE, Bowling RW, Tenhula JA. Evidence for use of an extension-mobilization category in acute low back syndrome: a prescriptive validation pilot study. *Phys Ther.* 1993;73(4):216–222.

99. Peterson T, Laslett M, Thorsen H, Manniche C, Ekdahl C, Jacobsen S. Diagnostic classification of non-specific low back pain. A new system integrating patho-anatomic and clinical categories. *Physiother Theory Pract.* 2003;19:213–237.

100. Peterson T, Laslett M, Thorsen H, Manniche C, Ekdahl C, Jacobsen S. Inter-tester reliability of a new diagnostic classification system for patients with non-specific low back pain. *Aust J Physiother.* 2004;50:85–94.

101. Werneke M, Hart D. Categorizing patients with occupational low back pain by use of the Quebec Task Force Classification system versus pain pattern classification procedures: discriminant and predictive validity. *Phys Ther.* 2004;84(3):243–254.

102. Bigos SJ, Davis GE. Scientific application of sports medicine principles for acute low back problems. The Agency for Health Care Policy and Research Low Back Guideline Panel (AHCPR, Guideline #14). *J Orthop Sports Phys Ther.* 1996;24(4):192–207.

103. Spitzer W. Diagnosis of the problem (the problem of diagnosis). In: Scientific approach to the assessment and measurement of activity related spinal disorders: A monograph for clinicians-Report of the Quebec Task Force on Spinal disorders. *Spine.* 1987;12(Suppl):S16–S21.

104. Werneke M, Hart D. Centralization phenomenon as a prognostic factor for chronic low back pain. *Spine.* 2001;25:758–764.

105. Frymoyer J. Predicting disability from low back pain. *Clin Orthop.* 1993;279:101–109.

106. Bogduk N. The sources of low back pain. In: Jayson M. *The lumbar spine and back pain.* 4th ed. Edinburg; Churchill Livingstone: 1992.

107. Bogduk N. Lumbar dorsal ramus syndrome. *Med J Aust.* 1980;2:537–541.

108. Bogduk N, Macintosh JE. The applied anatomy of the thoracolumbar fascia. *Spine.* 1984;9(2):164–170.

109. Bogduk N. The anatomical basis for spinal pain syndromes. *J Manipulative Physiol Ther.* 1995;18(9):603–605.

110. Laslett M. Breakout session. American Academy of Orthopedic Manual Physical Therapists. Reno, Nevada. 2003.

111. Cook C, Brismee JM, Sizer P. Subjective and objective descriptors of clinical lumbar spine instability: A Delphi study. *Man Ther.* 2006;11:11–21.

112. Granata KP, Wilson SE. Trunk posture and spinal stability. *Clin Biomech.* 2001;16:650–659.

113. Tubach F, Leclerc A, Landre M, Pietri-Taleb F. Risk factors for sick leave due to low back pain: A prospective study. *J Occup Environ Med.* 2002;44:451–458.

114. Fritz J, George S. Identifying psychosocial variables in patients with acute work-related low back pain: the importance of fear-avoidance beliefs. *Phys Ther.* 2002;82:973–983.

115. Roelofs J, Peters ML, Fassaert T, Vlaeyen JW. The role of fear of movement and injury in selective attentional processing in patients with chronic low back pain: a dot-probe evaluation. *J Pain.* 2005;6(5):294–300.

116. Childs JD, Piva SR, Erhard RE, Hicks G. Side-to-side weight-bearing asymmetry in subjects with low back pain. *Man Ther.* 2003;8(3):166–169.

117. Riddle D, Rothstein J. Intertester reliability of McKenzie's classifications of the syndrome types present in patients with low back pain. *Spine.* 1993;18(10):1333–1344.

118. Kilpikoski S, Airaksinen O, Kankaanpaa M, Leminen P, Videman T, Alen M. Interexaminer reliability of low back pain assessment using the McKenzie method. *Spine*. 2002;27(8):207–214.

119. Clare HA, Adams R, Maher CG. Reliability of detection of lumbar lateral shift. *J Manipulative Physiol Ther*. 2003;26(8):476–480.

120. Tenhula JA, Rose SJ, Delitto A. Tenhula et al Association between direction of lateral lumbar shift, movement tests, and side of symptoms in patients with low back pain syndrome. *Phys Ther*. 1990;70(8):480–486.

121. Young S. Personal communication. March 17, 2005.

122. Vroomen PC, de Krom MC, Wilmink JT, Kester AD, Knottnerus JA. Diagnostic value of history and physical examination in patients suspected of lumbosacral nerve root compression. *J Neurol Neurosurg Psychiatry*. 2002;72(5):630–634.

123. Boos N, Rieder R, Schade V, Spratt KF, Semmer N, Aebi M. 1995 Volvo Award in clinical sciences. The diagnostic accuracy of magnetic resonance imaging, work perception, and psychosocial factors in identifying symptomatic disc herniations. *Spine*. 1995;20(24):2613–2625.

124. Elfering A, Semmer NK, Schade V, Grund S, Boos N. Supportive colleague, unsupportive supervisor: the role of provider-specific constellations of social support at work in the development of low back pain. *J Occup Health Psychol*. 2002;7(2):130–140.

125. Luoma K, Riihimaki H, Luukkonen R, Raininko R, Viikari-Juntura E, Lamminen A. Low back pain in relation to lumbar disc degeneration. *Spine*. 2000;25(4):487–492.

126. Luoma K, Riihimaki H, Raininko R, Luukkonen R, Lamminen A, Viikari-Juntura E. Lumbar disc degeneration in relation to occupation. *Scand J Work Environ Health*. 1998;24(5):358–366.

127. Hasenbring M, Marienfeld G, Kuhlendahl D, Soyka D. Risk factors of chronicity in lumbar disc patients. A prospective investigation of biologic, psychologic, and social predictors of therapy outcome. *Spine*. 1994;19:2759–2765.

128. Young S, Aprill C, Laslett M. Correlation of clinical examination characteristics with three sources of chronic low back pain. *Spine J*. 2003;3(6):460–465.

129. O'Sullivan PB, Mitchell T, Bulich P, Waller R, Holte J. The relationship between posture and back muscle endurance in industrial workers with flexion-related low back pain. *Man Ther*. 2005.

130. Robinson J. Lower extremity pain of lumbar spine origin: differentiating somatic referred and radicular pain. *J Manual Manipulative Ther*. 2003;11:223–234.

131. Marks R. Distribution of pain provoked from lumbar facet joints and related structures during diagnostic spinal infiltration. *Pain*. 1989;39:37–40.

132. Mooney V, Robertson J. The facet syndrome. *Clin Orthop*. 1976;115:149–156.

133. Smyth MJ, Wright V. Sciatica and the intervertebral disc. An experimental study. *J Bone Joint Surg*. 1959;40A:1401–1418.

134. Kuslich S, Ulstrom CL, Michael CJ. The tissue origin of low back pain and sciatica: a report of pain response to tissue stimulation during operations on the lumbar spine using local anesthesia. *Ortho Clin North Am*. 1991;22:181–187.

135. Norlen G. On the value of the neurological symptoms in sciatica for the localization of a lumbar disc herniation. *Acta Chir Scadinav Supp*. 1944;95:1–96.

136. McCullough JA, Waddell G. Variation of the lumbosacral myotomes with bony segmental anomalies. *J Bone Joint Surg*. 1980;62:475–480.

137. Lauder T, Dillingham TR, Andary M. Effect of history and exam in predicting electrodiagnostic outcome among patients with suspected lumbosacral radiculopathy. *Am J Phys Med Rehabil*. 2000;79:60–68.

138. Kovacs FM, Abraira V, Zamora J, Teresa Gil del Real M, Llobera J, Fernandez C, Bauza JR, Bauza K, Coll J, Cuadri M, Duro E, Gili J, Gestoso M, Gomez M, Gonzalez J, Ibanez P, Jover A, Lazaro P, Llinas M, Mateu C, Mufraggi N, Muriel A, Nicolau C, Olivera MA, Pascual P, Perello L, Pozo F, Revuelta T, Reyes V, Ribot S, Ripoll J, Ripoll J, Rodriguez E; Kovacs-Atencion Primaria Group. Correlation between pain, disability, and quality of life in patients with common low back pain. *Spine*. 2004;29(2):206–210.

139. van Tulder MW, Koes BW, Bouter LM. Conservative treatment of acute and chronic nonspecific low back pain. A systematic review of randomized controlled trials of the most common interventions. *Spine*. 1997;22(18):2128–2156.

140. Resnik L, Dobrykowski E. Guide to outcomes measurement for patients with low back pain syndromes. *J Orthop Sports Phys Ther*. 2003;33(6):307–316.

141. White LJ, Velozo CA. The use of Rasch measurement to improve the Oswestry classification scheme. *Arch Phys Med Rehabil*. 2002;83(6):822–831.

142. Bomardier C. Outcome assessments in the evaluation of treatment of spinal disorders: summary and general recommendations. *Spine*. 2000;25(24):3100–3103.

143. Main CJ, Waddell G. Behavioral responses to examination. A reappraisal of the interpretation of "nonorganic signs." *Spine*. 1998;23(21):2367–2371.

144. Stroud MW, McKnight P, Jensen MP. Assessment of self-reported physical activity in patients with chronic pain: development of an abbreviated Roland-Morris disability scale. *J Pain*. 2004;5(5):257–263.

145. Lundberg M, Styf J, Carlsson S. A psychometric evaluation of the Tampa Scale for kinesiophobia: from a physiotherapeutic perspective. *Physiotherapy Theory Practice*. 2004;20:121–133.

146. Vlaeyen JW, Linton SJ. Fear-avoidance and its consequences in chronic musculoskeletal pain: a state of the art. *Pain*. 2000;85:317–332.

147. McKenzie R. *The lumbar spine: Mechanical diagnosis and therapy*. Waikanae, New Zealand; Spinal Publications: 1981.

148. Aina A, May S, Clare H. The centralization phenomenon of spinal symptoms—a systematic review. *Man Ther*. 2004;9:134–143.

149. Donelson R, Aprill C, Medcalf R, Grant W. A prospective study of centralization of lumbar and referred pain. A predictor of symptomatic discs and annular competence. *Spine*. 1997;22:1115–1122.

150. Erhard R, Delitto A, Cibulka M. Relative effectiveness of an extension program and a combined program of manipulation and flexion and extension exercises in patients with acute low back syndrome. *Phys Ther*. 1994;74:1093–1100.

151. Delitto A, Erhard R. Bowling R. A treatment-based classification approach to low back syndrome: identifying and staging patients for conservative treatment. *Phys Ther*. 1995;75:470–489.

152. Long A, Donelson R, Fung T. Does it matter which exercise? A randomized control trial of exercise for low back pain. *Spine*. 2004;29:2593–2602.

153. Parks KA, Crichton KS, Goldford RJ, McGill SM. A comparison of lumbar range of motion and functional ability scores in patients with low back pain: assessment for range of motion validity. *Spine*. 2003; 28(4):380–384.

154. Haswell K. Interexaminer reliability of symptom-provoking active sidebend, rotation, and combined movement assessments of patients with low back pain. *J Man Manipulative Ther*. 2004;12:11–20.

155. Donelson R, Silva G, Murphy K. Centralization phenomenon. Its usefulness in evaluating and treating referred pain. *Spine*. 1990;15:211–213.

156. Maitland GD. *Maitland's vertebral manipulation*. 6th ed. London; Butterworth-Heinemann: 2001.

157. Peterson C, Hayes K. Construct validity of Cyriax's selective tension examination: association of end-feels with pain at the knee and shoulder. *J Orthop Sports Phys Ther*. 2000;30(9):512–521.

158. Waddell G, Somerville D, Henderson I, Newton M. Objective clinical evaluation of physical impairment in chronic low back pain. *Spine*. 1992;17(6):617–628.

159. Wong TK, Lee RY. Effects of low back pain on the relationship between the movements of the lumbar spine and hip. *Hum Mov Sci*. 2004;23(1):21–34.

160. Sizer P, Phelps V, Dedrick G, Matthijs O. Differential diagnosis and management of root related pain. *Pain Prac* 2002;2:98–121.

161. Strender L, Sjoblom A, Ludwig R, Taube A, Sundell K. Interexaminer reliability in physical examination of patients with low back pain. *Spine*. 1997;22(7): 814–820.

162. Love R, Brodeur R. Inter- and intra-examiner reliability of motion palpation for the thoracolumbar spine. *J Manipulative Physio Ther*. 1987;19:261–266.

163. Jull G, Treleaven J, Versace G. Manual examination: is pain provocation a major cue for spinal dysfunction? *Aust J Physiother*. 1994;40:159–165.

164. Jull G, Bogduk N, Marsland A. The accuracy of manual diagnosis for cervical zygopophyseal joint pain syndromes. *Med J Aust*. 1988;148(5):233–236.

165. Boline P, Haas M, Meyer J, Kassak K, Nelson C, Keating J. Interexaminer reliability of eight evaluative dimensions of lumbar segmental abnormality: Part II. *J Manipulative Physiol Ther*. 1992;16(6): 363–373.

166. Sandmark H, Nisell R. Validity of five common manual neck pain provoking tests. *Scand J Rehabil Med*. 1995;27(3):131–136.

167. Bjornsdottir SV, Kumar S. Posteroanterior spinal mobilization: state of the art review and discussion. *Disabil Rehabil*. 1997;19(2):39–46.

168. Hestoek L, Leboeuf-Yde C. Are chiropractic tests for the lumbo-pelvic spine reliable and valid? A systematic critical literature review. *J Manipulative Physiol Ther*. 2000;23:258–275.

169. Macfadyen N, Maher CG, Adams R. Number of sampling movements and manual stiffness judgments. *J Manipulative Physiol Ther*. 1998;21(9): 604–610.

170. Maher C, Simmonds M, Adams R. Therapists' conceptualization and characterization of the clinical concept of spinal stiffness. *Phys Ther*. 1998;78: 289–300.

171. Anson E, Cook C, Comacho C, Gwilliam B, Karakostas T. The use of education in the improvement in finding R1 in the lumbar spine. *J Manipulative Manual Ther*. 2003;11(4):204–212.

172. Cook C, Turney L, Miles A, Ramirez L, Karakostas T. Predictive factors in poor inter-rater reliability among physical therapists. *J Manipulative Manual Ther*. 2002;10(4):200–205.

173. van Trijffel, Anderegg Q, Bossuyt P, Lucas C. Interexaminer reliability of passive assessment of intervertebral motion in the cervical and lumbar spine: a systematic review. *Man Ther*. 2005;10:256–269.

174. Phillips DR, Twomey LT. A comparison of manual diagnosis with a diagnosis established by a uni-level lumbar spinal block procedure. *Man Ther*. 2000;1(2): 82–87.

175. Dickey JP, Pierrynowski MT, Bednar DA, Yang SX. Relationship between pain and vertebral motion in chronic low-back pain subjects. *Clin Biomech*. 2002; 17(5):345–352.

176. Hicks G, Fritz J, Delitto A, Mishock J. Interrater reliability of clinical examination measures for identification of lumbar segmental instability. *Arch Phys Med Rehabil.* 2003;84(12):1858–1864.

177. Flynn T, Fritz J, Whitman J, Wainner R, Magel J, Rendeiro D, Butler B, Garber M, Allison S. A clinical prediction rule for classifying patients with low back pain who demonstrate short-term improvement with spinal manipulation. *Spine.* 2002;27(24): 2835–2843.

178. Childs JD, Fritz JM, Flynn TW, Irrgang JJ, Johnson KK, Majkowski GR, Delitto A. A clinical prediction rule to identify patients with low back pain most likely to benefit from spinal manipulation: a validation study. *Ann Intern Med.* 2004;141(12): 920–928.

179. Frtiz JM, Whitman J, Childs J. Lumbar spine segmental mobility assessment: an examination of validity for determining intervention strategies in patient with low back pain. *Arch Phys Med Rehabil.* 2005; 86:1745–1752.

180. Hicks G, Fritz JM, Delitto A, McGill S. Preliminary development of a clinical prediction rule for determining which patients with low back pain will respond to a stabilization exercise program. *Arch Phys Med Rehabil.* 2005;86:1753–1762.

181. Lee R, Evans J. An in vivo study of the intervertebral movements produced by posteroanterior mobilization. *Clin Biomech.* 1997;12:400–408.

182. Billis EV, Foster NE, Wright CC. Reproducibility and repeatability: errors of three groups of physiotherapists in locating spinal levels by palpation. *Man Ther.* 2003;8(4):223–232.

183. French SD, Green S, Forbes A. Reliability of chiropractic methods commonly used to detect manipulable lesions in patients with chronic low-back pain. *J Manipulative Physiol Ther.* 2000;23(4):231–238.

184. Niere K, Torney SK. Clinicians' perceptions of minor cervical instability. *Man Ther.* 2004;9(3): 144–150.

185. Lew PC, Briggs CA. Relationship between the cervical component of the slump test and change in hamstring muscle tension. *Man Ther.* 1997;2(2): 98–105.

186. Butler D, Jones M. *Mobilisation of the nervous system.* Melbourne; New York: Churchill Livingstone, 1991.

187. Johnson EK, Chiarello CM. The slump test: the effects of head and lower extremity position on knee extension. *J Orthop Sports Phys Ther.* 1997;26: 310–317.

188. Rebain R, Baxter GD, McDonough S. A systematic review of the passive straight leg raising test as a diagnostic aid for low back pain (1989 to 2000). *Spine.* 2002;27(17):E388–395.

189. Breig A, Troup JD. Biomechanical considerations in the straight-leg-raising test. Cadaveric and clinical studies of the effects of medial hip rotation. *Spine.* 1979;4(3):242–250.

190. Smith SA, Massie JB, Chesnut R, Garfin SR. Straight leg raising: anatomical effects on the spinal nerve root without and with fusion. *Spine.* 1993;18: 992–999.

191. Kobayashi S, Shizu N, Suzuki Y, Asai T, Yoshizawa H. Changes in nerve root motion and intraradicular blood flow during an intraoperative Straight-Leg-Raising Test. *Spine.* 2003;28(13):1427–1434.

192. Schnebel BE, Watckins RG, Dillin W. The role of spinal flexion and extension in changing nerve root compression in disc herniations. *Spine.* 1989;14: 835–837.

193. Scapillini R. Anatomic and radiologic studies on the lumbosacral meningovertebral ligaments of humans. *J Spinal Disorders.* 1990;3:6–15.

194. Wiltse LL. Anatomy of the extradural compartments of the lumbar spinal canal. Peridural membrane and circumneural sheath. *Radiol Clin North Am.* 2000;38(6):1177–1206.

195. Grimes PF, Massie JB, Garfin SR. Anatomical and biomechanical analysis of the lower lumbar foraminal ligaments. *Spine.* 2000;25:2009–2014.

196. Porchet F, Fankhauser H, de Tribolet N. Extreme lateral lumbar disc herniation: clinical presentation in 178 patients. *Acta Neurochir* (Wien). 1994;127 (3–4):203–209.

197. Estridge MN, Rouhe SA, Johnson NG. The femoral stretching test. A valuable sign in diagnosing upper lumbar disc herniations. *J Neurosurg.* 1982;57(6): 813–817.

198. Christodoulides AN. Ipsilateral sciatica on femoral nerve stretch test is pathognomonic of an L4/5 disc protrusion. *J Bone Joint Surg Br.* 1989;71(1):88–89.

199. Kreitz BG, Cote P, Yong-Hing K. Crossed femoral stretching test. A case report. *Spine.* 1996;21(13): 1584–1586.

200. Nadler SF, Malanga GA, Stitik TP, Keswani R, Foye PM. The crossed femoral nerve stretch test to improve diagnostic sensitivity for the high lumbar radiculopathy: 2 case reports. *Arch Phys Med Rehabil.* 2001;82(4):522–523.

201. Geraci MC, Alleva JT. Physical examination of the spine and its functional kinetic chain. In: Cole AJ, Herring SA (ed). *The low back handbook.* Philadelphia; Hanley and Belfus: 1996.

202. Stankovic R, Johnell O, Maly P, Willner S. Use of lumbar extension, slump test, physical and neurological examination in the evaluation of patients with suspected herniated nucleus pulposus. A prospective clinical study. *Man Ther.* 1999;4(1):25–32.

203. Charnley J. Orthopaedic signs in the diagnosis of disc protrusion with special reference to the straight-leg raising test. *Lancet.* 1951;1:186–192.

204. Knuttson B. Comparative value of electromyographic myelographic, and clinical-neurological examinations in diagnosis of lumbar root compression syndrome. *Acta Ortho Scand.* 1961;(Suppl 49):19–49.

205. Hakelius A, Hindmarsh J. The comparative reliability of preoperative diagnostic methods in lumbar disc surgery. *Acta Orthop Scand.* 1972;43:234–238.

206. Spangfort EV. The lumbar disc herniation: a computer aided analysis of 2504 operations. *Acta Orthop Scand.* 1972;11(Suppl 142):1–93.

207. Kosteljanetz M, Espersen O, Halaburt H, Miletic T. Predictive value of clinical and surgical findings in patients with lumbago-sciatica: a prospective study (part 1). *Acta Neurochirugiica.* 1984;73:67–76.

208. Kosteljanetz M, Bang F, Schmidt-Olsen S. The clinical significance of straight leg raising (Lasegue's sign) in the diagnosis of prolapsed lumbar disc. *Spine.* 1988;13:393–395.

209. Kerr RSC, Cadoux-Hudson TA, Adams CBT. The value of accurate clinical assessment in the surgical management of the lumbar disc protrusion. *J Neurol Neurosurg Psychiatr.* 1988;51:169–173.

210. Lauder TD, Dillingham TR, Andary MT, Kumar S, Pezzin LE, Stephens RT. Effect of history and exam in predicting electrodiagnostic outcome among patients with suspected lumbosacral radiculopathy. *Am J Phys Med Rehabil.* 2000;79:60–68.

211. Albeck M. A critical assessment of clinical diagnosis of disc herniation in patients with monoradicular sciatica. *Acta Neurochir.* 1996;138:40–44.

212. Gurdijian E, Webster J, Ostrowski, Hardy W, Lindner D, Thomas L. Herniated lumbar intervertebral discs: an analysis of 1176 operated cases. *J Trauma.* 1961;1:158–176.

213. Paris S. Physical signs of instability. *Spine.* 1985;10: 277–279.

214. Kirkaldy-Willis W, Farfan H. Instability of the lumbar spine. *Clinical Orthop.* 1982;165:289–295.

215. Fritz JM, Piva S, Childs J. Accuracy of the clinical examination to predict radiographic instability of the lumbar spine. *Eur Spine J.* 2005.

216. Cattrysse E, Swinkels R, Oostendorp R, Duquet W. Upper cervical instability: are clinical tests reliable? *Man Ther.* 1997;2(2):91–97.

217. Avery A. The reliability of manual physiotherapy palpation techniques in the diagnosis of bilateral pars defect in subjects with chronic low back pain. *Master of Science Thesis*, Curtin University of Technology, Western Australia.

218. Panjabi MM. The stabilizing system of the spine. Part 1 and Part 2. *J Spinal Disord.* 1992;5:383–397.

219. George S, Delitto A. Clinical examination variables discriminate among treatment-based classification groups: a study of construct validity in patients with acute low back pain. *Phys Ther.* 2005;85(4):306–314.

220. Heiss DG, Fitch DS, Fritz JM, Sanchez W, Roberts K, Buford J. The interrater reliability among physical therapists newly trained in a classification system for acute low back pain. *J Orthop Sports Phys Ther.* 2004;34(8):430–439.

221. Chiradejnant A, Maher C, Latimer J, Stepkovitch N. Efficacy of therapist selected versus randomly selected mobilization techniques for the treatment of low back pain: a randomized controlled trial. *Aust J Physiotherapy.* 2003;49:233–241.

222. Chiradejnant A, Latimer J, Maher C, Stepkovitch N. Does the choice of spinal level treated during posteroanterior (PA) mobilization affect treatment outcome? *Physiotherapy Theory Practice.* 2002;18: 165–174.

223. Dupuis P, Yong-Hing K, Cassidy J, Kirkaldy-Wills W. Radiologic diagnosis of degenerative lumbar spinal instability. *Spine.* 1985;10(3):262–276.

224. Takayanagi K, Takahashi K, Yamagata M, Moriya H, Kitahara H, Tamaki T. Using cineradiography for continuous dynamic-motion analysis of the lumbar spine. *Spine.* 2001;26:1858–1865.

225. Cook C, Brismee JM, Sizer P. Factor analysis. *Physiotherapy Research International.* 2005;10:59–71.

226. Cook C, Brismee JM, Sizer P. Suggestive identifiers of cervical lumbar spine instability. *Phys Ther.* 2005; 85(9):895–906.

227. Geertzen J, Van Wilgen C, Schrier E, Dijkstra P. Chronic pain in rehabilitation medicine. *Disabl Rehabil.* 2006;28:363–367.

228. Meloche W. Biopsychosocial multivariate predictive model of occupational low back disability. *Spine.* 2002;27:2720–2725.

229. Kendall N. Psychosocial approaches to the prevention of chronic pain: the low back paradigm. *Best Pract Res Clin Rheumatol.* 1999;13:545–554.

230. Valat J, Goupille P, Vedere V. (abstract). Low back pain: risk factors for chronicity. *Revue due Rhumatisme.* 1997;64:189–194.

231. Cats-Baril W, Frymoyer J. Identifying patients at risk of becoming disabled because of low back pain. The Vermont Rehabilitation Engineering Center predictive model. *Spine.* 1991;16:605–607.

232. Polatin P, Cox B, Gatchel R, Mayer T. A prospective study of Waddell signs in patients with chronic low back pain. When they may not be predictive. *Spine.* 1993;22:1618–1621.

233. Pincus T, Vlaeyen S, Kendall S, Von Korff M, Kalauokalani D, Reis S. Cognitive-Behavioral therapy and psychosocial factors in low back pain. *Spine.* 2002;27:133–138.

234. Ostelo R, De Vet H, Vlaeyen J. Behavioral graded activity following first-time lumbar disc surgery: 1-year results of a randomized clinical trial. *Spine.* 2003;28:1757–1765.

235. Crook J, Moldofsky H, Shannon H. Determinants of disability after a work related musculoskeletal injury. *J Rheumatol.* 1998;25:1570–1577.

236. Fritz JM, Delitto A, Erhard RE. Comparison of classification-based physical therapy with therapy based on clinical practice guidelines for patients with

acute low back pain: a randomized clinical trial. *Spine*. 2003;28(13):1363–1371.

237. Colle F, Rannou F, Revel M, Fermanian J, Poiraudeau S. Impact of quality scales on levels of evidence inferred from a systematic review of exercise therapy and low back pain. *Arch Phys Med Rehab*. 2002;83:1745–1752.

238. Van Tulder M, Furlan A, Bombardier C, Bouter L. Updated method guidelines for systematic reviews in the Cochrane Collaboration Back Review Group. *Spine*. 2003;28:1290–1299.

239. Faas A. Exercises: Which ones are worth trying, for which patients, and when? *Spine*. 1996;21:2874–2879.

240. Assendelft WJ, Morton SC, Yu EI, Suttorp MJ, Shekelle PG. Spinal manipulative therapy for low back pain. *Cochrane Database Syst Rev*. 2004;(1): CD000447.

241. Avery S, O'Driscoll ML. Randomized controlled trials on the efficacy of spinal manipulation therapy in the treatment of low back pain. *Physical Therapy Reviews*. 2004;9:146–152.

242. Ernst D, Canter P. Chiropractic spinal manipulation treatment for back pain? A systematic review of the randomized clinical trials. *Physical Therapy Reviews*. 2003;8:85–91.

243. Hurwitz EL, Morgenstern H, Harber P, Kominski GF, Belin TR, Yu F, Adams AH; University of California-Los Angeles. A randomized trial of medical care with and without physical therapy and chiropractic care with and without physical modalities for patients with low back pain: 6-month follow-up outcomes from the UCLA low back pain study. *Spine*. 2002;27(20):2193–2204.

244. Burton AK, McClune TD, Clarke RD, Main CJ. Long-term follow-up of patients with low back pain attending for manipulative care: outcomes and predictors. *Man Ther*. 2004;9(1):30–35.

245. Haas M, Goldberg B, Aickin M, Ganger B, Attwood M. A practice-based study of patients with acute and chronic low back pain attending primary care and chiropractic physicians: two-week to 48-month follow-up. *J Manipulative Physiol Ther*. 2004;27(3): 160–169.

246. Hoiriis KT, Pfleger B, McDuffie FC, Cotsonis G, Elsangak O, Hinson R, Verzosa GT. A randomized clinical trial comparing chiropractic adjustments to muscle relaxants for subacute low back pain. *J Manipulative Physiol Ther*. 2004;27(6):388–398.

247. Haas M, Nyiendo J, Aickin M. One-year trend in pain and disability relief recall in acute and chronic ambulatory low back pain patients. *Pain*. 2002;95 (1–2):83–91.

248. UK Beam Trial Team. United Kingdom back pain exercise and manipulation (UK BEAM) randomised trial: effectiveness of physical treatments for back pain in primary care. *BMJ*. 2004;329(7479):1377.

249. Niemisto L, Lahtinen-Suopanki T, Rissanen P, Lindgren KA, Sarna S, Hurri H. A randomized trial of combined manipulation, stabilizing exercises, and physician consultation compared to physician consultation alone for chronic low back pain. *Spine*. 2003;28(19):2185–2191.

250. Wand BM, Bird C, McAuley JH, Dore CJ, MacDowell M, De Souza LH. Early intervention for the management of acute low back pain: a single-blind randomized controlled trial of biopsychosocial education, manual therapy, and exercise. *Spine*. 2004;29 (21):2350–2356.

251. Niemisto L, Sarna S, Lahtinen-Suopanki T, Lindgren KA, Hurri H. Predictive factors for 1-year outcome of chronic low back pain following manipulation, stabilizing exercises, and physician consultation or physician consultation alone. *J Rehabil Med*. 2004;36(3):104–109.

252. Philadelphia Panel evidence-based clinical practice guidelines on selected rehabilitation interventions: overview and methodology. *Phys Ther*. 2001;81(10): 1629–1640.

253. van Tulder MW, Koes BW, Assendelft WJ, Bouter LM, Maljers LD, Driessen AP. [abstract] Chronic low back pain: exercise therapy, multidisciplinary programs, NSAID's, back schools and behavioral therapy effective; traction not effective; results of systematic reviews. *Ned Tijdschr Geneeskd*. 2000; 144(31):1489–1494.

254. Harte N, Baxter G, Gracey JH. The efficacy of traction for back pain: A systematic review of randomized clinical trials. *Arch Phys Med Rehabil*. 2003; 84:1542–1553.

255. Krause M, Refshauge KM, Dessen M, Boland R. Lumbar spine traction: evaluation of effects and recommended application for treatment. *Man Ther*. 2000;5(2):72–81.

256. White A, Panjabi M. The basic kinematics of the human spine: a review of past and current knowledge. *Spine*. 1978;3:12–20.

257. Pearcy MJ, Tibrewal SB. Axial rotation and lateral bending in the normal lumbar spine measured by three-dimensional radiography. *Spine*. 1984;9(6): 582–587.

258. Goel VK, Goyal S, Clark C, Nishiyama K, Nye T. Kinematics of the whole lumbar spine. Effect of discectomy. *Spine*. 1985;10(6):543–554.

259. Soni AH, Sullivan JA, Patwardhan AG, Gudavalli MR, Chitwood J. Kinematic analysis and simulation of vertebral motion under static load-part I: kinematic analysis. *J Biomech Eng*. 1982;104(2): 105–111.

# 12

# Manual Therapy of the Sacroiliac Joint and Pelvis

## Objectives

- Understand the biomechanics and gross movements of the sacroiliac joint.
- Understand the biomechanics of the pubic symphysis.
- Recognize the contributors to form and force closure of the pelvis.

- Identify the relationship between the lumbar and pelvic stabilization process.
- Outline an evidence-based examination process.
- Identify treatment methods that restore normal sacroiliac and pelvis function.

## PREVALENCE

In the past, the "incidence" of sacroiliac joint dysfunction (SIJ) was primarily clinician driven. The inaccessibility of the joint made the isolated manual evaluation of the sacroiliac joint difficult if not entirely impossible. Because clinicians had incomplete or erroneous knowledge of the contribution of the sacroiliac joint to lumbopelvic pain, and lacked complete knowledge of the specific anatomy of the SIJ joint, "guru-based" examination and treatment methods predominated many disciplines. While many authors and clinicians have written extensively on the subject, others have completely ignored the potential contribution of the joint.

Recent information has improved the understanding of the sacroiliac joint and the relationship to the lumbar spine. Although this textbook provides a separate chapter for sacroiliac and pelvic disorders, disassociation of the structures from the lumbar spine during the examination process is not advisable and generally not appropriate.[1] Of considerable importance to clinicians is the recent overwhelming evidence that suggests that because of anatomical, biomechanical, and neurophysiological considerations, loss of stability of the SIJ is crucial in the aetiology of non-specific low back pain.[1-4] Subsequently, when SIJ dysfunction is suspected, the clinician should consider instability a plausible culprit.

True SIJ dysfunction prevalence rates often reflect the method in which the investigators "defined" SIJ contribution and the population pool investigated. For example, Bernard and Kirkaldy-Willis[5] reported an incidence of contributing symptoms in 22.5% of patients with chronic low back pain (only history and examination). Additionally, it is known that pregnancy and post-pregnancy can lead to instability of the SIJ and **pubic symphysis.** Consequently, pelvic pain during pregnancy was reported to exist in 48–56% of females,[6-8] although others have reported lower values.[9,10] In an analysis of 12 studies on pelvic girdle pain, the *European Guidelines on the Diagnosis and Treatment of Pelvic Girdle Pain*[11] has reported incidence rates that have ranged from 4 to 76% of all pregnancies, depending on the inclusion criteria and the definition used in the study.

Others have reported lower prevalence rates of SIJ dysfunction, anywhere from 10 to 30%.[12-14] The strongest studies are those that use diagnostic blocks to confirm the presence of the SIJ as a pain generator: a double block more discriminative than a single block. In 1996, Dreyfuss et al.[15] reported a prevalence of 33% using single blocks.

Using **double injection blocks,** Maigne et al.[16] reported a prevalence of 18.5%. Later, Dreyfuss and colleagues[17] reported SIJ as a source of symptoms in 15% of the population. Worth noting is that each study looked for contribution of the SIJ to back pain, often finding concurrent symptoms with other pain generators.

## *Summary*

- Many textbooks and trade literature studies include nonscientific, guru-based literature to support hypothetical findings.
- Due to poor agreement regarding the symptoms associated with pelvic girdle pain, prevalence in the literature has ranged from 4 to nearly 80% of patients.
- It is likely that the true prevalence of SIJ pain in the nonpregnant, post-pregnant, and the pregnant population is approximately 20%.

# ANATOMY

## *Joint Anatomy*

The pelvic girdle consists of the two innominate bones, the sacrum and the bones of the coccyx. Six joints lie within the pelvic girdle, which includes the two sacroiliac joints, the sacrococcygeal, and in many cases the intercoccygeal and the pubic symphysis. The sacroiliac joint is a synovial joint with the sacral surface covered with hyaline cartilage and the iliac surface covered with a type of fibrocartilage.[18] The anterior portion is synovial and the posterior–superior portion is classified as a typical syndesmosis joint.[19] These articular surfaces are different from any other joint within the body.[20] The surfaces are designed for stability versus mobility; the persistence of selected furrows and ridges create an extremely rough, integrated surface of congruency (Figure 12.1).[21]

Wilder et al.[22] reported that the topography of the SIJ encourages the function of shock incorporation through energy absorption of the ligamentous structures. However, the topography of the SIJ includes flat joints that en-

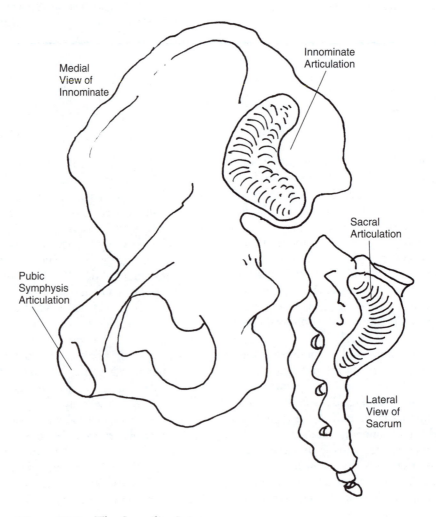

**Figure 12.1**    The Sacroiliac Joint

cumber very large forces, a recipe for shear-related insta-bility.[23] Without some form of external passive or active stabilization, the SIJ would allow considerable unorgan-ized movement.

It has long been noted that women have a greater prevalence of SIJ dysfunction than men, a problem that is theoretically associated with joint architecture and func-tional needs. Ebraheim et al.[24] reported that average fe-males exhibit 12.8% less joint surface contact than males, a finding that contrasted the report of Sgambati et al.[19] Other investigators have reported similar gross move-ments between males and females[25] but notable differ-ences in adolescent anatomy.[26] Age-related changes appear to be similar as well.[25]

The pubic symphysis (Figure 12.2) is a nonsynovial amphiarthrodial joint.[27] The joint exhibits a thick intrapu-bic fibrocartilaginous disc between the two hyaline-cov-ered pubis bones. Dysfunction to the symphysis pubis generally results in groin pain and/or inflammatory in-volvement with adjacent structures.[27,28] Like the cervical spine, most fibrocartilaginous discs exhibit a cavity within the structure, which is thought to be evidence of degener-ation of the disc.[18] Injury to the pubic symphysis may be the result of direct injurious force or micro-trauma related to repetitious activity.[28,29]

The sacrococcygeal joint is a synovial symphysis con-nection[18] and can be an origin site for coccygeal pain.[30] Like the pubic symphysis, a fibrocartilaginous disc be-tween the sacrum and the first coccyx bone develops and assists in allowing movement to the structures. When present, the intercoccygeal joint also presents with a fibro-cartilaginous disc.

## Osseous Structures

The sacroiliac joint consists of the articulations of sacrum and the innominate bones (Figure 12.3). The innominate

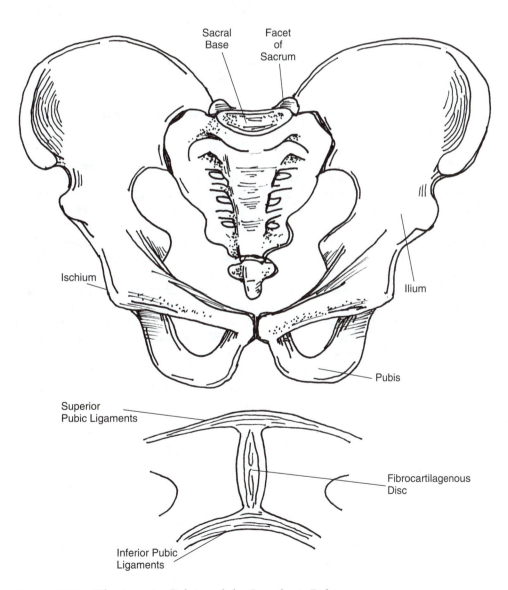

**Figure 12.2**    The Anterior Pelvis and the Symphysis Pubis

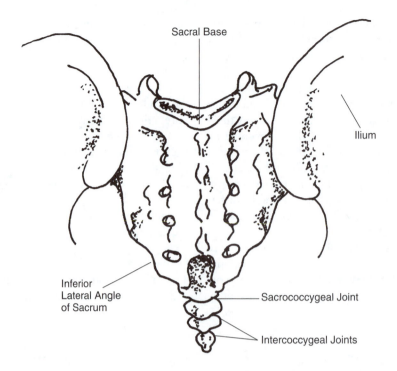

**Figure 12.3**    The Sacrococcygeal and Intercoccygeal Joints

bones are composed of the ilium, the pubis, and the is-chium (Figure 12.4). The ilium is the superior-most structure that forms the articulation with the sacrum and two-fifths of the surface of the acetabulum.[18] The pubis is the inferomedial aspect of the innominate and constitutes one-fifth of the articulation with the acetabulum of the hip. The ischium is the inferolateral aspect of the innominate, which provides the floor of the acetabulum and the posterior two-fifths of the articular surface of the acetabulum rim. The sacral–coccyx articulation (sacrococcygeal joint) includes the union of the coccyx and the sacrum.[18] The pubic symphysis includes the articulations of the two left and right pubic bones.

The sacrum is a triangular-shaped bone that articulates with the ilia of the innominates. The sacrum is formed by the fusion of five sacral vertebrae,[31] a process that results in a very strong and stable keystone. In addition to the articulation with the innominates, the sacrum articulates with the fifth lumbar process at the base and at the two superior articular processes. The sacrum serves as an attachment site for multiple ligaments such as the sacrotuberous ligament, the ventral sacroiliac ligament, the sacrospinous ligament, and the iliolumbar ligament and muscles including the piriformis, the multifidi, the erector spinae, and the gluteus maximus.

The triangular coccyx includes the complete or partial fusion of four bones.[31] Of the four segments, the first is the largest, and each vertebra progressively is smaller distally. The coccyx provides an attachment for the sacro-sciatic ligaments, the coccygeus muscles, and the tendon of the external sphincter muscle.

## Ligaments and Fascia

Several structures are involved in the control of movements and/or stabilization of the sacroiliac and pelvic complex. The primary ligaments associated with the sacroiliac joint include the ventral sacroiliac ligament, the interosseous sacroiliac ligament, the long dorsal sacroiliac ligament, the iliolumbar ligament, the sacrotuberous ligament, and the sacrospinous ligament.[18] The ligaments of the sacroiliac joint provide afferent output from the joint capsule and are innervated by the dorsal rami of the sacral nerves S1-S4.[32]

The ventral sacroiliac ligament and the interosseous sacroiliac ligament are less studied and are poorly understood. Bowen and Cassidy[33] report that the ventral sacroiliac ligament is primarily a thickening of the anterior aspect of the SIJ capsule. Although it is reported to be very strong, the interosseous ligament is not suspected as a cause of clinically determined lower back dysfunction.[33,34]

The sacrotuberous ligament has extensive connections posteriorly with the gluteus maximus, the long head of the biceps femoris, and the sacrospinous ligament and anteriorly with the iliococcygeus muscle.[35] During loading or tension to the sacrotuberous ligament, the amount of nutation (posterior rotation of the ilium to the sacrum or anterior rotation of the sacrum with relation to the ilium) is restricted. Conversely, counternutation (anterior rotation of the ilium to the sacrum or posterior rotation of the sacrum in relation to the ilium), a slackening of the sacrotuberous ligament, occurs, allowing freer movement and less stability contribution from this ligament.[35]

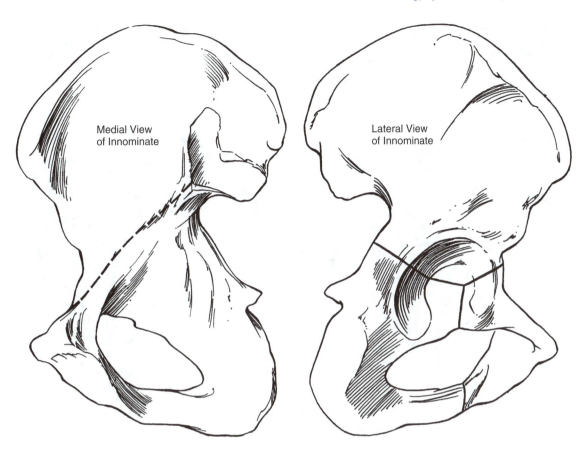

**Figure 12.4**    Medial and Lateral View of the Innominates

The long dorsal ligament can be palpated directly caudal to the posterior superior iliac spine. The long dorsal ligament is closely integrated with the erector spinae, the posterior layer of the thoracolumbar fascia, and the sacrotuberous ligament. The ligament contributes to the movement stability of the SIJ, specifically counternutation (Figure 12.5).[35] During counternutation, the tension is increased in the long dorsal ligament and is slackened during nutation, a finding in opposition to the sacrotuberous ligament. Although both ligaments are physiologically connected, they perform contradictory stabilization tasks for the SIJ.

The sacrospinous ligament originates on the sacrum and coccyx and inserts on the ischial spine of the innominate.[18] This ligament has been associated with numerous pelvic floor dysfunctions including pudendal nerve entrapment,[36] vaginal vault prolapse,[37] and urinary incontinence.[38]

The iliolumbar ligament is one of few structures that actually cross the sacroiliac joint.[4] Bodguk and Twomey[39] outlined five separate bands of the iliolumbar ligament, which traverse from the transverse process of L5 to the quadratus lumborum, the iliac crest, and the posterior aspect of the iliac tuberosity. The iliolumbar ligament ossifies by the fifth decade and is demarcated from the quadratus lumborum muscle.[40]

The iliolumbar ligament appears to restrict sagittal nutation and counternutation of the SIJ.[4,41] The ligament is able to perform a function of stabilization to the SIJ whenever the stability of L5 is intact. In situations where L5 is not stabilized the SIJ may demonstrate corresponding increased movement and decreased stability. This finding lends credence to the supposition that lumbar and pelvic stability are interrelated. It is proposed that the ventral bands provide greater SIJ stability in the sagittal plane versus the dorsal bands.[41]

The ligaments of the pubic symphysis and the sacrococcygeal joint are less studied. The ligaments associated with the pubic symphysis include the superior pubic ligament and the interior arcuate ligament. The stabilization contributions of these ligaments and the associated symphysis joint create a typically stable structure.[18] The ligaments associated with the sacrococcygeal joint are the ventral, dorsal, and lateral sacrococcygeal ligaments. The ventral sacrococcygeal ligament is a continuation of the anterior longitudinal ligament whereas the dorsal ligament is a continuation of the posterior longitudinal ligament of the spine.[18]

The thoracolumbar fascia envelopes the dorsal muscles of the trunk and forms an attachment for several upper limb and trunk muscles, including the latissimus dorsi, the gluteus maximus, the transverse abdominus, and internal oblique musculature.[42] The thoracolumbar fascia transmits forces between the spine, pelvis, and legs, and may

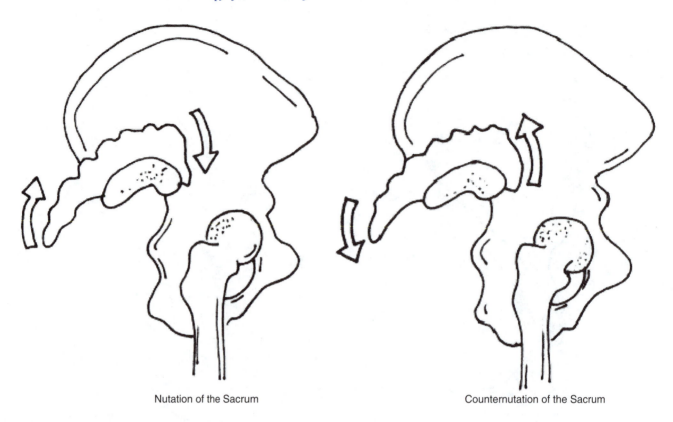

Nutation of the Sacrum                    Counternutation of the Sacrum

**Figure 12.5**   Nutation and Counternutation of the Sacrum

play a role in trunk stabilization during rotation and flexion-based activities.[3] Vleeming et al.[43] purported that increased tension within the thoracolumbar fascia leads to increased force closure and subsequent increased stability.

## Summary

- The pelvic girdle consists of the two innominate bones, the sacrum and the bones of the coccyx.
- The sacroiliac joint is a synovial joint with the sacral surface covered with hyaline cartilage and the iliac surface over with a type of fibrocartilage.
- The primary ligaments associated with the sacroiliac joint include the ventral sacroiliac ligament, the interosseous sacroiliac ligament, the long dorsal sacroiliac ligament, the iliolumbar ligament, the sacrotuberous ligament, and the sacrospinous ligament.

# BIOMECHANICS

## Movement Analysis

The mobile sacroiliac joints function as shock absorbers[3] even during middle ages (ages 40 and up). Mooney[20] suggests that the principle function of the SIJ is to "dissipate or attenuate the loads of the torso to the lower extremities and vice versa." Total movement is 3 degrees or less of rotation, 2 millimeters or less of translation in each of the three planes.[46] Zheng et al.[47] found translations of 0.5 millimeters (mm) in the lateral direction, 1.8 mm in the anterior-to-posterior direction, and 1.5 mm in the superior or interior direction with loads of 1,000 Newtons applied to the sacrum. Rotational movements were also very small, 1.6 degrees of axial rotation, about 1 degree of flexion or extension, and 1.1 degree of lateral bending.[47] In a seminal *in vivo* analysis, Sturesson et al.[42] found a mean rotation of 2.5 degrees (.8–3.9) and a mean translation of .7 mm (.1–1.6 mm).

Walheim and Selvik[48] indicated the pubic symphysis rotates 3 degrees and translates 2 degrees. During single-legged stance, the symphyseal can move vertically 2.6 mm and sagittally 1.3 mm on the weight-bearing side.[49] During walking, the pubic symphysis can piston (move up and down) up to 2.2. mm in the vertical direction and 1.3 mm in the sagittal direction. Since hypermobility beyond this normal range could lead to pubis instability, several investigators have examined the diagnostic utility of a standing x-ray to determine vertical displacement.[28,50,51] Berezine et al.[50] reported movements up to 5.9 mm (s.d. 3.3 mm) in a population of patients with pelvic pain versus only 2 mm in an asymptomatic population. Reiger and colleagues[52] reported that fail rates during externally applied loads generally resulted in disruption in a vertical direction, typically at the pubic symphysis.

Because the movements of the pelvis, even when displaced, are so small, the most discriminatory radiographic analysis appears to be the Chamberlain x-ray.[53,54] The **Chamberlain x-ray** involves an x-ray performed while the patient is standing on a box on the involved lower limb, while the other lower limb is non-weight-bearing. This maneuver allows a vertical migration of the weight-bearing side (pubic symphysis), and has been associated with pelvic instability.[51]

## *Summary*

- The mobile sacroiliac joints function as shock absorbers during younger and older ages (with a principle function to "dissipate or attenuate the loads of the torso to the lower extremities and vice versa").
- When a 1,000 N force is applied to the sacrum, rotational movements of the SIJ are approximately 1.6 degrees of axial rotation, 1 degree of flexion or extension, and 1.1 degree of lateral bending.[47] Sturesson et al. reported a mean rotation of 2.5 degrees (0.8–3.9) and a mean translation of .7 mm (0.1–1.6 mm); Walheim and Selvik indicated the pubic symphysis rotates 3 degrees and translates 2 degrees.
- During single-legged stance, the symphyseal can move vertically 2.6 mm and sagittally 1.3 mm on the weight-bearing side.

## *Muscular Contribution*

Thirty-five muscles attach to the pelvis and/or sacrum and have a direct or indirect role in stabilizing this region.[31] Muscular contribution is necessary for both form and force closure at the SIJ/pelvis. **Form closure** includes the passive stabilization contributions of interlocking ridges and grooves on the joint surfaces[3] and ligamentous stabilization. **Force closure** is a term that corresponds to increased SIJ/pelvis stiffness by isolated contraction of selected muscle groups. Key muscles of force closure are the gluteus maximus, biceps femoris, erector spinae, and latissimus dorsi.[1,3,21,43,55–57] Other muscles, commonly identified as local muscles, are responsible for the preset tension on the pelvis prior to initiation of movement. These muscles include the transverse abdominis, the multifidi, the piriformis, and the pelvic floor muscles.

The transverse abdominus is a key muscle for stabilization of the sacroiliac joint.[2,58] Others have found the feed-forward temporal contraction of the multifidus and obliquus internus abdominis a necessity prior to pelvic stabilization during hip flexion in standing.[59,60] Dysfunction of the SIJ resulted in delays of these muscles.

The multifidi originations of the lower lumbar spine insert onto the articular processes of the sacrum, the posterior thoracodorsal fascia, and the sacrotuberous ligament.[31] The deep fibers of the muscle span form one segment to the adjacent segment whereas the superficial fibers span three segmental levels. The deep fibers of the multifidi are considered the most significant stabilizers of the pelvis and lumbar spine.

The piriformis originates from the anterior aspect of the sacrum, the anterior aspect of the posterior inferior iliac spine, the upper aspect of the sacrotuberous ligament, and the capsule of the sacroiliac joint[31] and inserts on the greater trochanter of the femur. Snijders et al.[23] suggest that the piriformis plays an important part during force closure of the SIJ. The muscle is implicated as a contributor for chronic buttock pain[61] and can refer pain to the sacroiliac region.[31] Often, imaging of the pelvis and lumbar spine performed on patients with suspected piriformis syndrome is unremarkable.[62]

The pelvic floor muscles such as the levator ani and coccygeus muscles have shown to contribute considerably to pelvic ring stability. In a study by Pool-Goudzwaard et al.,[63] simulated tension in the pelvic floor muscles increase SIJ stiffness by 8.5%. Selected authors have outlined the contribution of the pelvic floor muscles to increasing intraabdominal pressure and an increase in lumbar spinal stiffness.[64,65] The muscle functions to stabilize the SIJ through force closure and the capacity to provide counterforce stiffness on the ligaments of the SIJ.[43] O'Sullivan et al.[66] outlined inappropriate pelvic floor descent (versus ascent) during altered motor control recruitment of the pelvic muscles in patients with SIJ pain during the active straight leg raise.

Hungerford et al.[59] indirectly lent evidence to the importance of the contribution of these muscles to stability through their report of delayed onsets of the multifidus, the obliques internals, and the gluteus maximus in patients with sacroiliac joint pain. Multiple authors[60,64,67,68] have reported that a feed-forward mechanism of selected pelvic stabilization exists in asymptomatic individuals and is absent in patients with lumbopelvic pain. O'Sullivan et al.[66] suggested abnormalities in stabilization of the diaphragm and the pelvic floor muscles during an active straight leg raise in patients with known pelvic dysfunction. This finding demonstrates the critical role these local muscles play in concert with ligamentous attachments for preset stability, a role very similar to the one played in the lumbar spine.

The erector spinae is a complex muscle group that originates on multiple lumbar segments and insert into the medial aspect of the PSIS bilaterally and the intermuscular aponeurosis.[31] The muscle can provide lumbar extension-based movements or unilateral side flexion when contracted on one side only.

The quadratus lumborum is thought to contribute to stability by increasing the tension of the iliolumbar ligament. The transverses abdominus, psoas, quadratus lumborum, and multifidus were each noted to have segmental attachment patterns in the lumbar spine.[69] As a group, these muscles surround the lumbar motion segments from the anterolateral aspect of a vertebral body to the spinous process. Generally, the quadratus lumborum is considered a strong ipsilateral flexor.[70] McGill et al.[71] suggest that electromyographic evidence, together with architectural features such as attachment location and activity during selected movements, make the quadratus lumborum a better stabilizer of the spine than the psoas.

Using surface EMG analysis, van Wingerden et al.[72] analyzed a battery of muscle groups to determine which muscles most significantly contributed to force closure. Their findings outlined the significant contribution of the erector spinae, the biceps femoris, and the gluteus maximus to increased stiffness and decreased shear at the SIJ. To a lesser extent, the latissimus dorsi also contributed. Notable were the contralateral and simultaneous contractions of the erector spinae with the gluteus maximus and the contractions of the biceps femoris ispilaterally, with the gluteus maximus. The aspect of the erector spinae that contributed most was the distal aspect, specifically the multifidus, hypothetically contributing with the attachments to the sacral ligamentous structures.

## Summary

- Stabilization of the SIJ occurs through form and force closure. Form closure includes the passive stabilization contributions of interlocking ridges and grooves on the joint surfaces and ligamentous stabilization. Force closure is a term that corresponds to increased SIJ/pelvis stiffness by isolated contraction of selected muscle groups.
- Thirty-five muscles attach to the pelvis and/or sacrum and have a direct or indirect role in stabilizing this region.[30] Muscular contribution is necessary for both form and force closure at the SIJ/pelvis.
- Key muscles of force closure are the gluteus maximus, biceps femoris, erector spinae, and latissimus dorsi, however, contribution of the local muscles, such as the transverses abdominis, the multifidi, the piriformis, and the pelvic floor muscles, are responsible for the preset tension on the pelvis prior to initiation of movement.

## Dysfunction

In essence, a dysfunction of the pelvic girdle occurs when stabilization is lost or when asymmetric stabilization is present between the two sides of the SIJ.[11,73] Normally, a predictable biomechanical sequence occurs in asymptomatic patients within the lumbopelvic region that stabilizes the pelvis and prepares the structure for weight bearing. This process occurs through two different methods: movement initiation and muscular contraction. Muscle contraction of the multifidi, the gluteus maximus, and the piriformis create initial tension in the sacrotuberous ligament and thoracolumbar fascia prior to nutation, preengaging the ligaments for stability.[3] During movement, nutation (posterior rotation of the ilium with respect to the sacrum) tenses the majority of the largest SIJ ligaments such as the sacrospinous and sacrotuberous ligaments.[35] The contact area of the sacroiliac joint is the lowest during posterosuperior displacement of the ilium on the sacrum,[24] thus requiring the greatest amount of form and force closure. Because of the muscle connections to the ligaments and due to the nature of nutation's increase in force closure during ligamentous tension, the SIJ demonstrates increased stiffness. Anterior rotation of the innominate on the sacrum (counternutation) appears to be a primary source of pain and instability in patients with chronic pelvic pain.[52] Causal displacement that occurs during counternutation (anterior rotation of the innominate on the sacrum) places stress on the long dorsal ligament, which is normally taut during neutral positions.[1]

Problems associated with feed-forward failures of ligament laxity discourage the process of form and force closure and lead to SIJ/pelvic instability. This is the primary dysfunction associated with SIJ and pubic symphysis pain. Instability is defined as the inability of the joint and surrounding structures to bear load without uncontrolled displacements.[4] Many patients report pain during movements of the lower extremity and describe a feeling of paralysis during painful provocation.[51] Additionally, an instable pelvis has been associated with the inability to move the lower limbs.[51]

Instability of the sacroiliac joints has long been suspected as a cause of low back pain and lumbopelvic dysfunction.[60,74] Stabilization of the SIJ is accomplished through increased friction throughout the joint during tension of selected muscles and ligaments.[72] More specifically, Pool-Goudzwaard et al.[3] suggests that the SIJ is protected from traumatic shear forces in three ways. First, because the joint is wedge shaped, the sacrum is stabilized during weight bearing by locking into the innominates like a keystone. Second, the cartilage surfaces of the SIJ are not smooth as in other synovial joints, thus this encourages stability, specifically in men. Men demonstrate more cartilage abnormalities than women, thus providing greater passive stability based on structural interface;[33] however, in situations that do not involve pregnancy, ranges are similar between sexes.[25] Third, multiple furrows and ridges within the joint itself encourage a locking function during weight bearing. This complementary system creates "form closure" secondary to a closely congruent passive locking system that is further enhanced during weight bearing.[21]

Force closure involves the active element of controlled stability.[3] Vleeming et al.[21] identified this process as a "self-locking" or "self-bracing" mechanism that allows enough functional movement but controlled stability to appropriately transfer large forces from the legs to the trunk. To accomplish this challenging task, several ligaments, muscles, and fascial elements are critical. As discussed previously, the force closure muscular contributions of the multifidi, transverse abdominus, and other surrounding musculature are critical.

In 2002, Damen et al.[73] reported that instability isn't necessarily a requisite for SIJ dysfunction, rather that asymmetric stability is more likely the cause. Normal subjects demonstrate large variations in laxity that is commonly stabilized by appropriate muscle contribution. Their study used a doppler imaging (DIV) method of measuring stiffness, which analyzes pelvic girdle mobility *in vivo*. However, selected muscle contractions can alter the findings of a DIV analysis, consequently changing the results of a given study.[72]

One notable consideration of the sacroiliac joint is the purported ability of the joint to assume a "subluxed" position. Because of the surface irregularities, Vleeming et al.[21] have proposed that it is theoretically possible for the joint to move and assume a new position that is "locked" into a position of displacement. Furthermore, the amount of displacement may be so minute that radiographic verification is unlikely.[21,75]

## Summary

- Dysfunction of the pelvic girdle occurs when stabilization is lost or when asymmetric stabilization is present between the two sides of the SIJ.
- Anterior rotation of the innominate on the sacrum (counternutation) appears to be a primary source of pain and instability in patients with chronic pelvic pain.
- A posterior-rotated innominate tends to be a more stable position as compared to anterior rotation.
- The SIJ is protected from traumatic shear forces in three ways: (1) through the wedge-shaped anatomy, (2) through the interlocking furrows and ridges, and (3) through the shape of the surface cartilage.
- Because of the surface irregularities, it is theoretically possible for the joint to move and assume a new position that is "locked" into a position of displacement, a position that is too small for radiographic verification.

# ASSESSMENT AND DIAGNOSIS

There are two apparent causes of SIJ/pelvis dysfunction: mechanical and nonmechanical. Huijbregts[76] outlines several nonmechanical pathologies that affect the SIJ including infections and inflammatory, metabolic, and iatrogenic conditions. These nonmechanical pathologies are not the focus of this textbook, but deserve mention. Relatively uncommon conditions that affect the SIJ such as ankylosing spondylitis, psoriatic arthritis, Reiter's syndrome, systemic lupus erythematosus, Sjoegren's syndrome, gout, Paget's disease, tuberculosis, and various bacterial infections are best addressed by a traditional medical physician. Generally, these disorders demonstrate nonmechanically based patterns and fail to respond to conservative care; however, all are difficult to diagnosis using traditional manual therapy evaluative methods.

Early osteopathic literature promoted clinical assessment methods that relied heavily on palpatory and observable phenomenon.[77,78] Many of these procedures were adopted by manual therapists, specifically physical therapists and osteopaths, with little questioning regarding their diagnostic value. Some of these methods are still used in clinical practice despite being shown to have questionable reliability and diagnostic value.[79-81] Examples of early emphases during assessment include objective assessment of "free movement," observation of displacement during sitting or standing, measurement of leg length change during supine to sit, and symptomatic identifiers such as buttock pain and groin pain.[77]

The current gold standard is a videofluoroscopy-guided anesthetic block injection into the SIJ.[82,83] Laslett et al.[84] described an alternate method where fluoroscopic-guided arthrographs were used to provoke concordant symptoms, followed by instillation of a small volume of anaesthetic for abolishment of symptoms. Both methods should result in an 80% reduction in pain for the test to be considered positive. Nonetheless, despite the rigor associated with these diagnostic clarification methods, there are some limitations associated with false positive rates,[83] and leaking outside the SIJ.[85] The *European Guidelines on the Diagnosis and Treatment of Pelvic Girdle Pain*[11] suggest that use of SIJ injections as a diagnostic tool are inappropriate in a number of conditions that could still qualify as SIJ or pelvic pain. For example, pain in the long dorsal ligament or pubic symphysis would not yield a positive test with double injections but is still considered an SIJ or pelvic disorder. Additionally, most SIJ injection methods are compared against clinical "reference standards" and vice versa. Some studies have been compared against questionable clinical tests and may yield inappropriate information.

Others have suggested the use of a clinical diagnosis to determine SIJ dysfunction. Cibulka et al.[80] suggested the use of a clinical diagnosis based on regional pain classification, the response of direct treatment techniques, and the restoration of pelvic symmetry as a diagnostic method. This method has yet to be compared against diagnostic blocks, thus the diagnostic value is unknown. Nonetheless, some of the diagnostic classification criteria are questionable specifically when diagnosing based on response to treatment. Since the SIJ and low back are highly integrated, the likelihood of applying a specific treatment that fails to address other regional anatomic sites is minute.

Additionally, restoration of pelvic symmetry is based on the theory that asymmetry is quantifiable, a theory that has yet to be enumerated within the literature. Additionally, such fine, precision-based assessments are at high risk for bias, and are certainly unproven for reliability.

There is some debate that both clinical examination findings and injections yield separate and beneficial findings. Maigne et al.[16] and Laslett[86] argue that pathological changes to soft tissue around the SIJ may serve as a pain generator and would not be identified during an interarticular injection. Laslett suggests the use of both a movement-based assessment that has demonstrated validity, such as the McKenzie assessment for directional preference, and the inclusion of an intraarticular block, performed together, are necessary for diagnosis of SIJ dysfunction. One of the hallmarks of the McKenzie approach is the theory that patients who demonstrate centralization behavior (centralizers) are low back pain injuries (typically associated with disc dysfunction),[87] and noncentralizers are generally "other" disorders. There is strong evidence that centralization is associated with a lumbar disc dysfunction,[88] thus the use of this assessment method is suggested during sacroiliac pelvic disorder assessment.

In a recent clinical trial, this hypothesis has shown to exhibit validity. In 2003, Laslett et al.[84] divided a population of chronic back patients into centralizers and noncentralizers. The centralizers were proposed low back dysfunction patients, purportedly associated with disc dysfunction, and were removed from the study. The noncentralizers were then examined with a battery of sacroiliac tests including an intraarticular block to further distill the findings. A large portion of these patients did present with positive findings and were considered to have SIJ dysfunction. Therefore, the traditionally lumbar examination method of repeated end range movements may prove useful to distill a subpopulation of SIJ dysfunction.

Lastly, recent evidence has suggested that SIJ dysfunction is best classified into homogenous entities. Albert et al.[13] reported that there are five classifications of pregnancy-related pelvic joint pain and provide prevalence rates for each classification. These authors identified pelvic girdle syndrome, symphysiolysis, one-sided sacroiliac pain, double-sided sacroiliac pain, and miscellaneous categories for pregnancy-related pain. Of the five, pelvic girdle syndrome displayed an incidence of 6%, symphysiolysis 2.3%, one-sided sacroiliac pain 5.5%, double-sided sacroiliac pain 6.3%, and miscellaneous categories 1.6%.

One notable concept of the Albert et al.[13,89] studies was the suggestions that not all SIJ dysfunctions are the same. In a 2000 study, various SIJ tests demonstrated differences in sensitivity and specificity values depending on the classification.[89] This suggests that some of the variability associated with clinical special tests may be associated with the variability of the diagnosis as well as the variability of testing and test methods selected. Subsequently, an understanding that various forms of SIJ dysfunction are probable and should inform the examiner that a very open-minded approach is necessary before condemning the likelihood of SIJ dysfunction based on the absence of selected findings.

## *Summary*

- There are two apparent causes of SIJ/pelvis dysfunction: mechanical and nonmechanical; mechanical causes are associated with instability and displacement. Nonmechanical causes are associated with infections and disease processes.
- Historic osteopathic methods of SIJ assessment lean heavily on palpation and observation, two methods that have not demonstrated reliability or validity.
- The current gold standard is a videofluroscopy-guided anesthetic block injection into the SIJ, although not all researchers agree with this selection.
- Some researchers have suggested the use of a clinical diagnosis for the "reference gold standard," mainly because many diagnostic methods compare the validity against clinical standards.
- There may be different "kinds" of pelvic disorders, thus many clinical special tests may present with different levels of sensitivity and specificity based on the "flavor" of the disorder.

## Subjective Considerations

The most important aspect of the subjective history is the identification of nonmechanical symptoms or risk factors associated with infections, and inflammatory, metabolic, and iatrogenic conditions. Peloso and Braun[90] indicate that many of the symptoms associated with Reiter's, ankylosing spondylitis, psoriatic arthritis, Reiter's syndrome (reactive arthritis), arthritis associated with inflammatory bowel disease, and undifferentiated spondyloarthropathies present with similar "symptoms" as mechanical SIJ/pelvis dysfunction. For example, these disorders commonly demonstrate pain with prolonged activity, tenderness over the SIJ or buttocks, potential involvement in the knees and hips, and restrictions in activities of daily living. However, selected symptoms are dissimilar to SIJ/pelvic dysfunction including involvement of the shoulders, restrictions in motion (specifically flexion and extension and side flexion), pain at the thoraco–lumbar junction, and improvement with moderate activity. Additionally, medical and laboratory work-up may find markers in the blood or tissue that identify these selected nonmechanical disorders. Medical screening is warranted in any situation where symptoms are contradictory to clinical reasoning.

Numerous authors have reported common subjective or patient history–based complaints that they have associated with sacroiliac pain.[83] Lateral buttock pain is the predominant symptom of patients with a sacroiliac joint dysfunction.[91] Nonetheless, the pain may also radiate down the posterior thigh, into the groin, into the anterior thigh, or transfer as distal as the foot or toes (Figure 12.6).[76] Slipman et al.[92] reported that the onset of pain occurs from a traumatic event such as a fall, or positional movements that generate force upon the SIJ such as torsion, heavy lifting, prolonged lifting, rising from a stooped position, or during a motor vehicle accident when the foot is depressed on the brake. Others have associated SIJ dysfunction with long-term positioning such as crossing the legs or assuming a slumped position.

## Pain Maps

**Pain maps** have been developed to outline the area of sensory change. Fortin et al.[93,94] suggested that SIJ-related pain results in an area approximately 3 cm wide and 10 cm long just inferior to the PSIS. These findings were determined after injecting asymptomatic individuals in the SIJ and determining areas of hyperesthesia using light touch. Others have reported the same finding, identifying that pain isolated to the PSIS region is specific for SIJ dysfunction.[95] Slipman et al.[96] reported contradictory findings in symptomatic subjects, pointing out that many patients reported symptoms into the lower lumbar, groin, thigh, ankle, and lower leg in patterns dissimilar to Fortin et al. Dreyfuss et al.[15] suggested the use of a pain map yields limited value for discriminating SIJ origin. Using intraarticular injections for patients with and without SIJ disorders, the authors compared pain patterns of several patients, and no specific pattern emerged for SIJ dysfunction versus a dysfunction of another origin.[15] Broadhurst and Bond[95] reported the absence of pain in the lumbar region was associated with SIJ dysfunction, and identified the presence of pain in the groin as significant. Groin pain was not considered a useful clinical tool in Dreyfuss's report.[16]

In a literature summary, Freburger and Riddle[83] and the *European Guidelines on the Diagnosis and Treatment of Pelvic Girdle Pain*[11] suggest that pain location should be considered but only in conjunction with other findings. These authors identified groin pain, pain below L5, pain in the region of the PSIS, and absence of pain in the lumbar spine as plausible albeit not discriminatory methods with some evidence-based support. Young et al.[97] reported that most of the patients with injection-confirmed SIJ had pain lateral and below L5, while discogenic patients presented with midline pain. Slipman et al.[92] theorize that variability in pain referral patterns exist because the joint's innervation is highly variable, pain may be referred from internal and external structures, and pain referral may be dependent on the distinct location of the SIJ injury. At best, location of pain offers limited assistance in isolating SIJ/pelvis dysfunction.

## Observation

The role of posture on pelvic pain is well studied. Abnormalities of anatomy[98] and posture[99] are not reliable predictors of cause of pain. Selected postures can alter SIJ motion and place tension on the stabilizing ligaments.

## Summary

- An effective history should include the dissemination of nonmechanical disorders of the pelvis.
- There is mixed evidence of the usefulness of pain maps in identifying SIJ disorders. It does appear that in most cases, SIJ pain tends to be unilateral, can refer to the lower extremity (as far as the foot), and does have significant overlap with referred patterns of the lumbar spine.
- SIJ pain is commonly lateral and caudal to L5 when compared with discogenic lumbar pain, but not in all cases.
- The variation in pain distribution may be reflective of the largeness of the joint and the different sensory groups that supply aspects of the joint.

Snijders et al.[100] reported that slumped sitting postures created a counternutation moment and tension upon the iliolumbar ligament and long dorsal ligament. It is proposed that the selected stress placed on these innervated ligaments may be a source of low back pain.[100]

Sturesson et al.[57] reported that the straddle position (stride standing) leads to primarily sagittal rotation and movement of the ilia on the sacrum. Others have reported that stabilization of the pelvis is enhanced during soft-seated sitting since this motion compliments the action of the oblique abdominal muscles and the contribution of these muscles for stability of the SIJ.[101]

One significant problem associated with using observation is the potential overfocus on movement "feel," postural position, or visual assessment.[102] Potter and Rothstein[103] examined intertester reliability among clinicians at determining appropriate pelvic symmetry. The percent agreement among clinicians was very poor, suggesting this tool has little transferability. Others[15,104] have demonstrated that asymmetric findings were not associated with low back pain or sacroiliac dysfunction. Levangie[104] found that leg length discrepancy, ASIS and PSIS bilateral comparisons, and iliac crest height determination presented diagnostic information that was actually more detrimental than beneficial to determine. Clearly, little evidence exists that asymmetry is an identifier of a pelvic dysfunction and even less evidence exists that clinicians can reliably see or feel palpation or visual-based structural observation. Subsequently, this textbook does not subscribe to observational methods that involve determination of asymmetry.

## Introspection

One critical finding to consider is the prevalence of SIJ/pelvic impairment in pregnant or post-pregnant females. Nearly 50% of pregnant females or females that have just conceived experience some iteration of pelvic pain.[6–8] With pre-examination odds this high, the likelihood of pelvic involvement in nonspecific low back pain is very high.

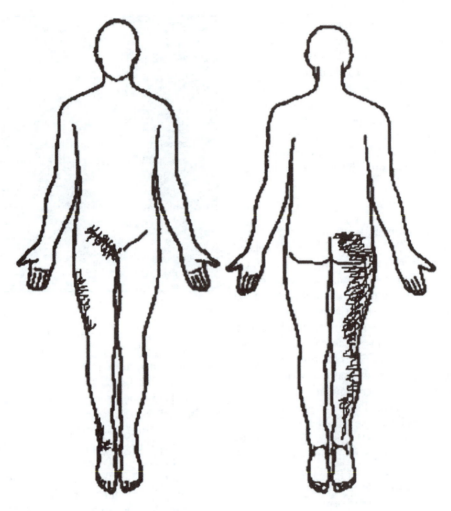

**Figure 12.6**    Commonly Reported Pain Map from Selected Studies

## Summary

- Various positions or postures do not appear to be effective for diagnosis of SIJ-related pain.
- Clearly, little evidence exists that asymmetry is an identifier of a pelvic dysfunction and even less evidence exists that clinicians can reliably see or feel palpation or visual-based structural observation.

# CLINICAL EXAMINATION

The sacroiliac joint is extremely complex and is difficult to appropriately examine and treat.[46,105] The complexity is further augmented by the paucity of clinical findings that are significantly associated with SIJ dysfunction.[15] Additionally, since the actual SIJ motion is so small and potentially subclinical, many manual examination means are simply not useful. Since injections are not routinely performed as part of manual therapy practice or diagnostic intervention, the likelihood of absolute identification of pain of sacroiliac origin based on traditional diagnostic principles is low.

## Active Physiological Movements

Some authors have reported a relationship of active physiological movements with SIJ dysfunction. Rost et al.[6] reported that most patients in a subclassification of pelvic pain during pregnancy reported pain during weight bearing such as walking. Schwarzer et al.[12] reported that no planar active physiological movements are associated with SIJ dysfunction—a finding also reported by Maigne et al.[16] Dreyfuss et al.[15] also reported no significant active physiological movements, such as lying down and sitting, that were associated with SIJ dysfunction. Their study did report that standing was associated with a 3.9 likelihood ratio versus nonstanding. Young et al.[97] reported that patients with confirmed SIJ dysfunction (through fluoroscopically guided double injections) significantly reported pain during rising from sitting. In their study, patients who reported pain during sit to stand were 28 times more likely to have SIJ dysfunction when concurrently positive with three of five clinical special tests. However, these findings in isolation are not significant enough to implicate SIJ-related pain. In Young's study, patients with discogenic pain also reported pain during rising from sitting, which suggests that the inclusion of a single active physiological examination finding provides little diagnostic value for the clinician.

Lastly, some clinicians continue to focus on and espouse the merits of palpatory assessment during active physiological movements.[31,80,106] For this textbook, these methods are not supported. This does not suggest that the palpatory methods used by other clinicians are not effective in the hands of selected practitioners and when combined with numerous other examination processes. However, there is a preponderance of evidence that, for the lay clinician, the reliability and diagnostic value of movement assessment techniques of the SIJ are fairly low.

Young et al.[97] reported that repeated movements are essential in detection of discogenic pain symptoms. Long et al.[87] and Laslett et al.[84] advocate that patients who centralize are most likely lumbar impairments and should be treated with directional preference exercises. Young does report that during the prepositioning of an innominate to allow specific anterior or posterior rotation, in some cases the patients will report a reduction of pain; however, this process does not occur during normal lumbar physiological assessment (Figures 12.7 and 12.8). The benefit of this finding is that it allows a discriminatory examination process in which low back impairments are separated from SIJ impairments. Patients who fail to centralize are classified as nonradiographic instability or sacroiliac impairment and require additional testing. Intentionally, the active physiological component of the SIJ examination is identical to the lumbar component.

"SIJ pain has no special distribution of features and is similar to symptoms arising from other lumbosacral structures. There are no provoking or relieving movements or positions that are unique or especially common to SIJ pain."[107] Subsequently, SIJ examination in absence of a lumbar spine screen may yield biased findings. This suggests that it is imperative to "rule out" the presence of lumbar spine pain prior to SIJ examination.

The reader is directed toward the lumbar spine examination, including active physiological movements with overpressures, and passive accessory movements outlined in Chapter Eleven. Any isolated pain provoking, reducing, or centralization-based movement performed in lumbar flexion, side flexion, extension, or rotation likely implicates the lumbar spine.

In cases where no centralization or abolition of pain results from active physiological movements of the lumbar spine, further active physiological movements are used to distill out a directional preference with repeated forces on the SIJ. Young[108] described two techniques to initiate anterior and posterior rotation of a single innominate. These methods are useful because they can lead the clinician toward a passive method for reducing pain.

## Lunge for Anterior Rotation

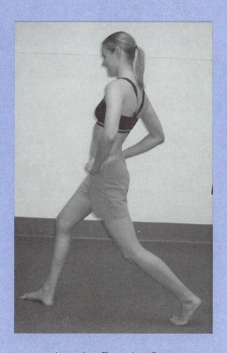

- Step One: The patient assumes a lunge position; the painful extremity assumes the posterior position.
- Step Two: The patient lunges forward until force is encountered on the posterior trial leg.
- Step Three: The patient repeats the anterior lunge maneuver to determine if pain is reduced with repeated movements.
- Step Four: Resting symptoms are reassessed upon completion.

**Figure 12.7**   Anterior Rotation Lunge

## Step and Bend for Posterior Rotation

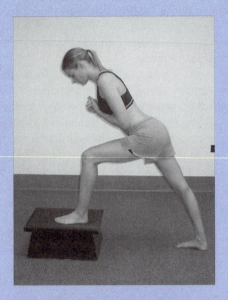

- **Step One:** The patient places the painful side extremity up on a 2- to 3-foot stool.
- **Step Two:** The patient then leans forward placing a backward or posterior torque on the innominate.
- **Step Three:** The patient repeats the posterior rotation technique to determine if pain is reduced with repeated movements.
- **Step Four:** Resting symptoms are reassessed upon completion.

**Figure 12.8**   Posterior Rotation Step and Bend

## Summary

- SIJ pain has no special distribution of features and is similar to symptoms arising from other lumbosacral structures.
- Patients with SIJ often report pain during unilateral weight bearing, sit to stand, and standing versus not standing.
- There is a preponderance of evidence that for the lay clinician, the reliability and diagnostic value of movement assessment techniques of the SIJ are poor.
- There is considerable evidence that patients who demonstrate centralization during a traditionally lumbar examination do not have SIJ disorders.

## Passive Movements

### Passive Physiological Movements

Cibulka et al.[79] reported that passive rotation asymmetry of the hip was positively associated with sacroiliac dysfunction, a finding that has been demonstrated *in vitro* by others.[109] Additionally, there is evidence that suggests that a relationship between free hip range of motion and the sacroiliac joint exists, although the direction of that relationship is uncertain. For example, Pollard and Ward[110] reported an improvement in hip range of motion after manipulation of the sacroiliac joint. This information may have questionable value. In the Cibulka study,[79] patients were classified as having sacroiliac pain only using regional pain classification, the response of the direct treatment technique, and after restoration of pelvic symmetry.

Others have advocated the use of physiological end range provocation movements of the innominates performed in sidelying.[74,111] Theoretically, these movements create torque on the intra- and extraarticular structures and could reproduce pain. Because of the complexity associated with both intra- and extraarticular structures, the ability to determine the required "direction" of the dysfunction based on feel, single movement provocation, or observation is evasive. For example, if anterior rotation of the right innominate on the sacrum is painful during end range movement, several structures could be at fault. Extraarticular structures such as the long dorsal ligament may be irritated or internal structures such as the capsule may be impinged. This dilemma is the most significant challenge associated with an examination because adequate carryover to treatment is difficult to hypothesize. This necessitates the use of repeated end range movements to outline whether the examination movement may be helpful as a treatment procedure.

## Passive Physiological Posterior Rotation (Nutation)

Physiological rotation is necessary to determine the direction of treatment for the impairment. Unfortunately, none of the palpation-based tests has demonstrated reliability and validity to the point where they are useful to determine treatment direction. Subsequently, pain provocation and the response to repeated movements will serve to dictate the type of innominate impairment and the direction needed for treatment such as manipulation. Posterior rotation of the innominate on the sacrum is considered **nutation.**

- Step One: The patient assumes a sidelying position, the painful side up. Resting symptoms are assessed.
- Step Two: The painful-sided leg is flexed beyond 90 degrees to engage the pelvis and to promote passive physiological flexion.
- Step Three: The clinician then situates his or her body into the popliteal fold of the painful-sided leg to "snug up" the position. The plinth-sided leg remains in an extended position.
- Step Four: The clinician then places his or her hands on the ischial tuberosity and the ASIS to promote further physiological rotation. The patient's pelvis is passively moved to the first sign of concordant pain.
- Step Five: The clinician then moves the patient beyond the first point of pain toward end range. The patient's symptoms are reassessed for concordance.
- Step Six: The clinician then applies repeated motions at the end range to determine if the patient's concordant pain abolishes or increases. It is imperative to determine a pattern during this step because this step will determine the direction selected for treatment.
- Step Seven: If concordant pain is bilateral, the process is repeated on the opposite side.

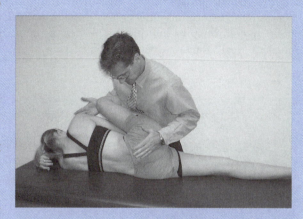

**Figure 12.9**   Passive Physiological Posterior Rotation: Nutation

## Passive Physiological Anterior Rotation (Counternutation)

Passive **counternutation** assessment is similar to nutation but requires selected changes in the pattern.

- Step One: The patient assumes a sidelying position, the painful side up. Resting symptoms are assessed.
- Step Two: The painful-sided leg is extended and the plinth-sided leg is flexed to 90 degrees. The motion is the mirror image of passive physiological nutation.
- Step Three: The clinician cradles the leg with the caudal-side hand and encourages further movement into hip extension. The cranial-side hand is placed on the PSIS and promotes anterior rotation of the innominate.
- Step Four: The patient's pelvis is passively moved to the first sign of concordant pain.
- Step Five: The clinician then moves the patient beyond the first point of pain toward end range. The patient's symptoms are reassessed for concordance.
- Step Six: The clinician then applies repeated motions at the end range to determine if the patient's concordant pain abolishes or increases. Again, it is imperative to determine a pattern during this step because this step will determine the direction selected for treatment.
- Step Seven: If concordant pain is bilateral, the process is repeated on the opposite side.

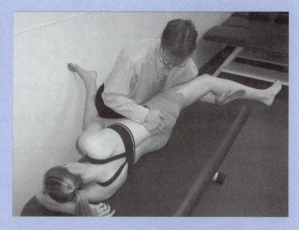

**Figure 12.10**   Passive Physiological Anterior Rotation; Counternutation

## *Passive Accessory Movements*

Essentially, there are no studies that have assessed the merit of passive accessory movements of the SIJ. Traditionally, clinicians have suggested that conventional PAs and APs may be beneficial in identifying "movement-related pain" and could be helpful in isolating the side of the lesion. In order to provide additional information, repeated passive accessory movements should cause a change in the concordant pain of the patient. In this manner, passive accessory movements may provide additional benefit or confirmatory information. When used in the context of "feel" for movement, in lieu of pain provoca-

tion, a passive accessory approach has diminished value because the range of motion and actual movements of the SIJ are so small.

As investigated with passive physiological movements, end range repeated movements might be helpful to determine if the examination movements are plausible treatment techniques. The passive accessory movements should be applied to the painful side of the SIJ/pelvis for maximum discriminatory value. A passive accessory movement may be beneficial if repeated passive physiological movements cause a reduction of pain during the examination process, otherwise the value is highly redundant to passive physiological movements.

### Unilateral and Bilateral Anterior–Posterior Movements of the Innominate

Both the unilateral and bilateral anterior–posterior (AP) of the innominate promotes posterior rotation of the innominate on the sacrum. Although both techniques should be examined, determination of which technique to use is based on the most complete reproduction of symptoms.

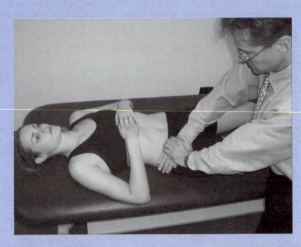

- Step One: The patient assumes a prone position. Resting symptoms are assessed.
- Step Two: For a unilateral AP, the clinician applies a light posterior pressure at the ASIS to promote posterior rotation of the innominate. The AP should be applied just to the first report of pain. (For a bilateral AP, the same process occurs with the contact points of both ASIS.)
- Step Three: The clinician then applies the force beyond the first point of pain and reassesses the patient's concordant sign.
- Step Four: The clinician then applies 5–30 seconds of repeated end range oscillations to determine the behavior of the concordant pain. Because the SIJ is a strong and irregular joint, a significant load may be required to produce symptoms.[90] A positive sign that would implicate this method as a treatment is reduction of pain with continuous oscillations.
- Step Five: If a unilateral AP is performed, the clinician can repeat on the opposite side.

**Figure 12.11**    Unilateral AP of the ASIS

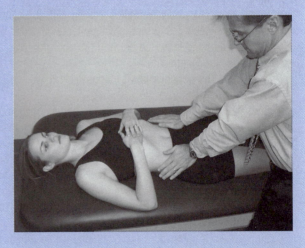

**Figure 12.12**    Bilateral AP of the ASIS

## Unilateral and Bilateral Posterior–Anterior Movements of the Innominate

Both the unilateral and bilateral posterior–Anterior (PA) of the innominate promotes anterior rotation of the innominate on the sacrum. Both techniques should be examined and determination of which technique to use is based on the most complete reproduction of symptoms.

- Step One: The patient assumes a supine position. Resting symptoms are assessed.
- Step Two: For a unilateral PA, the clinician applies a light posterior pressure at the PSIS to promote anterior rotation of the innominate. The PA should be applied just to the first report of pain. (For a bilateral PA, the same process occurs with the contact points of both PSIS.)
- Step Three: The clinician then applies the force beyond the first point of pain and reassesses the patient's concordant sign.
- Step Four: The clinician then applies 5–30 seconds of repeated end range oscillations to determine the behavior of the concordant pain. Because the SIJ is a strong and irregular joint, a significant load may be required to produce symptoms.[102] A positive sign that would implicate this method as a treatment is reduction of pain with continuous oscillations.
- Step Five: If a unilateral PA is performed, the clinician can repeat on the opposite side.

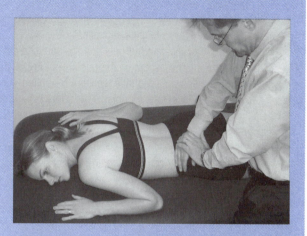

**Figure 12.13**    Unilateral PA of the PSIS

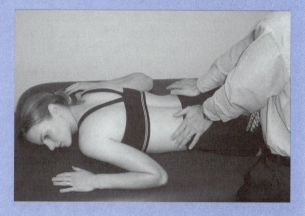

**Figure 12.14**    Bilateral PA of the PSIS

## Cephalic and Caudal Glide of the Pubis Rami

A unilateral cephalic glide of the pubis stresses the pubic symphysis by placing superior-to-inferior torque on the joint. Because the pubic symphysis is a strong and irregular joint, a significant load may be required to produce symptoms.[102]

- Step One: The patient assumes a supine position. Resting symptoms are assessed.
- Step Two: The clinician stands to the side opposite to the pubis rami he or she desires to glide cephalically.
- Step Three: After locating the pubis on the opposite side of the clinician, the inferior aspect of the pubis rami is palpated and by using the pisiform, a cephalic pressure is applied.
- Step Four: After locating the pubis on the same side of the clinician, the clinician palpates the superior aspect of the pubis rami and uses the pisiform to apply a caudal force.
- Step Five: The parallel antagonistic forces create a shear to the pubic symphysis. Concordant symptoms are assessed.
- Step Six: The clinician may apply the same force after switching sides.

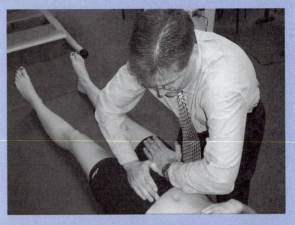

Figure 12.15　Concurrent Caudal and Cephalic Glide of the Pubis Rami

## Transverse Glide of the ASIS

Sturesson et al.[42] reported less than a millimeter of pure lateral translational movement of the SIJ during active movements. Nonetheless, it is possible that pain reproduction occurs during lateral translation of the innominate on the sacrum.

- Step One: The patient assumes a prone position. Resting symptoms are assessed.
- Step Two: The clinician applies a medial force to the PSIS while simultaneously applying a lateral force to the ASIS. The concurrent forces encourage a "lateral" glide of the pelvis.
- Step Three: The process is implemented using the same sequence of previous examinations. First, the pelvis is moved to the first point of pain. Second, the pelvis is moved beyond the first point of pain and finally an end range repeated movement is performed.
- Step Four: Since the movement associated with this examination is minimal, the clinician should not expect to "feel" actual translation. Pain provocation and/or abolishment are the targets of the examination.
- Step Five: The same procedure can be applied if the patient assumes a supine position. The contact points are reversed as is the direction of force. The process is also repeatable on both sides if the patient complains of bilateral pain.

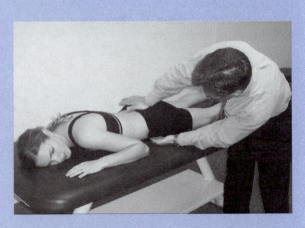

Figure 12.16　Transverse Glide of the ASIS

## Clinical Special Tests

A wealth of literature is dedicated to the examination of the diagnostic value associated with clinical special tests and diagnostic tests. Most investigators agree that the amount of displacement associated with an SIJ dysfunction make radiographic imaging inefficient.[4,21] Generally, traditional x-rays and CT scans are not beneficial in detecting SIJ dysfunction.[112,113] For pubic symphysis disorders, the Chamberlain x-ray is a valid method described by Mens et al.[51] Because of the limited value in these traditional diagnostic tests for the SIJ, the videofluroscopically guided intraarticular diagnostic block is the recognized gold standard,[15,61,114] but only for intraarticular disorders.[11]

Numerous "signs" of sacroiliac dysfunction are advocated by various clinicians including regional abnormalities in length tension relationships, leg length changes, static and dynamic osseous landmarks, provocation move-

## *Summary*

- Passive rotation asymmetry of the hip is positively associated with sacroiliac dysfunction, a finding that has been demonstrated *in vitro* by several investigators.
- Because palpation, observation, and single movement examination methods do not provide the examiner with credible criteria for assessment, the use of repeated end range movements are advocated as a diagnostic and treatment method.
- There are no studies that assess the merit of passive accessory–based movements. When used in the context of "feel" for movement, in lieu of pain provocation, a passive accessory approach has diminished value because the range of motion and actual movements of the SIJ are so small.

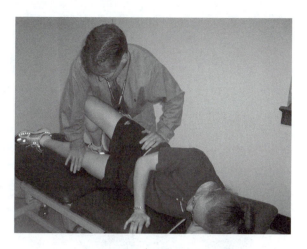

**Figure 12.17**    The Resisted Adduction Test

ments, and selected postures.[15] Despite the variety of suggested examination methods, few conclusive tests are accepted universally for their diagnostic value in isolating SI dysfunction. Some authors suggest there is no evidence to support the use of mobility testing for dysfunction of the sacroiliac joints.[102,115] Restrictive use of pain provocation tests used in isolation results in questionable outcomes.[16,105,114] Furthermore, some have promoted the use of pain provocation tests only when clustered together with other tests.[84,102,97,116]

## *Manual Muscle Testing*

Rost et al.[6] suggested that resisted sidelying adduction is symptomatic with patients experiencing hypermobility of the sacroiliac and pelvis. Mens et al.[117] reported that loss of hip adduction strength (Figure 12.17) (secondary to pain) was indicative of pelvic instability and was useful in implicating post-partum pelvic pain syndrome. Additionally, the nature of the active straight leg raise (ASLR) demonstrates pain during active hip flexion, which *may* also implicate pelvic instability. Although the ASLR is not a manual muscle test, the nature of the test mimics this procedure.

## *Palpation-Based Testing*

Deep palpation to the pubic symphysis is associated with osteitis pubis or instability of the pubic symphysis.[28] Vleeming et al.[1] suggests that painful palpation over the long dorsal ligament may implicate irritation of that ligament. Albert et al.[89] reported the usefulness of palpation directly on the pubic symphysis in patients experiencing symphysiolysis.

Levangie[104] reported poor diagnostic values of selected palpation-based assessment of symmetry for the pelvis. In this study, Levangie did not isolate SIJ patients through diagnostic block; therefore, the findings were associated with patients with long-term nonspecific low back pain that could include SIJ impairment (Figures 12.18–12.20).

The diagnostic value of each of the findings is very poor, suggesting that palpation-based methods are not helpful in identifying SIJ pain. If used in combination with other measures, the values may have use, but alone offer conflicting or very poor diagnostic value. Table 12.1 outlines the reliability and diagnostic value of these tests.

**TABLE 12.1    Diagnostic Value of Palpation-Based Clinical Special Tests**

| Clinical Test | Author | Reliability | Sensitivity | Specificity | +LR |
|---|---|---|---|---|---|
| Groin pain | Dreyfuss et al.[15] | 0.70 | 0.19 | 0.63 | 0.09 |
| Standing ASIS asymmetry | Levangie[104]** | 0.75 | 0.74 | 0.21 | .94 |
| Standing PSIS asymmetry | Levangie[104]** | 0.70 | 0.79 | 0.29 | 1.11 |
| Seated PSIS asymmetry | Levangie[104]** | 0.63 | 0.69 | 0.22 | .88 |
| Pubic symphysis palpation | Albert et al.[89] | 0.89 | 0.81* | 0.99 | 4.68 |

*For patients with symphysiolysis
**Patients had nonspecific low back pain but nonetheless nonverified sacroiliac pain
NR, Not reported; NT, Not tested

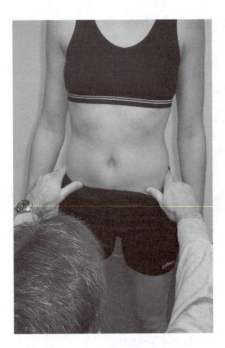

**Figure 12.18**    ASIS Symmetry in Standing

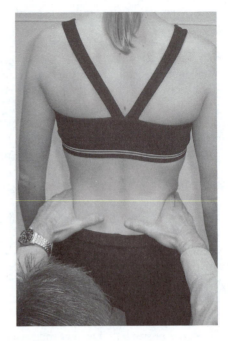

**Figure 12.20**    Iliac Crest Height during Standing

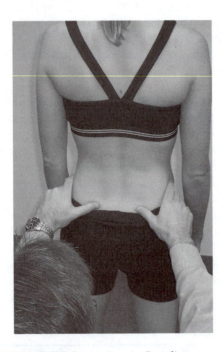

**Figure 12.19**    PSIS Symmetry in Standing

the reliability and diagnostic values of these selected tests. Comprehensively, these tests demonstrate poor reliability and very little diagnostic value. Levangie[118] used a mechanical device to improve the reliability of the movement-based assessments to avoid problems associated with poor consistency. In an earlier study, she reported limited diagnostic value. It is arguable whether the movement-based assessment provides any diagnostic value for detecting SIJ-related dysfunction.

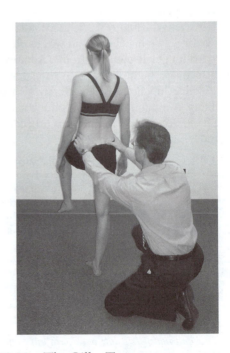

**Figure 12.21**    The Gillet Test

## Movement-Based Testing

Several movement-based assessments exist and have been studied for reliability and diagnostic value. Four of the movement-based assessments—the Gillet test (Figure 12.21), the long sit test (Figures 12.22 and 12.23), the standing flexion test (Figure 12.24), and the sitting flexion test (Figure 12.25)—involve measurement of asymmetry during selected movement procedures. Table 12.2 outlines

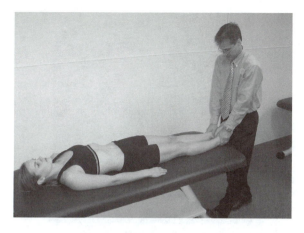

**Figure 12.22**    The Initial Step of the Long Sit Test

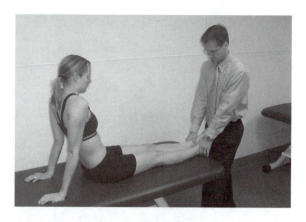

**Figure 12.23**    The Final Step of the Long Sit Test

**TABLE 12.2    Diagnostic Value of Selected Movement-Based Clinical Special Tests**

| Author | Reliability | Sensitivity | Specificity | +LR | −LR |
|---|---|---|---|---|---|
| **Gillet Test** | | | | | |
| Meigne et al[120] | 0.08 | NT | NT | NA | NA |
| Dreyfuss et al.[15] | 0.22 | 43 | 68 | 1.34 | 0.84 |
| Carmichael et al.[122] | 0.02 | NT | NT | NA | NA |
| Levangie[118] | NR | 8 | 93 | 1.07 | 0.99 |
| **Sitting Bend Over** | | | | | |
| Riddle and Freburger[119] | 0.37 | NT | NT | NA | NA |
| Dreyfuss et al.[15] | 0.22 | 3 | 90 | 0.30 | 1.08 |
| Levangie[104] | NR | 9 | 93 | 1.01 | 0.98 |
| **Standing Bend Over Test** | | | | | |
| Vincent and Smith[81] | 0.05 | NT | NT | NA | NA |
| Bowman and Gribbe[121] | 0.23 | NT | NT | NA | NA |
| Riddle & Freburger[119] | 0.32 | NT | NT | NA | NA |
| Levangie[118] | NT | 17 | 79 | 0.81 | 1.05 |
| **Long Sit (LS) Test or Leg Length (LL) Test** | | | | | |
| Riddle and Freburger[119] | 0.19 | NT | NT | NA | NA |
| Albert et al.[90] | 0.06 | NT | NT | NA | NA |
| Levangie[118] (LL) | 0.71* | NT | NT | 0.78 | NA |
| Levangie[104] (LS) | NR | 44 | 64 | 1.37 | 0.88 |

*Mechanical device used to improve reliability*
*NR, Not reported; NT, Not tested; LL, Leg length; LS, Long sit test*

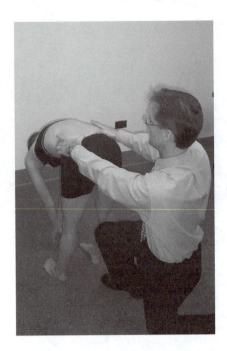

**Figure 12.24**    The Standing Flexion Test

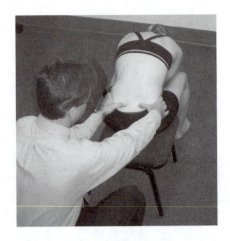

**Figure 12.25**    The Sitting Flexion Test

## Pain Provocation–Based Testing

Laslett and Williams[115] suggested that an efficient and effective method of examination consists of pain provocation-based maneuvers. Several studies that have analyzed pain provocation–based tests are outlined in Table 12.3. When compared to palpation and movement-based assessment, pain provocation tests yield much higher reliability and diagnostic value scores. Specifically, reliability is substantially better, often producing kappa and inter- and intraclass correlation values that qualify as "fair" to "good." Of the pain provocation tests examined, it appears that the active straight leg raise test, the thigh thrust, Patrick's test, and Gaenslen's test provide the best levels of reliability and diagnostic values.

**TABLE 12.3**    Diagnostic Value of Selected Pain Provocation-Based Clinical Special Tests

| Author | Reliability | Sensitivity | Specificity | +LR | −LR |
|---|---|---|---|---|---|
| **ASLR** | | | | | |
| Mens et al.[123] | NR | 87 | 94 | 14.5 | 0.13 |
| Damen et al.[73] | NR | 76 | 55 | 1.68 | 0.44 |
| **Thigh Thrust** | | | | | |
| Laslett and Williams[115] | 0.82 | NT | NT | NA | NA |
| Dreyfuss et al.[15] | 0.64 | 36 | 50 | 0.72 | 1.28 |
| Kokmeyer et al.[116] | 0.67 | NT | NT | NA | NA |
| Damen et al.[73] | NR | 61 | 72 | 2.17 | 0.54 |
| Ostgaard[124] | NR | 80 | 81 | 4.21 | 0.25 |
| Broadhurst et al.[61] | NR | 80 | 100 | NA | NA |
| Albert et al.[89] | 0.70 | 84–93* | 98 | 46.5 | 0.07–0.16 |
| **Gaenslen's** | | | | | |
| Laslett and Williams[115] | 0.72 | NT | NT | NA | NA |
| Dreyfuss et al.[15] | 0.61 | 71 | 26 | 1.02 | 1.11 |
| Kokmeyer et al.[116] | 0.60 | NT | NT | NA | NA |

**TABLE 12.3**   Diagnostic Value of Selected Pain Provocation-Based
Clinical Special Tests (Continued)

| Author | Reliability | Sensitivity | Specificity | +LR | −LR |
|--------|-------------|-------------|-------------|-----|-----|
| **Gapping Test** | | | | | |
| Blower et al.[125] | NR | 21 | 100 | NA | NA |
| Russell et al.[126] | NR | 11 | 90 | 1.1 | 0.98 |
| Laslett and Williams[115] | 0.69 | NT | NT | NA | NA |
| McCombe et al.[127] | 0.36 | NT | NT | NA | NA |
| Kokmeyer et al.[116] | 0.46 | NT | NT | NA | NA |
| Albert et al.[89] | 0.84 | 04–14 | 100 | NA | NA |
| **Compresion Test** | | | | | |
| Blower et al.[125] | NR | 0.00 | 100 | NA | NA |
| Russell et al.[126] | NR | 7 | 90 | 0.7 | 1.03 |
| Kokmeyer et al.[116] | 0.57 | NT | NT | NA | NA |
| Strender et al.[128] | 0.26 | NT | NT | NA | NA |
| Laslett and Williams[115] | 0.77 | NT | NT | NA | NA |
| McCombe et al.[127] | 0.16 | NT | NT | NA | NA |
| Albert et al.[89] | 0.79 | 25–38 | 100 | NA | NA |
| **Sacral Thrust** | | | | | |
| Laslett and Williams[115] | 0.32 | NT | NT | NA | NA |
| Dreyfuss et al.[15] | 0.30 | 53 | 29 | 0.74 | 1.62 |
| **Patrick's Test** | | | | | |
| Dreyfuss et al.[15] | 0.62 | 69 | 16 | 0.82 | 1.94 |
| Van Deursen et al.[129] | 0.38 | NR | NR | NA | NA |
| Broadhurst et al.[61] | NR | 77 | 100 | NA | NA |
| Albert et al.[89] | 0.54 | 42–40* | 99 | 41 | 0.58–0.60 |

*Reported for patients with one- and two-sided SIJ syndrome*
*NR, Not reported; NT, Not tested; NA, Not applicable*

## Active Straight Leg Raise

The active straight leg raise (ASLR) is considered an effective tool to determine dysfunction associated with pelvic pain with mobility dysfunction.[51] The test is associated with instability in counternutation. The greater the mobility of the pelvis, specifically in anterior rotation of the innominate on a fixed sacrum, the more marked the results from the ASLR.[51]

- Step One: The patient is positioned in supine. Resting symptoms are assessed.
- Step Two: The patient is instructed to raise the leg on his or her painful side (test both sides if both are painful) 6 inches above the mat. Concordant symptoms are assessed.
- Step Three: The clinician then stabilizes the pelvis of the patient by placing a SIJ belt around the pelvis or gripping the pelvis tightly with both hands.
- Step Four: The patient then lifts the leg again. Concordant symptoms are assessed.
- Step Five: The test is positive if the patient has pain during free lifting (step 2) but no pain during the stabilized lift (step 4).

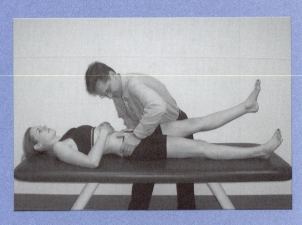

**Figure 12.26**    The Active Straight Leg Raise Test

## Gaenslen's Test

Gaenslen's test is considered an effective tool in isolating impairment that is irritated during anterior rotation of the innominate on the sacrum. Kokemeyer et al.[116] suggest that the test should be performed bilaterally allowing forced hip extension on the affected side if unilateral pain persists.

- Step One: The patient is positioned in supine with the painful leg resting very near the end of the treatment table. Resting symptoms are assessed.
- Step Two: The clinician sagitally raises the nonpainful side of the hip (with the knee bent) up to 90 degrees. Test both sides if the patient complains of pain bilaterally.
- Step Three: A downward force is applied to the lower leg (painful side) while a flexion-based counterforce is applied to the flexed leg (pushing the leg in the opposite direction). The effect causes a torque to the pelvis. Concordant symptoms are assessed.
- Step Four: The test is positive if the torque reproduces pain of the concordant sign.

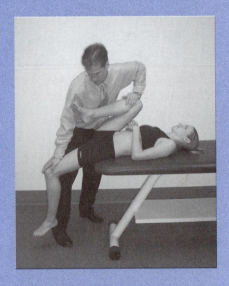

**Figure 12.27**    The Gaenslen's Test

## FABER's Test or Patrick's Test

Generally, FABER's test or Patrick's test does not provide the same level of diagnostic information that the other pain provocation tests do. However, the Patrick's test has been used frequently in studies and demonstrates acceptable value. In some cases, a patient may complain of pain in the anterior or lateral aspect of his or her hip. This finding is considered negative for SIJ dysfunction and positive for hip tightness.

- Step One: The patient is positioned in supine. Resting symptoms are assessed.
- Step Two: The painful-sided leg is placed in a "figure four" position. The ankle is placed just above the knee of the other leg.
- Step Three: The clinician provides a gentle downward pressure on both the knee of the painful side and the ASIS of the non-painful side. Concordant pain is assessed, specifically the location and type of pain.
- Step Four: A positive test is concordant pain that is posterior to the hip or near the SIJ.

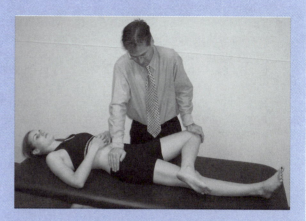

**Figure 12.28**    FABER's or Patrick's Test

## Thigh Thrust

The thigh thrust is a useful clinical test that has been included as part of a cluster of SIJ tests in recent studies. The thigh thrust is also known as the Ostgaard test, the 4P test, and the Sacrotuberous stress test, and involves a downward force of the thigh that causes a posterior translation of the innominate on the sacrum. Concordant pain reproduction is considered a positive test.

- Step One: The patient is positioned in supine. Resting symptoms are assessed.
- Step Two: The clinician stands on the opposite side of the painful side of the patient.
- Step Three: The painful-sided knee is flexed to 90 degrees.
- Step Four: The clinician places his or her hand under the sacrum to form a stable "bridge" for the sacrum.
- Step Five: A downward pressure is applied through the femur to force a posterior translation of the pelvis. The patient's symptoms are assessed to determine if they are concordant.
- Step Six: A positive test is concordant pain that is posterior to the hip or near the SIJ.

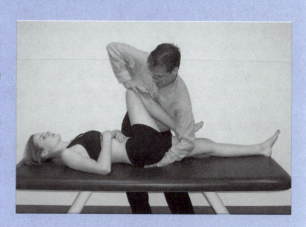

**Figure 12.29**    The Thigh Thrust

## Sacral Spring Test

The sacral spring test is one of the four pain provocation tests advocated by Laslett et al.[107] The test theoretically provides an anterior shearing force of the sacrum on both of the ilia.

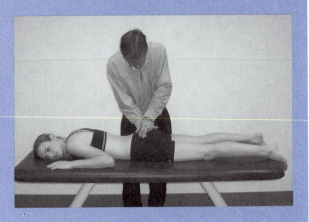

- Step One: The patient lies in a prone position. Resting symptoms are assessed.
- Step Two: The clinician palpates the second or third spinous process of the sacrum. Using the pisiform the clinician places a downward pressure on the sacrum at S3. By targeting the midpoint of the sacrum, the clinician is less likely to force the lumbar spine into hyperextension.
- Step Three: Vigorously and repeatedly, the clinician applies a strong downward force to the sacral in an attempt to reproduce the concordant sign of the patient.
- Step Four: A positive test is a reproduction of the concordant sign during downward pressure.

**Figure 12.30**    The Sacral Spring Test

## Sacroiliac Compression Test

The SIJ compression test is designed to apply bilateral compression to the posterior aspect of the SIJ and distraction to the anterior aspect of the SIJ.[31]

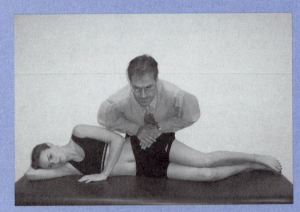

- Step One: The patient assumes a sidelying position with his or her painful side up superior to the plinth. Resting symptoms are assessed.
- Step Two: The clinician then cups the iliac crest of the painful side and applies a downward force through the ilium. As with the other SIJ tests, considerable vigor is required to reproduce the symptoms; in some cases repeated force is necessary.
- Step Three: A positive test is reproduction of the concordant sign of the patient.

**Figure 12.31**    The SI Compression Test

## SI Distraction Test

The Distraction test is similar in concept to the Compression test. Although the test has been described in supine, a more compelling version is performed unilaterally in a sidelying position.

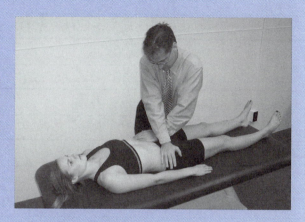

- Step One: The patient assumes a supine position. Resting symptoms are assessed.
- Step Two: The medial aspect of both anterior superior iliac spines is palpated by the clinician. The clinician crosses his or her arms, creating an X at the forearms, and a force is applied in a lateral–posterior direction. For comfort, it is often required that the clinician relocate his or her hands on the ASIS several times.
- Step Three: The clinician applies a vigorous force repeatedly in an attempt to reproduce the concordant sign of the patient.
- Step Four: A positive test is reproduction of the concordant sign of the patient.

**Figure 12.32**   The SI Distraction Test

## Combining Tests (Clusters)

Several studies have purported the benefit of combining selected SIJ tests to improve the reliability and diagnostic value. Kokmeyer et al.[116] showed improvement when three of five tests were positive, suggesting the findings were more discriminate than using only one test. Others have advocated the benefit of palpation or movement-based tests, although it is possible that the methods used to determine these results were methodologically flawed.[130] Recently, Laslett et al.[84] and Young et al.[108] used the discriminatory criteria of both centralization assessment and diagnostic blocks to determine patients with a sacroiliac dysfunction. The methodology used in this study assists in determining the true value of the testing procedures. Using a combination of three of five tests, the positive likelihood ratio improved to 4.16. Laslett et al. suggested that this cluster of tests is necessary versus one single test to rule out the potential for single tester error. Furthermore, Laslett et al. have outlined that finding two of four positive tests when testing the thigh thrust, distraction, compression, and sacral thrust, in the absence of centralization of the spine, is indicative of a positive SIJ dysfunction. The authors advocate testing the thigh thrust and distraction first and that any combination of two positive findings is indicative of SIJ dysfunction. Table 12.4 outlines the diagnostic value of the combined tests.

## Diagnosis and Treatment Decision Making

Indeed, isolation of the presence of a sacroiliac or pelvic impairment is a challenge. Further assessment of the homogenous category of SIJ impairment is all the more

## Summary

- The most useful palpation-based special test appears to be direct palpation of the pubic symphysis, but will only be positive in patients with pubic symphysis pain.
- Manual muscle testing appears to yield useful information, specifically resisted hip adduction and possibly resisted hip flexion.
- No observation or palpation for location-based tests appears to demonstrate acceptable reliability or validity.
- The active straight leg raise test appears to be useful in identifying patients with instability in movements of counternutation.
- A cluster of three of five clinical special tests has demonstrated strong validity for confirming injection-confirmed SIJ dysfunction. These tests include the Sacral Spring, the Compression and Distraction tests, Gaenslen's test, and the Thigh Thrust.

difficult. Nevertheless, the critical use of appropriate examination findings will improve the likelihood that one will not "miss" an SIJ/pelvic problem.

Palpation-based examination methods have long been a hallmark of diagnosing SIJ dysfunction. Unfortunately, there is little reliability or validity to these methods and

**TABLE 12.4    Diagnostic Value of Selected Combined SIJ Clinical Special Tests**

| Author | Reliability | Sensitivity | Specificity | +LR | −LR |
|---|---|---|---|---|---|
| **Supine to Sit Test and Sitting Flexion Test** | | | | | |
| Levangie[104] (2 of 2) | NT | NR | NR | NA | NA |
| **Distraction, Thigh Thrust, Gaenslen's Test, Compression, and Sacral Thrust** | | | | | |
| Laslett et al.[84] (3 of 5) | NT | 91 | 78 | 4.16 | 0.11 |
| **Standing Flexion, Sitting PSIS Palpation, Supine to Sit Test, Prone Knee Flexion Test** | | | | | |
| Cibulka & Koldehoff[80] (4 of 4) | NR | 82 | 88 | 6.83 | 0.20 |
| **Standing Flexion, Prone Knee Flexion, Supine Long Sitting Test, Sitting PSIS Test** | | | | | |
| Riddle & Freburger[119] (3 of 4) | 0.11–0.23 | NR | NR | NA | NA |
| **Gapping, Compression, Gaenslen's, Thigh Thrust, and Patrick's Test** | | | | | |
| Kokmeyer et al.[116] (3 of 5) | 0.71 | NT | NT | NA | NA |
| **Thigh Thrust, Distraction, Sacral Thrust, and Compression Tests** | | | | | |
| Laslett et al.[107] (2 of 4) | NR | 88 | 78 | 4.00 | 0.16 |

*NR, Not reported; NT, Not tested; NA, Not applicable*

they may serve only to bias the clinician to an incorrect diagnosis.

Numerous guru-based educators have suggested multitudes of various SIJ directional faults such as up-slips, down-slips, inflares, outflares, superior shears, and inferior shears, to name a few. Unfortunately, there is no literature that supports the absolute existence of these phenomena, nor are there diagnostic methods to support a positional diagnosis. Subsequently, most evidence-based studies have outlined dysfunction primarily associated with SIJ inflammatory disorders, anterior rotation of the innominate on the sacrum, posterior rotation of the innominate on the sacrum, and superior shear of the pubis with respect to the opposite side. Typically, superior shear of the pubis is associated with ipsilateral anterior rotation of the innominate on the sacrum.[51] Bilateral conditions of said disorders are plausible as well. By limiting our examination to these findings, the likelihood of correctly identifying the disorder is substantially improved. Because determining the correct side and the direction of the dysfunction is crucial for manual therapy and surgical treatment,[51,104] considerable effort should be dedicated to this exploration.

By using evidence-based information the chances of appropriately identifying the presence of an SIJ dysfunction is improved. The steps include (1) ruling out the presence of a disc-related lumbar spine impairment or an impairment that responds well to lumbar spine–related treatments, and (2) using evidence-based special tests to appropriately identify the presence of SIJ-related disorders.

Use of the criteria developed by Delitto and colleagues[131] allows the clinician is to segregate treatment responses of the lumbar spine into four primary categories (see Chapter Eleven). Positive treatment directed at traction, specific exercise, and mobilization groups is suggestive of a probable lumbar spine disorder. Failure to improve in any of the lumbar-directed responses is suggestive of clinical instability or SIJ dysfunction. Using centralization and other aspects of lumbar spine treatment to rule out back disorders versus others is a method designed to carefully discriminate and improve the likelihood of a correct diagnosis. By using the centralization phenomenon and 10% pretest prevalence, the likelihood of correctly identifying an SIJ dysfunction increases from 10 to 40%. Including other discriminatory factors such as gender, pregnancy, the results of an active straight leg raise, and incident of injury would provide even further conclusive information (Figure 12.33).

Laslett suggests the use of two of four positive tests to outline SIJ-related pain (Figure 12.34). A combination of two positive Thigh Thrust, Distraction, Compression, or Sacral Thrust tests, in the absence of centralization of the spine, is suggestive of an SIJ dysfunction. This finding is a modification from the original three of five tests suggested also by Laslett. Ruling "out" the lumbar spine and a positive two of four tests for SIJ is associated with a four times likelihood that SIJ dysfunction is truly present.

The last aspect of the evidence-based model involves treatment decision making. Although the findings of

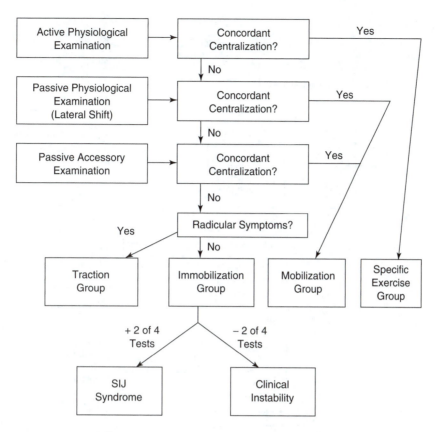

**Figure 12.33**    The Exercise Template for Examination of the Pelvis

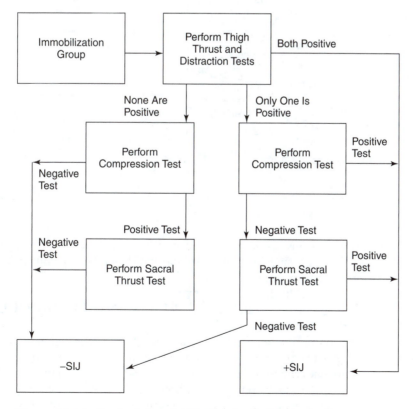

**Figure 12.34**    Laslett's Special Testing for Ruling in the Presence of SIJ Dysfunction

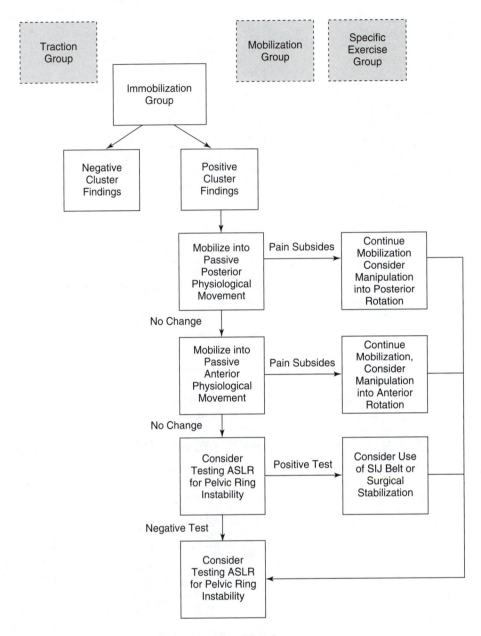

**Figure 12.35**    Treatment Template for SIJ Pelvis

ruling out lumbar spine and two of four positive tests increase the probability of accurately diagnosing SIJ pain, the tests do not outline what form of treatment is appropriate for the patient. Figure 12.35 outlines further refinement techniques to determine appropriate treatment decision making for care. Either the patient will respond to techniques that are counternutation or nutation based, or they will not respond to either. Positive response techniques should be continued or techniques should be associated with the positive movement pattern. However, if a patient does not response well to either direction of move-

ment, stabilization may be the appropriate treatment selection and should be implemented.

# TREATMENT TECHNIQUES

There may be no other region of the body that so much effort has been dedicated toward examination and diagnosis, yet so little study has been performed regarding treatment. At present, there are no studies that comprehensively and prospectively analyze the effectiveness of active stretching,

## *Summary*

- Theoretical position–based impairments are not well represented within the literature.
- One way to improve the diagnostic accuracy of detecting SIJ dysfunction is by ruling out the lumbar spine.
- Two of four positive SIJ tests after having ruled out the lumbar spine are indicative of SIJ dysfunction.
- Appropriate treatment is associated with desired patient response. Treatments that are associated with nutation or counternutation are appropriately administered if they reduce patient complaint of symptoms. If neither treatment is beneficial, stabilization may be the desired treatment approach.

muscle energy, manipulation, or mobilization for SIJ/pelvic treatment.[132] Numerous anecdotal findings suggest various forms of physical therapy and chiropractic treatment yield modest benefits for reduction of pain.[14] The *European Guidelines on the Diagnosis and Treatment of Pelvic Girdle Pain*[11] reports they cannot recommend the use of these methods because no single randomized clinical or pragmatic trial has been performed.

There may be several reasons for this finding. First, conclusive diagnosis of SIJ pain requires diagnostic blocks and is an expensive and time-consuming step, thus homogenizing groups in certain SIJ/pelvis groups is difficult. Second, few clinicians agree on the appropriate treatment for SIJ. Third, the understanding that instability is a common cause of SIJ/pelvis dysfunction is a relatively contemporary finding. Often, the appropriate design and production of a well-designed study takes years to occur.

Like other anatomical regions, the SIJ and pelvis may exhibit different forms of impairment. It is unfair to assume that all SIJ dysfunctions will exhibit the same set of symptoms, involve the same anatomical tissue, and will demonstrate a similar form of outcome. In 2002, Albert et al.[13] introduced five subgroups of posterior pelvic pain syndrome (PPPP), including SIJ pelvic girdle syndrome (pain in the SIJ and pubic symphysis), symphysiolysis, one-sided SIJ syndrome, double-sided SIJ syndrome, and mixed. Albert believes that although this finding that is based on clinical examination was from a population of 2,269 pregnant patients, the plausibility exists that nonpregnant patients may suffer from similar dysfunctions.[133] Anatomically and biomechanically, these disparate problems could represent clinically in very dissimilar ways.

### *Pelvic Girdle Syndrome (SIJ and Pubic Symphysis Pain)*

It is likely that pelvic girdle syndrome is a combined stabilization loss of the SIJ, low back, and pelvis joints. Consequently, the recovery rate for pelvic girdle syndrome tends to be poorer when compared to the other four classifications, with many patients reporting pain up to 2 years after the onset of this syndrome during pregnancy.[134]

### *Symphysiolysis*

Symphysiolysis is pain in the pubic symphysis. Albert reported an incidence of 2.3% of pregnant women, the lowest of the five classifications of PPPP (2002). Typically, pain associated with symphysiolysis disappears within a month after delivery, a recovery rate that is significantly better than those with pelvic girdle syndrome.[134] However, when compared to one-sided and double-sided SIJ syndrome, the pain may persist up to 6 months after delivery.

### *One-Sided SIJ Syndrome*

One-sided SIJ syndrome may be associated with asymmetric stabilization between the two SIJ joints or trauma/degeneration between innominates. Typically, when testing for end range repeated movements or provocation tests are performed, differences will be noted on each side, specifically if the test or movement provokes in the direction of dysfunction.

### *Double-Sided SIJ Syndrome*

Double-sided SIJ syndrome is commonly associated with stability loss and may be associated with hormone-related changes.[11] Generally, this dysfunction is self-resolving and tends to be isolated to the time of pregnancy.

### *Mixed*

Mixed models may be associated with various forms of instability, including both SIJ and pubic symphysis pain. Mixed models are most likely a reflection of instability, but may be a result of neuromuscular dysfunction as well.

## Active Physiological Movements

Self-correction methods of SIJ dysfunction allow the patient to "self-treat" in the absence of an attending clinician. Although there are numerous methods of self-treatment, those methods that are targeted toward the complimentary rotational displacements are the easiest for the patient to understand and perform in isolation.

*Methods for Anterior Displaced Innominate*

## Standing Rotation

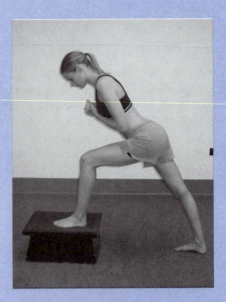

- Step One: The leg on the symptomatic side is placed on a box or some other structure approximately 2 to 3 feet high.
- Step Two: The patient then leans forward over the leg to encourage posterior pelvic rotation.
- Step Three: Repeated oscillations are used to "mobilize" the innominate.

**Figure 12.36**   Standing Rotation

## External Rotation with Trunk Flexion

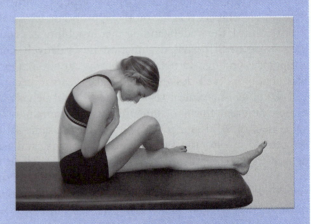

- Step One: The patient sits with the leg on the symptomatic side crossed at the knee. This movement promotes external rotation of the pelvis and corresponding posterior innominate movement.
- Step Two: The patient then leans forward to further the posterior rotation of the pelvis.

**Figure 12.37**   External Rotation with Flexion

## Method for Posterior Displaced Innominate: The Standing Rotation Stretch

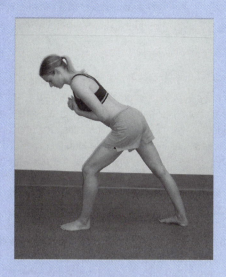

- Step One: The patient places the knee or foot of the sympto-matic leg posterior to the hip.
- Step Two: The patient extends backward by "sagging the pelvis" to promote anterior rotation of the innominate.

**Figure 12.38**    Standing Rotation Stretch

## Passive Physiological Movements

### Posterior Rotation of the Innominate on the Sacrum

This technique is selected if repeated physiological rotations led to pain relief or abolishment of symptoms during the clinical examination.

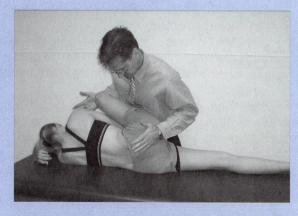

- Step One: The patient assumes a sidelying position, the painful side up. Resting symptoms are assessed.
- Step Two: The painful-sided leg is flexed beyond 90 degrees to engage the pelvis and to promote passive physiological flexion.
- Step Three: The clinician then situates his or her body into the popliteal fold of the painful-sided leg to "snug up" the position. The plinth-sided leg remains in an extended position.
- Step Four: The clinician then places his or her hands on the is-chial tuberosity and the ASIS to promote physiological rotation. The patient's pelvis is passively moved to the first sign of con-cordant pain, then the method is repeated at or near end range while respecting the patient's concordant sign.

**Figure 12.39**    Physiological Posterior Rotation of the Innominate

## Anterior Rotation of the Innominate on the Sacrum

This technique is selected if repeated physiological rotations led to pain relief or abolishment of symptoms during the clinical examination.

- Step One: The patient assumes a sidelying position, the painful side up. Resting symptoms are assessed.
- Step Two: The painful-sided leg is extended and the plinth-sided leg is flexed to 90 degrees. The motion is the mirror image of passive physiological nutation.
- Step Three: The clinician cradles the leg with the caudal-side hand and encourages further movement into hip extension. The cranial-sided hand is placed on the PSIS and promotes anterior rotation of the innominate.
- Step Four: The clinician then places his or her hands on the ischial tuberosity and the ASIS to further promote physiological rotation. The patient's pelvis is passively moved to the first sign of concordant pain, then the method is repeated at or near end range while respecting the patient's concordant sign.

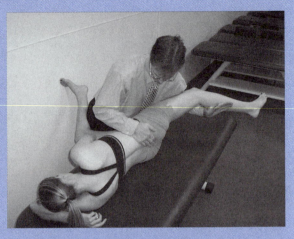

**Figure 12.40**   Physiological Anterior Rotation of the Innominate

## Passive Physiological Anterior Rotation in Prone

This technique is selected if repeated physiological anterior rotation of the innominate led to pain relief during the passive physiological examination, yet end range movements were contraindicated or inappropriate in the sidelying position.

- Step One: The patient assumes a prone position. Resting symptoms should be assessed.
- Step Two: The clinician stands to the same side as the leg where concordant symptoms are identified. The clinician places the cephalic hand on the PSIS while the caudal hand lifts the knee and thigh.
- Step Three: Using a sequential motion, the clinician then applies a downward glide to the PSIS (promoting anterior rotation of the innominate) at the same time he or she performs passive hip extension. The amount of force applied to the PSIS can be modulated.
- Step Four: The treatment should elicit the concordant sign of the patient.

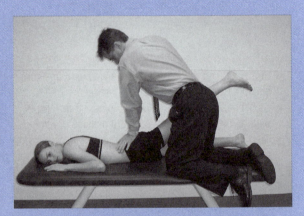

**Figure 12.41**   Passive Physiological Anterior Rotation in Prone

## Passive Accessory Movements (PAIVMS)

There are numerous methods of passive accessory techniques, many of which are redundant to the passive physiological procedures. Selection of a technique should distill out of the examination. For example, the use of a unilateral AP to the right ASIS should only be selected if pain reduces while performing repeated movements during the initial examination.

### Unilateral Gapping During Rotation

One method designed to encourage posterior glide is the unilateral gap. By placing the lumbar spine in a coupled position (meaning concurrent rotation and side flexion) the ligamentous and capsular system of the lumbar spine is in apposition and will demonstrate decreased movements. By using this setup, translation on the innominate should provide more isolated force to the pelvis versus the low back.

- Step One: The patient lies in a sidelying position. The painful side is placed up.
- Step Two: The clinician then rotates the lumbar spine (skyward) to L5 to couple the ligaments and facets.
- Step Three: The cephalic hand is placed flush against L5 to provide a block to the lumbar spine.
- Step Four: The caudal hand is placed on the ASIS to provide a force posteriorly.
- Step Five: Repeated movements should result in abolishing or diminishing symptoms.

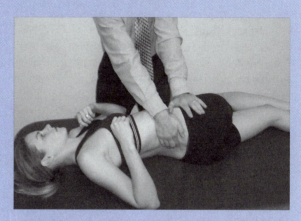

**Figure 12.42**    Unilateral Gapping of SIJ in Sidelying

### Posterior Shear of Innominate on Sacrum

The posterior shear of the innominate is very similar to the Thigh Thrust test and may be useful in cases of hypomobility (innominate is stuck in an incorrect position). The technique should only be used if posterior glide techniques such as an AP yield beneficial results during the examination.

- Step One: The patient is positioned in supine. Resting symptoms are assessed.
- Step Two: The clinician stands on the opposite side of the painful side of the patient.
- Step Three: The painful-sided knee is flexed to 90 degrees.
- Step Four: The clinician places his or her hand under the sacrum to form a stable "bridge" for the sacrum.
- Step Five: A downward pressure is applied through the femur to force a posterior translation of the pelvis. Repeated movements may be necessary and/or a thrust can be used for a manipulative procedure.

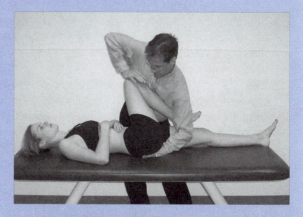

**Figure 12.43**    Posterior Shear of Innominate on Sacrum

## Manually Assisted Movements

Muscle energy techniques are commonly used as treatment techniques of the SIJ/pelvis. Since correct movement of a displaced pelvis is the goal of the treatment, three techniques will be discussed that theoretically correct an anteriorly rotated innominate, a posteriorly rotated innominate, and a displaced pubic symphysis.

---

### Adduction Isometric of the Pubic Symphysis

Mens et al.[51] point out that instability of the pelvis results in superior migration of the impaired (painful) sided pubis during weight bearing. One method to relocate this migrate is the adduction isometric treatment, commonly referred to as the "shot gun."

- Step One: The patient assumes a hooklying supine position. Resting symptoms are queried.
- Step Two: The clinician provides a series of resisted bilateral hip abduction bouts. The patient is requested to push out against the clinician-applied resistance for several bouts of 6-second holds.
- Step Three: Slowly, the clinician allows further hip abduction in the hooklying position until the knees are wide enough apart to allow the clinician to place his or her forearm, lengthwise, between their knees.
- Step Four: After the last abduction isometric bout, the clinician requests a strong and quick adduction isometric contraction against the forearm resistance.
- Step Five: Often, the patient experiences some discomfort and an audible with this activity.
- Step Six: Since the core of the problem is generally instability, the patient may benefit from the application of a SIJ belt directly after relocation.

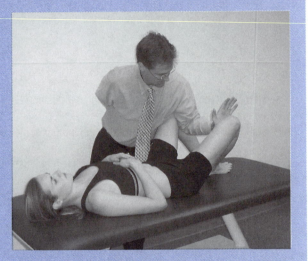

**Figure 12.44**   Correction of Displacement of Pubic Symphysis

---

### Muscle Energy Relocation of an Anterior Rotated Innominate

If the patient displays pain during physiological anterior rotation of the innominate in sidelying that is worsened with repeated movements into anterior rotation, he or she may be a good candidate for a muscle energy technique. The technique is efficient because the patient controls the amount of force applied through the SIJ.

- Step One: The patient assumes a supine position. Resting symptoms are queried.
- Step Two: The leg on the painful side is flexed at the knee and hip and raised into as much hip flexion as the patient can tolerate.
- Step Three: The opposite extremity is positioned in relative extension or neutral position.
- Step Four: Using his or her body weight, the clinician then leans into the flexed leg to provide a stable barrier for resistance. Often it is necessary for the clinician to use his or her arm closest to the painful side to hold on to the plinth for further stability.
- Step Five: The opposite arm is extended and placed on the knee of the patient.
- Step Six: The patient is instructed to push downward (in hip extension) against the resistance of the clinician while simultaneously flexing the opposite hip against the hand resistance. A series of three to five bouts of 5-second holds is beneficial.
- Step Seven: Upon completion, the concordant movement of the patient is reassessed.

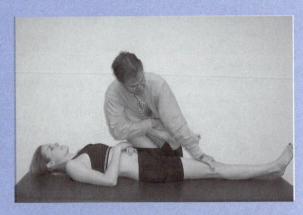

**Figure 12.45**   Muscle Energy Relocation of an Anterior Rotated Innominate

## Muscle Energy Relocation of a Posterior Rotated Innominate

If the patient displays pain during physiological posterior rotation of the innominate in sidelying that is worsened with repeated movements into posterior rotation, he or she may be a good candidate for a muscle energy technique.

- Step One: The patient assumes a supine position. Resting symptoms are queried.
- Step Two: The leg on the painful side is extended and the opposite leg is flexed at the hip and the knee. The position is the opposite of that in Figure 12.45.
- Step Three: It is best for the clinician to stand to the opposite side of the leg on the painful pelvis. Using his or her body weight, the clinician then leans into the flexed leg (nonpainful side) to provide a stable barrier for resistance. Often it is necessary for the clinician to use his or her arm closest to the painful side to hold on to the plinth for further stability.
- Step Four: The opposite arm is extended and placed on the knee of the patient.
- Step Five: The patient is instructed to lightly push downward (in hip extension) against the resistance of the clinician while simultaneously flexing the leg on the painful side against the hand resistance. A series of three to five bouts of 5-second holds is beneficial.
- Step Six: Upon completion, the concordant movement of the patient is reassessed.

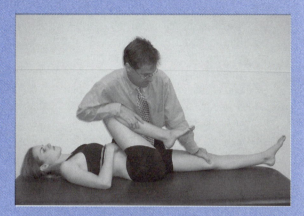

**Figure 12.46**  Muscle Energy Relocation of a Posterior Rotated Innominate

## Manipulation

Manipulation maneuvers are designed to provide correction of displacement and pain relief upon application.[135] Previously, using a purported SI technique, Flynn et al.[136] outlined that an audible was not necessary for a positive treatment outcome.[137] Using an innovative audiographic method to record cavitation sounds, Beffa and Mathews[138] indicated that the audible associated with a manipulation isn't always at the targeted segment of the adjustment.

Roentgen stereophotogrammetric analysis suggests that manipulation does not alter the position of the SIJ.[139] However, improvements in asymmetry do occur after manipulation, a finding also reported by Tullberg et al.[139] who hypothesized this response as associative soft tissue changes. Considerable evidence exists that manipulation does have the capacity to affect soft tissue around the SIJ, since the H-reflex is decreased after manipulation.[140]

The following techniques are described with the underlying assumption that repeated passive physiological or accessory movements do not provide pain relief. However, even if repeated movements provide pain relief, manipulation can be a treatment of choice. The manipulative procedures would be performed in the same direction that pain decreased with passive accessory movements versus the opposite direction, as described in the following examples.

## Sidelying Manipulation into Anterior Rotation

The sidelying manipulation into anterior rotation is a technique that may be beneficial if the patient had pain during repeated passive physiological posterior rotation of the innominate.

- Step One: The patient assumes a sidelying position, the painful side up. Resting symptoms are assessed.
- Step Two: The painful-sided leg is extended and the plinth-sided leg is flexed to 90 degrees. The motion is the mirror image of passive physiological nutation.
- Step Three: The clinician cradles the leg with the caudal-side hand and encourages further movement into hip extension. The cranial-side hand is placed on the PSIS and promotes anterior rotation of the innominate.
- Step Four: A quick but firm thrust is applied at end range. Rarely does an audible occur. The patient's concordant sign should be reassessed directly after the treatment.

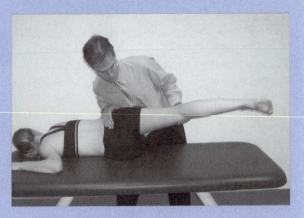

**Figure 12.47**   Sidelying, Manipulation into Anterior Rotation

## Sidelying Manipulation into Posterior Rotation

The sidelying manipulation into posterior rotation is a technique that may be beneficial if the patient had pain during repeated passive physiological anterior rotation of the innominate.

- Step One: The patient assumes a sidelying position, the painful side up. Resting symptoms are assessed.
- Step Two: The painful-sided leg is flexed beyond 90 degrees to engage the pelvis and to promote passive physiological flexion.
- Step Three: The clinician then situates his or her body into the popliteal fold of the painful-sided leg to "snug up" the position. The plinth-sided leg remains in an extended position.
- Step Four: The clinician then places his or her hands on the ischial tuberosity and the ASIS to promote further physiological rotation. The patient's pelvis is passively moved to end range.
- Step Five: A quick but firm thrust is applied at end range. Rarely does an audible occur. The patient's concordant sign should be reassessed directly after the treatment.

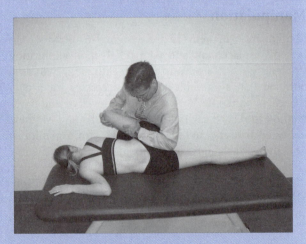

**Figure 12.48**   Sidelying, Manipulation into Posterior Rotation

## The Anterior Innominate Thrust

The anterior innominate thrust is well described in previous studies.[141] The technique has been characterized in the clinical prediction rule criteria for the lumbar spine developed by Flynn and colleagues.[137] There is some question whether the procedure actually manipulates the SIJ or the fifth facet of the lumbar spine. Nonetheless, a patient who demonstrates pain with repeated anterior rotation of the innominate may be a good candidate for this procedure.

- Step One: The patient lies supine. Resting symptoms are assessed.
- Step Two: The patient interlocks his or her fingers behind the neck. The elbows are pulled together.
- Step Three: The clinician side flexes the patient's body away and rotates the body toward them (in opposition). The patient is rolled until end range.
- Step Four: The clinician then applies a quick thrust at end range.

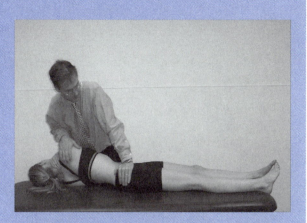

**Figure 12.49**    The Anterior Innominate Thrust

## Anterior–Posterior PSIS Thrust

The anterior PSIS thrust may be beneficial in patients that report increased pain with repeated passive physiological posterior rotation.

- Step One: The patient assumes a prone position. Resting symptoms should be assessed.
- Step Two: The clinician stands to the same side as the leg where concordant symptoms are identified. The clinician places the cephalic hand on the PSIS while the caudal hand lifts the knee and thigh.
- Step Three: Using a sequential motion, the clinician then applies a downward glide to the PSIS (promoting anterior rotation of the innominate) at the same time he or she performs passive hip extension. At end range, the clinician provides a quick thrust.

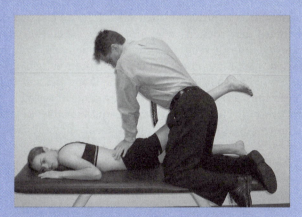

**Figure 12.50**    Anterior Thrust (patient prone, thrust to PSIS)

## Cyriax Grade V SIJ Manipulation

Cyriax[142] described a procedure in which the lower limb of the painful-sided pelvis is distracted quickly, thus causing a manipulative force throughout the pelvis. Because a patient who exhibits pubic symphysis dysfunction often displays superior displacement of one pubis on the other, this method may demonstrate benefit. Thus, this technique is appropriate for a patient who has a positive Chamberlain x-ray, or has pain with repeated anterior rotation of the innominate.

- Step One: The patient lies supine and resting symptoms are evaluated.
- Step Two: The clinician elevates the extended leg approximately 30 degrees. Tension is applied on the lower extremity to remove any slack.
- Step Three: The lower leg is gently oscillated (up and down) to relax the patient.
- Step Four: Once the patient has relaxed and allowed the full weight of their leg to fall into the clinician's hands, a quick longitudinal thrust is applied.

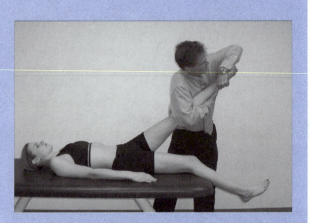

**Figure 12.51**   Long Leg Lever Thrust-Cyriax Grade V

## Stabilization

Most textbooks and some journal articles have outlined the importance of recognizing the "side" of the sacroiliac dysfunction prior to performing a selected manual therapy intervention.[142–146] Determination of the symptomatic side has included palpation, asymmetry palpatory assessment, pain-provocation maneuvers, a long-sit test that determines the "rotated" side, hip rotation alterations, and reported side of symptoms. Of these methods, only reported side of symptoms and pain-provocation maneuvers have fared reasonably well within the literature, and since uncertainty exists regarding the discriminatory value of the other diagnostic methods, it is questionable whether treatment based on specific questionable findings would yield satisfactory results.

Mens et al.[51] report that the active straight leg raise is a provocative test because it forces the same-side innominate into anterior rotation (with respect to the sacrum) and subsequently causes alignment dysfunction at the SIJ and pubic symphysis. Gaenslen's test functions similarly on the leg, which moves into extension. If these two tests are positive for patients who fall into this classification, innominate manipulation (either through a thrust procedure or muscle energy technique) implementing movement into the opposite direction is beneficial. In some instances, if pain is reproduced during surface palpation over just inferior to the posterior superior iliac spine, one can establish the involvement of the long dorsal ligament as a pain generator, specifically if counternutation reproduces the concordant pain of the patient.[1]

Posterior rotation of the innominate on the sacrum (nutation) places tension on the sacrotuberous ligament and various intraarticular structures. If the concordant pain occurs during posterior rotation, then one may suspect a nutation-based dysfunction. Determining which direction to treat into requires the same type of logical deduction as pain reproduced during counternutation. First, in conditions where repeated posterior rotation decreases, treatment may include repeated mobilization or manipulation "into" the direction where repeated movements caused decreased pain. Second, in conditions where repeated posterior rotation caused increased concordant symptoms, manipulation into the opposite direction as that produced by repeated movements is necessary.

For confirmation, Laslett et al.'s[84] cluster of clinical special tests to isolate SIJ dysfunction may be the most effective selection. Although these tests do not outline the "direction" of SIJ impairment, they do assist in determining that the SIJ is a pain generator of the concordant sign. If one finds at least two of four positive tests during examination, treatment may consist of a manipulation followed by stabilization with a belt and/or exercises or the directional approaches discussed earlier.

Overwhelming evidence suggests that the majority of underlying SIJ/pelvis disorders are instability related. Subsequently, stabilization is an essential part of a manual therapist's treatment of SIJ/pelvic disorders. Two approaches exist, passive and active, the passive approaches further subdivided into an SI belt and surgery.

Several active approaches exist, each designed to target the muscles that provide force closure of the pelvis. Two particular activities involve the contraction of the transverse abdominus, internal oblique, and the multifidi. The exercises are similar to those performed for the lumbar spine.

## Transverse Abdominis

- Step One: The patient assumes a supine hooklying position.
- Step Two: A blood pressure cuff is placed behind the back (proximal to the base of the sacrum) and is inflated to 20 mm/Hg. The gauge of the blood pressure cuff is given to the patient for viewing.
- Step Three: The clinician instructs the patient to lift their naval up toward their chin while compressing the naval downward toward his or her spine. The patient is instructed to perform this activity without increasing the pressure gauge under his or her back.
- Step Four: A correct contraction allows a hollowing of the abdominals and an inward drift of the ASIS. The inward drift ensures that SIJ force closure is occurring.

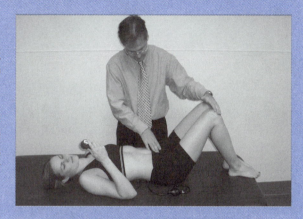

**Figure 12.52**    Transverse Abdominis Contraction and Internal Obliquis

## Multifidi

- Step One: The patient assumes a four-point kneeling posture (quadruped).
- Step Two: The clinician palpates the multifidi bilaterally just distal to the L4 spinous process.
- Step Three: The patient is first instructed to tighten their pelvic floor muscles. This is performed by instructing the patient to pull their anus inward toward his or her naval. Other directions such as pulling the scrotum into the body (if male) or tightening and pulling up on the vagina (if female) are also useful cues.
- Step Four: The patient is then instructed to swell the multifidi under the clinician's fingers without allowing movement of the pelvis. This motion is palpated by the clinician.
- Step Five: Because these techniques are difficult to produce, the use of a real-time ultrasound is advocated.
- Step Six: If the patient is able to master these isometric contractions, progressions include pistoning the lower leg or small movements of hip extension during quadruped.

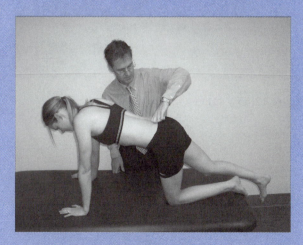

**Figure 12.53**    Multifidi Contraction

### Global Muscles, Force Coupling

Numerous muscles have been identified that stiffen the SIJ during contraction. These muscles are often identified as global muscles and are frequently associated with movement generation. Although the literature does not outline time-based criteria of when to target these muscle groups, it is plausible to consider training these muscles when local muscles have been appropriately isolated during exercise. Figures 12.54 through 12.58 identify potential force coupling exercises.

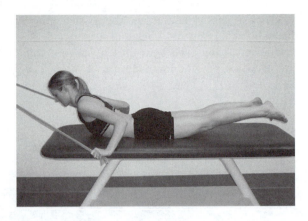

**Figure 12.57**    Force Couple—Gluteus Maximus

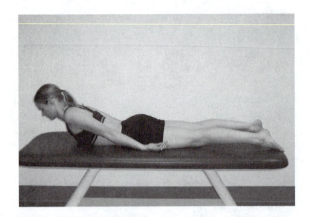

**Figure 12.54**    Force Couple—Erector Spinae

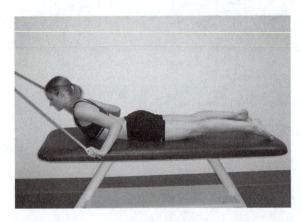

**Figure 12.55**    Force Couple—Latissimus Dorsi

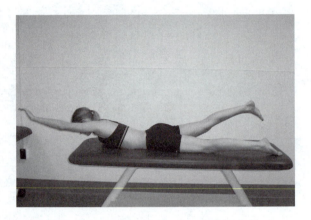

**Figure 12.58**    Combined Force Couple Using Contralateral Maneuvers

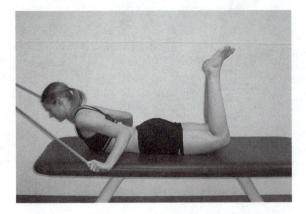

**Figure 12.56**    Force Couple—Biceps Femoris

## Summary

- Five known iterations of pelvic SIJ pain have been reported.
- The outcome for the five are mixed: those with pelvic girdle syndrome, a combined stabilization loss of the SIJ, low back, and pelvis joints, tends to be poorer than other forms of disorders.
- Many of the documented SIJ disorders are associated with pain during pregnancy because this is where the research has been performed.
- More research is needed on this area of classification.
- A cornucopia of manual therapy methods exists for pelvic treatment; the benefit of these methods is still unknown, but is supported by anecdotal evidence.
- Numerous stabilization methods have been investigated and are supported by the literature.

# TREATMENT OUTCOMES

Anecdotally, manual therapy has provided promising findings. In a study by Galm et al.[147] manual therapy led to more rapid improvements in a two-sample comparison of patients classified as SIJ dysfunction with documented concurrent herniated disc. Manual therapy was the only treatment difference between the two groups. Prone position mobilization and manipulation procedures were selected because these methods were considered safe for a patient with disc impairment.[148] Additionally, Lukban et al.[149] suggested, "Manual physical therapy may be a useful therapeutic modality for patients diagnosed with IC, high-tone pelvic floor dysfunction, and sacroiliac dysfunction." Intervention seems to be most useful in patients with primary complaints of urinary frequency, suprapubic pain, and dyspareunia.

Stuter et al.[150] reported that quadriceps inhibition occurred after manipulation to the SIJ in sidelying. Others have reported reductions in the H-reflex after manipulation,[140] changes in hormone levels directly post-treatment,[151] reduction of lower extremity symptoms,[140] and improvement of pain[135,152] after SIJ manipulation, despite the likelihood that the manipulation does not substantially change the position of the innominate on the sacrum.[139] However, these studies identify the short-term effects of manipulation and none has analyzed the benefits comparatively versus other treatment methods.

Stabilization has been investigated and has been shown to have benefit. Stuge et al.[153] performed an RCT that included 81 women with pelvic pain within 6–16 weeks of pregnancy. The study included two groups: a general-exercise group or stabilization-specific exercise group. The treatment group received 30–60 minutes of specific stabilization exercise, 3 days a week for 18–20 weeks plus mobilization. The control group received modalities, mobilization, and general exercises every other week for 20 weeks. The assessments at baseline, after 20 weeks of intervention and at 1-year post-partum of the outcomes measure that included the SF-36, Oswestry, and visual analog scale were statistically significantly better in the specific stabilization group. These findings are in contrast of those by Mens et al.[154] On the same population classification of patients, Mens et al. reported no significant differences between exercise groups that performed diagonal exercises designed to target force coupling versus a placebo group. The *European Guidelines on the Diagnosis and Treatment of Pelvic Girdle Pain*[11] advocate the use of an individualized stabilization program as part of a multifactorial treatment for post-partum pelvic pain.

An SIJ stabilization belt is a passive approach for stabilization. The belt compresses the ASIS of the innominate, medially producing a countertorque on the ligamentous structures. The success of this stabilization method has been reported and described by numerous investigators for short-term use.[8,23,53,124,154] Mens et al.[154] reported that tightening an SIJ belt around 13 of 14 patients reduced the radiographic-identified impairment. Depledge et al.[155] compared a soft SIJ belt (with standard exercise), rigid SIJ belt (with standard exercise), and no use (with standard exercise) for patients with pubic symphysis dysfunction in a randomized trial. The authors reported equivocal improvement in all three groups, questioning the superiority of one belt versus another or no use. However, since the preponderance of SIJ dysfunction involves hypermobility, an SIJ belt should always be considered as a possible temporary treatment option.

Surgical fusion of the SIJ and/or pubic symphysis is another passive procedural method that has yielded fair results for abolishment of pain.[28] Typically, SIJ/pelvic fusion consists of plates to the upper and lower aspects of the pubic rami or large screws placed through the SIJ.

## Summary

- No randomized or pragmatic trials have investigated the benefit of muscle energy, stretching, mobilization, or manipulation for confirmed SIJ-related pain.
- Stabilization of the SIJ has demonstrated benefit within the literature. The most effective stabilization methods appear to be very similar to local stabilization of the lumbar spine, targeting segmental stabilizers for long-term benefit.
- Stabilization tools such as a belt have shown minimal long-term benefit but good short-term benefit.

# Chapter Questions

1. Describe why the majority of sacroiliac dysfunction involves the tendency of the joint to succumb toward hypermobility.
2. Describe the biomechanical relationship between the pelvis joints and the lumbar spine. Indicate the difficulties in separating the two areas during an examination.
3. Outline the five suggested classification groups for pelvic girdle pain.
4. Describe the use of clusters for clinical special tests of the sacroiliac spine.
5. Outline an effective treatment mechanism for SIJ pain.

# *References*

1. Vleeming A, Pool-Goudzwaard AL, Hammudoghlu D, Stoeckart R, Snijders CJ, Mens JM. The function of the long dorsal sacroiliac ligament: its implication for understanding low back pain. *Spine*. 1996;21(5):556–562.

2. Richardson C, Snijders C, Hides J, Damen L, Pas M, Storm J. The relation between the transverse abdominis muscles, sacroiliac joint mechanics, and low back pain. *Spine*. 2002;27:399–405.

3. Pool-Goudzwaard AL, Vleeming A, Stoeckart R, Snijders CJ, Mens JM. Insufficient lumbopelvic stability: a clinical, anatomical and biomechanical approach to 'a-specific' low back pain. *Man Ther*. 1998;3(1):12–20.

4. Pool-Goudzwaard A, van Dijke G, Mulder P, Spoor C, Snijders C, Stoeckart R. The iliolumbar ligament: its influence on stability of the sacroiliac joint. *Clin Biomech*. 2003;18:99–105.

5. Bernard T, Kirkaldy-Willis H. Recognizing specific characteristics of non specific low back pain. *Clin Orthop*. 1987;217:266–280.

6. Rost CC, Jacqueline J, Kaiser A, Verhagen AP, Koes BW. Pelvic pain during pregnancy: a descriptive study of signs and symptoms of 870 patients in primary care. *Spine*. 2004;29(22):2567–2572.

7. Sturesson B, Uden G, Uden A. Pain pattern in pregnancy and "catching" of the leg in pregnant women with posterior pelvic pain. *Spine*. 1997;22(16):1880–1883.

8. Berg G, Hammar M, Moller-Jensen J. Low back pain during pregnancy. *Obstet Gynecol*. 1998;1:71–75.

9. Ostgaard H, Zetherstrom G, Roos-Hansson E, Svanberg B. Reduction of back and posterior pelvic pain in pregnancy. *Spine*. 1994;19:894–900.

10. Larsen E, Wilken-Jensen C, Hansen A. Symptom-giving pelvic girdle relaxation in pregnancy: Prevalence and risk factors. *Acta Obstet Gynecol Scand*. 1999;78:105–110.

11. Vleeming A, Albert H, Ostgaard H, Stuge B, Sturesson B. *European Guideline on the Diagnosis and Treatment of Pelvic Girdle Pain*. February 2, 2005.

12. Schwarzer A, Aprill CN, Bogduk N. The sacroiliac joint in chronic low back pain. *Spine*. 1995;20:31–37.

13. Albert HB, Godskesen M, Westergaard JG. Incidence of four syndromes of pregnancy-related pelvic joint pain. *Spine*. 2002;27(24):2831–2834.

14. Bogduk N. Management of chronic low back pain. *Med J Aust*. 2004;180(2):79–83.

15. Dreyfuss P, Michaelsen M, Pauza K, McLarty J, Bogduk N. The value of medical history and physical examination in diagnosing sacroiliac joint pain. *Spine*. 1996;21(22):2594–2602.

16. Maigne JY, Aivaliklis A, Pfefer F. Results of sacroiliac joint double block and value of sacroiliac pain provocation tests in 54 patients with low back pain. *Spine*. 1996;21(16):1889–1892.

17. Dreyfuss P, Dryer S, Griffin J, Hoffman J, Walsh N. Positive sacroiliac screening tests in asymptomatic adults. *Spine*. 1994;19(10):1138–1143.

18. Lee D. The pelvic girdle. *An approach to the examination and treatment of the lumbo-pelvic-hip region*. Edinburgh; Churchill Livingstone: 1989.

19. Sgambati E, Stecco A, Capaccioloi L, Brizzi E (Abstract). Morphometric análisis of the sacroiliac joint. *Ital J Anat Embryol*. 1997;102:33–38.

20. Mooney V. Sacroiliac joint dysfunction. In: Vleeming A, Mooney V, Dorman T, Snijders C, Stoeckart R. *Movement stability and low back pain: the essential role of the pelvis*. New York; Churchill Livingstone: 1997.

21. Vleeming A, Stoeckart R, Volkers C, Snijders C. Relation between form and function in the sacroiliac joint. Part 1: Clinical anatomic aspects. *Spine*. 1990;15:130–132.

22. Wilder DG, Pope MH, Frymoyer JW. The functional topography of the sacroiliac joint. *Spine*. 1980;5:575–579.

23. Snijders C, Vleeming A, Stoeckart R. Transfer of lumbosacral load to iliac bones and legs. 1. Biomechanics of self-bracing of the sacro-iliac joints and its significance for treatment and exercise. *Clin Biomech*. 1993;8:285–294.

24. Ebraheim NA, Madsen TD, Xu R, Mehalik J, Yeasting RA. Dynamic changes in the contact area of the sacroiliac joint. *Orthopedics*. 2003;26(7):711–714.

25. Jacobs H, Kissling R. The mobility of the sacroiliac joints in healthy volunteers between 20 and 50 years of age. *Clin Biomech*. 1995;10:352–361.

26. Bollow M, Braun J, Kannenberg J, Bierdermann T, Schauer-Petrowskaja C, Paris S, Mutze S, Hamm B. Normal morphology of sacroiliac joints in children: magnetic resonance studies related to age and sex. *Skeletal Radiol*. 1997;26:697–704.

27. Gamble J, Simmons S, Freedman M. The symphysis pubis. Anatomic and pathologic considerations. *Clin Orthop*. 1986;203:261–272.

28. Williams P, Thomas D, Downes E. Osteitis pubis and instability of the pubic symphysis. When nonoperative measures fail. *Am J Sports Med*. 2000;28: 350–355.

29. Phieffer L, Lundberg W, Templeman D. Instability of the posterior pelvic ring associated with disruption of the pubic symphysis. *Orthop Clin North Am*. 2004;35:445–449.

30. Traycoff RB, Crayton H, Dodson R. Sacrococcygeal pain syndromes: diagnosis and treatment. *Orthopedics*. 1989;12(10):1373–1377.

31. Lee D. The pelvic girdle. *An approach to the examination and treatment of the lumbo-pelvic-hip region*. 2nd ed. Edinburgh; Churchill Livingstone: 1999.

32. Grob KR, Neuhuber WL, Kissling RO. (abstract). Innervation of the sacroiliac joint of the human. *Z Rheumatol.* 1995;54(2):117–122.

33. Bowen V, Cassidy J. Macroscopic and microscopic anatomy of the sacroiliac joint from embryonic life until the eight decade. *Spine.* 1985;6:620–628.

34. MacAvoy MC, McClellan RT, Goodman SB, Chien CR, Allen WA, van der Meulen MC. Stability of open-book pelvic fractures using a new biomechanical model of single-limb stance. *J Orthop Trauma.* 1997;11(8):590–593.

35. Vleeming A, de Vries H, Mens J, van Wingerden JP. Possible role of the long dorsal sacroiliac ligament in women with peripartum pelvic pain. *Acta Ostet Gynecol Scand.* 2002;81:430–436.

36. Ramsden CE, McDaniel MC, Harmon RL, Renney KM, Faure A. Pudendal nerve entrapment as source of intractable perineal pain. *Am J Phys Med Rehabil.* 2003;82(6):479–484.

37. Silva-Filho AL, Santos-Filho AS, Figueiredo-Netto O, Triginelli SA. Uncommon complications of sacrospinous fixation for treatment of vaginal vault prolapse. *Arch Gynecol Obstet.* 2005;271(4):358–362.

38. Boukerrou M, Lambaudie E, Collinet P, Lacaze S, Mesdagh H, Ego A, Cosson M. (Abstract). Mechanical resistance of pelvic ligaments used for incontinence or prolapse surgery. *Gynecol Obstet Fertil.* 2004;32(7–8):601–606.

39. Bogduk N, Twomey L. *Clinical anatomy of the lumbar spine.* Melbourne; Churchill Livingstone: 1987.

40. Luk K, Ho H, Leong J. The iliolumbar ligament: a study of its anatomy, development and clinical significance. *J Bone Joint Surg.* 1986;68:197–200.

41. Pool-Goudzwaard AL, Kleinrensink GJ, Snijders CJ, Entius C, Stoeckart R. The sacroiliac part of the iliolumbar ligament. *J Anat.* 2001;199(Pt 4):457–463.

42. Sturesson B, Selvik G, Uden A. Movements of the sacroiliac joints. A roentgen stereophotogrammetric analysis. *Spine.* 1989;14(2):162–165.

43. Vleeming A, Pool-Goudzwaard AL, Stoeckart R, van Wingerden J, Snijders C. The posterior layer of the thoracolumbar fascia. Its function in load transfer from spine to legs. *Spine.* 1995;20:753–758.

44. Miller JA, Schultz AB, Andersson GB. Load-displacement behavior of sacroiliac joints. *J Orthop Res.* 1987;5(1):92–101.

45. Vleeming A, Buyruk HM, Stoeckart R, Karamursel S, Snijders CJ. An integrated therapy for peripartum pelvic instability: a study of the biomechanical effects of pelvic belts. *Am J Obstet Gynecol.* 1992;166(4):1243–1247.

46. Harrison DE, Harrison DD, Troyanovich SJ. The sacroiliac joint: a review of anatomy and biomechanics with clinical implications. *J Manipulative Physiol Ther.* 1997;20(9):607–617.

47. Zheng N, Watson LG, Yong-Hing K. Biomechanical modelling of the human sacroiliac joint. *Med Biol Eng Comput.* 1997;35(2):77–82.

48. Walheim GG, Selvik G. Mobility of the pubic symphysis. In vivo measurements with an electromechanic method and a roentgen stereophotogrammetric method. *Clin Orthop.* 1984;(191):129–135.

49. Meissner A, Fell M, Wilk R, Boenick U, Rahmanzadeh R. (abstract). Biomechanics of the pubic symphysis. Which forces lead to mobility of the symphysis in physiological conditions? *Unfallchirurg.* 1996;99:415–421.

50. Berezin D. Pelvic insufficiency during pregnancy and after parturition. *Acta Obst Gynecol Scand.* 1954;23:1–130.

51. Mens J, Vleeming A, Snijders C, Stam H, Ginai A. The active straight leg raising test and mobility of the pelvic joints. *Eur Spine J.* 1999;8:468–473.

52. Rieger H, Winckler S, Wetterkamp D, Overbeck J. Clinical and biomechanical aspects of external fixation of the pelvis. *Clin Biomech.* 1996;11:322–327.

53. Abramson D, Sumner MR, Wilson PD Relaxation of the pelvic joints in pregnancy. *Surg Gynecol Obst.* 1934;58:595–613.

54. Death A, Kirby R, MacMillan C. Pelvic ring mobility: assessment by stress radiography. *Arch Phys Med Rehabil.* 1982;63:204–206.

55. Vleeming A, Mooney V, Dorman T, Snijders C, Stoeckart R. *Movement stability and low back pain: the essential role of the pelvis.* New York; Churchill Livingstone: 1997.

56. Sturesson B, Uden A, Vleeming A. A radiostereometric analysis of movements of the sacroiliac joints during the standing hip flexion test. *Spine.* 2000;25(3):364–368.

57. Sturesson B, Uden A, Vleeming A. A radiostereometric analysis of the movements of the sacroiliac joints in the reciprocal straddle position. *Spine.* 2000;25(2):214–217.

58. Kidd AW, Magee S, Richardson CA. Reliability of real-time ultrasound for the assessment of transversus abdominis function. *J Gravit Physiol.* 2002;9(1):P131–132.

59. Hungerford B, Gilleard W, Hodges P. Evidence of altered lumbopelvic muscle recruitment in the presence of sacroiliac joint pain. *Spine.* 2003;28(14):1593–1600.

60. Hodges P. Is there a role for transverses abdominus in lumbo-pelvic stability? *Man Ther.* 1999;4:74–86.

61. Broadhurst NA, Bond MJ. Pain provocation tests for the assessment of sacroiliac joint dysfunction. *J Spinal Disord.* 1998;11(4):341–345.

62. Lee EY, Margherita AJ, Gierada DS, Narra VR. MRI of piriformis syndrome. *AJR Am J Roentgenol.* 2004;183(1):63–64.

63. Pool-Goudzwaard A, van Dijke G, van Gurp M, Mulder P, Snijders C, Stoeckart R. Contribution of

pelvic floor muscles to stiffness of the pelvic ring. *Clin Biomech*. 2004;19:564–571.

64. Hodges P, Richardson R. Contraction of the abdominal muscles associated with movement of the lower limb. *Phys Ther*. 1997;77:1132–1144.

65. Shirley D, Hodges P, Eriksson A, Gandevia S. Spinal stiffness changes throughout the respiratory cycle. *J Appl Physiol*. 2003;95:1467–1475.

66. O'Sullivan P, Beales D, Beetham J, Cripps J, Graf F, Lin I, Tucker B, Avery A. Altered motor control strategies in subjects with sacroiliac joint pain during the active straight leg raise test. *Spine*. 2002;27:E1–E8.

67. Hodges P, Richardson C. Feedforward contraction of transverses abdominus is not influenced by the direction of arm movement. *Exp Brain Res*. 1997;114:362–370.

68. Moseley G, Hodges P, Gandevia S. Deep and superficial fibers of the lumbar multifidus muscle are differentially active during voluntary arm movements. *Spine*. 2002;27:29–36.

69. Jemmett RS, Macdonald DA, Agur AM. Anatomical relationships between selected segmental muscles of the lumbar spine in the context of multi-planar segmental motion: a preliminary investigation. *Man Ther*. 2004;9(4):203–210.

70. Andersson EA, Oddsson LI, Grundstrom H, Nilsson J, Thorstensson A. EMG activities of the quadratus lumborum and erector spinae muscles during flexion-relaxation and other motor tasks. *Clin Biomech*. 1996;11(7):392–400.

71. McGill S, Juker D, Kropf P. Quantitative intramuscular myoelectric activity of quadratus lumborum during a wide variety of tasks. *Clin Biomech*. 1996;11(3):170–172.

72. van Wingerden JP, Vleeming A, Buyruk HM, Raissadat K. Stabilization of the sacroiliac joint in vivo: verification of muscular contribution to force closure of the pelvis. *Eur Spine J*. 2004;13(3):199–205.

73. Damen L, Buyruk HM, Guler-Uysal F, Lotgering FK, Snijders CJ, Stam HJ. The prognostic value of asymmetric laxity of the sacroiliac joints in pregnancy-related pelvic pain. *Spine*. 2002;27(24):2820–2824.

74. Wang M, Dumas GA. Mechanical behavior of the female sacroiliac joint and influence of the anterior and posterior sacroiliac ligaments under sagittal loads. *Clin Biomech*. 1998;13(4-5):293–299.

75. Mooney V, Puzos R, Vleeming A, Gulick J, Swenski D. Exercise treatment for sacroiliac pain. *Orthopedics*. 2001;24:29–32.

76. Huijbrets P. Sacroiliac joint dysfunction: Evidence-based diagnosis. *Orthopaedic Division Review*. 2004;8:18–44.

77. Johnson W. Sacroiliac strain. *J Am Osteopathic Association*. 1964;63:1015–1029.

78. Stoddard A. Conditions of the sacroiliac joint and their treatment. *Physiotherapy*. 1958;44:97–101.

79. Cibulka MT, Sinacore D, Cromer G, Delitto A. Unilateral hip rotation range of motion asymmetry in patients with sacroiliac joint regional pain. *Spine*. 1998;23:1009–1015.

80. Cibulka MT, Koldehoff R. Clinical usefulness of a cluster of sacroiliac joint tests in patients with and without low back pain. *J Orthop Sports Phys Ther*. 1999;29(2):83–89.

81. Vincent-Smith B, Gibbons P. Inter-examiner and intra-examiner reliability of the standing flexion test. *Man Ther*. 1999;4(2):87–93.

82. Saal JS. General principles of diagnostic testing as related to painful lumbar spine disorders: a critical appraisal of current diagnostic techniques. *Spine*. 2002;27(22):2538–2545.

83. Freburger JK, Riddle D. Using published evidence to guide the examination of the sacroiliac joint region. *Phys Ther*. 2001;81:1135–1143.

84. Laslett M, Young SB, April CN, McDonald B. Diagnosing painful sacroiliac joints: A validity study of a McKenzie evaluation and sacroiliac provocation tests. *Aust J Physiotherapy*. 2003;49:89–97.

85. Hogan QH, Abram SE. Neural blockade for diagnosis and prognosis. A review. *Anesthesiology*. 1997;86(1):216–241.

86. Laslett M. The value of the physical examination in diagnosis of painful sacroiliac joint pathologies. *Spine*. 1998;23(8):962–964.

87. Long A, Donelson R, Fung T. Does it matter which exercise? A randomized control trial of exercise for low back pain. *Spine*. 2004;29(23):2593–2602.

88. Werneke M, Hart D, Cook D. A descriptive study of the centralization phenomenon. *Spine*. 1999;24:676–683.

89. Albert H, Godskesen M, Westergaard J. Evaluation of clinical tests used in classification procedures in pregnancy-related pelvic joint pain. *Eur Spine J*. 2000;9(2):161–166.

90. Peloso PM, Braun J. Expanding the armamentarium for the spondyloarthropathies. *Arthritis Res Ther*. 2004;6 Suppl 2:S36–43.

91. Chan KF. Musculoskeletal pain clinic in Singapore—sacroiliac joint somatic dysfunction as cause of buttock pain. *Ann Acad Med Singapore*. 1998;27(1):112–115.

92. Slipman C, Patel P, Whyte W. Diagnosing and managing sacroiliac pain. *J Musculoskeletal Med*. 2001;18:325–332.

93. Fortin JD, April CN, Ponthieux B, Pier J. Sacroiliac joint: pain referral maps upon applying a new injection/arthrography technique. Part II: Clinical evaluation. *Spine*. 1994;19(13):1483–1489.

94. Fortin JD, Dwyer AP, West S, Pier J. Sacroiliac joint: pain referral maps upon applying a new injec-

tion/arthrography technique. Part I: Asymptomatic volunteers. *Spine.* 1994;19(13):1475–1482.

95. Broadhurst NA, Simmons DN, Bond MJ. Piriformis syndrome: Correlation of muscle morphology with symptoms and signs. *Arch Phys Med Rehabil.* 2004;85 (12):2036–2039.

96. Slipman C, Jackson H, Lipetz J. Sacroiliac joint pain referral zones. *Arch Phys Med Rehab.* 2000;81: 334–338.

97. Young S, Aprill C, Laslett M. Correlation of clinical examination characteristics with three sources of chronic low back pain. *Spine J.* 2003;3(6):460–465.

98. Jensen M, Brant-Zawadzki M, Obuchowski N, Modic M, Malka S, Ross J. Magnetic resonance imaging of the lumbar spine in people without back pain. *New England J Med.* 1994;331:69–73.

99. Dieck GS, Kelsey JL, Goel VK, Panjabi MM, Walter SD, Laprade MH. An epidemiologic study of the relationship between postural asymmetry in the teen years and subsequent back and neck pain. *Spine.* 1985;10(10):872–877.

100. Snijders C, Hermans P, Niesing R, Spoor C, Stoekart R. The influence of slouching and lumbar support on iliolumbar ligaments, intervertebral discs, and sacroiliac joints. *Clin Biomech.* 2004;19: 323–329.

101. Snijders C, Bakker M, Vleeming A, Stoeckart R, Stam H. Oblique abdominal muscle activity in standing and in sitting on hard and soft seats. *Clin Biomech.* 1995;10:73–78.

102. Laslett M. Keynote address. Annual conference of the *American Academy of Orthopaedic Manual Physical Therapists.* Reno, NV. 2003.

103. Potter NA, Rothstein JM. Intertester reliability for selected clinical tests of the sacroiliac joint. *Phys Ther.* 1985;65(11):1671–1675.

104. Levangie P. The association between static pelvic asymmetry and low back pain. *Spine.* 1999;24(12): 1234–1242.

105. Walker JM. The sacroiliac joint: a critical review. *Phys Ther.* 1992;72(12):903–916.

106. Cibulka MT, Aslin K. How to use evidence-based practice to distinguish between three different patients with low back pain. J Orthop Sports *Phys Ther.* 2001;31(12):678–688.

107. Laslett M, Aprill C, McDonald B, Young S. Diagnosis of sacroiliac joint pain: validity of individual provocation tests and composites of tests. *Man Ther.* 2005;10:207–218.

108. Young S. Personal communication. March 17, 2005.

109. Smidt G, Wei S, McQuade K, Barakatt E, Sun T, Stanford W. Sacroiliac motion for extreme hip positions. A fresh cadaver study. *Spine.* 1997;15: 2073–2082.

110. Pollard H, Ward G. The effect of upper cervical or sacroiliac manipulation on hip flexion range of

motion. *J Manipulative Physiol Ther.* 1998;21(9): 611–616.

111. Winkle D. Diagnosis and Treatment of the Spine: *Nonoperative orthopaedic medicine and manual therapy.* Denver, CO: Aspen Publishing: 1996.

112. Moore M. *Diagnosis and surgical treatment of chronic painful sacroiliac dysfunction.* In: Vleeming A, Mooney V, Dorman T, Snijders C. Second interdisciplinary world congress on low back pain. San Diego, CA, 9–11 November.

113. Ribeiro S, Prato-Schmidt A, van der Wurff P. sacroiliac dysfunction. *Acta Orthop Bras.* 2003;11: 118–125.

114. van der Wurff P, Meyne W, Hagmeijer RH. Clinical tests of the sacroiliac joint. *Man Ther.* 2000;5(2): 89–96.

115. Laslett M, Williams M. The reliability of selected pain provocation tests for sacroiliac joint pathology. *Spine.* 1994;19(11):1243–1249.

116. Kokmeyer DJ, Van der Wurff P, Aufdemkampe G, Fickenscher TC. The reliability of multitest regimens with sacroiliac pain provocation tests. *J Manipulative Physiol Ther.* 2002;25(1):42–48.

117. Mens J, Vleeming A, Snijders C, Koes B, Stam H. Validity of the active straight leg test for measuring disease severity in patients with posterior pelvic pain after pregnancy. *Spine.* 2002;27:196–200.

118. Levangie PK. Four clinical tests of sacroiliac joint dysfunction: the association of test results with innominate torsion among patients with and without low back pain. *Phys Ther.* 1999;79(11):1043–1057.

119. Riddle DL, Freburger JK. Evaluation of the presence of sacroiliac joint region dysfunction using a combination of tests: a multicenter intertester reliability study. *Phys Ther.* 2002;82(8):772–781.

120. Meijne W, van Neerbos K, Aufdemkampe G, van der Wurff P. Intraexaminer and interexaminer reliability of the Gillet test. *J Manipulative Physiol Ther.* 1999;22:4–9.

121. Bowman C, Gribbe R. The value of the forward flexion test and three tests of leg length changes in the clinical assessment of the movement of the sacroiliac joint *J Orthopaedic Med.* 1995;17:66–67.

122. Carmichael J. Inter- and intra-examiner reliability of palpation for sacroiliac joint dysfunction. *J Manipulative Physiol Therapeutics.* 1987;10:164–171.

123. Mens JM, Vleeming A, Snijders CJ, Ronchetti I, Stam HJ. Reliability and validity of hip adduction strength to measure disease severity in posterior pelvic pain since pregnancy. *Spine.* 2002;27(15): 1674–1679.

124. Ostgaard H, Andersson G. Previous back pain and risk of developing back pain in future pregnancy. *Spine.* 1991;16:432–436.

125. Blower P, Griffin A. (abstract). Clinical sacroiliac tests in ankylosing spondylitis and other causes of

low back pain-2 studies. *Annales of Rheumatic Disorders.* 1984;43:192–195.

126. Russell A, Maksymovich W, LeClerq S. Clinical examination of the sacroiliac joints: A prospective study. *Arthritis Rheumatism.* 1981;24:1575–1577.

127. McCombe P, Fairbank J, Cockersole B, Pynesent P. Reproducibility of physical signs in low back pain. *Spine.* 1989;14:908–917.

128. Strender L, Sjoblom A, Sundell K, Ludwig R, Taube A. Interexaminer reliability in physical examination of patients with low back pain. *Spine.* 1997;22: 814–820.

129. Van Deursen L, Oatijn J, Ockhuysen A, Vortman B (abstract). The value of some clinical tests of the sacroiliac joint. *Man Med.* 1990;5:96–99.

130. Fritz JM. How to use evidence-based practice to distinguish between three different patients with low back pain. *J Orthop Sports Phys Ther.* 2001;31(12): 689–695.

131. George S, Delitto A. Clinical examination variables discriminate among treatment-based classification groups: a study of construct validity in patients with acute low back pain. *Phys Ther.* 2005;85(4):306–314.

132. Dreyfuss P, Dreyer SJ, Cole A, Mayo K. Sacroiliac joint pain. *J Am Acad Orthop Surg.* 2004;12:255–265.

133. Albert H. Personal Communication. March 28, 2005.

134. Albert H, Godskesen M, Westergaard J. Prognosis in four syndromes of pregnancy-related pelvic pain. *Acta Obstet Gynecol Scand.* 2001;80(6):505–510.

135. Michaelsen M. Manipulation under joint anesthesia/analgesia: a proposed interdisciplinary treatment approach for recalcitrant spinal axis pain of synovial joint region. *J Manipulative Physiol Ther.* 2000;23: 127–129.

136. Flynn T, Fritz J, Whitman J, Wainner R, Magel J, Rendeiro D, Butler B, Garber M, Allison S. A clinical prediction rule for classifying patients with low back pain who demonstrate short-term improvement with spinal manipulation. *Spine.* 2002;27: 2835–2843.

137. Flynn T, Fritz J, Wainner R, Whitman J. The audible pop is not necessary for successful spinal high-velocity thrust manipulation in individuals with low back pain. *Arch Phys Med Rehabil.* 2003;84: 1057–1067.

138. Beffa R, Mathews R. Does the adjustment cavitate the targeted joint? An investigation into the location of cavitation sounds. *J Manipulative Physiol Ther.* 2004;27:e2.

139. Tullberg T, Blomberg S, Branth B, Johnsson R. Manipulation does not alter the position of the sacroiliac joint. A roentgen stereophotogrammetric analysis. *Spine.* 1988;23:1124–1128.

140. Murphy B, Dawson N, Slack J. Sacroiliac joint manipulation decreases the H-reflex. *Electromyogr Clin Neurophysiol.* 1995;35:87–94.

141. Childs JD, Fritz JM, Flynn TW, Irrgang JJ, Johnson KK, Majkowski GR, Delitto A. A clinical prediction rule to identify patients with low back pain most likely to benefit from spinal manipulation: a validation study. *Ann Intern Med.* 2004;141(12):920–928.

142. Cyriax JH. *Textbook of orthopaedic medicine.* 11th ed. London: Baillière Tindall, 1984.

143. Bernard TN, Cassidy JD. The sacroiliac joint syndrome, pathophysiology, diagnosis, and management. In: Frymoyer JW, eds. *The adult spine: Principles and practice.* 2nd ed. Philadelphia. Lippincott-Raven, 1997:2343–2366.

144. Dontigny RL. Anterior dysfunction of the sacroiliac joint as a major factor in the etiology of idiopathic low back pain syndrome. *Phys Ther.* 1990;70: 250–265.

145. Mitchell FL Jr, Moran PS, Pruzzo NA. *An evaluation and treatment: Manual of osteopathic muscle energy techniques.* Valley Park, MO: Mitchell, Moran and Pruzzo Associates, 1979.

146. Hertling D. The sacroiliac joint and the lumbar-pelvic-hip complex. In: Hertling D, Kessler RM, eds. *Management of common musculoskeletal disorders: Physical therapy principles and methods.* 3rd ed. Philadelphia: JB Lippincott Co, 1990.

147. Galm R, Frohling M, Rittmeister M, Schmitt E. Sacroiliac joint dysfunction in patients with imaging-proven lumbar disc herniation. *Eur Spine J.* 1998;7(6):450–453.

148. Lee K, Carlini W, McCormick G, Albers G. Neurologic complications following chiropractic manipulation: a survey of California neurologists. *Neurology.* 1995;45:1213–1215.

149. Lukban J, Whitmore K, Kellogg-Spadt S, Bologna R, Lesher A, Fletcher E. The effect of manual physical therapy in patients diagnosed with interstitial cystitis, high-tone pelvic floor dysfunction, and sacroiliac dysfunction. *Urology.* 2001;57(6 Suppl (1):121–122.

150. Suter E, McMorland G, Herzog W, Bray R. Decrease in quadriceps inhibition after sacroiliac joint manipulation in patients with anterior knee pain. *J Manipulative Physiol Ther.* 1999;22:149–153.

151. Kokjohn K, Schmid D, Triano JJ, Brennan P. The effect of spinal manipulation on pain and prostaglandin levels in women with primary dysmenorrhea. *J Manipulative Physiol Ther.* 1992;15:279–285.

152. Fickel TE. 'Snapping hip' and sacroiliac sprain: example of a cause–effect relationship. *J Manipulative Physiol Ther.* 1989;12(5):390–392.

153. Stuge B, Hilde G, Vollestad N. Physical therapy for pregnancy-related low back and pelvic pain: a systematic review. *Acta Obstet Gynecol Scand.* 2003;82: 983–990.

154. Mens JM, Snijders CJ, Stam HJ. Diagonal trunk muscle exercises in peripartum pelvic pain: a randomized clinical trial. *Phys Ther.* 2000;80(12):1164–1173.

155. Depledge P, McNair P, Keal-Smith C, Williams M. Management of symphysis pubis dysfunction during pregnancy using exercise and pelvic support belts. *Phys Ther.* 2005;85:1290–1300.

# 13

# Manual Therapy of the Hip

## Objectives

- Identify the pertinent structures and biomechanics of the hip.
- Demonstrate the appropriate and responsive hip examination sequence.
- Identify plausible mobilization and manual therapy treatment techniques.
- Discuss the effect of mobilization and manual therapy on recovery for hip patients in randomized trials.

## PREVALENCE

There are numerous forms of hip-related pathologies including conditions such as tendonitis, osteoarthritis, osteoporosis, bursitis, and hip fractures. Pathological conditions of the hip result from degeneration and/or trauma. There does seem to be a relationship between age and the incidence of a hip pathology, although trauma is commonly associated with injuries such as **hip labrum** tears.[1]

The most common form of hip pathology encountered by manual therapists is osteoarthritis. In previous studies, manual therapists have demonstrated success in treating osteoarthritis of the knee.[2,3] Although the majority of adults at 55 years of age show radiographic evidence of osteoarthritis, the actual diagnostic standings for a definitive prevalence and incidence rate of hip osteoarthritis is rarely agreed upon.[4] By age 75 approximately 80% of individuals have radiographic evidence of osteoarthritis,[5] although radiographic evidence does not directly relate to severity of pain. In an 8-year longitudinal study showed within that time span approximately 13% of women underwent a total joint replacement for corresponding symptoms.[6]

There is a very high relationship between osteoporosis and hip fracture, affecting nearly 8.2 persons per 1,000 annually.[7] In 1996, there were 340,000 hospitalizations for hip fractures among individuals who were 65 years or older, an increase of 23% during the 10-year period; nearly 80% of these were women.[8]

### Summary
- The most common form of hip dysfunction is osteoarthritis, which affects nearly 80% of individuals by the age of 75 years.
- Osteoporosis can lead to hip fractures and hospitalization for older individuals.

## ANATOMY

### The Joint

The hip or coxafemoral joint includes the concave acetabulum of the innominate of the pelvis and the head of the femur.[9] Structurally, the hip is a very stable joint supported by one of the strongest ligament systems in the body and a very deep acetabulum. Further stability is added by the contribution of the fibrocartilaginous acetabular labrum,[9] which deepens the acetabulum for greater congruency. The semi-circular-shaped acetabular labrum is a fibrocartilaginous rim that attaches to the outer border of the acetabulum, an element that decreases the friction of the joint surfaces.[10] The transverse ligament completes the "circle" of the labrum and functions as an attachment site for the ligamentum teres. The labrum is much thicker medially, superiorly, and posteriorly than anteriorly, thus predisposing the anterior labrum to tears. The joint capsule attaches to the labrum, is integrated with the ligamentous structures, and has an attachment to the rectus femoris muscle.[10]

The hip is unlike the shoulder in the fact that the amount of accessory motion outside of distraction is minimal.[11] Normal arthrokinematic movements such as those associated with glide and slide are finite, a consequence of structure and function.

## Osseous Structures

Four bones make up the coxofemoral joint: (1) the femur, (2) the pubis, (3) the ischium, and (4) the ilium. The innominate bones are composed of the ilium, the pubis, and the ischium. The ilium is the superior-most osseous structure of the innominate that forms the articulation with the sacrum and two-fifths of the surface of the acetabulum.[12] The pubis is the inferomedial aspect of the innominate and constitutes one-fifth of the articulation with the acetabulum of the hip. The ischium is the inferolateral aspect of the innominate that provides the floor of the acetabulum and the posterior two-fifths of the articular surface of the acetabulum rim. The acetabulum is covered in hyaline cartilage.

The femur is a very large and stable long bone that is further subdivided into the head, neck, and trochanteric regions. The spherical head is directed cranially and medially, and slightly anterior. The surface of the head of the femur is covered with hyaline cartilage for smooth contact with the acetabulum. The neck of the femur connects the head of the femur with the shaft and is angled about 125 degrees in an adult. Over time during growth, the angle decreases and varies greatly among individuals.

The trochanteric region includes the greater and lesser trochanters, attachment sites for several muscles of the hip region. The greater trochanter is situated lateral and posterior and is caudal to the neck of the femur. The tendons of the gluteus medius, and to some extent the gluteus maximus, inserts on the lateral aspect of the greater trochanter that also serves as the location for the intertrochanteric bursae. The medial aspect is the attachment site for the tendons of the obturator externus, the obturator internus, the gemelli, the gluteus minimus, and the piriformis. The inferior aspect of the medial greater trochanter gives origin to the upper part of the vastus lateralis. The lesser trochanter serves as the insertion site for the iliacus and the psoas major.[13]

## Ligaments and Capsule

There are several major ligaments of the hip (Figure 13.1), the most prominent being the **Y ligament of Bigelow.** The Y ligament of Bigelow provides anterior ligamentous support and originates from the anterior inferior iliac spine of the pelvis and attaches to the intertrochanteric line of the femur. The ligament was given the name "Y" because the bifurcation of the two ligaments looks like an inverted Y. The ligaments support the anterior aspect of the capsule and provide stabilization against excessive extension-based movements. The Y ligament of Bigelow is considered the strongest single ligament within the body.

The pubofemoral ligament connects the pubic ramus to the intertrochanteric line and limits abduction while providing some extension support.[14] The ligament extends across the antero-inferior aspect of the joint to blend with the iliolumbar ligament. Because of the orientation of the fibers, the ligament also assists in preventing excess abduction.[14] This ligament reinforces the hip capsule and adds to the strength during end range movements.

The ischiofemoral ligament, the thinnest of the hip ligaments, extends from the posterior acetabular rim to the inner surface of the greater trochanter of the femur.[14] Primarily, the ligament stabilizes the hip in full extension. Like the iliolumbar ligament and the pubofemoral ligament, the ischiofemoral ligament is tightened during internal rotation and reinforces the hip capsule.

The ligamentum teres is a flat, triangular-shaped ligament that arises from the base of the transverse acetabular ligament of the acetabulum and inserts into the head of the femur. In conjunction with the hip capsule, the ligamentum teres limits functional distraction of the hip joint, and may have some stabilizing effect. The ligament is tensioned when the thigh is semi-flexed, adducted, or externally rotated, and is relaxed when the limb is abducted. The teres ligament provides a conduit for the medial and lateral circumflex arteries and supplies the femur with blood and nutrients.

The hip capsule is fibrous and encloses the hip joint. The anterior attachment sites include the acetabulum and the neck of the femur at the intertrochanteric line. Posteriorly, the lateral aspect of the femoral neck is extracapsular and medial. The posterior capsule is attached to the acetabulum and pubic ramis. The anterior ligament, which arises above the ASIS and adjacent to the acetabulum, reinforces the capsule with a component of the iliofemoral ligament and the aforementioned ischiofemoral and pubofemoral ligaments. The contribution of the ligaments to the capsule often tightens the ligament during extension and occasionally during internal rotation.

## Muscles

The largest forces at the hip are a result of muscular contraction,[15] specifically those required during single leg stance. Crowninshield and Brand[16] report that an activity such as the single leg stance, in which the ipsilateral gluteus medius is forced to contract to stabilize the pelvis, leads to compression forces three to four times the body weight. Others have projected the force at six times the person's body weight.[9]

Dividing the muscle into regions more effectively aids in describing the multiple muscles of the hip. The regions are subdivided into the anterior, medial, lateral, and posterior musculature. The anterior musculature includes the rectus femoris, sartorius, and the iliopsoas group. Medially, the musculature consists of the adductor group, the pectineus and the gracilis. Numerous muscles comprise the lateral musculature of the hip, including the gluteus medius, tensor fasciae latae (TFL), piriformis, quadratus

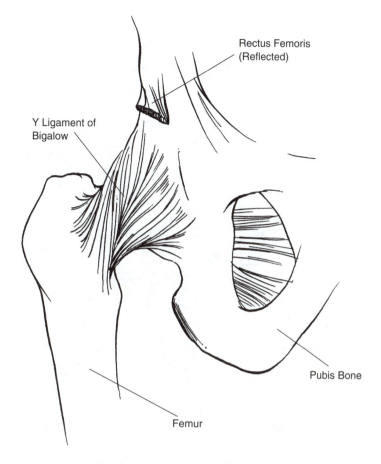

Rectus Femoris
(Reflected)

Y Ligament of
Bigalow

Pubis Bone

Femur

**Figure 13.1**    The Ligaments of the Hip

femoris, obturator internus, obturator externus, gemellus superior, and gemellus inferior. Lastly, the posterior muscles include the primary muscle group responsible for hip extension such as the gluteus maximus and hamstrings. Table 13.1 outlines the functions of these muscles.[17,18]

## *Bursae*

Primarily there are four bursae at the hip (Figure 13.2). Two bursae are of special interest since these bursae are commonly involved in pathology. The trochanteric bursa is located on the side of the hip near the posterior aspect

**TABLE 13.1**    The Muscles of the Hip

| Location | Muscle | Function |
|---|---|---|
| Anterior | Sartorius | Hip flexion, abduction, and external rotation |
| | Rectus femoris | Hip flexion and knee extension |
| | Psoas major | Hip flexion and lumbar compression |
| | Iliacus | Hip flexion |
| Posterior | Gluteus maximus | Hip extension |
| | Hamstrings | Hip extension and knee flexion |
| Medial | Gracilis | Primarily hip adduction |
| | Hip adductor group | Hip adduction |
| Lateral | Gluteus medius | Hip abduction and pelvic stabilization during unilateral stance |
| | Gluteus minimus | Hip abduction |

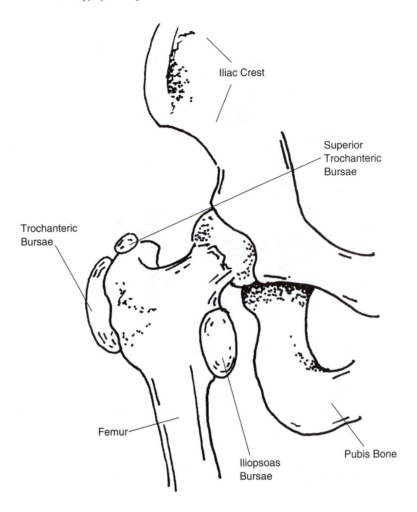

**Figure 13.2**   Anterior and Lateral Bursae of the Hip

### *Summary*

- The hip joint consists of the femur, the three bones that make up the innominate, and the surrounding ligaments and muscles.
- The hip joint is a deep-set ball and socket joint that sacrifices mobility for stability.
- The capsular-ligamentous system of the hip creates the most stable synovial joint system within the body.
- Of the numerous muscles that surround the hip, two primary stabilizers, the gluteus medius and the gluteus maximus, play a considerable role during gait and function.

of the greater tubercle. The trochanteric bursa normally functions to increase lubrication of the hip abductors, but when pathological, may cause a dull, burning pain on the outer hip that is worsened with abduction or squatting. The ischial bursa (not pictured) is located in the posterior buttock region and lies over the ischial tuberosity. The ischial bursa may cause dull pain in the buttock region that is most noticeable climbing uphill and is generally worsened during sitting, specifically in firm-seated chairs.[13]

## Biomechanics

Cyriax[19] and Kaltenborn[20] outlined the existence of a **capsular pattern** during early stages of osteoarthritis and other forms of hip capsule trauma. Cyriax[19] proposed the loss of internal rotation typically proceeded flexion, abduction, then extension, and that external rotation loss was rare. He and Kaltenborn,[20] as well as other manual therapy disciplines, have advocated the use of capsular patterns for both examination and treatment. These theories were based on clinical experience and "perception" versus experimental analyses.

Recently, two experimental studies[21,22] have refuted the existence of a definable hip capsular pattern, suggesting that the existence of a single capsular pattern in patients with early or progressive stages of osteoarthritis does not exist.

Others have also reported gross range-of-motion losses, nonpatterned in external and internal rotation, as well as abduction in osteoarthritis conditions.[23] Based on these findings, examination and treatment based on capsular pattern could provide inconsistent, unreliable, and subsequently invalid results. Although the use of a capsular pattern has been documented as helpful in a series of case studies, this method is excluded as a component of this chapter since it appears highly variable. Additionally, even though occasional range-of-motion variations (i.e., internal range-of-motion loss with osteoarthritis) provide some benefit during examination for selected pathologies, this pattern appears to lack reliability to overlay all like-type disorders.

Using the NHANES database, Roach and Miles[24] reported normative values for the combined age groups of 25 through 74. The following values of 121 degrees of hip flexion, 19 degrees of hip extension, 42 degrees of hip abduction, 32 degrees of internal rotation, and 32 degrees of external rotation closely reflect those of Hoppenfeld,[25] but differ from those of Kendall et al.[26] and Daniels and Worthingham.[27] What was interesting regarding the findings was that the values associated with all ranges declined with age, although those with hip flexion declined only minimally.

Along with planar movements, the hip can also move in combined motions of circumduction, which is a movement combination of variations of plane-based motions. The benefit of combined motions during examination and treatment is that the structures assume a more compromised and tightened position and may provide more discriminatory results. Specifically, combined movements should be examined if no mechanically based painful findings are extracted from the initial examination.

## *Summary*

- Little evidence exists to support Cyriax's theory of capsular pattern. To date, there are no studies that have verified a consistent pattern of range-of-motion loss at the hip.
- Roach and Miles outlined the following normative values for range of motion at the hip: 121 degrees of hip flexion, 19 degrees of hip extension, 42 degrees of hip abduction, 32 degrees of internal rotation, and 32 degrees of external rotation.

# ASSESSMENT AND DIAGNOSIS

Effective clinical examination of the hip requires differentiation of causal pain originators from other structures such as the lumbar spine, pelvis, and in some occasions the knee. Often, the location, frequency, and pattern of pain closely represent that of lumbar spine or pelvic origin. Although there is considerable overlap, most pain-reproducing procedures of the hip demonstrate pain of intraarticular origin and often exhibit symptoms in the groin with occasional radiation to the knee (Figure 13.3).[28,29] Thigh and buttock pain and pain that refers below the knee is *generally* associated with structures of the low back or pelvis, not the hip.[28] Nonetheless, documented situations in which hip pain caused radiating pain below the knee and pain into the back have occurred.[30]

Recently, Brown et al.[30] outlined significant signs and symptoms that differentiated low back and hip pain for diagnostic clarity. The authors reported that for a hip-only diagnosis (hip pain and no low back pain), limited internal rotation, groin pain, and/or a limp during gait were positive predictors of a hip-only origin. The absence of a short leg, decreased range of motion, and a negative femoral nerve stress test (prone knee flexion) were negatively associated with a hip-only diagnosis. In other words, common examination methods such as leg length, range-of-motion losses, and the femoral nerve stress test were less likely to implicate the hip as the causal factor, thus suggesting the origin is from another structure. Examination items such as a lumbar "list," pain on internal rotation, an antalgic limp, and weakness were not discriminatory predictors of hip versus back pain.

Lauder[31] produced one of the most comprehensive discussions of pain patterns associated with various forms of hip dysfunction in 2002. She reported that disorders of the hip frequently mimic lumbar dysfunction from L1 to L3. Additionally, pain from trochanteric bursitis may refer to the buttock and slightly anterior to the bursae, occasionally resulting in leg parathesia.[32] Often low back pain and trochanteric bursitis are concurrently reported, although not directly related (Lauder 2002).

## Subjective Considerations

### *Observation*

Sims[15] recommends a comprehensive lower extremity observational assessment to determine abnormalities of the hip. He suggests that excessive motions at other joints, most notably the foot, could affect the hip. Additionally, visual cues such as decreased stance time or lurching toward the affected hip during the stance phase are signs of an antalgic gait.[33]

Although visual markers such as Q-angle are controversially associated with knee problems, no studies outline a relationship with potential for hip pain. Loss of passive extension during standing is indicative of age-related posture and is sometimes associated with osteoarthritis and low back pain. Although obesity is not directly associated with hip bursitis, the relationship has been suggested in a single case study.[34]

### *Behavior of Pain*

Groin pain is typically associated with intraarticular hip conditions such as capsulitis, chondritis, and osteoarthritis.

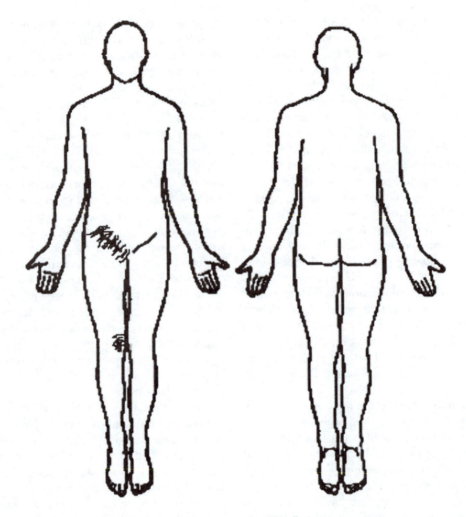

**Figure 13.3**    Pain Drawing of Intraarticular Hip Pain

In all three of these conditions, referral of pain to the anterior medial knee and lateral knee are commonly reported.[30] Lateral, pinpoint hip pain is generally associated with trochanteric bursitis.[31] Often, pain worsens upon weight bearing or inactivity for intraarticular pain and worsens with compression or stretching in extraarticular conditions such as trochanteric bursitis.[35]

### Gait

One of the six determinants of gait, the controlled lateral shift of the center of gravity, is a function of the hip musculature, specifically the hip abductors.[36] Additionally, pelvic rotation is designed to lengthen the stride of an individual, improving economy by covering greater length with similar energy efforts. This process is designed to reduce the total energy expenditure in human locomotion, and is typically altered only when dysfunction is present. For optimum efficiency, these determinants require full extension, 30 degrees of flexion, at least 10 degrees of external rotation, and approximately 7 degrees of internal rotation. These movements are typical ranges found during joint play.[37] Severe damage to the hip that eliminates these movements can reduce the efficiency of gait up to 47%.[36] Subsequently, gait analysis may identify selected hip pathology, specifically when reports of problems with endurance during propulsion are prominent.

### Alignment

As stated in Chapter 11, variation in alignment of the hip and pelvis demonstrates very little diagnostic value. Levangie[38] found that leg length discrepancy, ASIS and PSIS bilateral comparisons, and iliac crest height determination presented diagnostic information that was actually more detrimental than beneficial.

Measuring leg length is used to conclude if predisposing biomechanical disadvantages may result in increased pain. Various leg length measures using a tape measure have demonstrated acceptable reliability when compared with radiographic methods.[39] A common method includes a measure from the inferior border of the greater trochanter to the inferior aspect of the medial malleolus (Figure 13.4). However, variable correlations to actual impairment or biomechanical dysfunctions exist and the clinician should be wary of direct cause-and-effect relationship.[40–42]

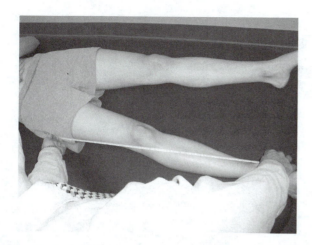

**Figure 13.4**    Leg Length Tape Measure: Greater Trochanter to Medial Malleolus

## Functional Scales

### Harris Hip Score

The *Harris Hip Score* is a disease-specific scale (osteoarthritis) containing eight items representing pain, walking, function, activities of daily living, and range of motion of the hip joint.[43] The scale has a numerical rating system from 0 to 100, in which pain and function receive the heaviest weighting (44 and 47 points).[44] The scale is not self-administered[44] and a value of below 70 is considered a poor score, indicative of problems. Scores from 70 to 80 are considered a fair score, 81 to 90 good, and 91 to 100 excellent. The instrument has been shown to be reliable,[45] and valid for use in various populations of hip injuries.[44] At present, the scale has been validated in German,[46] English, Dutch,[47] and Swedish.[48]

### WOMAC

The WOMAC is also a disease-specific scale, but is self-administered.[44,49–51] The index also contains specific domains such as pain, stiffness, and physical function, physical function having the highest weighting. The WOMAC has been shown to be valid and responsive for osteoarthritis conditions.[44] The instrument includes a Likert-type scale with a maximum score of 96. The WOMAC and Harris Hip scale are more responsive to change than generic scales such as the SF-36[52] and may be more effective in measuring change over time. Like the Harris Hip scale, the WOMAC has been validated in several languages including German and Dutch.[47,53]

### Lower Extremity Functional Scale

The Lower Extremity Function Scale (LEFS) is a region-specific scale but, unlike the WOMAC and the Harris Hip score, is not limited to use with osteoarthritis. The LEFS is a self-report mechanism, primarily designed as a performance-based measure.[54] The LEFS is reliable (ICC = 0.95),[55] demonstrates construct validity, and is more sensitive to change than the SF-36.[56] The LEFS is a functional scale that can measure multiple joints[55] and can be used conjunctively with measures of pain and physical exertion.

## Summary

- Many of the pain distribution patterns exhibited by hip conditions are similar to those of the pelvis and lumbar spine.
- The most common pain distribution pattern of the hip is lateral hip pain and/or groin pain.
- A lurching gait and gluteus medius stance is indicative of either pain or osteoarthritis of the hip.
- Little evidence exists to support the use of alignment to identify selected hip dysfunction.
- Three functional scales are beneficial for hip assessment. Two of the scales, the WOMAC and the Harris Hip scale, are disease-specific instruments. The Lower Extremity Function Scale is nondisease specific and can be used on lower extremity joints outside the hip.

# CLINICAL EXAMINATION

## Active Movements

A relationship between hip range of motion, specifically internal rotation and low back dysfunction, has been suggested in the literature.[57] Flynn et al.[58] reported that the clinical prediction rule for identifying patients who benefit from manipulation was partially based on hip internal rotation findings of greater than 35 degrees. Sjoile[59] reported that low back pain in adolescents was related to decreased hip mobility in flexion and internal rotation. Vad et al.[60] reported a relationship between hip internal rotation and low back pain in professional golfers. Conversely, McConnell[61] proposes that limited hip extension and external rotation negatively affect the functional mobility of the lumbar spine.

## Active Physiological Movements

There are two methods of active physiological testing. One method involves the planar movement of the hip to ascertain the effects of active movement on selected directions. The second involves **functional testing** to determine which functional activities most closely reproduce the concordant sign of the patient. It is rare that both methods are required during a general examination.

## Supine Hip Flexion

Hip flexion requires the contractile capability of the anterior hip musculature and causes concurrent tension on the posterior structures of the hip.[62] Injuries to the hamstrings or posterior hip structures are often reported as pain during end range hip flexion.[62] Others have reported that the loss of a complete hip flexion arc is commonly associated with patients diagnosed with hip pathology.[63]

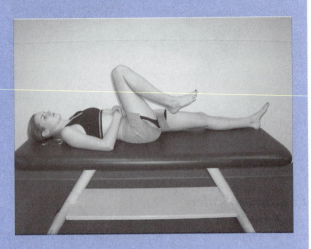

- Step One: The patient lies supine. Resting symptoms are assessed.
- Step Two: The patient is instructed to raise his or her hip into flexion to the first point of pain.
- Step Three: The patient is instructed to move beyond the first point of pain toward end range.
- Step Four: Upon completion, pain is reassessed for the concordant sign.

**Figure 13.5**   Supine Hip Flexion

## Sidelying Hip Abduction

Active sidelying abduction may be painful in conditions such as a gluteus medius tear, trochanteric bursitis, and abductor tendinopathy.[64] Weaknesses in active range of motion are found concurrently with **Trendelenburg's sign** and during gait deviations that demonstrate a limp. Commonly, patients attempt to compensate for hip weakness by substituting the hip flexors during a request for hip abduction movements.

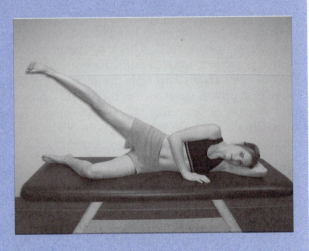

- Step One: The patient lies in sidelying. Resting symptoms are assessed.
- Step Two: The patient is instructed to raise his or her non-plinth-sided lower extremity to the first point of pain (in abduction).
- Step Three: The patient is instructed to move beyond the first point of pain toward end range.
- Step Four: Upon completion, pain is reassessed for the concordant sign.

**Figure 13.6**   Sidelying Hip Abduction

## Sidelying Hip Adduction

Pain with hip adduction may be associated with adductor tendonitis, pelvic instability, or a pubic rami fracture. Because the movement is not wholly discriminative for ruling in a pelvic instability, the movement should never be used in isolation.

- Step One: The patient lies in sidelying. Resting symptoms are assessed.
- Step Two: The patient is instructed to raise his or her plinth-sided lower extremity into hip adduction to the first point of pain.
- Step Three: The patient is instructed to move beyond the first point of pain toward end range.
- Step Four: Upon completion, pain is reassessed for the concordant sign.

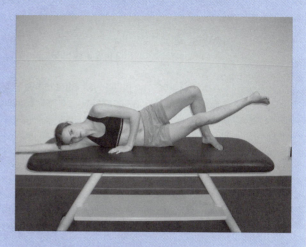

**Figure 13.7**  Sidelying Hip Adduction

## Prone Hip Extension

Perry et al.[65] suggest that the prone extension position more accurately isolates hip extension musculature and advocate this position for testing of extensor muscles. Findings have shown that hip extension loss is related to increased risk for falls, low back pain, and capsular range-of-motion losses in the hip. Hip extension loss is purported to be a cause of altered lumbopelvic rhythm and lower quarter dysfunction.[66]

- Step One: The patient lies prone. Resting symptoms are assessed.
- Step Two: The patient is instructed to raise his or her lower extremity into hip extension to the first point of pain.
- Step Three: The patient is instructed to move beyond the first point of pain toward end range.
- Step Four: Upon completion, pain is reassessed for the concordant sign.

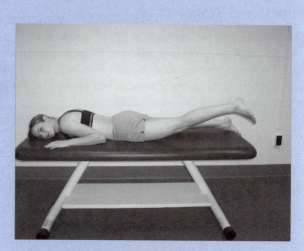

**Figure 13.8**  Prone Hip Extension

## Sitting Internal Rotation

Hip internal rotation measures are considered sensitive tools for assessing intraarticular symptoms.[67,68] Two studies have reported an association between diminished internal range of motion associated with the failure to improve from manipulation to the low back.[67,68] Pain during active internal rotation may result from placing tension on the active external rotators such as the piriformis.[69]

- Step One: The patient sits upright. Resting symptoms are assessed.
- Step Two: The patient is instructed to rotate his or her lower extremity internally to the first point of pain.
- Step Three: The patient is instructed to move beyond the first point of pain toward end range.
- Step Four: Upon completion, pain is reassessed for the concordant sign.

## Sitting External Rotation

Sitting external rotation requires the contraction of the external rotators such as the piriformis. Although rarely linked to dysfunction, the sitting external rotation motion is generally thought of as extracapsular tightness and may implicate extraarticular structures more so than intraarticular. Although it would seem that active external rotation would elicit pain in some conditions such as a gluteus medius tear, no studies have confirmed or supported this assumption.

- Step One: The patient sits upright. Resting symptoms are assessed.
- Step Two: The patient is instructed to rotate his or her lower extremity externally to the first point of pain.
- Step Three: The patient is instructed to move beyond the first point of pain toward end range.
- Step Four: Upon completion, pain is reassessed for the concordant sign.

## Functional Tests

Functional tests are commonly called **quick tests**[70] and are designed to provide a glimpse of pain provocation with various activities. Additionally, functional tests may be helpful in serving as the concordant movement for examination and reexamination of the patient.

### *Summary*

- Pain during active range of motion of the hip is indicative of selected dysfunctions and may prove useful during collection of data.
- Functional testing of the hip can serve as a baseline measure or may reproduce pain during combined movements.

## Deep Squat

A deep squat may be effective in determining the contribution of posterior extraarticular hip structures such as the gluteus maximus, or, if pain is reproduced anteriorly, may be associated with acetabular impingement syndrome. In patients with an antalgic gait, the load and shift requirements of a deep squat may also reproduce intraarticular pain.

- Step One: The patient is asked to stand. Resting symptoms are assessed.
- Step Two: movement is painful, the clinician should determine if the movement is concordant.
- Step Three: The patient is instructed to move beyond the first point of pain.
- Step Four: Symptoms are assessed to determine if the movement is concordant.

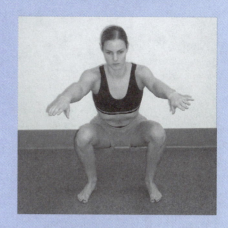

**Figure 13.9**    Deep Bilateral Squat

## Trendelenburg's Stance

Trendelenburg's stance is often used to evaluate weakness or pain in the hip abductors.[28] Weakness of the hip abductors has been linked to knee problems, iliotibial band syndrome, and gait and running abnormalities.[71] Patients with pain or weakness will demonstrate a dropping of the contralateral pelvis during unilateral stance.[28] This movement differs from a lumbar list, a visual finding that is frequently observed in patients with a lumbar dysfunction.

- Step One: The patient is instructed to stand. Resting symptoms are assessed.
- Step Two: The patient is instructed to stand on one leg, while bending the knee of the opposite leg.
- Step Three: The clinician should evaluate for opposite-sided (to the weight-bearing leg) pelvic drop and concordant symptoms on the weight-bearing leg.

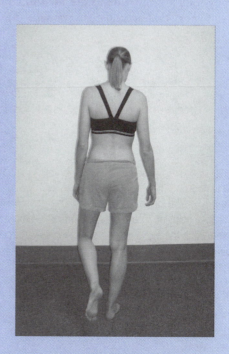

**Figure 13.10**    Trendelenburg's Stance

### Unilateral Step-Up

Arokoski et al.[23] found differences in the ability of symptomatic and asymptomatic patients in climbing stairs. The unilateral step-up also leads to compression forces three to six times the body weight of the individual; therefore, in the presence of intraarticular pain, this procedure may be very sensitive.[9]

- Step One: The patient is instructed to stand with one leg on a 4- to 8-inch step. The lower extremity that is on the step should continue to weight bear through the bent knee. Resting symptoms are assessed.
- Step Two: The patient is instructed to straighten the leg on the step, thus lifting the opposite lower extremity from the ground and eliminating weight bearing.
- Step Three: The clinician should evaluate the weight-bearing side for concordant symptoms.

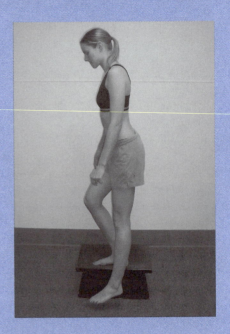

**Figure 13.11**    Unilateral Step Up

## Passive Movements

### *Passive Physiological Movements*

Passive physiological movements are used to confirm active physiological finding and to reproduce the concordant sign. These movements include the motions of abduction, adduction, flexion, internal rotation, external rotation, and extension.

### Abduction

Passive abduction may be restricted in patients with demonstrable osteoarthritis of the hip. Additionally, some evidence exists that lateral hip labrum tears may produce pain during passive contact of the femoral head to the lesion site of the hip.[73]

- Step One: The patient assumes a supine position. The clinician assesses resting symptoms.
- Step Two: The clinician passively glides the hip into abduction to the first point of reported pain. One hand blocks the pelvis just cephalic to the hip joint to prevent excessive lumbar motion. The clinician queries to determine if the pain is concordant.
- Step Three: The clinician passively moves the leg toward end range. Pain is again queried accordingly.
- Step Four: If no pain is present, the clinician applies an overpressure to rule out the specific passive movement of the joint.
- Step Five: Upon completion, resting symptoms are again assessed.

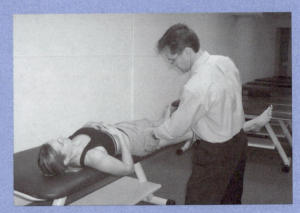

**Figure 13.12**    Passive Hip Abduction

## Adduction

Passive hip adduction, iliotibial band stretching, and other stretch-related maneuvers may reproduce symptoms in patients who experience trochanteric bursitis.[31] Rarely does passive hip adduction reproduce symptoms in patients with hip osteoarthritis.

- Step One: The patient assumes a supine position. The clinician assesses resting symptoms.
- Step Two: The clinician passively pulls the opposite hip into adduction to the first point of reported pain. One hand blocks the opposite knee of the patient to prevent excessive lumbar side flexion. The clinician queries to determine if the pain is concordant.
- Step Three: The clinician passively moves the leg toward end range. Pain is again queried accordingly.
- Step Four: If no pain is present, the clinician applies an overpressure to rule out that specific passive movement of the joint.
- Step Five: Upon completion, resting symptoms are again assessed.

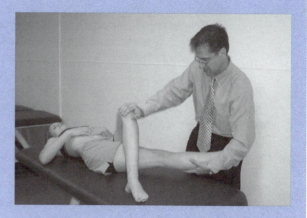

**Figure 13.13**    Passive Hip Adduction

## Flexion

There are numerous types of dysfunction associated with hip flexion. Lauder[31] reported that often ischial bursitis is reproduced with movements such as passive hip flexion along with resisted hip extension. Cyriax described the "sign of the buttock" as pain during hip flexion that is similar in range to pain during a straight leg raise. A positive "sign of the buttock" is indicative of a sinister pathology in the pelvis, hip, or lumbar spine. Greenwood et al.[72] have reported the benefit of the "sign of the buttock" during differentiation of hip and low back pain. Flexion is occasionally painful in patients with femoroacetabular impingement.

- Step One: The patient assumes a supine position. The clinician assesses resting symptoms.
- Step Two: The clinician passively lifts the hip into flexion to the first point of reported pain. The clinician queries to determine if the pain is concordant.
- Step Three: The clinician passively moves the leg toward end range. Pain is again queried accordingly.
- Step Four: If no pain is present, the clinician applies an overpressure to rule out the specific passive movement of the joint.
- Step Five: Upon completion, resting symptoms are again assessed.

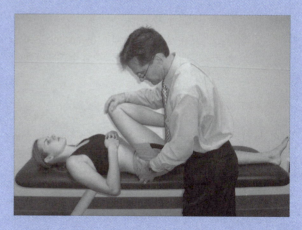

**Figure 13.14**    Passive Hip Flexion

## Internal Rotation

Like hip flexion, internal rotation has been linked with numerous hip-related pathologies.[74,75] Loss of internal rotation is a direct predictor of whether or not a patient with hip pain receives a total hip replacement in the future.[76] This finding is consistent with patients diagnosed with hip osteoarthritis and is strongly associated with hip pain and loss of joint space on an x-ray.[77] Internal rotation is also a criterion of osteoarthritis using the criteria developed by Altman et al.[78] Lastly, patients with piriformis syndrome may complain of reproduction of symptoms with end range passive internal rotation while the hip maintains an extended position.[79]

- Step One: The patient assumes a supine position. The clinician assesses resting symptoms.
- Step Two: The clinician passively cradles the lower leg below the knee and slowly internally rotates the hip to the first point of reported pain. The other hand squeezes the femur and provides a rotational movement in order to reduce the stress placed upon the knee. The clinician queries to determine if the pain is concordant.
- Step Three: The clinician passively moves the leg toward end range. Pain is again queried accordingly.
- Step Four: If no pain is present, the clinician applies an overpressure to rule out the targeted passive movement of the joint.
- Step Five: Upon completion, resting symptoms are again assessed.

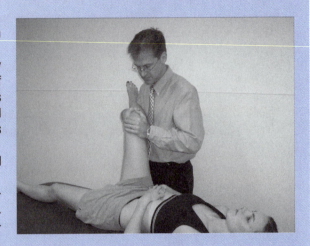

**Figure 13.15**    Passive Internal Rotation

## External Rotation

Arokoski et al. suggested a relationship between hip osteoarthritis and loss of passive external rotation. Additionally, external rotation is occasionally painful when the passive end range force is applied to internal rotator musculature.

- Step One: The patient assumes a supine position. The clinician assesses resting symptoms.
- Step Two: The clinician passively cradles the lower leg below the knee and slowly externally rotates the hip to the first point of reported pain. The other hand squeezes the tibia and provides a rotational movement in order to reduce the stress placed upon the knee. The clinician queries to determine if the pain is concordant.
- Step Three: The clinician passively moves the leg toward end range. Pain is again queried accordingly.
- Step Four: If no pain is present, the clinician applies an overpressure to rule out that specific passive movement of the joint.
- Step Five: Upon completion, resting symptoms are again assessed.

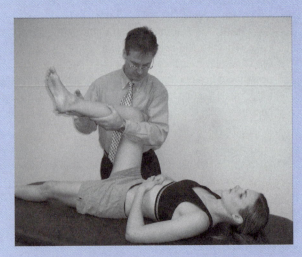

**Figure 13.16**    Passive External Rotation

### Hip Extension

Like active hip extension loss, passive hip extension restrictions are associated with capsular restrictions and long-term pain. Passive hip extension may place tension on the anterior aspect of the hip capsule and labrum, thus reproducing symptoms in that select population.

- Step One: The patient assumes a prone position. The clinician assesses resting symptoms.
- Step Two: The clinician passively lifts the hip into extension to the first point of reported pain. One hand blocks just cephalically to the hip joint to reduce the amount of lumbar extension that occurs with this procedure. The clinician queries to determine if the pain is concordant.
- Step Three: The clinician passively moves the leg toward end range. Pain is again queried accordingly.
- Step Four: If no pain is present, the clinician applies an overpressure to rule out that specific passive movement of the joint.
- Step Four: Upon completion, resting symptoms are again assessed.

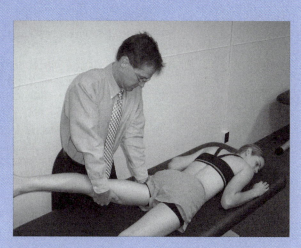

**Figure 13.17**    Passive Hip Extension

## *Passive Accessory Movements*

Kaltenborn[20] proposed that the close-packed position of the hip joint is extension, internal rotation, and slight abduction. Sims[15] suggested that accessory movement in the proposed "close-packed" position is highly limited. Furthermore, Williams[11] argues that no accessory motion exists even within the open-packed position.

### Anterior–Posterior Glide

An anterior–posterior glide of the hip may identify pain associated with cartilage compression and will most likely consist of very small movements.

- Step One: The patient assumes a sidelying position. The clinician assesses resting symptoms.
- Step Two: The clinician applies a passive glide of the hip joint using the thumb to lock anterior to the greater trochanter and the heel of the hand to apply the force to the thumb contact point.
- Step Three: The clinician passively moves toward a posterior direction. Any reproduction of pain that is concordant implicates this assessment method as a possible treatment technique.
- Step Four: Upon completion, resting symptoms are again assessed.

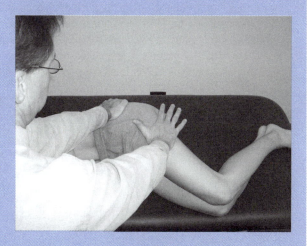

**Figure 13.18**    Anterior Posterior Glide

## Posterior–Anterior Glide

A posterior–anterior glide of the hip may identify pain associated with cartilage compression and represents very small movements.

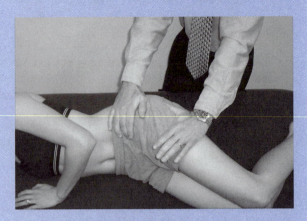

- Step One: The patient assumes a sidelying position. The clinician assesses resting symptoms.
- Step Two: The clinician applies a passive glide of the hip joint using the thumb to lock posterior to the greater trochanter and the heel of the hand to apply the force to the thumb contact point.
- Step Three: The clinician passively glides toward an anterior direction. Any reproduction of pain that is concordant implicates this assessment method as a possible treatment technique.
- Step Four: Upon completion, resting symptoms are again assessed.

**Figure 13.19**    Posterior Anterior Glide

## Sidelying Distraction

In cases where the patient's pain is significant, gentle techniques such as the sidelying distraction maneuver may be useful.

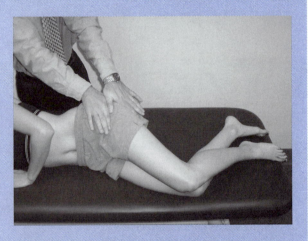

- Step One: The patient assumes a sidelying position lying on the asymptomatic side. The clinician assesses resting symptoms.
- Step Two: The clinician applies an inferior passive glide of the hip by using the web space of his or her hand. The contact point of the hip includes the surrounding tissue of the greater trochanter.
- Step Three: The clinician passively glides the extremity toward a caudal direction. If the patient's upper leg is placed anterior to the tableside leg, the force applied is more substantial. Any reproduction of pain that is concordant implicates this assessment method as a possible treatment technique.
- Step Four: Upon completion, resting symptoms are again assessed.

**Figure 13.20**    Sidelying Distraction

## Indirect Distraction

The indirect distraction method involves displacement of the knee and ankle as well as the hip. The technique has been shown to generate up to 200–600 Newtons of distraction force[37], which is required for distraction of the hip. Because more than one joint is distracted, indirect traction requires greater intensity during application than direct traction.

- Step One: The patient assumes a supine position. The clinician assesses resting symptoms.
- Step Two: The clinician queries the patient for a history of knee or ankle dysfunction that would contraindicate the use of this method. If none, the clinician cradles the ankle of the patient into both of his or her hands.
- Step Three: The clinician then takes up the slack to preposition the hip into targeted motion. Generally, resting position of the hip includes a moderate degree of flexion and abduction with slight external rotation.[37]
- Step Four: The clinician then provides an inferior force by leaning backward while holding the ankle.
- Step Five: Upon completion, resting symptoms are again assessed.

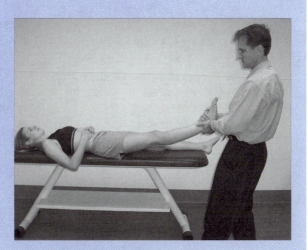

**Figure 13.21**    Indirect Distraction

## Direct Distraction

The direct distraction maneuver mimics the indirect method in application. This procedure, however, allows the majority of force to transfer through the hip joint.

- Step One: The patient assumes a supine position. The clinician assesses resting symptoms. A belt may be used to assist in the technique.
- Step Two: The clinician places the lower extremity over his or her shoulder. The clinician places his or hands (ulnar border) near the hip joint for an appropriate contact.
- Step Three: Using the shoulder as a fulcrum, the clinician pulls inferiorly with the hands at the hip and pushes cephalically with the shoulder for an inferior distraction. The clinician passively glides the joint toward the projected end range. Pain is again queried accordingly.
- Step Four: Upon completion, resting symptoms are again assessed.

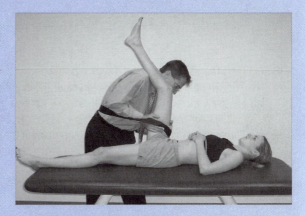

**Figure 13.22**    Direct Distraction

## Combined Movements

Maitland[70] advocates the use of combined movements, specifically if all other hip accessory and physiological movements are pain-free. Most combined movements are performed passively for improved efficiency and control. For the hip, combined movements typically include flexion and internal or external rotation, external rotation and abduction, or internal rotation and adduction. When a combined movement is initiated, the periarticular tissue such as the capsule and ligaments are taut and engaged more effectively than during lax positions. Adding compression and/or distraction further engages the tissue, thus sensitizing the examination method.

## Internal Rotation and Adduction

Internal rotation and adduction may increase the tension placed upon the capsule and ligaments and may provide greater stress during a mobilization or stretching method. Often, this movement is associated with pain in patients with hip osteoarthritis and/or synovitis.

- Step One: The patient assumes a supine position.
- Step Two: At 90 degrees of flexion, the clinician passively moves the hip into full internal rotation concurrently while applying an adduction force.
- Step Three: Symptoms are evaluated to determine if the movement produces a concordant response.

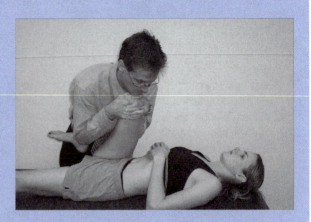

**Figure 13.23**   Internal Rotation, Adduction

## External Rotation, Flexion, and Abduction

DeAngelis and Busconi[28] suggest that the hip capsule is most lax in external rotation, flexion, and abduction, and report that the patient will often hold his or her hip into this combined movement when an inflammatory process is present.

- Step One: The patient assumes a supine position.
- Step Two: The hip is moved to 90 degrees of flexion, the clinician passively moves the hip into full external rotation concurrently while applying an abduction force.
- Step Three: Symptoms are evaluated to determine if the movement produces a concordant response.

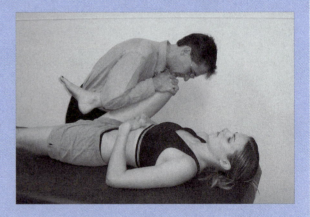

**Figure 13.24**   External Rotation, Flexion, and Abduction

## Summary

- Of the passive hip movements, the movements most often related to dysfunction include internal rotation, flexion, and occasionally external rotation.
- It is questionable whether passive accessory movements such as anterior-to-posterior and posterior-to-anterior glide create movement within the hip joint.
- Traction techniques generate the greatest amount of displacement at the hip.
- Combined movements may be effective in targeting capsular and ligamentous tissue by prepositioning in tightened positions.

## Clinical Special Tests

Unlike other body regions, few hip clinical special tests have been diagnostically validated. Less publication interest has been demonstrated on this topic, possibly since the findings are not as controversial as other body regions (i.e., SIJ, low back). Consequently, many of the clinical special tests lack testing and demonstrate unknown diagnostic value.

### Palpation

No studies were found that measured the reliability or validity of palpation of the hip. Selected authors[35,80,81] purport the benefit of palpation of the hip, primarily for ruling in or out trochanteric, hip flexor muscle pain, and ischial tuberosity bursitis. No studies were found that measured the sensitivity or specificity of palpation so the diagnostic value remains unknown.

### Muscle Testing

There are mixed findings regarding the benefit of muscle testing. Generally, the reliability of manual muscle testing at the hip is good for supine hip extensor strength testing.[65] Hip abduction yields variable results since the angle the hip is placed in may bias the results of the muscle assessment.[66] The use of an external tool such as a dynamometer may improve muscle testing.

### Diagnostic Testing

Common diagnostic tests of the hip include the Ober test, FABER test, Thomas test, prone hip extensor test, hip scour, and posterior hip labrum test.

### Ober Test

The Ober test was first described in 1936.[82] Typically, the test is used to measure the "tightness" of the iliotibial band (ITB). The Ober test was originally designed as a sidelying maneuver, in which the clinician moves the "knee-flexed, lower extremity" (the non-plinth-sided leg) from flexion to extension (at the hip), while stabilizing the pelvis. The adduction or abduction angle of the hip joint is measured with an inclinometer or a goniometer to determine the "length" of the ITB.[82] Nonetheless, there are varieties of described methods and none provides normative standards for scoring.[82] Gajdosik et al.[82] did find greater "tightness" of the lateral structures during knee flexed testing and provided normative values of six degrees of abduction for women and four degrees of abduction for men.

- Step One: The patient lies sidelying with the asymptomatic leg placed on the plinth side.
- Step Two: The clinician prepositions the knee into flexion.
- Step Three: The clinician then stabilizes the pelvis at the iliac crest.
- Step Four: The clinician then guides the lower extremity (at the hip) into extension.
- Step Five: Using a goniometer, the clinician then measures the degree of abduction or adduction.
- Step Six: A comparison of both sides is warranted.

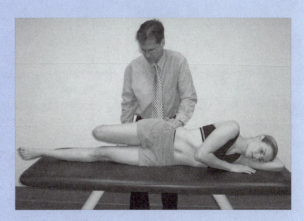

**Figure 13.25** The Ober Test

## FABER Test

The FABER test (flexion, abduction, external rotation) is a sensitive and specific test for determining range-of-motion loss with osteoarthritis.[83] For patients who display three planes of joint restriction (based on the **Altman criteria**), the sensitivity was 54% and the specificity was 88% (+LR = 4.4) for the FABER test. Mitchell et al.[29] also reported high specificity but lower sensitivity. The test is also used for detecting range losses in patients who have osteoarthritis and is differentiated from the sacroiliac joint by location of pain. The test is occasionally referred to as Patrick's test.

- Step One: The patient is positioned in supine. Resting symptoms are assessed.
- Step Two: The painful side leg is placed in a "figure four" position. The ankle is placed just above the knee of the other leg.
- Step Three: The clinician provides a gentle downward pressure on both the knee of the painful side and the ASIS of the nonpainful side. Concordant pain is assessed, specifically the location and type of pain.
- Step Four: A positive test is concordant pain that is lateral or anterior to the hip joint.

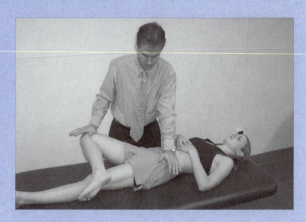

**Figure 13.26**    The FABER Test

## Thomas Test

The Thomas test was designed as a method to measure hip flexor or knee extensor tightness.[84] The original method proposed by Thomas involved pulling the asymptomatic hip into full flexion and measuring the amount of resultant extension of the opposite extremity. Staheli[85] claims that this test is flawed because lumbar extension can alter the position of the pelvis. Harvey[86] has modified the approach by applying a volitional posterior pelvic tilt during the test to ensure lumbar stability. Measurements are taken at both the hip and the knee to determine tightness in the iliopsoas and rectus femoris, respectively.

- Step One: The patient sits at the edge of the plinth. The patient is then instructed to roll back, pulling both knees to his or her chest.
- Step Two: One knee (the asymptomatic side) is held to the chest and the other is slowly lowered into extension of the hip. The knee is allowed to extend.
- Step Three: The patient is instructed to pull his or her pelvis into posterior rotation.
- Step Four: The clinician then measures the extension angle of the hip and/or the knee.

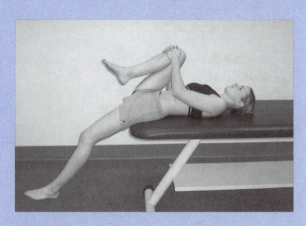

**Figure 13.27**    The Thomas Test

## Prone Hip Extensor Test

Staheli[85] suggested the use of the prone hip extensor test in lieu of the Thomas test for measurement of hip flexor structures. Because lumbar extension is still possible, the use of belts reduces the likelihood of unwanted extension by stabilizing the pelvis.

- Step One: The patient is instructed to lie prone.
- Step Two: The clinician then places two belts around the patient: one just distal to the PSIS, the other just proximal to the gluteal fold. A special effort to unencumber hip extension should be made.
- Step Three: The clinician then passively moves the hip into extension.
- Step Four: The extension angle at the hip is measured with a goniometer.

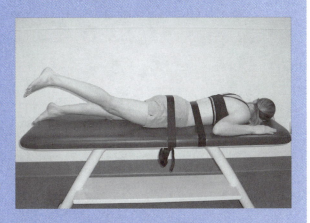

**Figure 13.28**    Prone Hip Extension Test

## Hip Scour

The hip scour, often called the hip quadrant[70] or flexion-internal rotation test,[87] is frequently used to identify hip labrum tears. Suenaga et al.[87] reported a sensitivity of 79% and a specificity of 50% (+LR = 1.5) with the internally rotated position of the hip scour and posterosuperior complete labral tears of the hip. Narvani et al.[1] reported a sensitivity of 75% and a specificity of 43% (+LR = 1.3). The authors suggested this method forces abutment of the femoral head upon the labrum tear, thus eliciting pain and apprehension of the patient.

- Step One: The patient assumes a supine position.
- Step Two: The clinician flexes the patient's knee, loads through the knee, then performs a sweeping compression and rotation from external rotation to internal rotation.
- Step Three: A positive test is pain or apprehension at a given point during the examination.

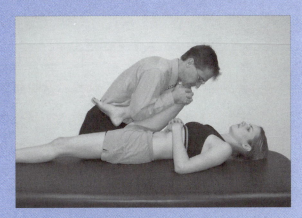

**Figure 13.29**    The Hip Scour

### Posterior Hip Labrum Test

Fitzgerald[88] reported that although rare, a posterior hip labrum tear is possible in patients who have incurred a traumatic event. The author noted that the clinical finding most notably associated with the operative verification was a clinical maneuver that involved concurrent extension and external rotation of the hip. Fitzgerald[88] did not report the sensitivity and specificity of the findings, but did note that nearly all of the patients who had a labrum tear reported pain with this test.

- Step One: The patient lies in a prone position.
- Step Two: The hip on the painful side is slowly moved near full extension.
- Step Three: The clinician then applies a concurrent external hip rotation while completing the final degrees of full extension.
- Step Four: A positive test is identified by reproduction of the patient's concordant pain.

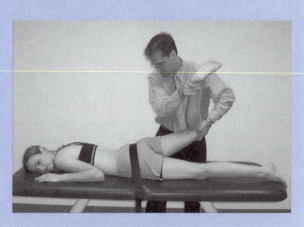

**Figure 13.30**   The Posterior Hip Labrum Test

## *Summary*

- The special clinical tests of the hip have been less investigated for diagnostic accuracy as compared to many other regions of the body.
- The FABER test appears to demonstrate fair diagnostic accuracy in detecting hip osteoarthritis, yet none of the other special clinical tests has been exhaustively investigated. Many of the clinical special tests appear to measure more than one construct.

## TREATMENT TECHNIQUES

Generally, manual therapy treatments associated with the hip involves some mechanism of stretching to improve range of motion that were concordant during the examination. Techniques designed to improve range of motion includes stretching, manually assisted stretching, and mobilization.

### Hip Extension Stretch

- Step One: The patient is placed in prone. Resting symptoms are assessed by the clinician.
- Step Two: Using one hand the clinician blocks the hip joint just cephalic to the gluteal crease.
- Step Three: The other hand applies a passive stretch into extension while stabilizing with the blocking hand.
- Step Four: The position is held for approximately 10–15 seconds.

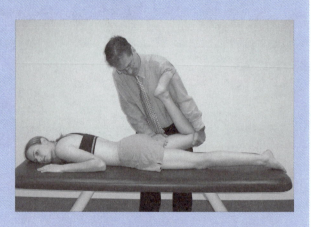

**Figure 13.31**   Passive Hip Extension Stretch

## Internal Rotation Stretch

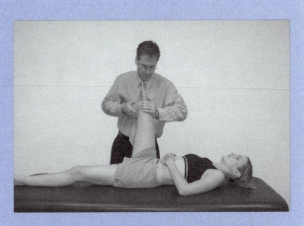

- Step One: The patient assumes a supine position. The clinician assesses resting symptoms.
- Step Two: The clinician passively cradles the lower leg below the knee and slowly internally rotates the hip toward end range. The other hand squeezes the femur and provides a rotational movement in order to reduce the stress placed upon the knee.
- Step Three: The position is held for approximately 10–15 seconds.

**Figure 13.32**    Passive Internal Rotation Stretch

## External Rotation Stretch

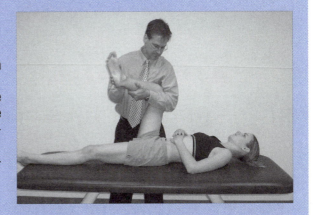

- Step One: The patient assumes a supine position. The clinician assesses resting symptoms.
- Step Two: The clinician passively cradles the lower leg below the knee and slowly externally rotates the hip toward end range. The other hand squeezes the femur and provides a rotational movement in order to reduce the stress placed upon the knee.
- Step Three: The position is held for approximately 10–15 seconds.

**Figure 13.33**    Passive External Rotation Stretch

## Flexion Stretch

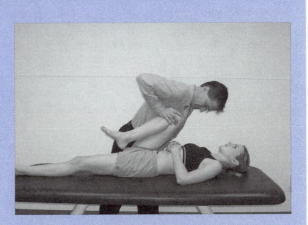

- Step One: The patient assumes a supine position. The clinician assesses resting symptoms.
- Step Two: The clinician passively glides the lower extremity into hip flexion. One hand palpates the ASIS of the pelvis to determine if movement is purely from the hip or if lumbar flexion is contributing to the quantity of motion.
- Step Three: The position is held for approximately 10–15 seconds.

**Figure 13.34**    Passive Flexion Stretch

## *Muscle Energy Methods*

Active assist stretching using muscle energy techniques is also a method that is effective for range-of-motion gains.

### Hip Extension Muscle Energy

- Step One: The patient is placed in prone. The clinician assesses resting symptoms.
- Step Two: Using one hand the clinician blocks the hip joint just cephalic to the gluteal crease.
- Step Three: The other hand applies a passive stretch into extension while stabilizing with the blocking hand.
- Step Four: The patient is instructed to push lightly into hip flexion against the counterforce of the clinician.
- Step Five: The position is held for approximately 6 seconds.

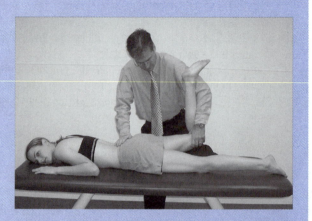

**Figure 13.35**    Muscle Energy Stretch to Gain Hip Extension

### Hip Internal Rotation, Muscle Energy

- Step One: The patient assumes a supine position. The clinician assesses resting symptoms.
- Step Two: The clinician passively cradles the lower leg below the knee and slowly internally rotates the hip toward end range. The other hand squeezes the femur and provides a rotational movement in order to reduce the stress placed upon the knee.
- Step Three: The patient is instructed to turn lightly his or her hip into external rotation.
- Step Four: The position is held for approximately 6 seconds.

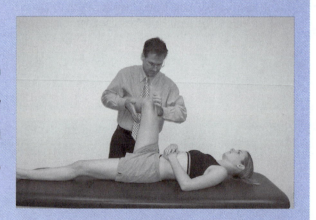

**Figure 13.36**    Muscle Energy Stretch to Gain Internal Rotation

## Hip External Rotation, Muscle Energy

- Step One: The patient assumes a supine position. The clinician assesses resting symptoms.
- Step Two: The clinician passively cradles the lower leg below the knee and slowly externally rotates the hip toward end range. The other hand squeezes the femur and provides a rotational movement in order to reduce the stress placed upon the knee.
- Step Three: The patient is instructed to turn lightly his or her hip into internal rotation.
- Step Four: The position is held for approximately 6 seconds.

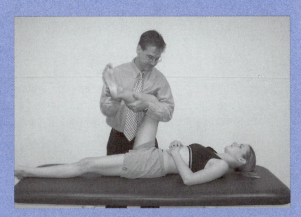

**Figure 13.37**    Muscle Energy Stretch to Gain External Rotation

## *Mobilization and Traction*

Prepositioning in the "close-packed" position of extension, abduction, and internal rotation reduces the quantity of traction at the hip joint when compared against similar forces placed during a "loose-packed position" (external rotation, slight flexion, and abduction).

## Indirect Traction Treatment

- Step One: The patient assumes a supine position. The clinician assesses resting symptoms.
- Step Two: The clinician queries the patient for a history of knee or ankle dysfunction that would contraindicate the use of this method. If none, the clinician cradles the ankle of the patient into both of his or her hands.
- Step Three: The clinician then takes up the slack to preposition the hip into targeted motion. Generally, resting position of the hip includes a moderate degree of flexion and abduction with slight external rotation.[37]
- Step Four: The clinician then provides an inferior force by leaning backward while holding the ankle.
- Step Five: Upon completion, resting symptoms are again assessed.

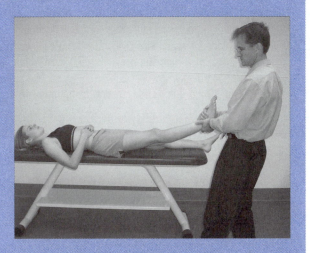

**Figure 13.38**    Indirect Caudal Glide

*(continued)*

- Step Six: On some occasions, the use of a belt may increase the amount of force applied during direct traction. When the belt is placed in a figure-eight fashion, it will cinch up to the lower extremity during traction and will create a very stable contact.

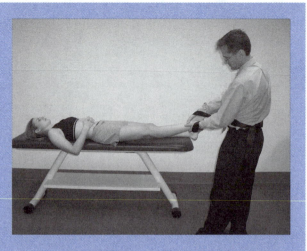

**Figure 13.39**　Indirect Caudal Glide with Belt

## Direct Traction

- Step One: The patient assumes a supine position. The clinician assesses resting symptoms.
- Step Two: The clinician places the lower extremity over his or her shoulder. The clinician places his or hands (ulnar border) near the hip joint for an appropriate contact.
- Step Three: Using the shoulder as a fulcrum, the clinician pulls inferiorly with the hands at the hip and pushes cephalically with the shoulder for an inferior distraction. The clinician passively glides the joint toward the projected end range. Pain is again queried accordingly.
- Step Four: Upon completion, resting symptoms are again assessed.

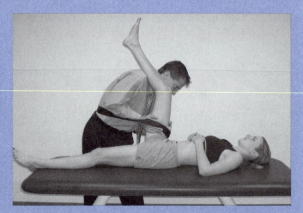

**Figure 13.40**　Direct Caudal Glide with Belt

Sims[15] outlines the benefit of selected accessory glides during planar mobilization. He suggests these methods are effective for pain relief and range-of-motion gains. It is arguable whether significant movement actually occurs during the treatment application. However, some evidence does exist for the use of a posterior-to-anterior technique. Yerys et al.[89] reported that mobilization methods such as a posterior-to-anterior mobilization (PA) provided a significant improvement in hip extension strength.

## Anterior-to-Posterior Glide

- Step One: The patient assumes a sidelying position. The clinician assesses resting symptoms.
- Step Two: The clinician applies a passive glide of the hip joint using the thumb to lock anterior to the greater trochanter and the heel of the hand to apply force to the thumb contact point.
- Step Three: The clinician passively moves toward a posterior direction. The clinician applies a series of 30-second bouts.
- Step Four: Upon completion, resting symptoms are again assessed.

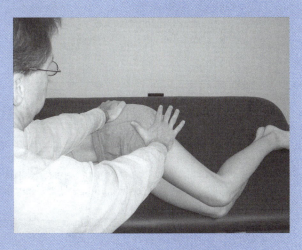

**Figure 13.41**    Anterior-Posterior Glide

## Posterior-to-Anterior Glide

- Step One: The patient assumes a sidelying position. The clinician assesses resting symptoms.
- Step Two: The clinician applies a passive glide of the hip joint using the thumb to lock posterior to the greater trochanter and the heel of the hand to apply force to the thumb contact point.
- Step Three: The clinician passively glides toward an anterior direction. The clinician applies a series of 30-second bouts.
- Step Four: Upon completion, resting symptoms are again assessed.

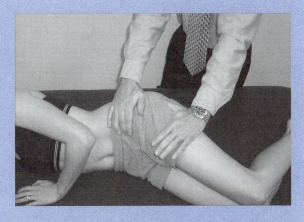

**Figure 13.42**    Posterior-Anterior Glide

## Modification of the Posterior-to-Anterior Glide

A treatment modification of the posterior-to-anterior glide that is frequently used is called the military crawl mobilization. This method allows greater vigor during a mobilization by prepositioning the patient in a tightened capsular position.

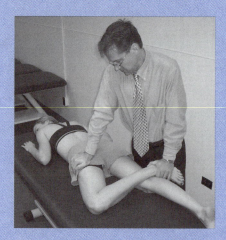

- Step One: The patient assumes a prone position with a preposition of flexion, abduction, and external rotation of the hip. The position is analogous to a soldier crawling under barbed wire.
- Step Two: The clinician applies a passive glide of the hip joint using the thumb to lock posterior to the greater trochanter and the heel of the hand to apply the force to the thumb contact point.
- Step Three: The clinician passively glides toward an anterior direction. The clinician applies a series of 30-second bouts.
- Step Four: Upon completion, resting symptoms are again assessed.

**Figure 13.43**    Posterior-Anterior Glide (Preposition of Military Crawl)

## Lateral Glide

The lateral glide is a mobilization method that most likely yields little range-of-motion improvement but may be effective in reducing the pain of the patient. The use should be restricted to patients who are pain dominant, who do not tolerate the more aggressive movement-based mobilizations.

- Step One: The patient assumes a supine position.
- Step Two: Using a belt and judicious hand placement provides a greater contact point for mobilization anterior and medial to the hip joint.
- Step Three: The clinician places his or her shoulder against the knee of the patient to create a counterforce during the mobilization.
- Step Four: The mobilization procedure includes a lateral glide of the hip joint at the contact of the medial and anterior hip concurrently with the medial glide of the knee.
- Step Five: The clinician should perform a series of bouts lasting approximately 30 seconds.
- Step Six: Upon completion, resting symptoms are again assessed.

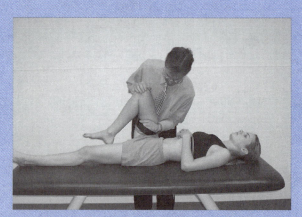

**Figure 13.44**    Lateral Glide with Belt

## Curvilinear Glide

- Step One: The patient assumes a supine position. The hip is prepositioned in flexion, abduction, and external rotation.
- Step Two: The clinician places his or her web space of the hand near the lateral crease of the hip joint.
- Step Three: The mobilization is targeted medially, anteriorly, and inferiorly.
- Step Four: The clinician should perform a series of bouts lasting approximately 30 seconds.
- Step Five: Upon completion, resting symptoms are again assessed.

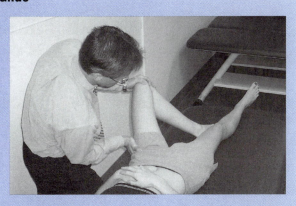

**Figure 13.45**  Posterior-Anterior Glide (Preposition of Curvilinear Glide)

## Mobilization with Compression

Maitland[70] advocates the use of compression of the hip to stimulate synovial fluid production.[15] The size of the joint dictates that a lot of force is warranted during application.

## Passive Internal Rotation with Compression

- The patient assumes a supine position. The clinician assesses resting symptoms.
- Step Two: The clinician passively cradles the lower leg below the knee and slowly internally rotates the hip toward end range. The other hand squeezes the femur and provides a rotational movement in order to reduce the stress placed upon the knee.
- Step Three: The clinician performs a series of passive physiological movements into internal rotation.
- Step Four: Concurrently, the clinician places a compressive load through the femur into the hip joint of the patient.
- Step Five: The technique is performed for about 30 seconds and symptoms are reassessed upon completion of three bouts.

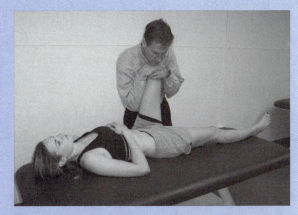

**Figure 13.46**  Passive Internal Rotation with Compression

## Compression with an Anterior–Posterior Glide

- Step One: The patient assumes a sidelying position. The clinician assesses resting symptoms.
- Step Two: The clinician placed one palm anterior to the greater trochanter for the AP force. The other hand is placed over the trochanter of the patient and applies a compressive force.
- Step Three: The clinician passively moves toward a posterior direction while concurrently providing a compressive force through the trochanter. The clinician applies a series of 30-second bouts.
- Step Four: Upon completion, resting symptoms are again assessed.

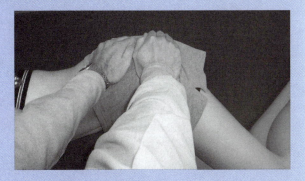

**Figure 13.47**  Compression with an AP

## Passive Hip Flexion with Concurrent Compression

- Step One: The patient assumes a supine position. The clinician assesses resting symptoms.
- Step Two: The clinician passively glides the lower extremity into hip flexion. One hand palpates the ASIS of the pelvis to determine if movement is purely from the hip or if lumbar flexion is contributing to the quantity of motion.
- Step Three: The clinician's hand responsible for passive flexion applies a concurrent load through the femur of the patient.
- Step Four: The repeated movements into flexion are targeted at three bouts of 30 seconds.

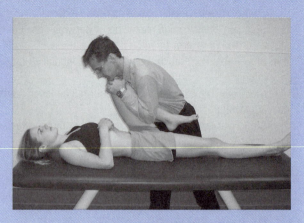

**Figure 13.48**   Hip Flexion with Compression

## *Manipulation*

Like other joints, manipulation can be targeted at the hip joint. Because of the force required at this joint the most effective manipulation strategies generally include indirect techniques.

## Indirect Manipulation

- Step One: The patient assumes a supine position. The clinician assesses resting symptoms.
- Step Two: The clinician queries the patient for a history of knee or ankle dysfunction that would contraindicate the use of this method. If none, the clinician cradles the ankle of the patient into both of his or her hands.
- Step Three: The clinician then takes up the slack to preposition the hip into targeted motion. Generally, resting position of the hip includes a moderate degree of flexion and abduction with slight external rotation.[37]
- Step Four: The clinician then provides an inferior force by leaning backward while holding the ankle.
- Step Five: At end range, the clinician applies a rapid and quick distraction force to manipulate the hip.

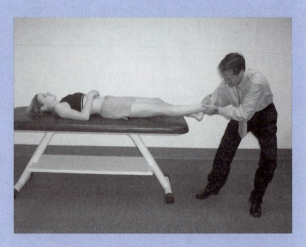

**Figure 13.49**   Indirect Manipulation

### Indirect Manipulation (Cyriax Grade V)[19]

Cyriax described a technique designed to manipulate the SIJ in which the leg is manually thrust into distraction while in a loose-packed position. This method may also manipulate the hip joint as well.

- Step One: The patient assumes a supine position. The lower extremity of the patient is prepositioned into flexion, slight external rotation, and slight abduction.
- Step Two: Using the arm cephalic to the patient, the clinician cradles the lower leg of the patient and grips the ankle posteriorly.
- Step Three: The caudal arm to the patient is flexed at the elbow and the patient's anterior ankle is gripped.
- Step Four: A premovement of circumduction allows the patient to relax prior to the manipulation procedure.
- Step Five: The manipulation involves a quick distraction into full extension of the knee, thus providing a vacuum-like force through the hip.
- Step Six: Patients with ankle, knee, or pelvic disorders are not good candidates for this procedure.

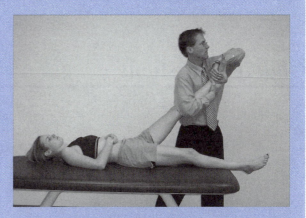

**Figure 13.50**    Indirect Manipulation (Cyriax grade V)

## *Summary*

- Treatment techniques for the hip include stretching, mobilization, manipulation, and variations and combinations of these methods.
- Traction may be the most effective technique for joint distraction.
- Manipulation methods generally involve some mechanism of traction indirectly applied to increase the force input.

# TREATMENT OUTCOMES

Passive stretching, manually assisted stretching, and mobilization have demonstrated equivocal value for range-of-motion gains. Kerrigan et al.[90] suggest that the more vigorous the hip flexor stretching, the more beneficial the gains, despite the age of the individual. Winter et al.[66] found similar results in a comparison of passive and manually assistive stretching to improve hip flexor mobility.

Manually assistive stretching in the form of muscle energy techniques may be used in patients that demonstrate fear or pain during passive stretching. Medeiros et al.[91] report similar outcomes when comparing two groups that received isometric contraction and passive stretch procedures.

Mobilization with traction has been used in many studies and may result in increased joint distraction. In selected case reports, traction and mobilization methods lead to improvement in internal rotation range of motion,[92] although most studies demonstrated reduction in subjective pain but no changes in range of motion,[37] in one case, as quickly as one visit.[93] Past studies that used radiographic quantification during traction have reported movement up to 10–20 cm during distraction.[37,94] Arvidsson[37] identified that an increase in applied force created a direct increase of displacement.

In the most comprehensive study to date, Hoeskma et al.[43] reported statistically significant improvements of hip function and pain in a group that received manual therapy, versus a group that was limited to exercise alone. After 5 weeks, patients in the manual therapy group had significantly better outcomes for pain, stiffness, hip function, and range of motion. Improvements of pain, hip function, and range-of-motion values were still present after 29 weeks. Hoeksma et al.[43] used hip traction and a traction

## *Summary*

- There is moderate evidence within the literature that static stretching is beneficial for range-of-motion gains of the hip.
- There is good evidence within the literature that manipulation and traction are beneficial for pain and range of motion at the hip.
- There is limited evidence within the literature to support mobilization of the hip.

manipulation performed in the limited positions during their clinical trial.

Lastly, a method known as strain–counterstrain, or positional release, is a passive positional technique designed to relieve pain and dysfunction by placing the muscular tissue in a shortened position for a reduction of the tender point.[95] The reliability of assessing the tender points was poor but pain was significantly reduced post-treatment.[96] Another study has demonstrated significantly improved response to a manual muscle test using a dynamometer, possibly associated with reducing pain in the targeted segment. Further studies are needed for additional analysis.[95]

# Chapter Questions

1. Describe the biomechanics of the hip. Identify which physiological movement demonstrates the greatest potential for mobility.
2. Discuss the capsular pattern theory of the hip. Debate the value of Altman's selection of internal rotation as an osteoarthritis factor.
3. Outline the most common techniques used to increase hip range of motion. Compare the similarities of the techniques.

# References

1. Narvani A, Tsiridis E, Kendall S, Chaudhuri R, Thomas P. A preliminary report on prevalence of acetabular labrum tears in sports patients with groin pain. *Knee Surg Traumatol Arthrosc.* 2003;11:403–408.
2. Deyle G, Henderson N, Matekel R, Ryder M, Garber M, Allison S. Effectiveness of manual physical therapy and exercise in osteoarthritis of the knee. A randomized controlled trial. *Ann Intern Med.* 2000;132:173–181.
3. Marks R, Cantin D. Symptomatic osteoarthritis of the knee: the efficacy of physiotherapy. *Physiother.* 1997;83:306–312.
4. D'Ambrosia RD. Epidemiology of osteoarthritis. *Orthoped* 2005;28(2 Suppl):s201–5.
5. Schlesinger N. Osteoarthritis: pathology, epidemiology, and risk factors. *Phys Med Rehabil.* 2001;15:1–9.
6. Lane NE, Nevitt MC, Hochberg MC, Hung YY, Palermo L. Progression of radiographic hip osteoarthritis over eight years in a community sample of elderly white women. *Arthritis Rheum.* 2004;50(5):1477–1486.
7. Kern LM, Powe NR, Levine MA, Fitzpatrick AL, Harris TB, Robbins J, Fried LP. Association between screening for osteoporosis and the incidence of hip fracture. *Ann Intern Med.* 2005;142(3):173–181.
8. Stevens JA, Olson S. Reducing falls and resulting hip fractures among older women. *MMWR Recomm Rep.* 2000;49(RR-2):3–12.
9. Anderson, MK; Hall, SJ; Martin M. *Sports injury management.* Philadelphia; Lippincott Williams & Wilkins: 2000.
10. Starkey C, Ryan J. *Evaluation of orthopedic and athletic injuries.* Philadelphia; F.A. Davis Company: 1996.
11. Williams P, Bannister L. In: Berry M, Collins P, Dyson M, Dussek J, Ferguson M (eds) *Gray's anatomy.* 38th ed. Churchill Livingstone; Edinburgh: 1995.
12. Lee D. The pelvic girdle. *An approach to the examination and treatment of the lumbo-pelvic-hip region.* Edinburgh; Churchill Livingstone: 1989.
13. Gross J. *Musculoskeletal examination.* Malden, Mass; Blackwell Pub: 2002.
14. Nicholas J, Hershman E. *The lower extremity and spine in sports medicine.* Vol 2. St. Louis, MO; Mosby: 1986.
15. Sims K. Assessment and treatment of hip osteoarthritis. *Man Ther.* 1999;4:136–144.
16. Crowninshield R, Brand R. A physiologically based criterion of muscle force prediction in locomotion. *J Biomechanics.* 1981;14:793–801.
17. Bogduk N, Macintosh JE, Pearcy MJ. A universal model of the lumbar back muscles in the upright position. *Spine.* 1992;17(8):897–913.
18. Delp S, Hess W, Hungerford D, Jones L. Variation of rotation moment arms with hip flexion. *J Biomech.* 1999;32:493–501.
19. Cyriax J. *Textbook of Orthopaedic Medicine.* 7th ed. Vol. 1. London; Baillierre Tindall: 1978.
20. Kaltenborn F. *Manual mobilization of the extremity joints.* 4th ed. Olaf Norlis Bokhandel, Oslo: 1989.
21. Klassbo M, Harms-Ringdahl K, Larsson G. Examination of passive ROM and capsular patterns in the hip. *Physiother Res Int.* 2003;8(1):1–12.
22. Bijl D, Dekker J, van Baar ME, Oostendorp RA, Lemmens AM, Bijlsma JW, Voorn TB. Validity of Cyriax's concept capsular pattern for the diagnosis of osteoarthritis of hip and/or knee. *Scand J Rheumatol.* 1998;27(5):347–351.

23. Arokoski MH, Haara M, Helminen HJ, Arokoski JP. Physical function in men with and without hip osteoarthritis. *Arch Phys Med Rehabil.* 2004;85(4): 574–581.

24. Roach K, Miles T. Normal hip and knee active range of motion: The relationship to age. *Phys Ther.* 1991; 71:656–665.

25. Hoppenfeld S. *Physical examination of the spine and extremities.* New York; Appleton-Century-Crofts: 1976.

26. Kendall H, Kendall F, Wadsworth G. *Muscles: Testing and function.* 2nd ed. Baltimore; Williams & Wilkens: 1971.

27. Daniels L, Worthingham C. *Muscle testing techniques of manual examination.* 3rd ed. Philadelphia; WB Saunders: 1972.

28. DeAngelis NA, Busconi BD. Assessment and differential diagnosis of the painful hip. *Clin Orthop Relat Res.* 2003;(406):11–18.

29. Ordeberg G. Characterization of joint pain in human OA. *Novartis Found Symp.* 2004;260:105–115.

30. Brown MD, Gomez-Marin O, Brookfield KF, Li PS. Differential diagnosis of hip disease versus spine disease. *Clin Orthop Relat Res.* 2004;(419):280–284.

31. Lauder T. Musculoskeletal disorder that frequently mimic radiculopathy. *Phys Med Clinics North Am.* 2002;13:469–485.

32. Collee G, Dijkmans B, Vanderbroucke J, Rozing P, Cats A. A clinical epidemiological study in low back pain: description of two clinical syndromes. *Br J Rheum.* 1990;29:354–357.

33. Vidigal EC, da Silva OL. Observation hip. *Acta Orthop Scand.* 1981;52(2):191–195.

34. Kandemir U, Bharam S, Philippon M, Fu F. Endoscopic treatment of calcific tendonitis of gluteus medius and minimus. *Arthroscopy.* 2003;19:E1–E4.

35. Jones D, Erhard R. Diagnosis of trochanteric bursitis versus femoral neck stress fracture. *Phys Ther.* 1997; 77:58–67.

36. Waters RL, Mulroy S. The energy expenditure of normal and pathologic gait. *Gait Posture.* 1999;9(3): 207–231.

37. Arvidsson I. The hip joint: forces needed for distraction and appearance of the vacuum phenomenon. *Scand J Rehabil Med.* 1990;22:157–161.

38. Levangie P. The association between static pelvic asymmetry and low back pain. *Spine.* 1999;24(12): 1234–1242.

39. Beattie P, Isaacson K, Riddle DL, Rothstein JM. Validity of derived measurements of leg-length differences obtained by use of a tape measure. *Phys Ther.* 1990;70(3):150–157.

40. Krawiec CJ, Denegar CR, Hertel J, Salvaterra GF, Buckley WE. Static innominate asymmetry and leg length discrepancy in asymptomatic collegiate athletes. *Man Ther.* 2003;8(4):207–213.

41. Friberg O. Clinical symptoms and biomechanics of lumbar spine and hip joint in leg length inequality. *Spine.* 1983;8(6):643–651.

42. Goel A, Loudon J, Nazare A, Rondinelli R, Hassanein K. Joint moments in minor limb length discrepancy: a pilot study. *Am J Orthop.* 1997;26(12):852–856.

43. Hoeksma HL, Dekker J, Ronday HK, Heering A, van der Lubbe N, Vel C, Breedveld FC, van den Ende CH. Comparison of manual therapy and exercise therapy in osteoarthritis of the hip: a randomized clinical trial. *Arthritis Rheum.* 2004;51(5):722–729.

44. Soderman P, Henrik M. Is the Harris Hip Score system useful to study the outcome of total hip replacement? *Clin Orthop.* 2001;384:189–197.

45. Shields R, Enloe L, Evans R, Smith K, Steckel S. Reliability, validity, and responsiveness of functional tests in patients with total joint replacements. *Phys Ther.* 1995;75:169–176.

46. Kirschner S, Walther M, Mehling E, Faller H, Konig A. (abstract). Reliability, validity and responsiveness of the German short musculoskeletal function assessment questionnaire (SMFA-D) in patients with osteoarthritis of the hip undergoing total hip arthroplasty. *Z Rheumatol.* 2003;62:548–554.

47. Roorda L, Jones C, Waltz M, Lankhorst G, Bouter M, van der Eijken J, Willems W, Heyligers I, Voaklander D, Kelly K, Suarez-Almazor M. Satisfactory cross cultural equivalence of the Dutch WOMAC in patients with hip osteoarthritis waiting for arthroplasty. *Ann Rheum Dis.* 2004;63:36–42.

48. Soderman P. On the validity of the results from the Swedish National Total Hip Arthoplasty Register. *Acta Orthop Scand Suppl.* 2000;296:1–33.

49. Bellamy N, Buchanan WW, Goldsmith CH, Campbell J, Stitt LW. Validation study of WOMAC: a health status instrument for measuring clinically important patient relevant outcomes to antirheumatic drug therapy in patients with osteoarthritis of the hip or knee. *J Rheumatol.* 1988;15(12):1833–1840.

50. Sun Y, Sturmer T, Gunther KP, Brenner H. Reliability and validity of clinical outcome measurements of osteoarthritis of the hip and knee—a review of the literature. *Clin Rheumatol.* 1997;16(2):185–198.

51. Salaffi F, Leardini G, Canesi B, Mannoni A, Fioravanti A, Caporali R, Lapadula G, Punzi L. Reliability and validity of the Western Ontario and McMaster Universities (WOMAC) Osteoarthritis Index in Italian patients with osteoarthritis of the knee. *Osteoarthritis Cartilage.* 2003;11(8):551–560.

52. Wright JG, Young NL. A comparison of different indices of responsiveness. *J Clin Epidemiol.* 1997;50(3): 239–246.

53. Wollmerstedt N, Kirschner S, Wolz T, Ellssel J, Beyer W, Faller H, Konig A. (abstract). [Evaluating the reliability, validity and responsiveness of the German short

musculoskeletal function assessment questionnaire, SMFA-D, in inpatient rehabilitation of patients with conservative treatment for hip osteoarthritis]. *Rehabilitation* (Stuttg). 2004;43(4): 233–240.

54. Stratford P, Kennedy D, Pagura S, Gollish J. The relationship between self-report and performance-related measures: Questioning the content validity of timed tests. *Arthritis Rheum.* 2003;49:535–540.

55. Watson C, Propps M, Ratner J, Zeigler D, Horton P, Smith S. Reliability and responsiveness of the Lower Extremity Functional Scale and the anterior knee pain scale in patients with anterior knee pain. *J Orthop Sports Phys Ther.* 2005;35:136–146.

56. Binkley J, Stratford P, Lott S, Riddle D. The Lower Extremity Functional Scale (LEFS): scale development, measurement properties, and clinical application. North American Orthopaedic Rehabilitation Research Network. *Phys Ther.* 1999;79:371–383.

57. Childs JD, Fritz JM, Flynn TW, Irrgang JJ, Johnson KK, Majkowski GR, Delitto A. A clinical prediction rule to identify patients with low back pain most likely to benefit from spinal manipulation: a validation study. *Ann Intern Med.* 2004;141(12):920–928.

58. Flynn T, Fritz J, Whitman J, Wainner R, Magel J, Rendeiro D, Butler B, Garber M, Allison S. A clinical prediction rule for classifying patients with low back pain who demonstrate short-term improvement with spinal manipulation. *Spine.* 2002;27(24):2835–2843.

59. Sjolie AN. Low-back pain in adolescents is associated with poor hip mobility and high body mass index. *Scand J Med Sci Sports.* 2004;14(3):168–175.

60. Vad VB, Bhat AL, Basrai D, Gebeh A, Aspergren DD, Andrews JR. Low back pain in professional golfers: the role of associated hip and low back range-of-motion deficits. *Am J Sports Med.* 2004;32(2):494–497.

61. McConnell J. Recalcitrant chronic low back and leg pain—a new theory and different approach to management. *Man Ther.* 2002;7(4):183–192.

62. Lee RY, Munn J. Passive moment about the hip in straight leg raising. *Clin Biomech.* 2000;15(5):330–334.

63. Woods D, Macnicol M. The flexion-adduction test: an early sign of hip disease. *J Pediatr Orthop.* Part B 2000;10:180–185.

64. Kagan A. Rotator cuff tears of the hip. *Clin Orthop Relat Res.* 1999(368):135–140.

65. Perry J, Weiss WB, Burnfield JM, Gronley JK. The supine hip extensor manual muscle test: a reliability and validity study. *Arch Phys Med Rehabil.* 2004;85(8):1345–1350.

66. Winters MV, Blake CG, Trost JS, Marcello-Brinker TB, Lowe LM, Garber MB, Wainner RS. Passive versus active stretching of hip flexor muscles in subjects with limited hip extension: a randomized clinical trial. *Phys Ther.* 2004;84(9):800–807.

67. Heikkila S, Viitanen JV, Kautiainen H, Kauppi M. Sensitivity to change of mobility tests; effect of short term intensive physiotherapy and exercise on spinal, hip, and shoulder measurements in spondyloarthropathy. *J Rheumatol.* 2000;27(5):1251–1256.

68. Fritz JM, Whitman JM, Flynn TW, Wainner RS, Childs JD. Factors related to the inability of individuals with low back pain to improve with a spinal manipulation. *Phys Ther.* 2004;84(2):173–190.

69. Huber HM. (abstract). The piriformis syndrome—a possible cause of sciatica. *Schweiz Rundsch Med Prax.* 1990;79(9):235–236.

70. Maitland GD. *Peripheral manipulation* 3rd ed. London; Butterworth-Heinemann: 1986.

71. Fredericson M, Cookingham CL, Chaudhari AM, Dowdell BC, Oestreicher N, Sahrmann SA. Hip abductor weakness in distance runners with iliotibial band syndrome. Hip abductor weakness in distance runners with iliotibial band syndrome. *Clin J Sport Med.* 2000;10(3):169–175.

72. Greenwood MJ, Erhard RE, Jones DL. Differential diagnosis of the hip vs. lumbar spine: five case reports. *J Orthop Sports Phys Ther.* 1998;27(4):308–315.

73. Ito K, Leunig M, Ganz R. Histopathologic features of the acetabular labrum in femoroacetabular impingement. *Clin Orthop Relat Res.* 2004;(429):262–271.

74. Warren P. Management of a patient with sacroiliac joint dysfunction: a correlation of hip range of motion asymmetry with sitting and standing postural habits. *J Man Manip Ther.* 2003;11:153–159.

75. Cibulka MT, Threlkeld J. The early clinical diagnosis of osteoarthritis of the hip. *J Orthop Sports Phys Ther.* 2004;34(8):461–467.

76. Birrell F, Croft P, Cooper C, Hosie G, Macfarlane G, Silman A; PCR Hip Study Group. Predicting radiographic hip osteoarthritis from range of movement. *Rheumatology* (Oxford). 2001;40(5):506–512.

77. Reijman M, Hazes JM, Koes BW, Verhagen AP, Bierma-Zeinstra SM. Validity, reliability, and applicability of seven definitions of hip osteoarthritis used in epidemiological studies: a systematic appraisal. *Ann Rheum Dis.* 2004;63(3):226–232.

78. Altman R, Alarcon G, Appelrouth D, Bloch D, Borenstein D, Brandt K, Brown C, Cooke TD, Daniel W, Feldman D, et al. The American College of Rheumatology criteria for the classification and reporting of osteoarthritis of the hip. *Arthritis Rheum.* 1991;34(5):505–514.

79. Beatty R. The piriformis muscle syndrome: a single diagnostic maneuver. *Neurosurgery.* 1994;34:512–514.

80. Caruso F, Toney M. Trochanteric bursitis. A case report of plain film, scintigraphic, and MRI correlation. *Clin Nucl Med* 1994;19:393–395.

81. Adkins S, Figler R. Hip pain in athletes. *Am Fam Physician.* 2000;61:2109–2118.

82. Gajdosik R, Sandler M, Marr H. Influence of knee positions and gender on the Ober test for length of the iliotibial band. *Clin Biomech.* 2003;18:77–79.

83. Margo K, Drezner J, Motzkin D. Evaluation and management of hip pain: an algorithmic approach. *J Fam Pract*. 2003;52(8):607–617.

84. Thurston A. Assessment of fixed flexion deformity of the hip. *Clin Orthop Relat Res*. 1982;169:186–189.

85. Staheli L. The prone hip extension test: a method of measuring hip flexion deformity. *Clin Orthop Relat Res*. 1977;123:12–15.

86. Harvey D. Assessment of the flexibility of elite athletes using the modified Thomas test. *Br J Sport Med*. 1998;32:68–70.

87. Suenaga E, Noguchi Y, Jingushi S, Shuto T, Nakashima Y, Miyanishi K, Iwamoto Y. Relationship between the maximum flexion-internal rotation test and the torn acetabular labrum of a dysplastic hip. *J Orthop Sci*. 2002;7:26–32.

88. Fitzgerald R. Acetabular labrum tears. Diagnosis and treatment. *Clin Orthop Relat Res* 1995;311:60–68.

89. Yerys S, Makofsky H, Byrd C, Pennachio J, Cinkay J. Effect of mobilization of the anterior hip capsule on gluteus maximus strength. *J Man Manip Ther*. 2002;10:218–224.

90. Kerrigan DC, Xenopoulos-Oddsson A, Sullivan MJ, Lelas JJ, Riley PO. Effect of a hip flexor-stretching program on gait in the elderly. *Arch Phys Med Rehabil*. 2003;84(1):1–6.

91. Medeiros JM, Smidt GL, Burmeister LF, Soderberg GL. The influence of isometric exercise and passive stretch on hip joint motion. *Phys Ther*. 1977;57(5):518–523.

92. Angstrom L, Lindstrom B. (abstract). Treatment effects of traction and mobilization of the hip joint in patients with inflammatory rheumatological diseases and hip osteoarthritis. *Nordisk Fysioterapi*. 2003;7:17–27.

93. Whipple T, Plafcan D, Sebastianelli W. Manipulative treatment of hip pain in a ballet student: a case study. *J Dance Med Science*. 2004;8:53–55.

94. Insulander B. (abstract). Some findings regarding manual traction on hip joints. *Sjukgymnasten*. 1973;4:289–296.

95. Wong C, Schauer-Alvarez C. Effect of strain counterstrain on pain and strength in hip musculature. *J Man Manip Ther*. 2004;12:215–223.

96. Wong C, Schauer C. Reliability, validity, and effectiveness of strain counterstrain techniques. *J Man Manip Ther*. 2004;12:107–112.

# 14

# Manual Therapy of the Knee

CHAD E. COOK AND ROBERT FLEMING

## Objectives

- Identify the pertinent structure and biomechanics of the knee.
- Demonstrate the appropriate sequential knee examination.
- Identify plausible mobilization and manual therapy treatment techniques.

- Outline the special tests of the knee and the diagnostic accuracy of each of the tests.

## PREVALENCE

Knee pain is present in approximately 20% of the adult population.[1] Jackson et al.[1] report that acute knee pain accounts for up to 1 million emergency room visits yearly and 1.9 million primary care visits. Knee fractures occur in less than 7% of emergency room visits.[2] A form of knee pain known as **patellofemoral pain syndrome** (PFPS) is common, accounting for 25.6% of knee-related problems.[3] A meniscal tear makes up approximately 9–11% of knee-related impairments[4] and is much less common than knee pain associated with osteoarthritis.

Selected knee injuries are variable in frequency and depend greatly on the activity level and age of the patient. Osteoarthritis significantly affects the functional capacity of knee joints in nearly 10% of adults age 60 and over.[5] Prevalence increases in individuals that are overweight,[6,7] have a history of an anterior cruciate ligament injury[8] and/or total **meniscectomy**,[7] and are females,[7] or have a genetic predisposition.[9] Nearly 44% of individuals with osteoarthritis report knee instability that is associated with a decreased ability to function during activities of daily living.[10]

Soft tissue–related injuries are common in patients who have experienced tibial plateau fractures.[11] Soft tissue injuries such as an anterior cruciate ligament tear are common during trauma or sports-related activities. Tears that are not surgically repaired run a greater risk of meniscus damage, disability, osteoarthritis, and future surgery over time.[12]

PFPS generally affects younger patients, particularly those that participate in athletic activities.[3] PFPS conditions may range from mild irritations to traumatic dislocations. Nearly half of patellofemoral dislocations occur without a first-time, predisposing incident.[13] Recurrent patellofemoral pain is uncommon (less than 15% recurrence rate) but can cause disability.[14]

## Summary

- Knee problems are prevalent in up to 20% of the general population.
- Problems such as osteoarthritis are more common in individuals with previous knee injuries, are female, and have a genetic history.
- Conditions such as patellofemoral pain syndrome typically affect younger individuals who are active.

## ANATOMY

### Osseous Structures

The osseous structures of the knee include the femur, the tibia, and the patella. At the distal end of the femur lie the femoral condyles that are responsible for the articulation with the patella and the tibial plateau (Figure 14.1).[5] The femoral condyles are covered with articular cartilage, are convex in nature, and demonstrate two separate articulation points, one medial and one lateral.[15] The superior division of the medial and lateral condyles within the femoral groove is primarily flat. The groove deepens as distally toward the tibia.[5] The angle of the femoral groove has been associated with patellofemoral stability.[16]

The tibia (Figure 14.2) gives birth to the tibial plateau and contributes significantly to knee stability.[5] The medial and lateral plateaus are concave, a tendency that is enhanced by the inclusion of the medial and lateral menisci.[15] The lateral tibial plateau is larger to account for the movement of the lateral femoral condyle.

Between the two tibial plateaus is the pyramid-shaped intercondylar eminence. This eminence serves as a pivot point for the femur and stabilizes the knee from excessive extension.[5] This region also serves as an attachment site of the menisci.

The patella is a triangular-shaped sesamoid bone designed to improve the extensor mechanism of the knee (Figure 14.3). The inferior (posterior) surface of the patella has a medial and lateral facet but does exhibit three and occasionally four concave surfaces of articulation.[15] The medial facet typically demonstrates the greatest anatomical variation.[17] Generally, the medial facet is subdivided into two facets to more appropriately articulate with the condyle of the femurs.[17] The lateral facet is

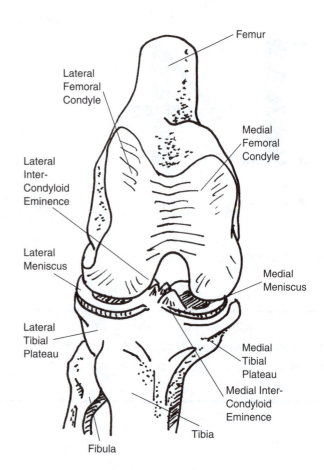

**Figure 14.2**    The Proximal Articulation Components of the Tibia

longer and wider than the medial facet and is concave in both longitudinal and medial–lateral directions.[17] Occasionally, a transverse ridge subdivides the lateral facet, creating a superior and inferior face for articulation.

The inferior aspect of the patella articulates with the superior femoral groove during extension and the superior aspect of the patella articulates with the inferior aspect of the femoral groove during flexion.[17] The contact surface of the patella with the femur is greatest during flexion and least during full extension.[15]

## Joints

### *The Tibiofemoral Joint*

The tibiofemoral joint is the largest joint of the body (Figure 14.4). The femoral condyles are cam-shaped and circular in structure. The medial condyle of the femur is larger than the lateral condyle[15] and encounters greater weight-bearing forces than the lateral aspect.[18] Although the lateral condyle is smaller than the medial condyle, the lateral condyle projects anteriorly and acts as a stabilizer of the patella. The anterior part of the lateral condyle is flattened and provides a contact surface with the anterior horn and the anterior part of the tibial articular surface during full extension. Generally, the lateral component of the tibial

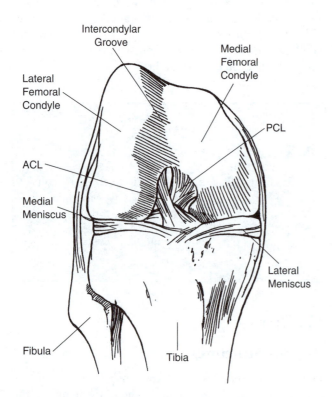

**Figure 14.1**    The Distal Articulation Components of the Femur

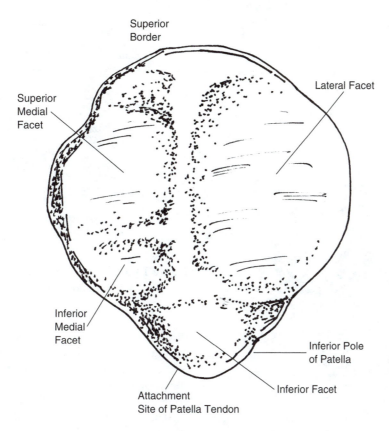

Superior
Border

Superior
Medial
Facet

Lateral Facet

Inferior
Medial
Facet

Inferior Pole
of Patella

Inferior Facet

Attachment
Site of Patella Tendon

**Figure 14.3**    Inferior (Posterior) Surface of the Patella

## Summary

- The osseous structures of the knee include the femur, the patella, and the tibia.
- The femur provides for the articulation of the patellofemoral joint and the tibiofemoral joint.
- The posterior surface of the patella promotes movement and stability within the condyle of the femur.

femoral joints allows greater mobility and is less stabile and prone to laxity more so than the medial compartment.

The femur articulates with the tibial plateau, which is inclined laterally and posteriorly and promotes stability during extension. The medial and lateral menisci, both of which contribute to stability during various degrees of extension and flexion, significantly enhance this articulation. Both menisci absorb ground reaction forces across the knee and redistribute those forces to all aspects of the femoral condyle and tibial plateau.[15]

### The Patellofemoral Joint

The patellofemoral joint is the articulation of the patella within the femoral groove. During flexion and extension, the patella moves up to 7 or 8 centimeters in relation to the femoral condyles.[5] The primary function of the patella is to improve the mechanical advantage of the quadriceps during movements of flexion and extension. The patella moves in a C-shaped pattern from extension to flexion and back. Additionally, the patella tilts medially from knee flexion to laterally during knee extension. This is most likely a mechanism associated with the concurrent rotation of the tibia and the shape and congruence of the femoral condyles.

When dysfunction of the patella occurs, it may dislocate, sublux, fracture, degenerate, or develop a tracking problem.[19] Pain associated with the patellofemoral joint is typically diffuse, generally involves crepitus and locking, and may lead to decreased functional activities.[19] The tracking problem may result in a number of consequences including abnormal loading, abnormal pressures at the femur and patella, and pain.[20]

## Summary

- The tibiofemoral joint is the largest joint of the body.
- The medial aspect of the femur bears more weight than the lateral aspect.
- The extremely mobile patellofemoral joint moves up to 7 or 8 centimeters in relation to the femoral condyles.

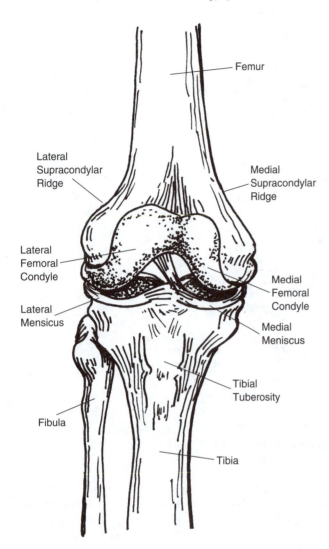

**Figure 14.4**    Anterior View of the Tibiofemoral Joint

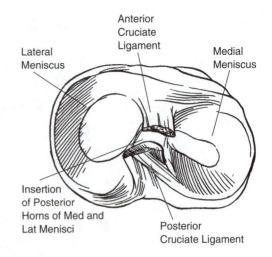

**Figure 14.5**    The Tibial Attachments of the Medial and Lateral Menisci

## Intraarticular Structures

The most prominent nonligamentous intraarticular structures are the medial and lateral menisci (Figure 14.5). The menisci's primary role is stabilization, shock absorption, proprioception, and improvement in lubrication and sequencing of the knee.[18,21] The menisci actually absorb the majority of compressive force at the knee because the combined mass is greater than that of the surrounded articular cartilage.[21] Like discs at other regions of the body, the knee menisci help to distribute contact forces over the articular surfaces by increasing the contact surface of the joint.[18]

The medial meniscus attaches anterior to the articulating surface of the tibia, to the medial aspect of the capsule of the knee and at the intercondyler tubercle. The medial meniscus also has an attachment posterior with the semimembranosus.[5] The lateral meniscus attaches (both the anterior and posterior horn) near a common attachment posterior to the intercondylar tubercle of the tibia and near the attachment of the posterior horn of the medial

meniscus. The posterior aspect of the lateral meniscus generally is attached to two meniscofemoral ligaments and is thought to be significantly altered biomechanically by the cooperative action of the popliteus and the meniscofemoral ligaments.[22,23] Both the anterior aspects of the medial and lateral meniscus are attached via the ligamentum transversum, also known as the transverse meniscal ligament.[5]

The medial meniscus is C-shaped and the lateral meniscus is primarily circular-shaped. Both menisci distort significantly (elongate in a sagittal plane) and move posteriorly during flexion and move anteriorly during extension. This distortion is greatest during higher loads.[18] During rotation, such as during the screw home mechanism, the menisci follow the movements of the femur.[15] Actions such as weight bearing increase the mobility of the menisci. Of the two menisci, the medial meniscus encounters more forces during weight bearing than the lateral meniscus.

The menisci are damaged occasionally during weight-bearing activities and during normal processes of degeneration. Recently, studies have shown that degeneration and tears often occur synonymously.[21] Damage to the cartilage generally begins at the surface then extends through the thickness of the cartilage.[18] Meniscal damage leads to cartilage thinning and subsequent loss of joint space.[21]

The outer aspect of the menisci is innervated and is capable of producing pain when torn or degenerated.[18] Historically, damage to the menisci involved removal of the menisci to avoid the painful consequences associated with knee locking. Nonetheless, when the menisci are removed, forces along the femur and the tibia are significantly increased, specifically at the contact points of articulation.[21] Furthermore, removal of the menisci commonly leads to articular surface breakdown of the femur and tibia within a few years.[18,21,24] Articular breakdown may result in flattening of the femur at the compression site, fibrillation, sclerosis, and further narrowing of the joint space.[25]

## Muscles

Several muscles contribute to normal knee motion. The quadriceps femoris muscles include the rectus femoris, vastus lateralis, vastus medialis, and the vastus intermedialis. Much of the efficiency of the knee extensor mechanism depends on the timing and position of the patella during muscular contraction. The maximal quadriceps contraction occurs at 60 degrees of knee flexion.[15]

The knee flexors include the hamstrings, sartorius, gracilis, popliteus, and the gastronemius muscles. The popliteus muscle also contributes to knee flexion concurrently while initiating internal rotation.

## Summary

- The medial and lateral menisci's primary role is stabilization, shock absorption, proprioception, and improvement in lubrication and sequencing of the knee.
- Both menisci distort significantly (elongate in a sagittal plane) and move posteriorly during flexion and move anteriorly during extension.
- The outer aspect of the menisci is innervated and is capable of becoming a pain generator.
- The collective output of the muscles in the knee work in concert to increase the stability during static and dynamic activities.

## Ligaments and Capsule of the Knee

### The Anterior Cruciate Ligament

The anterior cruciate ligament (ACL) is the primary structure responsible to counter anterior tibial transfer with respect to the femur (Figure 14.6).[5] The ACL is a broad helical ligament that allows for appropriate tibia-to-femur rotation during movement but still supports the transfer of the tibia and side-to-side stabilization of the knee. The femoral attachment of the ACL is at the posterior aspect of the medial surface of the lateral femoral condyle.[5] The tibial attachments are at the anterior aspect of the tibial spine.[5]

Like other ligaments of the knee, the ACL is actually two distinct bands, an anterior-medial and a posterolateral band, based on the origins of the tibia. The anterior-medial band is taut in flexion and the posterolateral band is taut in extension.[5] Subsequently, the bands change tension throughout movement of the knee from flexion to extension. Since the ligaments are relatively horizontal during flexion, the ligaments serve to stabilize tibial translation mostly at nearly 90 degrees. Nonetheless, the liga-

ment is also a secondary restraint to varus and valgus forces and internal rotation of the tibia.

The ligament is commonly injured when the tibia is driven anteriorly on the femur but a large portion of ACL injuries are nontraumatic, occurring commonly in female athletes during cutting or pivoting activities.[26] Damage to the ACL may lead to increased risk of meniscus, chondral, and subchondral injury within 5 to 10 years.[12]

### The Posterior Cruciate Ligament

The posterior cruciate ligament (PCL) has a relatively compact tibial attachment, located posteriorly between the posterior horn of the medial and lateral menisci.[27] The femoral attachment is extensive adjacent to the condylar cartilage and near the medial femoral condyle.[27] Most researchers agree that the PCL is made of two separate systems of fibers that function separately based on the forces provided to the knee joint.[28] The PCL fibers run anterior and proximal and are designed to counter tibial posterior translation. It is projected that the PCL is strongest while one is younger, slowly weakening with age.[27]

The PCL is the primary restraint of the tibia on the femur when the knee is flexed from 30 to 90 degrees.[27] Isolated cutting of the PCL minimally affects posterior tibial translation while the knee is in extension.[29] Structures other than the PCL are responsible for stability of

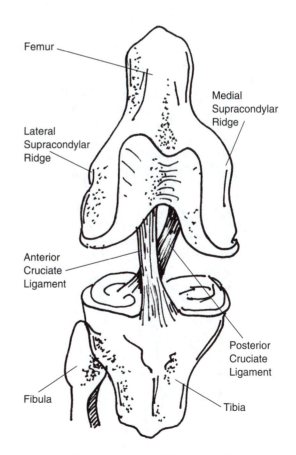

**Figure 14.6**    The Anterior and Posterior Cruciate Ligaments

the knee from 20 degrees of flexion to extension.[27] The PCL is a secondary restraint to tibial internal and external rotation and valgus and varus forces.[27]

The condition of the ACL affects the PCL as does the condition of the PCL affect the ACL. A stiffer ligament leads to increased force across both ligaments and a more flexible or lax ligament leads to diminished forces along both ligaments.[30] The ligaments function in concert to control anterior and posterior tibial translation.

### The Lateral Collateral Ligament

The lateral collateral ligament is tightened during extension and is slackened during approximately 30 degrees of knee flexion (Figure 14.7).[29] The popliteofibular ligament (not pictured) contributes to posterior–lateral stability during all angles of flexion and contributes as a deterrent to varus forces during extension and flexion.[29]

### The Medial Collateral Ligament Complex

The medial collateral ligament complex (MCL) (Figure 14.8) consists primarily of three main structures: the longitudinal fibers of the superficial medial collateral liga-

ment (sMCL), the deep medial collateral ligament (dMCL), and the posteromedial capsule (PMC).[31] At present, the true function of these fibers and whether the fibers function together or independently is unknown.

The MCL structures provide coronal shear stability and reduce the forces associated with valgus. In additional to the passive structures, the contribution of the muscles of the pes anserine aid in stabilizing the knee. Passively, the posteromedial capsule provides passive support during extension of the knee and provides some stability at extension. The MCL contributes more toward valgus stability of the knee during flexion.

### The Meniscofemoral Ligaments

The **meniscofemoral ligaments** connect to the posterior horn of the lateral meniscus to the intercondylar area of the femur.[32] Less common are meniscofemoral ligaments that attach to the anterior horn of the medial meniscus. These ligaments are present in approximately 90% of individuals. MFLs are considered stabilizers of the knee, specifically stabilizers in rotation. Others[33] indicate that MFLs are responsible for moving the posterior horn

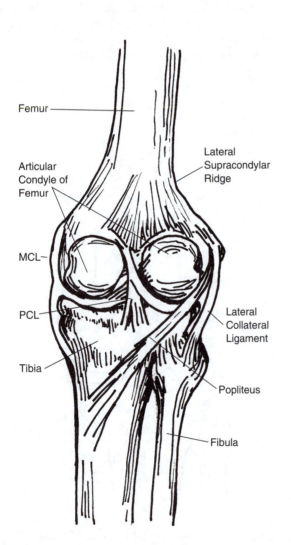

**Figure 14.7**   The Lateral Collateral Ligament

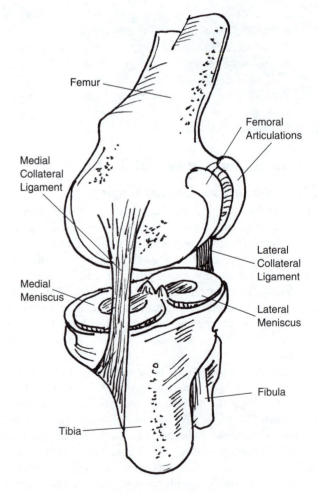

**Figure 14.8**   The Medial Collateral Ligament Complex

of the meniscus during movement of the knee. The ligaments keep the meniscus moving consistently with the movement of the femur, thus preventing the meniscus from being "ground" between the femur and the tibia.

Since the popliteus muscle also contributes to movement of the posterior horn of the meniscus, some have proposed that the MFLs function to counter the pull of the popliteus muscle.[34] The anterior and posterior MFLs may serve to move the meniscus during extension and flexion movement, each being responsible for the movement of the menisci depending on the position of the femur relative to the tibia. Additionally, the MFLs are considered secondary restraints to a posterior drawer of the knee.

### The Posterolateral Knee Structures

The posterolateral knee structures include the lateral collateral ligament, the arcuate ligament, the popliteofibular ligament, and variably the fibellofibular ligament.[35] Isolated injuries to the posterolateral corner are rare,[35] but may occur during contact to the anterior-medial aspect of the extended knee during weight bearing[27] or forced external rotation during a loaded and extended knee.[36] When injured, patients report a sensation of knee instability during extension. Movements such as hyperextension are vague clinical findings during examination and may not be definitive of posterolateral knee instability.[35] Posterolateral knee instability is rotational in nature and may involve displacement of the tibia posteriorly on the femur.

Because the PCL couples with external rotation of the tibia during posterior translation, the PCL ligament contributes poorly to the stability of the posterior lateral corner, specifically in extension. Isolated rupture of the posterior–lateral corner has a significant effect on the rotational and translatory stability of an extended knee.[27] Because of this, posterior drawer tests performed in flexion are not sufficient to determine posterior–lateral instability. Generally, to determine posterior–lateral corner instability, the clinician must examine tibial external rotation during 30–90 degrees of knee flexion.[27,37]

Posterolateral instability may involve an injury to the popliteus tendon since this structure is considered an important restraint to tibial external rotation.[37] The popliteus tendon originates on the posterolateral aspect of the femur and inserts on the anterior–lateral aspect of the fibular head, just distal to the lateral joint line. The tendon tightens during extension and external rotation.

### Posterior Ligaments and Structures

The most important posterior stabilizing structures of the knee are the deep posterior capsule, the lateral condylar ligament, the oblique popliteal ligament, the semimembranosus muscle, and the arcuate ligament. The deep posterior capsule is tightened during knee extension and blends nicely with the tendinous insertions of the gastronemius muscles. The lateral condylar ligament, oblique popliteal ligament, and the arcuate ligament assist in stabilizing the structure of the posterolateral knee. The semimembranosus

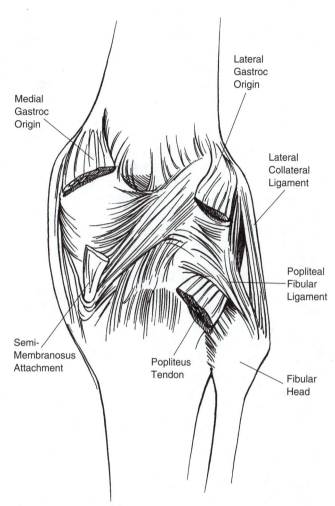

**Figure 14.9**  The Posterior Structures of the Knee

## Summary

- There are multiple ligamentous structures responsible for stability of the knee.
- Damage to one of the ligaments may negatively affect other ligaments.
- The most common outcome to damaged ligaments is instability.

can contract and tighten the oblique popliteal ligament that is considered a continuation of the tendon (Figure 14.9).

# BIOMECHANICS

## Movement and Stability

### Tibial Femoral Joint

In a normal knee, approximately 0 to 140 degrees of extension to flexion are present.[15] Most individuals also exhibit some degree of knee hyperextension during passive weight bearing and non–weight bearing. In normal individuals, the combined contribution of the muscles, ligaments, and menisci serve to increase the stiffness and stability of the knee and allow the action of transmission of large loads throughout the joint.[30]

Tibiofemoral translation is somewhat predictable during movements of extension to flexion. As a whole, during knee flexion, the tibia moves posteriorly on a fixed femur and the menisci move posteriorly as well. During knee extension, the tibia moves anteriorly on the fixed femur and the menisci move anteriorly. Movements in weight bearing initiate structures such as the cruciate ligaments and the menisci to balance the shear and compression forces at the tibial femoral joint.[38] Anterior forces are restrained primarily by the ACL whereas posterior forces are restrained by the PCL.

Von Eisenhart-Rothe et al.[39] reported that the femur translates posteriorly on the tibia at 30–90 degrees of knee flexion during co-contraction of the extensors and flexors in a simulated loading response. However, isolated contraction on healthy subjects demonstrates anterior translation of the tibia with respect to the femur during extensor contraction and posterior translation of the tibia with respect to the femur during flexor contraction.[40] Individuals with a damaged ACL demonstrated posterior translation during isolated extensor and flexor contractions.[39] These findings are supported by other studies[41] that also found posterior migration of the femur on the tibia during flexion.

Although the lateral condyle is often considered to translate more so than the medial condyle, research results are mixed.[39,40] Rolling is a fundamental movement of most articular surfaces and the femur does roll significantly on the fixed tibia. During flexion, the femur rolls and slides posteriorly to the tibia to allow the distal and posterior aspects of the femoral condyle to interface with the flattened tibial plateau. Much of this movement is guided by the posterior translation of the menisci and the control supplied by the cruciate ligaments and can be disrupted significantly during damage to these structures.[39] The ACL pulls on the femur and encourages anterior slide during knee flexion while it rolls in a posterior direction. The PCL encourages the femoral condyle to slide posterior during active extension and roll in an anterior direction.

During extension and flexion, the knee exhibits coupled knee internal and external rotation and sagittal motions.[30] This concurrent action of coupled tibial rotation, called the **screw home mechanism,** occurs to enhance the stability of the knee. When the knee is flexed in a closed chain, the tibia moves internally, in some cases up to 6.5–36 degrees.[42,43] During knee extension in a closed chain, the tibia moves into external rotation. Conversely, the femur appears to translate posteriorly, rotate laterally, and migrate proximally during flexion with respect to the tibia.[30] To some extent, coupled varus and valgus motion

occurs in conjunction with the sagittal and transverse plane movements. Nonetheless, these motions do not appear to be as compelling as rotations, flexion, and extension.[30]

During flexion beyond 120 degrees, the femoral condyles lose congruency with the tibial plateau and have contact points at the posterior horn of the menisci.[38] This is because the rolling of the femur outdistances the concurrent slide of the tibiofemoral complex. The external rotation that occurs at the femur increases the surface area for roll since it mimics the translatory aspect at the joint. Martelli and Pinskerova[44] advocate that the medial condyle is congruent and rounded and the lateral surface is flattened, allowing the lateral condyle to roll and slide at a greater quantity than the medial surface.

## Screw Home Mechanism

The screw home mechanism appears to be guided by the location of the joint axis and by the passive action of the posterior and anterior cruciate ligaments.[45] This mechanism is altered when damage is incurred to the anterior and posterior cruciate ligaments or when the stress–tension relationship of this ligament has in some way been altered.[45]

The popliteus plays a vital role in the screw home mechanism and initiates rotation of the tibia at 0–20 degrees of flexion. During this rotation, the menisci follow the movements of the femur.[15] The popliteus is situated and well adapted to prevent tibial external rotation during knee flexion.[30] During active extension, the popliteus functions actively to initiate knee flexion and retraction of the lateral meniscus.[30]

## Summary

- During an extension contraction, the tibia translates anteriorly.
- During a flexion contraction, the tibia translates posteriorly.
- During flexion, the tibia follows the convex–concave rule and rolls posteriorly. During extension, the tibia rolls anteriorly.
- The popliteus plays a vital role in the screw home mechanism and initiates rotation of the tibia at 0–20 degrees of flexion.
- During screw home rotation, the menisci follow the movements of the femur.

## Patella Femoral Joint

Movement of the patellofemoral joint is a complex kinematic process. Numerous *in vitro* studies have investigated patellofemoral movements and have reported significant variations of patterns.[46,47] One study attempted to load

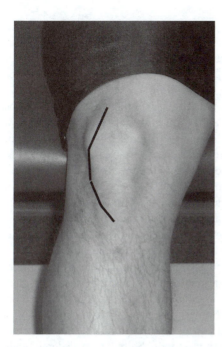

**Figure 14.10**   Movement of the Patella during Extension to Flexion of the Knee

the knee during 90 degrees of flexion to extension and found consistency of the patella during movement on the femur. During movement from flexion to extension, the patella starts in a medially tilted position, and then shifts to neutral, lastly shifting to a laterally tilted position while in extension (Figure 14.10).[48]

Recently, an *in vivo* study demonstrated variability in patellofemoral movements during extension to flexion movements. Laprade and Lee[3] reported that the patella typically moves distally during progressive extension to flexion, variably moves from anterior to posterior movement (in many cases the patella just moved posteriorly), and variably moves progressively laterally during knee flexion. In some cases, the kneecap moved medially first, then laterally as knee flexion progressed.

## *Summary*

- The articulation pattern of the patella may be variable during flexion and extension movements.
- The patella typically moves distally during progressive extension to flexion, variably moves from anterior to posterior movement (in many cases the patella just moved posteriorly), and variably moves progressively laterally during knee flexion.
- Abnormalities in patellofemoral biomechanics generally manifest at 0–30 degrees of flexion because of the deepening of the trochlear groove of the femur.

Abnormalities in patellofemoral biomechanics generally manifest at 0–30 degrees of flexion because of the deepening of the trochlear groove of the femur. Increases in knee flexion increase the weight-bearing aspect of the patellofemoral joint.[49] As the tibia continues to flexion, the iliotibial band pulls posteriorly on the patella, promoting posterior displacement against the femur.[17] If the patella lies too far laterally during this motion, this process can cause abnormal lateral forces, tracking problems, and lateral dislocations. Powers[16] reported that the depth of the trochlear groove is highly correlated with abnormal patellar kinematics, with increased shallowness of the trochlear groove being predictive of lateral patellar tilt and abnormal tracking.

# ASSESSMENT AND DIAGNOSIS

## Subjective Considerations

The primary approach to the subjective exam should first include the possible determination of nonmechanical disorders of the knee and isolation of the type of mechanical disorder if present. With knee disorders, identifying the mechanism of injury and/or onset of pain can aid in determining if the presenting disorder may have involved possible tearing or rupturing of structures or, if the onset of pain is more insidious, a more degenerative or sinister condition may be present. Additionally, the subjective exam will serve to identify potential movements or activities that are related to the concordant signs. For example, patients with meniscal injuries often report knee pain after twisting their leg while bearing full weight and often will experience a popping or tearing sensation, followed by severe pain. Swelling can take several hours to appear. Ligamentous injuries may occur with a similar mechanism to meniscal tears, and often will be the result of a direct blow to the knee, but swelling often occurs immediately.[1] Manske and Davies[50] noted the subjective variables of pain in the region of the patellofemoral joint while ascending or descending stairs may be indicative of PFPS.

Based on criteria of the *American College of Rheumatology*, osteoarthritis of the knee may be suspected if the following criteria are present: age older than 50, knee stiffness for less than 30 minutes, crepitus, bony tenderness, bony enlargement, and no palpable warmth.[1,51] If four criteria are present, the sensitivity of the characteristics is 84% with a specificity of 89%. If at least three of the criteria are present, the chance of osteoarthritis being present is 62%. Of the five criteria, two of the criteria are considered aspects of a subjective examination (age and stiffness) and two of five criteria increase the probability of osteoarthritis to 4%.[1] With this said, at least one physical exam variable would need to be present to bring probability to acceptable levels. This is in line with the fact that the clinical history alone, related to the diagnosis of meniscus or ligamentous tears, can only heighten suspicion and help formulate tentative management strategies and not necessarily differentiate between the two. The physical exam will be more helpful in determining the pathology associated with these disorders.[1]

Nonmechanical disorders such as septic arthritis will present as an acute onset of knee pain with effusion and warmth; signs and symptoms of infection will be present as well. There will most likely be no history of trauma to correlate to the effusion. Patients with this presentation should immediately be referred to a medical physician for appropriate consultation.[1,52]

Functional scales are designed to measure the outcomes of an intervention. The *Lower Extremity Function Scale* (LEFS) is a region-specific scale that is not limited to use with osteoarthritis. The LEFS is a self-report mechanism, primarily designed as a performance-based measure.[53] The LEFS is reliable (ICC = 0.95),[54] demonstrates construct validity, and is more sensitive to change than the SF-36.[55] The LEFS is a functional scale that can measure multiple joints[54] and is used conjunctively with measures of pain and physical exertion.

## Summary

- The purpose of the subjective examination is to identify the concordant mechanical disorders associated with the knee.
- Based on criteria of the *American College of Rheumatology*, osteoarthritis of the knee may be suspected if the following criteria are present: age older than 50, knee stiffness for less than 30 minutes, crepitus, bony tenderness, bony enlargement, and no palpable warmth.
- Nonmechanical disorders often include acute onset of knee pain with effusion, warmth, and signs and symptoms of infection.
- The *Lower Extremity Functional Scale* is a valid, self-report, region-specific questionnaire that measures problems associated with activities of daily living.

# CLINICAL EXAMINATION

## Observation

Observation of gait parameters and static alignment of the lower extremities are often key components to the clinical examination of the knee. The current literature regarding static alignment focuses on alignment at the foot and ankle. Selfe[56] reviewed the effect of correction of foot and ankle asymmetries and found that patients experienced an average of 67% reduction in patellofemoral knee pain following the dispensation of foot orthotics. Additionally,

rear foot posting produced an immediate and statistically significant medial glide in the patellofemoral joint. Selfe[56] noted that while the rear foot posting produced the medial glide, there was not an analysis of the association to reduction in symptoms.

Gross et al.[57] reviewed the effect of foot orthoses on the patellofemoral joint and their findings indicate that a significant amount of patients report improvement in their pain; however, there is less clear evidence of how correction of foot and ankle symmetry affects the patellofemoral joint. Hinterwimmer[58] found no difference in patellar kinematics in individuals with lower extremity asymmetries of genu varum and mild medial compartment osteoarthritis. Livingston et al.[59] found that the magnitude of right to left rear foot asymmetries was no different between symptomatic and asymptomatic patellofemoral pain groups.

Observational analysis of gait deviations is another component to assessment of the patient with knee pain. In the absence of obvious deviations that occur during significant trauma and swelling, minor gait deviations often are concurrent with knee pain. Selfe[56] reviewed gait analysis in patients with patellofemoral pain and found that men and women have similar torque generation at the knee during gait, wider-soled shoes increased knee flexor torque by 30%, and patients have a decreased walking velocity and more extended knees during gait than healthy controls. Additional studies[60,61] have demonstrated similar findings. A limitation of many of these studies is that they are laboratory based or utilize special equipment to measure gait deviations. This technology is not readily available in clinical practice, thus gait deviations may need to be observable and subjectively related to the patient's complaint.

## Summary

- Posture and foot alignment may suggest knee pain associated with other factors; however, in isolation, asymmetry does not implicate the causal problem.
- A gait analysis is helpful to outcome PFPS and other related knee anomalies.

## Active Physiological Movements

Active movements during a clinical examination are utilized to identify physical impairments that are relevant to the concordant signs. By determining the behavior of the concordant signs to selected active movements, the clinician can effectively identify potential active physiological treatment approaches.

### Plane-Based Active Range of Motion

Assessment of active range of motion of the knee can be assessed in different manners that will help not only determining objective range of motion of the knee, but also the

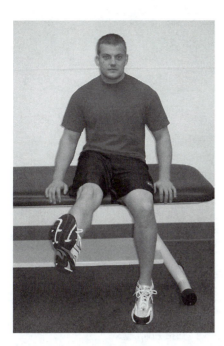

**Figure 14.11**    Active Physiological Knee Extension in Sitting

lows for a closer replication of functional positions and movements that are relevant to the concordant signs. For example, pain-reproducing movements for the knee may often include ascending and descending stairs and squatting. Cliborne et al.[62] used a *functional squat test* as one outcome measure following a program of hip mobilization in patients with knee osteoarthritis. The procedure included having the patient stand with their feet comfortably apart, then squat down until either pain limits the range or the heels come off the floor (Figure 14.13).

A single step-down test (Figure 14.14) is used to measure functional control of the knee during eccentric and concentric knee movements. The single step-down test is useful for patients who lack the range of motion to perform the functional squat test.

*Hop tests* (Figure 14.15) are often used with patients that are post-ACL reconstruction as a means to determine functional activity tolerance and predict dynamic knee stability and possible future injury. The *Hop tests* appear to have potential to predict dynamic knee stability, but currently the literature suggests that the predictive capability of these tests is questioned.[63]

relativity of the impairment to the concordant signs. Non–weight bearing active range-of-motion movements (AROM) can be performed in sitting (Figures 14.11 and 14.12) or supine position. These positions will influence the stressing of tissues surrounding the knee in different ways.

### Functional Active Range-of-Motion Testing

AROM performed in a weight-bearing position, while less convenient to attain objective measurements of ROM, al-

## Summary

- Active range-of-motion techniques should include functional activities and plane-based movements.
- Functional tests should be geared toward the concordant reproduction of the patient's complaint.

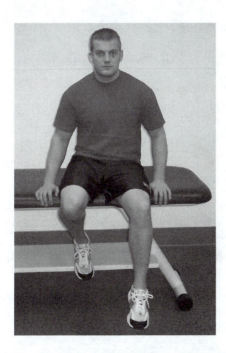

**Figure 14.12**    Active Physiological Knee Flexion in Sitting

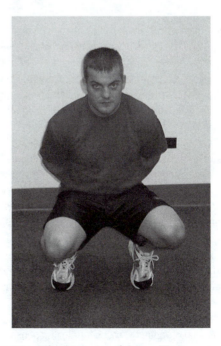

**Figure 14.13**    The Functional Squat Test

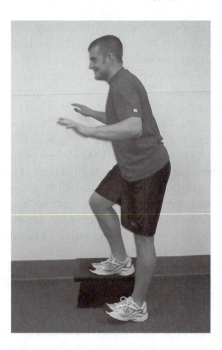

Figure 14.14    The Single Step Down Test

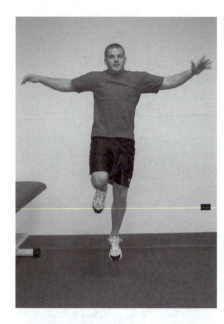

Figure 14.15    The Hop Test

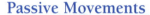

## Passive Movements

### *Passive Physiological Movements*

Passive physiological movements of the knee are similar to active physiological movements and are used to confirm the relationship to the concordant signs. Additionally, passive physiological movements of the knee allow for a more complete examination of component movements (i.e., tibial rotation) that are difficult to actively replicate and occur during functional movement. Abnormal "end feels" of movement have been found to be associated with a patient's concordant sign.[64,65] The clinician should strive to correlate any detection of abnormal movement to the concordant signs.

## Passive Physiological Knee Flexion

- Step One: The patient assumes the supine position.
- Step Two: The clinician grasps the patient's leg just proximal to the knee with one hand and just distal to the mid-tibia with the other. The clinician may find it necessary to use a portion of his or her chest to support the leg while applying movement. Additionally, the clinician should strive to maintain the lower extremity/hip in a consistent neutral position (this can be modified as needed to correlate to the concordant signs).
- Step Three: The clinician gently moves the knee into the flexion (sagittal) plane, stopping at the first point of pain.
- Step Four: The clinician will assess for symmetry of motion and assess for reproduction of concordant signs while moving the knee beyond the first point of pain, progressing toward end range as the patient's complaint of pain allows.
- Step Five: Repeated movements or sustained holds into knee flexion are then performed to the point of flexion range that pain allows to assess the response of the repeated movements on the patient's pain (or like symptoms).
- Step Six: As needed, the clinician can apply force (overpressure) to the end of range to assess for pain response.

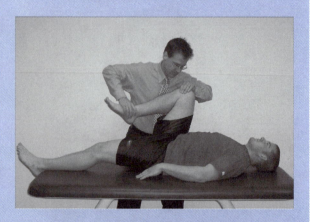

Figure 14.16    Passive Physiological Knee Flexion

## Knee Flexion with Abduction and Adduction

Combined passive movements are used to examine further available physiological range in an effort to find concordant signs and improve the sensitivity of the examination.

- Step One: The clinician follows the procedures above and flexes the knee to 10–20 degrees short of end of available range.
- Step Two: The clinician firmly grasps the distal femur with one hand while holding the lateral femur against his or her chest. This handling will help ensure that the clinician *does not allow femoral rotation* during this phase of the examination. The clinician's other hand will grasp the distal tibia.
- Step Three: As the clinician flexes the knee, he or she directs the heel toward the direction of the greater trochanter of the hip (producing abduction movement of the tibia). Movement will occur up until pain is reproduced, then gently past this point as tolerated. If the concordant sign is not reproduced, this movement can then be repeated with the tibia held in various degrees of available tibia internal rotation.

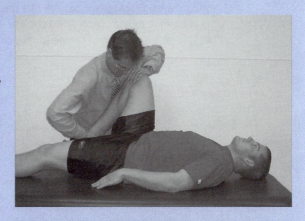

**Figure 14.17** Knee Flexion and Abduction

- Step Four: As needed, the clinician can apply force (overpressure) to the end of range to assess for pain response.
- Step Five: As the clinician flexes the knee, he or she directs the heel toward the direction of the groin (producing adduction movement of the tibia). Movement will occur up until pain is reproduced, then gently past this point as tolerated. If the concordant sign is not reproduced, this movement can then be repeated with the tibia held in various degrees of available tibia external rotation.
- Step Six: As needed, the clinician can apply force (overpressure) to the end of range to assess for pain response.

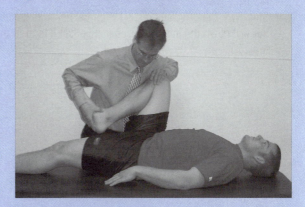

**Figure 14.18** Knee Flexion with Adduction

## Passive Physiological Extension

Range of extension ROM is often much smaller than flexion, thus handling procedures are very different.

- Step One: The patient assumes the supine position.
- Step Two: The clinician grasps the lateral ankle with one hand, while the interthenar eminence of the other hand is placed on the tibial tubercle.
- Step Three: Using side bending of the trunk and a simultaneous force on the above-noted contact areas with the hands, the clinician then produces an extension movement of the knee, stopping at the first point of pain.
- Step Four: The clinician will assess for symmetry of motion and assess for reproduction of concordant signs while moving the knee beyond the first point of pain, progressing toward end range as the patient's complaint of concordant pain allows.
- Step Five: Repeated movements into knee extension are then performed to the point of extension range that pain allows to assess the response of the repeated movements on the patient's pain (or like symptoms).
- Step Six: As needed, the clinician can apply force (overpressure) to the end of range to assess for pain response.

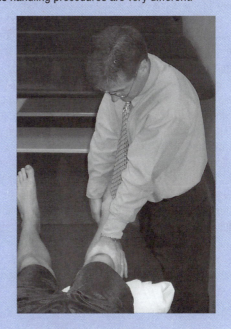

**Figure 14.19** Passive Knee Extension

## Knee Extension with Adduction and Abduction

As noted previously, combined passive movements are used to examine further available physiological range in an effort to find concordant signs and improve the sensitivity of the examination. The following example is for knee extension combined movements:

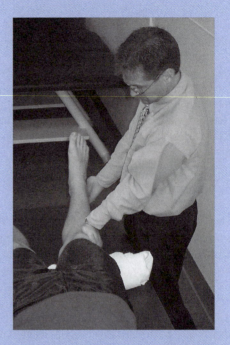

- Step One: The clinician follows the procedures above and extends the knee to 10–15 degrees short of end of available range.
- Step Two: The clinician grasps the lateral ankle as noted above, but will move the interthenar eminence just lateral to the tibial tubercle.

**Figure 14.20**    Knee Extension with Abduction

- Step Three: As the clinician extends the knee, using side bending of the trunk and a simultaneous force on these contact areas with the hands, the clinician then produces an extension–abduction movement of the knee (abduction movement of the tibia). Movement will occur up until pain is reproduced, then gently past this point as tolerated.
- Step Four: As needed, the clinician can apply force (overpressure) to the end of range to assess for pain response.
- Step Five: The clinician grasps the lateral ankle as noted above, but will move the interthenar eminence just medial to the tibial tubercle.
- Step Six: As the clinician extends the knee, using side bending of the trunk and a simultaneous force on these contact areas with the hands, the clinician then produces an extension–adduction movement of the knee (adduction movement of the tibia). Movement will occur up until pain is reproduced, then gently past this point as tolerated.
- Step Seven: As needed, the clinician can apply force (overpressure) to the end of range to assess for pain response.

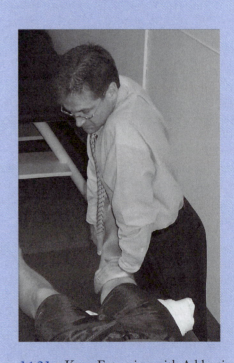

**Figure 14.21**    Knee Extension with Adduction

## Tibial Internal and External Rotation

Approximately 20 degrees of rotation occurs at the tibial femoral joint. Restrictions are common and may require physiological intervention.

- Step One: The patient assumes a supine position. The clinician cradles the tibia on his or her forearm and grasps the foot distally at the heel.
- Step Two: The ankle of the patient is passively dorsiflexed to create a stable lever during rotation. The knee is flexed to approximately 90 degrees.
- Step Three: The clinician applies a passive internal rotation to the first point of pain. Repeated movements or sustained holds are applied to determine if the movements reduce pain. The activity is repeated toward end range.

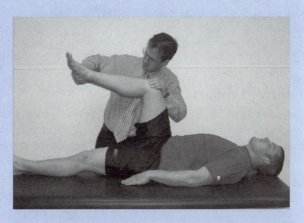

**Figure 14.22**    Tibial Internal Rotation at 90 Degrees of Knee Flexion

- Step Four: The clinician applies a passive external rotation to the first point of pain. Repeated movements or sustained holds are applied to determine if the movements reduce pain. The activity is repeated toward end range.

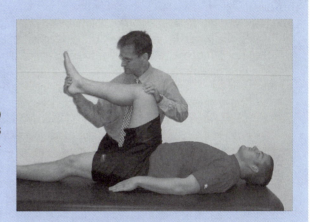

**Figure 14.23**    Tibial External Rotation at 90 Degrees of Knee Extension

## Summary

- The purpose of passive physiological testing is to reproduce the concordant sign of the patient.
- By incorporating adduction, abduction, and rotations in the plane-based movements of flexion and extension, the clinician may more accurately isolate the disorder of the patient.

### Passive Accessory Movements

Assessment of passive accessory movements is used to assess component motion of a joint segment/region, including the relevance to the patient's impairment and concordant signs. As we have repeated throughout this text, assessment of position, orientation, or movement of the body/joint segments without inclusion of the relevance to the concordant signs will yield less reliable clinical information and will limit the clinician's ability to analyze further the patient's response to movements.

The following describes the procedures of passive accessory movement testing of the knee. It is important to note that the assessment of accessory glides necessitates movements in varying ranges of physiological ROM. Careful analysis will allow the clinician to establish the relevance of an impairment of accessory motion to physiological ROM and to the concordant signs that may have been established in the active and/or passive physiological components of the examination.

### Tibiofemoral Joint—Posterior to Anterior

- **Step One:** The patient assumes the supine position. The knee is prepositioned at 60–80 degrees of flexion.
- **Step Two:** The clinician will grasp the proximal tibia with both hands, wrapping the fingers around to the posterior tibia.
- **Step Three:** The clinician then gently moves the tibia on the femur in a posterior-to-anterior direction, stopping at the first point of pain. The pain is assessed for the concordant sign. In knee flexion ranges of less than approximately 60 degrees, the clinician will need to ensure he or she moves his or her body from posterior to anterior and slightly caudal to attempt not to passively flex the patient's knee. Additionally, the clinician will need to ensure to maintain a consistent position of the hip for all ranges assessed.
- **Step Four:** The clinician will assess for quality of motion and assess for reproduction concordant signs while moving the knee beyond the first point of pain, progressing toward end range as the patient's complaint of pain allows.
- **Step Five:** Repeated movements are then performed to the point of range/movement that pain allows, to assess the response of the repeated movements on the patient's pain (or like symptoms).

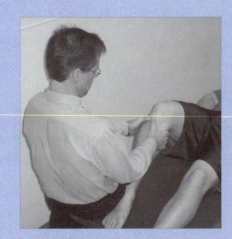

**Figure 14.24**    Posterior-Anterior Mobilization of the Tibiofemoral Joint

## Anterior-to-Posterior Mobilization of the Tibiofemoral Joint

- Step One: The patient assumes the supine position. The clinician can place a small bolster behind the femur to allow the knee to rest in approximately 10–30 degrees of flexion.
- Step Two: The clinician will place both thumbs on the tibial tubercle and allow the fingers to rest on the postero-lateral aspects of the tibia.
- Step Three: Pushing with the thumbs, the clinician then gently moves the tibia on the femur in an anterior-to-posterior direction, stopping at the first point of pain.
- Step Four: The clinician will assess for quality of motion and assess for reproduction of concordant signs while moving the knee beyond the first point of pain, progressing toward end range as the patient's complaint of pain allows.
- Step Five: Repeated movements are then performed to the point of range/movement that pain allows, to assess the response of the repeated movements on the patient's pain (or like symptoms).

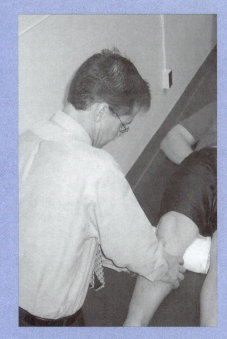

**Figure 14.25**    Anterior to Posterior Mobilization of the Tibiofemoral Joint

## Medial and Lateral Shear of the Tibiofemoral Joint

- Step One: The patient assumes the supine position. The clinician can place a small bolster behind the femur to allow the knee to rest in approximately 10–20 degrees of flexion.
- Step Two: For medial shear, the clinician uses one hand to grasp the medial aspect of the distal femur, in the region of the condyles, while with the other hand the clinician grasps the lateral aspect of the proximal tibia.
- Step Three: The clinician will stabilize the femur while applying a medially directed movement of the tibia on the femur, stopping at the first point of pain.

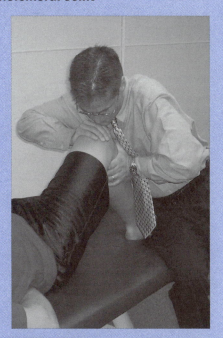

**Figure 14.28**    Medial Glide of the Tibia on the Femur

*(continued)*

- Step Four: The clinician will assess for quality of motion and assess for reproduction of concordant signs while moving the knee beyond the first point of pain, progressing toward end range as the patient's complaint of pain allows.
- Step Five: Repeated movements are then performed to the point of range/movement that pain allows, to assess the response of the repeated movements on the patient's pain (or like symptoms).
- Step Six: For lateral shear, the clinician uses one hand to grasp the lateral aspect of the distal femur, in the region of the condyles, while with the other hand the clinician grasps the lateral aspect of the proximal tibia.
- Step Seven: The clinician will stabilize the femur while applying a laterally directed movement of the tibia on the femur, stopping at the first point of pain.

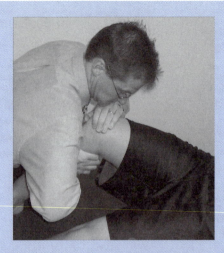

**Figure 14.29**    Lateral Glide of the Tibia on the Femur

The movement of the tibia on the femur may isolate the outer horns of the menisci and force movement of the menisci. Movement of the tibia posteriorly on the femur results in anterior movement of the menisci on the femur. Figure 14.26 illustrates this process.

The movement of the tibia anteriorly on the femur in a flexed position may force posterior migration of the meniscus with respect to the tibia. Figure 14.27 illustrates this phenomenon.

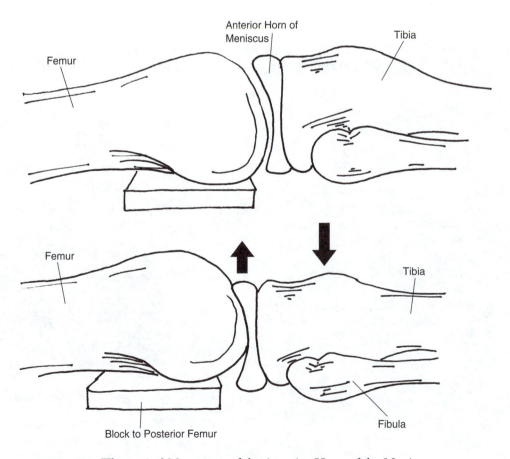

**Figure 14.26**    Theoretical Movement of the Anterior Horn of the Meniscus

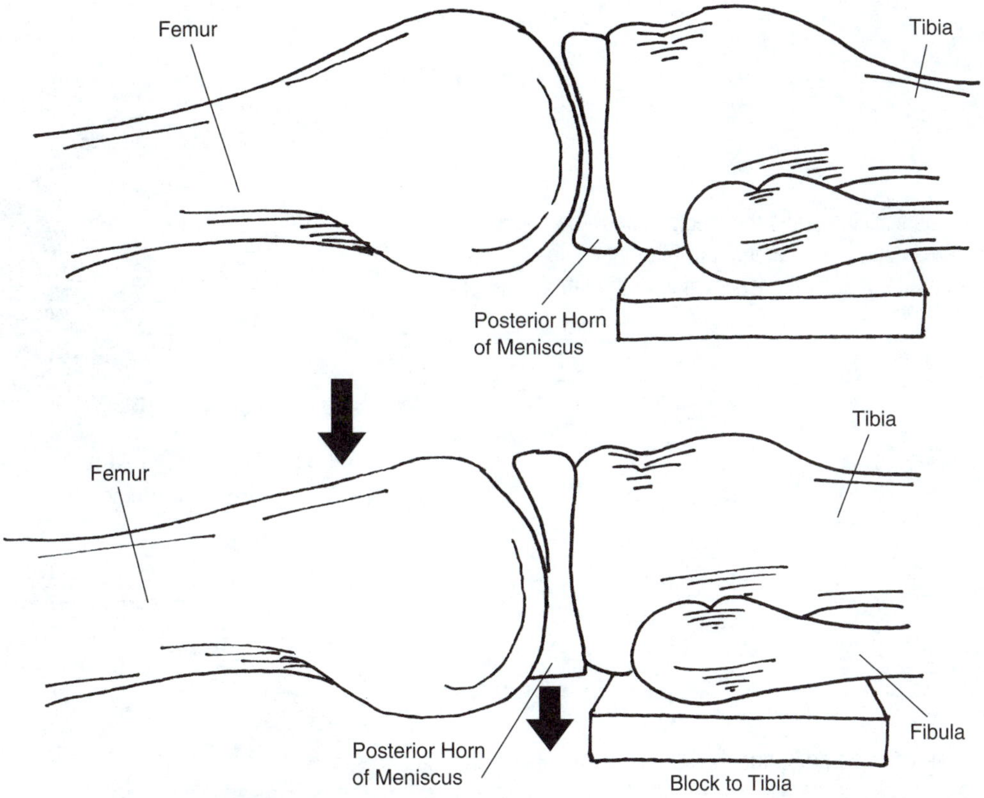

Femur

Tibia

Posterior Horn
of Meniscus

Femur

Tibia

Posterior Horn
of Meniscus

Fibula

Block to Tibia

**Figure 14.27**    Theoretical Movement of the Posterior Horn of the Meniscus

## Rotations of the Tibiofemoral Joint

- Step One: The patient assumes a hooklying position. The clinician stabilizes the foot by sitting on the dorsum.
- Step Two: The clinician grabs the lateral half of the tibia with one hand and stabilizes the femur with the other. The clinician then applies a medially directed and anterior rotation to the lateral half of the tibia.

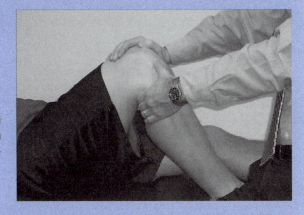

**Figure 14.30**    Medial and Anterior Rotation of the Tibia on the Femur

(*continued*)

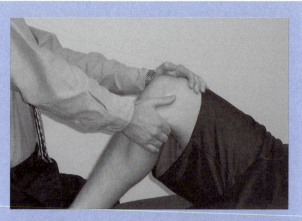

**Figure 14.31**    Lateral and Anterior Rotation of the Tibia on the Femur

- Step Three: The clinician grabs the medial half of the tibia with one hand and stabilizes the femur with the other. The clinician then applies a lateral and anterior rotation to the lateral half of the tibia.

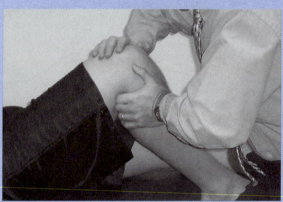

**Figure 14.32**    Medial and Posterior Rotation of the Tibia on the Femur

- Step Four: The clinician grabs the lateral half of the tibia with one hand and stabilizes the femur with the other. The clinician then applies a medial and posterior rotation to the lateral half of the tibia.

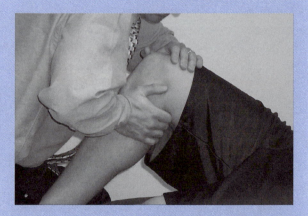

**Figure 14.33**    Lateral and Posterior Rotation of the Tibia on the Femur

- Step Five: The clinician grabs the medial half of the tibia with one hand and stabilizes the femur with the other. The clinician then applies a lateral and posterior rotation to the lateral half of the tibia.
- Step Six: Movements are repeated or sustained (at the first point of pain and at end range) to determine if concordant and whether the pain abolishes with movements.

During movement from flexion to extension, the patella starts in a medially tilted position and then shifts to neutral, lastly shifting to a laterally tilted position while in extension.[48] Additionally, the patella moves distally during progressive extension to flexion, variably moves from anterior to posterior movement (in many cases the patella just moved posteriorly), and variably moves progressively laterally during knee flexion.[3] Consequently, it is important to assess the numerous ranges of patella mobility.

## Cephalad and Caudal Movements of the Patellofemoral Joint

- **Step One:** The patient assumes the supine position. The knee is placed in approximately 30 degrees of flexion.
- **Step Two:** The clinician places the apex of the patella in their interthenar groove, cupping the hand slightly. Additionally, the clinician will lean forward and align his or her forearm with the shaft of the tibia.
- **Step Three:** With his or her other hand, the clinician places the web space of his or her hand across the superior aspect of the patella. Additionally, the clinician will lean forward and align his or her forearm with the shaft of the femur.
- **Step Four:** The clinician then gently glides the patella in cephalad direction, stopping at the first point of pain.
- **Step Five:** The clinician will assess for quality of motion and assess for reproduction of concordant signs while moving the patella beyond the first point of pain, progressing toward end range as the patient's complaint of pain allows.
- **Step Six:** Repeated movements are then performed to the point of range/movement that pain allows, to assess the response of the repeated movements on the patient's pain (or like symptoms).

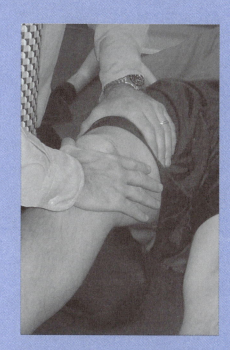

**Figure 14.34**    Cephalic Glide of the Patella

- **Step Seven:** *Caudal Movement.* The clinician can follow the steps for cephalad movement of the patella, but will move the patella in a caudal direction.

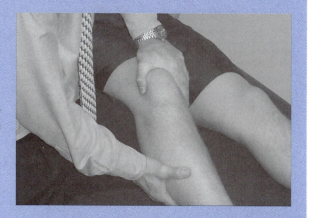

**Figure 14.35**    Caudal Glide of the Patella

## Medial and Lateral Movements of the Patellofemoral Joint

- Step One: The patient assumes the supine position. The knee is placed in approximately 30 degrees of flexion.
- Step Two: *Lateral Movement.* The clinician will stand on the lateral side of the knee and place the fingers against the medial border of the patella.
- Step Three: The clinician will produce a laterally directed movement of the patella, stopping at the first point of pain.
- Step Four: The clinician will assess for quality of motion and assess for reproduction concordant signs while moving the patella beyond the first point of pain, progressing toward end range as the patient's complaint of pain allows.
- Step Five: Repeated movements are then performed to the point of range/movement that pain allows, to assess the response of the repeated movements on the patient's pain (or like symptoms).

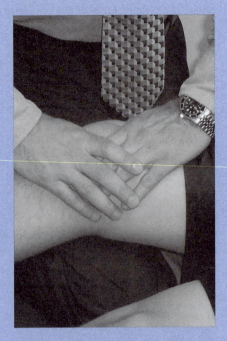

**Figure 14.36**    Lateral Glide of the Patella

- Step Six: *Medial Movement.* The clinician can follow the above steps for lateral movement of the patella (although the thumbs and web space now provide the contact force), but produce movement in a medially directed direction.

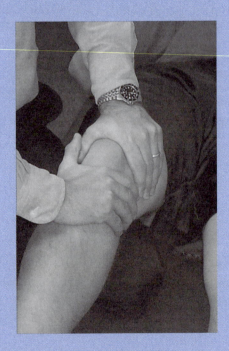

**Figure 14.37**    Medial Glide of the Patella

## Medial and Lateral Tilt Movements of the Patellofemoral Joint

Based on the posterior facet anatomy of the patella, medial and lateral "tilting" or rotation of the patella in the transverse plane is an accessory movement of the patellofemoral joint.

- Step One: The patient assumes the supine position. The knee is placed in approximately 30 degrees of flexion.
- Step Two: To create a medial tilt, the clinician will place one of his or her thumbs or thenar eminences on the medial half of the patella, while the other thumb or thenar eminence blocks the lateral aspect of the patella (to limit the patella from moving laterally).
- Step Three: The clinician will produce a medial "tilting" movement of the patella by pushing on the medial half of the patella in an anterior-to-posterior direction, stopping at the first point of pain.
- Step Four: The clinician will assess for quality of motion and assess for reproduction of concordant signs while moving the patella beyond the first point of pain, progressing toward end range as the patient's complaint of pain allows.
- Step Five: Repeated movements are then performed to the point of range/movement that pain allows, to assess the response of the repeated movements on the patient's pain (or like symptoms).

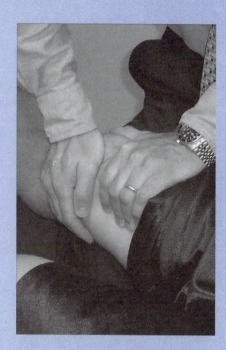

**Figure 14.38**    Medial Tilt of the Patella

- Step Six: To create a lateral tilt, the clinician can follow the above steps, but will produce lateral tilting movement by producing movement in an anterior-to-posterior direction on the lateral half of the patella. The clinician should also be sure to block the medial border of the patella to prevent a medial movement of the patella during the lateral tilting movement.

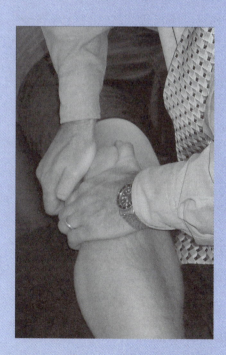

**Figure 14.39**    Lateral Tilt of the Patella

## Medial and Lateral Rotation Movements

The medial and lateral rotation described in this section refers to rotation in the frontal plane (i.e., the apex [superior border] of the patella directed medially is medial rotation).

- Step One: The patient assumes the supine position. The knee is placed in approximately 30 degrees of flexion.
- Step Two: *Medial Rotation.* The clinician, standing on the lateral side of the knee, will grasp the patella with both hands, placing the apex of the patella in the web space of the caudal hand and the superior aspect of the patella in the web space of the cephalad hand.
- Step Three: To produce a medially directed rotation, the clinician will rotate the apex of the patella medially, stopping at the first point of pain. The clinician may find it helpful when producing these movements to take up tissue slack around the knee. This can be accomplished by placing the hands on the patella as described in Step Two (the following describes medially directed movement) but place the cephalic hand medially (about the 2 o'clock position) and the caudal hand just opposite the cephalad hand (about the 8 o'clock position). Now firmly grasping the soft tissues move your hands back to the original position. This technique should allow the clinician to feel more localized movement of the patella versus the surrounding soft tissues.
- Step Four: The clinician will assess for quality of motion and assess for reproduction of concordant signs while moving the patella beyond the first point of pain, progressing toward end range as the patient's complaint of pain allows.

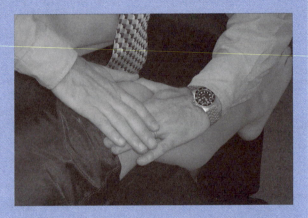

**Figure 14.40**    Medial Rotation of the Patella

- Step Five: Repeated movements are then performed to the point of range/movement that pain allows, to assess the response of the repeated movements on the patient's pain (or like symptoms).
- Step Six: *Lateral Rotation.* The clinician can follow the above steps but produce movement of the patella in a lateral direction.

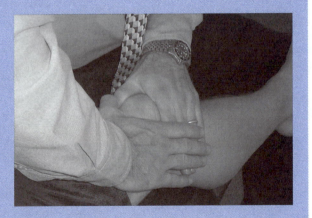

**Figure 14.41**    Lateral Rotation of the Patella

### Patellar Compression

Compression of joint surfaces in examination is purported to aid in determining if a patient's symptoms are from a "joint surface disorder"; that is, possible changes to the joint surfaces that may contribute to a patient's symptoms.[66] There is no known validity to the fact that pain from just compression of a joint surface correlates to tissue changes of the joint surfaces. With this in mind, the reader is encouraged to consider compression as an additional examination technique that may reveal concordant signs. Additionally, compression can be used to aid in ruling out the involvement of a joint region when examination movements are assessed with strong compression without symptom provocation.[66]

Common clinical findings that suggest examination with compression include:[66]

1. The standard examination movements do not clearly correlate to the patient's symptoms.
2. The patient complaint of pain through range of movement.
3. Crepitus of the joint with movement.
4. Heavy work or activity causes minor symptoms ("compressive loads").
5. Lying on the involved joint provokes symptoms.

There are varieties of joint regions that require examination with compression, the patellofemoral joint being one of them. For the patellofemoral joint, cephalad/caudal, medial/lateral, medial/lateral tilt, and medial/lateral rotation movements are performed with compression. The clinician can perform the previously described examination movements of the patellofemoral joint with compression then assess for relevance to concordant signs.

Compression is achieved by moving the patella toward the femur, gently at first, then producing the previously described movements. As with any other accessory examination techniques, the clinician should consider assessing with the knee positioned in various ranges of physiological ROM.

### Patellar Distraction

Patellar distraction is basically the opposite of compression. Gently, the clinician will need to use the pads of the fingers to grasp the lateral and medial posterior facet-region of the patella and produce a movement of the patella away from the femur. Assessment then includes producing cephalad/caudal, medial/lateral, medial/lateral tilt, medial/lateral rotation movements while sustaining distraction. The clinician's goals will remain the same of relating the relevance of provoking movements to concordant signs.

---

### Posterior-to-Anterior Glide of Superior Tibial–Fibular Joint

The superior tibial–fibular joint region should be included in a comprehensive evaluation of the knee as this structure can contribute to pain and dysfunction in the knee region and plays an integral role in the interaction between the foot/ankle and the knee.

- Step One: The patient assumes the sidelying position with the area examined facing upward. The clinician should aim to position the lower extremity in a relatively neutral position (i.e., pillow between knees, etc.)
- Step Two: The clinician will stand behind the patient and palpate for the posterior margin of the head of the fibula.
- Step Three: The clinician will then place the pads of his or her thumbs against the posterior margin of the head of the fibula.
- Step Four: Using the thumbs, produce a posterior-to-anterior directed movement, stopping at the first point of pain.
- Step Five: The clinician will assess for quality of motion and assess for reproduction of concordant signs while moving the fibula beyond the first point of pain, progressing toward end range as the patient's complaint of pain allows.
- Step Six: Repeated movements are then performed to the point of range/movement that pain allows, to assess the response of the repeated movements on the patient's pain (or like symptoms).
- Step Seven: The above-described movement should then be performed with compression. This is achieved by leaving one thumb on the posterior margin of the fibula and taking the interthenar groove of the other hand and placing it on top of the thumb. Compression is achieved by pushing downward toward the table while simultaneously producing the posterior-to-anterior movement. Steps Five and Six are then followed while using compression.

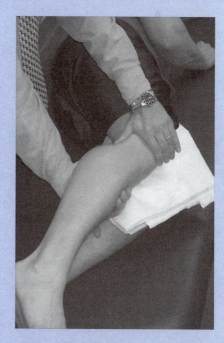

**Figure 14.42** Posterior to Anterior Glide of the Tibial-Fibular Joint

## Anterior-to-Posterior Glide of the Tibial–Fibular Joint

- Step One: The patient assumes the sidelying position with the area examined facing upward. The clinician should aim to position the lower extremity in a relatively neutral position (i.e., pillow between knees, etc.).
- Step Two: The clinician stands in front of the patient and palpates for the posterior margin of the head of the fibula.
- Step Three: The clinician then places the pads of his or her thumbs against the anterior margin of the head of the fibula.
- Step Four: Using the thumbs, produce a posterior-to-anterior directed movement, stopping at the first point of pain.
- Step Five: The clinician will assess for quality of motion and assess for reproduction of concordant signs while moving the fibula beyond the first point of pain, progressing toward end range as the patient's complaint of pain allows.
- Step Six: Repeated movements are then performed to the point of range/movement that pain allows, to assess the response of the repeated movements on the patient's pain (or like symptoms).
- Step Seven: The previously described movements should then be performed with compression. This is achieved by leaving one thumb on the anterior margin of the fibula and taking the interthenar groove of the other hand and placing it on top of the thumb. Compression is achieved by pushing downward toward the table while simultaneously producing the anterior-to-posterior movement. Steps Five and Six are then followed while using compression.

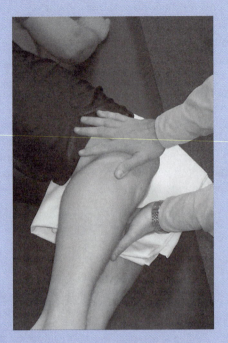

**Figure 14.43**   Anterior to Posterior Glide of the Tibial Fibular Joint

## Cephalad and Caudal of the Tibial–Fibular Joint

- Step One: The patient assumes the sidelying position with the area examined facing upward. The clinician should aim to position the lower extremity in a relatively neutral position (i.e., pillow between knees, etc.)
- Step Two: The clinician will stand behind the patient and palpate for the anterior and posterior margins of the head of the fibula.
- Step Three: The clinician then grasps the rear-foot of the same lower extremity. The clinician will ensure that the rear-foot is clear of the table to produce movement of the rear-foot.

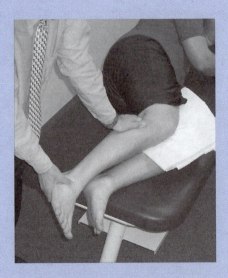

**Figure 14.44**   Cephalic Glide of the Fibula

- **Step Four:** The clinician will indirectly produce cephalad and caudal movements of the fibula by producing inversion (caudal fibula) or eversion (cephalad fibula) of the rear-foot. Simultaneous palpation of the superior fibula occurs during these movements. Movement occurs up to the first point of pain.
- **Step Five:** The clinician will assess for quality of motion and assess for reproduction of concordant signs while moving the fibula beyond the first point of pain (by moving the rear-foot), progressing toward end range as the patient's complaint of pain allows.
- **Step Six:** Repeated movements are then performed to the point of range/movement that pain allows, to assess the response of the repeated movements on the patient's pain (or like symptoms).

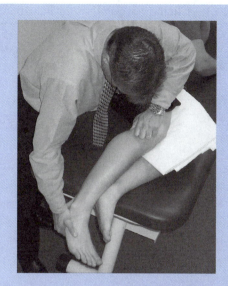

**Figure 14.45**　Caudal Glide of the Fibula

## Summary

- The purpose of passive accessory testing is to reproduce the concordant sign of the patient.
- Appropriate isolation of passive accessory testing may require prepositioning of the knee to implicate symptoms.
- Strategies such as compression are effective in isolating painful conditions.
- Combined accessory movements may tighten structures and further implicate casual problems.

## Clinical Special Tests

### *Palpation*

Palpation tests for the knee are best divided into two main categories: (1) palpation for the presence of **intraarticular disorders** and (2) palpation for the presence of a fracture. Table 14.1 outlines the diagnostic value of palpation.

#### *Joint Line Tenderness*

Palpation for joint line tenderness (Figure 14.46) is a basic maneuver used to implicate meniscal injuries or general effusion of the knee.[79] Since the anterior–medial aspect of the medial meniscus becomes prominent during internal rotation and flexion, it may be advantageous to preposition the knee during the palpation procedure. Extension of the knee may further improve the sensitivity of this palpation procedure.

#### *Joint Effusion*

The benefit of palpation for joint effusion highly depends on the timing and the amount of effusion noted. Calmbach and Hutchens[67] suggest that a "rapid onset"

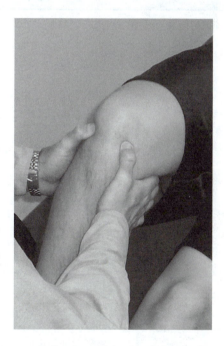

**Figure 14.46**　Palpation of the Medial Tibial Joint Line

(within 2 hours) of a large, tense effusion suggests rupture of the anterior cruciate ligament or fracture of the tibial plateau with resultant hemarthrosis, whereas a slower onset (24–36 hours) of a mild-to-moderate effusion is consistent with meniscal injury or ligamentous sprain.

#### *Palpation Tests for Knee Fractures*

The **Ottawa Knee Rules** are a prospective set of clinical findings that are designed to assist in determining the use of a radiograph. There are five components to the Ottawa Knee Rules: (1) age > 55, (2) tenderness at the head of the fibula, (3) isolated tenderness of patella during

**TABLE 14.1**    Clinical Special Tests for Palpation

| Clinical Test | Author | Sensitivity | Specificity | +LR | −LR |
|---|---|---|---|---|---|
| Joint Line Tenderness | Barry et al.[103] | 86 | 43 | 1.5 | 0.32 |
| | Noble & Erat[104] | 73 | 13 | 0.8 | 2.1 |
| | Fowler & Lubliner[105] | 85 | 30 | 1.2 | 0.5 |
| | Saengnipanthkul et al.[106] | 58 | 74 | 2.2 | 0.6 |
| | Kurosaka et al.[107] | 55 | 67 | 1.6 | 0.67 |
| | Anderson & Lipscomb[108] | 77 | NR | NA | NA |
| | Akseki et al. Medial Meniscus[109] | 88 | 44 | 1.6 | 0.27 |
| | Akseki et al. Lateral Meniscus[109] | 67 | 80 | 3.4 | 0.41 |
| | Karachalios et al. Medial Meniscus[110] | 71 | 87 | 5.5 | 0.33 |
| | Karachalios et al. Lateral Meniscus[110] | 78 | 90 | 7.8 | 0.24 |
| | Eren Medial Meniscus[111] | 86 | 67 | 2.6 | 0.20 |
| | Eren Lateral Meniscus[111] | 92 | 97 | 30.7 | 0.08 |
| Joint Effusion | Noble & Erat[104] | 53 | 54 | 1.1 | 0.87 |
| | Barry et al.[103] | 30 | 100 | NA | NA |

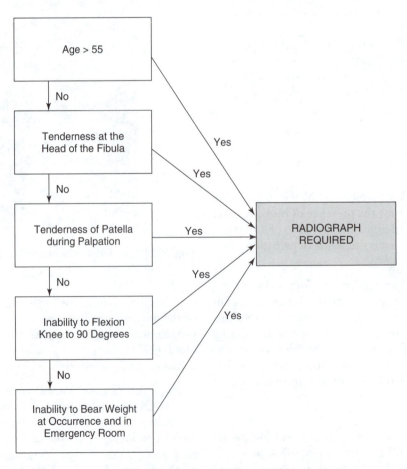

**Figure 14.47**    The Ottawa Knee Rules Diagram[114]

**TABLE 14.2**    Clinical Special Tests for Detection of Knee Fractures

| Clinical Test | Author | Sensitivity | Specificity | +LR | −LR |
|---|---|---|---|---|---|
| Ottawa Ankle Rules | Stiell et al.[112] | 100 | 49.5 | NA | NA |
| | Richman et al.[113] | 84.6 | 45.2 | 1.54 | 0.34 |
| | Emparanza & Aginage[114] | 100 | 52 | NA | NA |
| | Szucs et al.[115] | 100 | 46.6 | NA | NA |
| | Stiell et al.[116] | 100 | 48 | NA | NA |
| | Ketelslegers et al.[117] | 100 | 31.6 | NA | NA |
| | Seaberg et al.[118] | 96.6 | 26.5 | 1.31 | 0.12 |
| | Tigges et al.[119] | 97.7 | 19.1 | 1.71 | 0.12 |
| | Khine et al.[120] | 92.3 | 48.9 | 1.80 | 0.15 |

palpation, (4) inability to flex knee to 90 degrees, and (5) inability to bear weight both immediately and in the emergency department. The Ottawa Knee Rules are recognized as the most valid mechanism to determine whether plain film radiographs are necessary in the event of trauma (Figure 14.47 and Table 14.2).[1]

## Manual Muscle Testing

Manual muscle testing of knee flexion and/or extension with a hand-held dynamometer has demonstrated good reliability in studies: (1) that have used children as subjects,[68] (2) subjects status post hip fracture,[69] (3) patients with cerebral palsy,[70] (4) patients with spinal muscular atrophy,[71] and (5) the community-dwelling elderly.[72] However, manual muscle testing was considered poor when tested using subjects that were healthy.[73] The inclined squat strength test is considered an alternative to the break test and is considered more functional. The test has demonstrated good reliability using subjects with no known pathology.[74]

## Clinical Special Tests for Intraarticular Disorders

### McMurray's Test

McMurray's test for meniscal tears was first described by McMurray in 1942.[75] Since the development of the test, numerous iterations have been demonstrated, all with the name "McMurray's test".[76] Nonetheless, the true McMurray's test has rarely been studied for diagnostic accuracy and instead several variations are reported as homogeneous adaptations. According to McMurray, external tibial rotation tests the internal (medial) cartilage and internal rotation tests the external (lateral) cartilage. Variations of knee flexion purportedly alter the effect on the anterior and posterior cartilage horns. In theory, greater flexion affects the posterior horn while less knee flexion targets the anterior horn. A positive test is the concordant pain and a click during rotation of the tibia on the femur. Table 14.3 (page 527) outlines the diagnostic value of the test.

- Step One: The patient lies in a supine position. The knee is fully flexed to end range.
- Step Two: The clinician grasps the foot of the patient at the heel to guide tibial rotation. The other hand of the clinician is placed on the top of the patient's knee to counter the force through the heel.
- Step Three: While maintaining knee flexion, the clinician applies medial and lateral rotation of the tibia on the femur. This position purportedly tests the posterior horns of the medial and lateral meniscus.
- Step Four: The clinician may vary the angle of knee flexion to target different regions of the meniscus. The more the knee is placed in extension the greater the chance of targeting the anterior horn of the meniscus (purportedly).
- Step Five: A positive test includes concordant pain and a clicking sound either heard or felt.

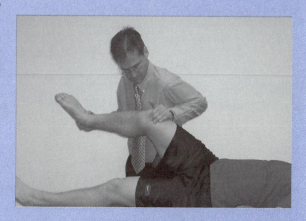

**Figure 14.48**    McMurray's Test

## Apley's Compression Test

Apley first described Apley's compression, also known as Apley's grind test, in 1947.[77] The test originally described by Apley involves several motions that involve both compression and distraction forces. The Apley's compression test described by Hoppenfield[78] involves compression and twisting forces performed at the knee in absence of the flexion and extension movements. Distraction forces described by Apley are followed to differentiate between meniscal and capsuloligamentous injuries. For simplicity, the compression test as described by Hoppenfield is reported.[78] Table 14.3 outlines the diagnostic value of the test.

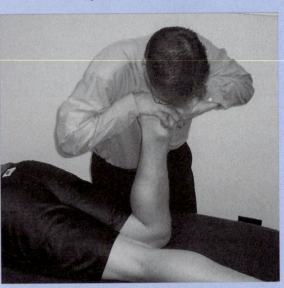

- Step One: The patient lies in a prone position. The knee is flexed to approximately 90 degrees.
- Step Two: The clinician grasps the foot of the patient and applies a compressive force through the shaft of the tibia.
- Step Three: While maintaining the compressive force, the clinician applies a medial and lateral twist of the tibia on the stabilized femur.
- Step Four: The clinician determines if the compression force is concordant and painful.

**Figure 14.49** Apley's Compression Test

- Step Five: The clinician then places his or her knee on the patient's thigh to support it to the table. A distraction force is then applied.
- Step Six: During the maintained distraction force, the clinician applies medial and lateral twisting to the knee to determine if the action is painful and concordant.
- Step Seven: According to Apley, if the knee is painful and concordant during compression and twisting, the problem is associated with the meniscus. If the knee is painful and concordant during the distraction and twisting, the problem is capsuloligamentous.

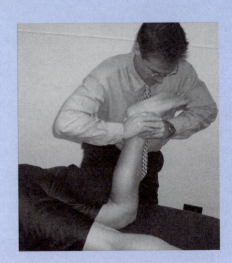

**Figure 14.50** Apley's Distraction Test

TABLE 14.3    Clinical Special Tests for Detection of Intraarticular Disorders

| Clinical Test | Author | Sensitivity | Specificity | +LR | −LR |
|---|---|---|---|---|---|
| McMurray's Test | Kurosaka et al.[107] | 37 | 77 | 1.61 | 0.81 |
| | Noble et al.[104] | 63 | 57 | 1.5 | 0.65 |
| | Fowler & Lubliner[105] | 29 | 96 | 7.8 | 0.73 |
| | Evans et al.[121] | 20 | 91 | 2.3 | 0.87 |
| | Saengnipanthkul et al.[106] | 47 | 94 | 7.8 | 0.56 |
| | Anderson and Lipscomb[108] | 58 | NR | NA | NA |
| | Akseki et al. Medial Meniscus[109] | 67 | 69 | 2.16 | 0.47 |
| | Akseki et al. Lateral Meniscus[109] | 53 | 88 | 4.41 | 0.53 |
| | Karachalios et al. Medial Meniscus[110] | 48 | 94 | 8 | 0.55 |
| | Karachalios et al. Lateral Meniscus[110] | 65 | 86 | 4.64 | 0.40 |
| Apley's Compression Test | Fowler & Lubliner[105] | 16 | 80 | 0.8 | 1.1 |
| | Grifka et al.[122] | 58 | 80 | 2.9 | 0.5 |
| | Kurosaka et al.[107] | 13 | 90 | 1.3 | 0.96 |

## *Clinical Tests for Anterior Cruciate Instability*

### Anterior Drawer Test

Numerous studies have investigated the diagnostic accuracy of the anterior drawer test. The majority have noted usefulness of the test, although the diagnostic figures are not as strong as the Lachman's test. The test was originally described by Segund in 1879.[79] It is notable that the sensitivity of the anterior drawer test is affected by concomitant injuries.[79] A positive test is considered as "abnormal" displacement of the tibia on the femur when compared to the opposite extremity.[79] Table 14.4 (page 529) outlines the diagnostic value of the test.

- Step One: The patient lies in a supine position. The hip is flexed to 45 degrees and the knee is flexed to 90 degrees.
- Step Two: The clinician sits at the foot of the patient, stabilizing the lower extremity by sitting slightly on the foot. The hands of the clinician are placed behind the tibia of the patient. The thumbs are placed superiorly to the joint line, on the femur.
- Step Three: The clinician applies a superior force to the hamstring tendons to inhibit contraction and to feel for relaxation.
- Step Four: The clinician applies quick posterior-to-anterior movements to determine the displacement of the tibia on the fixed femur.
- Step Five: The opposite extremity is evaluated for comparison.

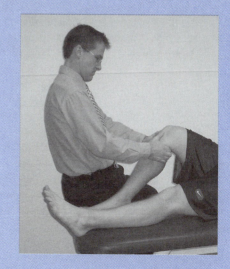

**Figure 14.51**    The Anterior Drawer Test

## Lachman's Test

Torg et al.[80] first described Lachman's test. The test is also a clinical assessment for anterior cruciate ligament disruption. The test demonstrates very good diagnostic values, although some examiners with small hands may have difficulties performing the procedure. Additionally, the procedure is difficult to perform on patients with large thigh girths. A positive test is also considered "abnormal" displacement of the tibia on the femur when compared to the opposite extremity.[79] Table 14.4 outlines the diagnostic value of the test.

- Step One: The patient lies in a supine position. The knee is placed in approximately 15 degrees of knee flexion.
- Step Two: The clinician sits to the outside of the patient's knee. The femur is stabilized caudally with one hand while the other cradles the tibia proximally and posteriorly. For smaller clinicians, it may be helpful to plant the elbow of the tibial-hand on the mat for a counterforce.
- Step Three: The clinician applies quick posterior-to-anterior thrust to determine the displacement of the tibia on the fixed femur.
- Step Four: The opposite extremity is evaluated for comparison.

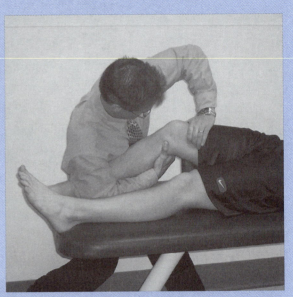

**Figure 14.52**    Lachman's Test

## Pivot Shift Test

The action of the pivot shift is similar to the movement of the lower extremity during giving way of the knee.[79] The pivot shift movement includes an anterior subluxation of the lateral tibial plateau on the femur when the knee is in full flexion and a reduction of the translation when the knee approaches full extension. A positive test is the clunking and the pain that occurs during the reduction at approximately 30 degrees short of extension. Table 14.4 outlines the diagnostic value of the test.

- Step One: The patient lies in a supine position. The affected leg is picked up by the clinician at the ankle with one hand and the knee is supported with the other at the head of the fibula.
- Step Two: The clinician places the knee in at least 90 degrees of flexion. The knee is guided into extension with both hands while the clinician places a slight valgus force at the fibular head.
- Step Three: The valgus force is increased as the knee approaches full extension.
- Step Four: If positive, the displaced tibia will reduce at approximately 30 degrees of extension.
- Step Five: The opposite extremity is evaluated for comparison.

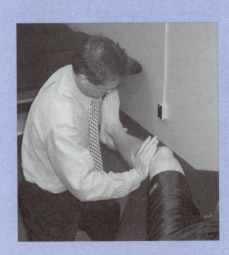

**Figure 14.53**    The Pivot Shift Test

**TABLE 14.4**    Clinical Special Tests for Detection of Anterior Cruciate Ligament Instability

| Clinical Test | Author | Sensitivity | Specificity | +LR | −LR |
|---|---|---|---|---|---|
| Anterior Drawer Test | Hardaker et al.[123] | 18 | NR | NA | NA |
| | Tonino et al.[124] | 27 | 98 | 13.5 | 0.74 |
| | Boeree & Ackroyd[125] | 56 | 92 | 7 | 0.47 |
| | Richter et al.[126] | 67 | 88 | 5.6 | 0.37 |
| | Steinbruck & Wiehmann[127] | 92 | 91 | 10.2 | 0.08 |
| | Sandberg et al.[128] | 39 | 78 | 1.8 | 0.78 |
| | Braunstein[129] | 91 | 89 | 8.27 | 0.10 |
| | DeHaven[130] | 9 | NR | NA | NA |
| | Donaldson et al.[131] | 70 | NR | NA | NA |
| | Hughston et al.[81] | 65 | 23 | 0.84 | 1.52 |
| | Jonsson et al.[132] | 93 | NR | NA | NA |
| | Lee et al.[133] | 78 | 100 | NA | NA |
| | Lui et al.[134] | 63 | NR | NA | NA |
| | Mitsou & Vallianatos[135] | 72 | NR | NA | NA |
| Lachman's Test | Gurtler et al.[136] | 100 | NR | NA | NA |
| | Donaldson et al.[131] | 99 | NR | NA | NA |
| | Hardaker et al.[123] | 74 | NR | NA | NA |
| | Tonino et al.[124] | 89 | 98 | 44.5 | 0.11 |
| | Boeree & Ackroyd[125] | 63 | 90 | 6.3 | 0.41 |
| | Lee et al.[133] | 90 | 99 | 90 | 0.10 |
| | Richter et al.[126] | 93 | 88 | 7.7 | 0.07 |
| | Steinbruck & Wiehmann[127] | 86 | 95 | 17.2 | 0.14 |
| | Lui et al.[134] | 89 | 100 | NA | NA |
| Pivot Shift Test | Hardaker et al.[123] | 29 | NR | NA | NA |
| | Tonino et al.[124] | 18 | 98 | 9 | 0.83 |
| | Boeree & Ackroyd[125] | 31 | 97 | 10.3 | 0.71 |
| | Richter et al.[126] | 48 | 97 | 16 | 0.53 |
| | Steinbruck & Wiehmann[127] | 22 | 99 | 22 | .78 |
| | Dahlstedt & Dalen[137] | 37 | NR | NA | NA |
| | Dehaven[130] | 27 | NR | NA | NA |
| | Donaldson et al.[131] | 35 | NR | NA | NA |
| | Liu et al.[134] | 95 | NR | NA | NA |

## Clinical Tests for Posterior Cruciate Instability

Injuries of the posterior cruciate ligament (PCL) are uncommon but when present lead to significant dysfunction and disability. The PCL restricts posterior translation of the tibia on the femur during weight bearing. Most PCL injuries occur during impact to the tibia and resultant anterior deceleration of the femur on the stationary tibia.

## Posterior Drawer Test

The posterior drawer test was originally described by Noulis in 1875.[79] The test is designed to measure posterior displacement of the tibia on a fixed femur and is considered positive if one leg translates posteriorly more so than the other noninvolved side. The test is prone to false positives if the ACL is torn and the tibia normally sits in an anteriorly translated position. Table 14.5 outlines the diagnostic value of the test.

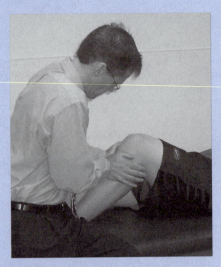

- Step One: The patient lies in a supine position. The hip of the patient is flexed to 45 degrees and the knee of the patient is flexed to 70 degrees.
- Step Two: The clinician sits at the foot of the patient. Both palms lie flush on the anterior surface of the tibia. The fingers wrap posteriorly to stabilize the tibia.
- Step Three: Stabilizing the foot by sitting on it, the clinician then applies a posterior force of the tibia on the fixed femur in quick thrusts.
- Step Four: A positive test is represented by more tibial translation on one side versus another.
- Step Five: The opposite extremity is evaluated for comparison.

**Figure 14.54**    The Posterior Drawer Test

## Posterior Sag Sign

The posterior sag sign was originally described by Robson in 1903.[79] The test is designed to allow visual confirmation of the posterior tibial translation that occurs during a PCL injury. A positive test is significant visual posterior translation during a non-weight-bearing assessment. Table 14.5 outlines the diagnostic value of the test.

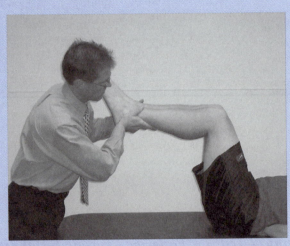

- Step One: The patient lies in a supine position. The hip of the patient is flexed to 45 degrees and the knee of the patient is flexed to 70–90 degrees. Both feet are lifted and held in a neutral position from the mat by the clinician.
- Step Two: There are two possible follow-up steps. The clinician may visually assess the tibial translation without force or the clinician may apply a posterior translation of the tibia through the tibia to enhance the sag.
- Step Three: A positive test is when the tibia translates more posteriorly on one side versus another.
- Step Four: Both legs are assessed at the same time.

**Figure 14.55**    The Posterior Sag Sign

## Quadriceps Active Test

The quadriceps active test was recently described by Daniel et al. in 1988.[79] The test measures anterior translation of the tibia during an active quadriceps contraction while in the "drawer position." Anterior translation during the active quadriceps contraction of 2 millimeters or more is considered a positive test. The excellent diagnostic values of Daniel were most likely inflated secondary to the lack of blinding in the study. Table 14.5 outlines the diagnostic value of the test.

- Step One: The patient lies in a supine position. The hip is flexed to 45 degrees and the knee is flexed to 90 degrees.
- Step Two: The clinician sits at the foot of the patient, stabilizing the lower extremity by sitting slightly on the foot.
- Step Three: The patient is directed to actively contract his or her quadriceps. The clinician looks for anterior displacement of the tibia on the femur comparatively to the opposite side.
- Step Four: The clinician applies quick posterior-to-anterior movements to determine the displacement of the tibia on the fixed femur.
- Step Five: The opposite extremity is evaluated for comparison.

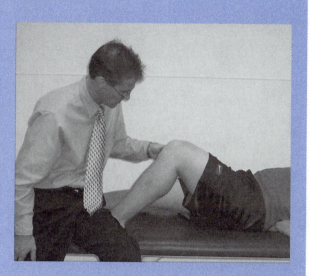

**Figure 14.56**   The Quadriceps Active Test

**TABLE 14.5**    Clinical Special Tests for Detection of Posterior Cruciate Ligament Instability

| Clinical Test | Author | Sensitivity | Specificity | +LR | −LR |
|---|---|---|---|---|---|
| Posterior Drawer Test | Baker et al.[138] | 86 | NR | NA | NA |
| | Loos et al.[139] | 51 | NR | NA | NA |
| | Rubenstein et al.[140] | 90 | 99 | 90 | 0.10 |
| Posterior Sag Sign | Rubenstein et al.[140] | 79 | 100 | NA | NA |
| Quadriceps Active Test | Rubenstein et al.[140] | 54 | 97 | 18 | 0.47 |
| | Daniel et al.[141] | 98 | 100 | NA | NA |

## Dial Test

The Dial test is designed to determine isolated posterolateral corner instability and to differentiate the laxity from a PCL tear. The Dial test is performed at 30 degrees of knee flexion. If one side exhibits 10–15 degrees more external rotation than the other, the patient most likely exhibits posterolateral corner laxity. However, if this laxity is only present at 30 degrees and not 90 degrees, the injury is concurrent with a PCL rupture.[81]

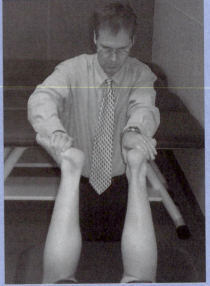

- Step One: The patient lies in prone. Both knees are flexed to approximately 30 degrees.
- Step Two: Both knees are passively rotated into external rotation. External rotation is compared bilaterally.
- Step Three: Both knees are moved to 90 degrees of flexion and passively externally rotated. The test can be performed in supine as well.

**Figure 14.57**    The Dial Test Performed in Prone at 90 Degrees

## Varus Stress Test

The varus stress test is designed to measure the integrity of structures to stabilize against varus forces. These structures may include the lateral collateral ligament (LCL) and selected internal ligaments such as the PCL and ACL. Typically, the test is performed in both 0 and 30 degrees of flexion. According to Hughston et al.,[82] lateral instability at 0 degrees of flexion is usually associated with a PCL, arcuate ligament, ACL, or some other disruption. The stress test in slight flexion is more associated with an LCL tear. A positive test is considered greater laxity than the opposite extremity. Table 14.6 outlines the diagnostic value of the test.

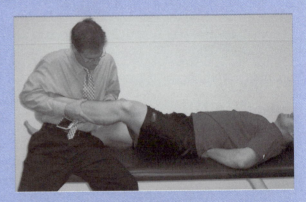

- Step One: The patient lies in a supine position. The affected leg is flexed to approximately 30 degrees. The clinician then places the foot in his or her axilla for stability.
- Step Two: The clinician places one hand on the lateral aspect of the tibia and the other hand on the medial aspect of the femur. The clinician then preloads the joint into varus.
- Step Three: Further varus force is applied by twisting the body in the direction of more varus.
- Step Four: A positive test is excess gapping into varus.
- Step Five: The test is repeated at 0 degrees of flexion.

**Figure 14.58**    The Varus Stress Test at 30 Degrees of Knee Flexion

### Valgus Stress Test

The valgus stress test is designed to measure the integrity of structures to stabilize against valgus forces. These structures may include the medial collateral ligament (LCL) and similar selected internal ligaments such as the PCL and ACL as the varus stress test. The test is also performed in both 0 and 30 degrees of flexion with findings in the different positions associated with difference structures. According to Hughston et al.,[82] a positive stress test at 30 degrees and a negative test at 0 indicate a MCL tear with a posterior capsule injury. A positive valgus stress test at 0 degrees may suggest a PCL tear and a tear within the posterior capsule but does not usually indicate an ACL tear.[82] A positive test is considered greater laxity than the opposite extremity. Table 14.6 outlines the diagnostic value of the test.

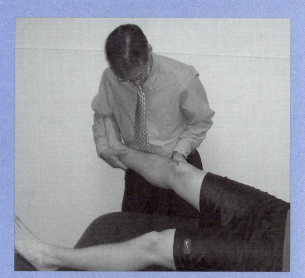

**Figure 14.59**   The Valgus Stress Test at 0 Degrees of Knee Flexion

- Step One: The patient lies in a supine position. The affected leg is flexed to approximately 30 degrees. The clinician then places the foot in his or her axilla for stability.
- Step Two: The clinician places one hand on the medial aspect of the tibia and the other hand on the lateral aspect of the femur. The clinician then preloads the joint into varus.
- Step Three: Further varus force is applied by twisting the body in the direction of more valgus. The body motion is opposite of the varus movement.
- Step Four: A positive test is excess gapping into valgus.
- Step Five: The test is repeated at 0 degrees of flexion.

**TABLE 14.6**   Clinical Special Tests for Varus and Valgus Laxity

| Clinical Test | Author | Sensitivity | Specificity | +LR | −LR |
|---|---|---|---|---|---|
| Valgus Stress Test | Harilainen et al.[142] | 86 | NR | NA | NA |
| | Garvin et al.[143] | 96 | NR | NA | NA |
| Varus Stress Test | Harilainen et al.[142] | 25 | NR | NA | NA |

## *Clinical Special Tests for Patellofemoral Disorders*

### Vastus Medialis Coordination Test

The vastus medialis coordination test was originally described by Souza.[79] A test is considered positive if coordinated knee extension is poor during terminal knee extension. The region assumed responsible is the vastus medialis. Table 14.7 (page 536) outlines the diagnostic value of the test.

- Step One: The patient lies in a supine position. The clinician places his or her fist or thigh under the knee so that the knee is slightly flexed.
- Step Two: The patient is instructed to extend the knee slowly.
- Step Three: The clinician observes for full extension and a full coordinated movement.
- Step Four: A test is considered positive if the knee is not fully extended or if control of the knee was not apparent during the movement.
- Step Five: The opposite extremity is evaluated for comparison.

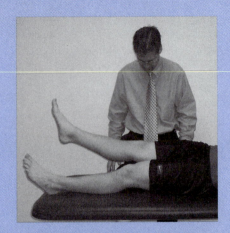

**Figure 14.60**    The Vastus Medialis Coordination Test

### Patellar Apprehension Test

The patellar apprehension test is designed to determine whether pain and/or apprehension are present during a lateral glide of the patella. Reproduction of pain or apprehension identifies a positive test. Table 14.7 outlines the diagnostic value of the test.

- Step One: The patient lies in a supine position. The clinician places a lateral glide on the knee cap.
- Step Two: The movement is started at 30 degrees. At that range and during concurrent lateral patellar glide, the knee and the hip are flexed together.
- Step Three: A test is considered positive if the knee is not fully extended secondary to fear or if control of the knee was not apparent during the movement.

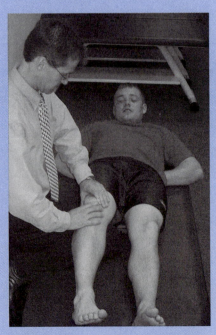

**Figure 14.61**    The Patella Apprehension Test

## Clarke's Test

Clarke's test for patellofemoral grinding is designed to measure whether the origination of the pain occurs at the articulation of the patella and the femur. Because the test can provide false positives during full extension, the test is best performed in a slight degree of flexion. A positive test is considered concordant reproduction of pain by the patient. Table 14.7 outlines the diagnostic value of the test.

- Step One: The patient lies in a supine position. The affected leg is placed in slight flexion.
- Step Two: The clinician provides an inferior force to the patella. Slight compression is administered.
- Step Three: The patient is instructed to contract his or her quadriceps. A positive test is pain during the quadriceps contraction concurrently during inferior glide and compression of the patella.

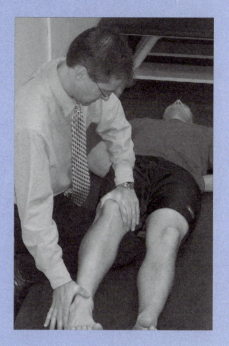

**Figure 14.62**   Clarke's Test for Patella Grinding

## Eccentric Step Test

The eccentric step test involves an eccentric load to the knee during a controlled step down. The test is considered positive if pain is reproduced during the activity. Table 14.7 outlines the diagnostic value of the test.

- Step One: The patient stands on a 15 cm step. The patient is instructed to place his or her arms on his or her hips.
- Step Two: The patient is instructed to lower his or her nonaffected leg slowly to the floor. The affected leg eccentrically controls the lowering.
- Step Three: A positive test is concordant reproduction of symptoms.

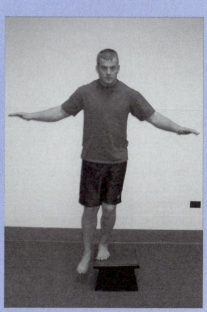

**Figure 14.63**   The Eccentric Step Test

**TABLE 14.7**    Clinical Special Tests for Patellofemoral Syndrome

| Clinical Test | Author | Sensitivity | Specificity | +LR | −LR |
|---|---|---|---|---|---|
| Vastus Medialis Coordination Test | Nils et al.[83] | 16.1 | 92.9 | 2.26 | 0.90 |
| Patellar Apprehension Test | Nils et al.[83] | 32.3 | 85.7 | 2.26 | 0.78 |
| | Sallay et al.[144] | 39 | NR | NA | NA |
| Clarke's Test | Nils et al.[83] | 48.4 | 75 | 1.94 | 0.68 |
| Eccentric Step Test | Nils et al.[83] | 41.9 | 82.1 | 2.34 | 0.70 |

## Summary

- The purpose of a clinical special test is for confirmation of the examination findings.
- Palpation-based tests may be useful in isolating intraarticular disorders or fractures.
- In general, tests for anterior and posterior laxity demonstrate better likelihood ratios than tests for meniscal involvement.
- Few tests have been studied for the effectiveness of outlining PFPS.

# TREATMENT TECHNIQUES

Treatment of knee disorders should focus on identifying physical impairments that are relative to concordant signs. Physical impairments can range from disorders associated with motor control, active and passive mobility, and passive structure competence of the systems of the knee.

Mobilization, active or passive, in any direction may be beneficial for the patient with osteoarthritis.[84] Activities such as active quadriceps contractions have been shown to reduce negative biochemical parameters within the knee.[84] Compression-based mobilizations may be most effective at producing these changes and have been shown to lead to better outcomes than treatments with no compression.[85] As with the previous chapters, the examination methods are often similar to the treatment procedures.

## Compression Mobilization of the Tibial–Femoral Joint

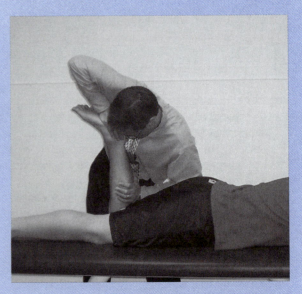

- Step One: The patient assumes a prone position. The clinician stabilizes the tibia by applying a perpendicular grip to the tibia and fibula with his or her mobilizing arm.
- Step Two: The knee is bent toward the concordant region of pain. The clinician applies a compressive load through the tibiofemoral joint by loading the heel of the patient with the nonmobilizing hand.
- Step Three: The clinician applies oscillations during compression for treatment of the patient with the mobilizing hand (contact hand of the tibia and fibula).

**Figure 14.64**    Prone Compression Mobilization of the Tibiofemoral Joint

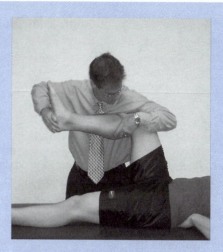

**Figure 14.65**   Supine Compression Mobilization of the Tibiofemoral Joint

- Step Four: The procedure can also be performed using similar hand-holds with the patient in a supine position.

## Scoop Mobilization for the Posterior Horn

Because the menisci of the knee are frequently injured or fail to move during knee flexion and extension, the menisci are often targeted for treatment. Anterior–posterior mobilizations of the tibia and femur, respectively, should assist in differentiating the anterior and posterior horn of the meniscus. Posterior horn injuries are typically worse during flexion of the knee and functional activities such as squatting. The scoop mobilization is used to target the posterior horn of the meniscus.

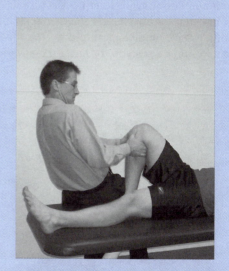

- Step One: The patient is placed in a sitting position or a supine, hooklying position.
- Step Two: The clinician flexes the patient to the first point of pain or toward end range flexion.
- Step Three: The clinician places his or her hands at the joint line posteriorly to the knee of the patient. The clinician then further flexes the knee toward end range flexion.
- Step Four: The mobilization procedure is a curvilinear posterior-to-anterior pull that targets the menisci. The technique is most effective near end range flexion.

**Figure 14.66**   Posterior Anterior Scoop Mobilization

## Compression Mobilization of the Patellofemoral Joint

- Step One: The patient assumes a supine position. The knee is flexed slightly by placing a bolster under the knee.
- Step Two: The clinician applies a load to the patella by placing his or her hand on top of the knee cap.
- Step Three: The tibiofemoral joint is oscillated during the load to the knee cap.

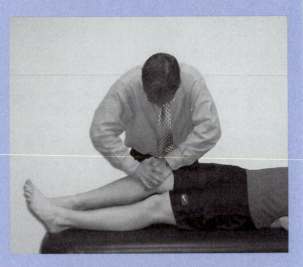

**Figure 14.67**    Compression Mobilization of the Patellofemoral Joint

### Tibial Shear at Multiple Ranges

The tibial shear mobilization is performed at various ranges throughout the knee. Because the capsule is engaged at greater degrees of flexion (Figure 14.68), the tibial shear mobilization in flexion tends to target the capsule. The tibial shear in extension may target the menisci. Concordant pain during passive physiological testing typically identifies the most appropriate position for linear mobilization of the tibia.

### Tibial Rotation at Multiple Ranges

Occasionally, rotation is more sensitive at reproducing the concordant sign than the linear shear methods. Subsequently, rotational mobilization may be effective at various ranges as well (Figure 14.69). Like the tibial shear methods, concordant pain during passive physiological testing typically identifies the most appropriate position for rotational mobilization of the tibia.

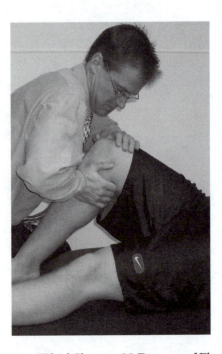

**Figure 14.68**    Tibial Shear at 90 Degrees of Flexion

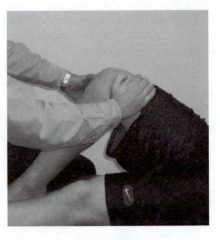

**Figure 14.69**    Rotation Mobilization at 90 Degrees of Flexion

## Hamstring Stretches

Several studies have described various hamstring stretching methods. It appears that any form of hamstring stretching (i.e., hold–relax, static hold) tends to provide the same level of range improvement, with only minimal carryover.[86–88] A hold–relax stretch is an effective method that allows a patient to govern the amount of stretch force provided.[87]

- Step One: The patient assumes a supine position. The hamstrings are prepositioned in a 90/90 posture (hip and knee at 90 degrees).
- Step Two: The clinician places the heel of the patient under his or her shoulder. The patient is instructed to push downward into the shoulder at his or her first point of perceived tightness. Hold times vary, but in most cases, a hold time of 10–15 seconds of a submaxial contraction is appropriate.
- Step Three: The clinician slowly moves the tibia into further extension after each isometric contraction of the patient.

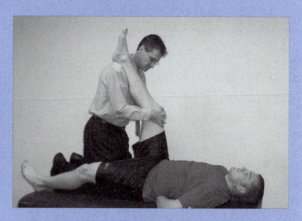

**Figure 14.70**    Isometric (Hold-Relax) Hamstring Stretching of the Patient

## Manipulation of the Tibial Femoral Joint

Meyer et al.[89] describe a tibiofemoral manipulation in which the tibia is rapidly distracted from the femur. The technique was used concurrently with patellofemoral mobilization and leads to a positive consequence in a single case study.

- Step One: The patient assumes a prone position. The clinician uses a belt to stabilize the femur.
- Step Two: The knee is slightly flexed to the targeted range of discomfort. The clinician can preposition the knee in internal or external rotation, depending on the concordant pain of the patient.
- Step Three: The manipulation includes a rapid distraction of the tibia on the femur.

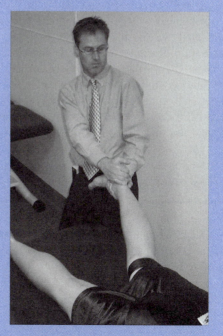

**Figure 14.71**    Tibiofemoral Distraction Manipulation of the Knee

## Summary

- The majority of manual therapy treatment methods are distilled from the examination process.
- Adding components such as compression, end range movements, and distraction may increase the usefulness of manual therapy treatment.

# TREATMENT OUTCOMES

The literature appears to be lacking in data regarding passive accessory movements of the tibio-femoral joint. Assessment of patellar mobility does appear in the literature as a common component to the treatment of PFPS. Studies have examined the assessment of static patellar orientation, particularly medial and lateral orientation and mobility assessment. With the exception of one study, these assessments demonstrated poor reliability.[50,90–92] One study that did demonstrate acceptable levels of reliability included experienced manual therapists and a single subject.[93]

Evidence exists that rehabilitation, including a variety of methods, is beneficial in the treatment of knee osteoarthritis.[84,94–97] The majority of studies analyzed the effects of various forms of strengthening and stretching exercises. Only a few examined the benefits associated with manual therapy of the knee.[84,94,98]

Noel et al.[85] reported that mobilization with compression, a long axis compression technique of the tibia in a flexed position, led to significantly greater preset range-of-motion goals versus the comparative group who did not receive mobilization with compression. Mobilizations were performed at end range, were concordantly painful, and were rated as unpleasant by more recipients.

Deyle et al.[94] found that treatment that included manual therapy and exercise was more effective than exercise alone. Their findings demonstrated significant improvements in self-perceptions of pain, stiffness, and functional ability as well as the distance walked in 6 minutes when compared to placebo. This implies that these treatment methods have merit and may be beneficial for treatment of patients with osteoarthritis of the knee. It also implies that these treatment methods demonstrate credibility and may lead to faster and more beneficial outcomes. In a follow-up study, Deyle and colleagues[99] reported that an in-clinic program consisting of manual therapy and exercise led to better outcomes than a home-based exercise program in a sample of patients with knee arthritis. The manual therapy included a variety of tibial–femoral and patella mobilizations in conjunction with stretching exercise.

Less evidence exists that manual therapy is beneficial for patients with patellofemoral pain syndrome.[100] Crossley et al.[101] reported improvements in knee flexion during stair climbing compared to placebo treatment. Manual therapy mobilization was a component of treatment but was combined with taping, biofeedback, and strengthening exercises. The *Philadelphia Panel Guidelines* found no evidence to support any form of manual or nonmanual treatment of patellofemoral pain syndrome, specifically friction massage, that demonstrated no benefits in numerous studies.[102]

## Summary

- Outside the use of manual therapy for the treatment of arthritis, few studies have examined the effectiveness of treatment for the knee.
- Little evidence exists to support the use of manual therapy for PFPS, although when combined with other treatments, the technique may be beneficial.
- Some evidence exists that include compression with mobilization increases the return of range of motion quicker than an absence of compression.

# Chapter Questions

1. How does the biomechanics of the knee factor into the selection of the manual therapy treatment approach?
2. Describe how the femoral condyle dictates the likelihood of PFPS.
3. Outline the method in which a mobilization to the tibia or femur can isolate the menisci.
4. Describe how compression may positively affect a condition during manual therapy of the knee.
5. Describe three variations of a plane-based mobilization that may alter the outcome of the technique.

# References

1. Jackson JL, O'Malley PG, Kroenke K. Evaluation of acute knee pain in primary care. *Ann Intern Med.* 2003;139(7):575–588.

2. Bachmann l, Haberzeth S, Steurer J, ter Riet G. The accuracy of the Ottawa knee rule to rule out knee fractures. *Ann Intern Med.* 2004;140:121–124.

3. Laprade J, Lee R. Real-time measurement of patellofemoral kinematics in asymptomatic subjects. *Knee.* 2005;12:63–72.

4. Ellis M, Griffin K. For knee pain, how predictive is physical examination for meniscal injury? *J Fam Pract.* 2004;53:918–920.

5. Larson R, Grana W. The knee: *Form, function, pathology, and treatment.* Philadelphia; W.B. Saunders Co: 1992.

6. Holmberg S, Thelin A, Thelin N. Knee osteoarthritis and body mass index: A population-based case-control study. *Scand J Rheumatol.* 2005;34:59–64.

7. Englund M, Lohmander LS. Risk factors for symptomatic knee osteoarthritis fifteen to twenty-two years after meniscectomy. *Arthritis Rheum.* 2004;50: 2811–2819.

8. Lohmander LS, Ostenberg A, Englund M, Roos H. High prevalence of knee osteoarthritis, pain, and functional limitations in female soccer players twelve years after anterior cruciate ligament injury. *Arthritis Rheum.* 2004;50:3145–3152.

9. Neame RL, Muir K, Doherty S, Doherty M. Genetic risk of knee osteoarthritis: A sibling study. *Ann Rheum Dis.* 2004;63:1022–1027.

10. Fitzgerald GK, Piva S, Irrgang JJ. Reports of joint instability in knee osteoarthritis: its prevalence and relationship to physical function. *Arthritis Rheum.* 2004;51:941–946.

11. Shepherd L, Abdollahi K, Lee J, Vangsness CT. The prevalence of soft tissue injuries in nonoperative tibial plateau fractures as determined by magnetic resonance imaging. *J Orthop Trauma.* 2002;16:628–631.

12. Fithian D, Paxton LW, Goltz DH. Fate of the anterior cruciate ligament-injured knee. *Orthop Clin North Am.* 2002;33:621–636.

13. Hawkins RJ, Bell RH, Anisette G. Acute patellar dislocations: the natural history. *Am J Sports Med.* 1986;14:117–120.

14. Fithian D, Paxton E, Stone ML, Silva P, Davis D, Elias D, White L. Epidemiology and natural history of acute patellar dislocation. *Am J Sports Med.* 2004; 32:1114–1121.

15. Neumann D. *Kinesiology of the musculoskeletal system: Foundations for physical rehabilitation.* St Louis; Mosby: 2002.

16. Powers C. Patellar kinematics, part II: the influence of the depth of the trochlear groove in subjects with and without patellofemoral pain. *Phys Ther.* 2000;80 (10):965–978.

17. Fulkerson J. *Disorders of the patellofemoral joint.* 4th ed. Philadelphia; Lippincott Williams & Wilkins: 2004.

18. Pena E, Calvo MA, Martinez D, Palanca M, Doblare M. Finite element analysis of the effect of meniscal tears and mensicectomies on human knee biomechanics. *Clin Biomech.* 2005;20:498–507.

19. Loudon J, Wiesner D, Goist-Foley H, Asjes C, Loudon K. Intrarater reliability of functional performance tests for subjects with patellofemoral pain syndrome. *J Athletic Training.* 2002;37:256–261.

20. Upadhyay N, Vollans S, Seedhom B, Soames R. Effect of patellar tendon shortening on tracking of the patella. *Am J Sports Med.* 2005;33:1–10.

21. Bennett LD, Buckland-Wright JC. Meniscal and articular cartilage changes in knee osteoarthritis: A cross sectional double-contrast macroradiographic study. *Rheumatology.* 2002;41:917–923.

22. Gupta C, Smith A, McDermott ID, Bull A, Thomas R, Amis A. Meniscofemoral ligaments revisited. *J Bone Joint Surg Br.* 2002;84:846–851.

23. Gupta C, Bull A, Thomas R, Amis A. The meniscofemoral ligaments: secondary restraints to the posterior drawer. *J Bone Jnt Surg Br.* 2003;85:765–773.

24. Macnicol M, Thomas N. The knee after meniscectomy. *J Bone Joint Surg Br.* 2000;82(2):157–159.

25. Wilson W, van Rietbergen B, van Donkelaar CC, Huiskes R. Pathways of load-induced cartilage damage causing cartilage degeneration in the knee after meniscectomy. *J Biomech.* 2003;36:845–851.

26. Kernozek TW, Torry MR, Van Hoof H, Cowley H, Tanner S. Gender differences in frontal and sagittal plane biomechanics during drop landings. *Med Sci Sports Exerc.* 2005;37:1003–1012;

27. Amis A, Bull AM, Gupte CM, Hijazi I, Race A, Robinson JR. Biomechanics of the PCL and related structures: Posterolateral, posteromedial, and meniscofemoral ligaments. *Knee Surg Sports Traumatol Arthors.* 2003;11:271–281.

28. Hughston JC, Bowden JA, Andrews JR, Norwood LA. Acute tears of the posterior cruciate ligament. Results of operative treatment. *J Bone Joint Surg Am.* 1980;62:438–450.

29. Girgis FG, Marshall JL, Monajem ARS. The cruciate ligaments of the knee joint. Anatomical, functional and experimental analysis. *Clin Orthop.* 1975; 106:216–231.

30. Moglo K, Shirazi-Adl A. Cruciate coupling and screw home mechanism in passive knee joint during extension-flexion. *J Biomech.* 2005;28:1075–1083.

31. Robinson JR, Bull AM, Amis AA. Structural properties of the medial collateral ligament complex of the human knee. *J Biomech.* 2005;38(5):1067–1074.

32. Gupta C, Bull A, deW T, Amis A. A review of the function and biomechanics of the meniscofemoral ligament. *Arthroscopy.* 2003;19:161–171.

33. Last RJ. Some anatomical details of the knee joint. *J Bone Joint Surg Br.* 1948;30:683–688.

34. Heller L, Langman J. The meniscofemoral ligaments of the human knee. *J Bone Joint Surg Br.* 1964; 46:307–313.

35. Lee J, Papakonstantinou O, Brookenthal K, Trudell D, Resnick D. Arcuate sign of posterolateral knee

injuries: Anatomic, radiographic, and MR imaging data related to patterns of injury. *Skeletal Radiol.* 2003;32:619–627.

36. Munshi M, Pretterklieber M, Kwak S, Antonio G, Trudell D, Resnick D. MR imaging, MR arthrography, and specimen correlation of the posterolateral corner of the knee. An anatomic study. *AJR.* 2003; 180:1095–1101.

37. Ferrari D. Arthroscopic evaluation of the popliteus: clues to posterolateral laxity. *Arthroscopy.* 2005;21(6): 721–726.

38. Escamilla R. Knee biomechanics of the dynamic squat exercise. *Med Sci Sports Ex.* 2001;33:127–141.

39. von Eisenhart-Rothe R, Bringmann C, Siebert M, Reiser M, Englmeier KH, Eckstein F, Graichen H. Femoral-tibial and menisco-tibial translation patterns in patients with unilateral anterior cruciate ligament deficiency—a potential cause of secondary meniscal tears. *J Orthop Research.* 2004;22:275–282.

40. Isaac DL, Beard SJ, Price AJ, Rees J, Murray DW, Dodd C. In-vivo sagittal plane knee kinematics: ACL intact deficient and reconstructed knees. *Knee.* 2005;12:25–31.

41. Bylski-Austrow DI, Ciarelli MJ, Kayner DC, Matthews LS, Goldstein SA. Displacements of the menisci under joint load: an in vitro study in human knees. *J Biomech.* 1994;27:421–431.

42. Blankevoort L, Huiskes R, de Lange A. The envelope of passive knee joint motion. *J Biomech.* 1988; 21:705–720.

43. Kurosawa H, Walker PS, Abe S, Garg A, Hunter T. Geometry and motion of the knee for implant and orthotic design. *J Biomech.* 1985;18(7):487–499.

44. Martelli S, Pinskerova V. The shapes of the tibial and femoral articular surfaces in relation to tibiofemoral movement. *J Bone Joint Surg Br.* 2002; 84:607–613.

45. Piazza SJ, Cavanagh PR. Measurement of the screw-home motion of the knee is sensitive to errors in axis alignment. *J Biomech.* 2000;33(8):1029–1034.

46. Nagamine R, Otani T, White SE, McCarthy DS, Whiteside LA. Patellar tracking measurement in the normal knee. *J Orthop Res.* 1995;13:115–122.

47. van Kampen A, Huiskes R. The three-dimensional tracking pattern of the human patella. *J Orthop Res.* 1990;8:372–382.

48. Ahmed AM, Duncan NA, Tanzer M. in vitro measurement of the tracking pattern of the human patella. *J Biomed Eng.* 1999;121:222–228.

49. Besier T, Draper C, Gold G, Beaupre G, Delp S. Patellofemoral joint contact area increases with knee flexion and weight bearing. *J Orthop Res.* 2005; 23:345–350.

50. Manske RC, Davies DJ. A non-surgical approach to examination and treatment of the patellofemoral joint., part 1. Examination of the patellofemoral

joint. *Critical Reviews in Physical & Rehabilitation Medicine.* 2003;15(2):141–166.

51. Altman R, Asch E, Bloch D, Bole G, Borenstein D. Development of criteria for the classification and reporting of osteoarthritis. Classification of osteoarthritis of the knee. Diagnostic and Therapeutic Criteria Committee of the American Rheumatism Association. *Arthritis Rheu.* 1986;29:1039–1049.

52. Chu S, Yang S, Lue K, Hsieh Y. Clinical significance of gelatinases in septic arthritis of native and replaced knees. *Clin Orthop Rel Res.* 2004;427:179–183.

53. Stratford P, Kennedy D, Pagura S, Gollish J. The relationship between self-report and performance-related measures: Questioning the content validity of timed tests. *Arthritis Rheum.* 2003;49:535–540.

54. Watson C, Propps M, Ratner J, Zeigler D, Horton P, Smith SS. Reliability and responsiveness of the Lower Extremity Functional Scale and the anterior knee pain scale in patients with anterior knee pain. *J Orthop Sports Phys Ther.* 2005;35:136–146.

55. Binkley J, Stratford P, Lott S, Riddle D. The Lower Extremity Functional Scale (LEFS): scale development, measurement properties, and clinical application. North American Orthopaedic Rehabilitation Research Network. *Phys Ther.* 1999;79: 371–383.

56. Selfe J. The patellofemoral joint: A review of primary research. *Critical Reviews in Physical & Rehabilitation Medicine.* 2004;16(1):1–30.

57. Gross MT, Foxworth JL. The role of foot orthoses as an intervention for patellofemoral pain. *J Orthop Sports Phys Ther.* 2003;33(11):661–670.

58. Hinterwimmer S, von Eisenhart-Rothe R, Siebert M, Welsch F, Vogl T, Graichen H. Patella kinematics and patellofemoral contact areas in patients with genu varum and mild osteoarthritis. *Clin Biomech.* 2004;19(7):704–710.

59. Livingston LA, Mandigo JL. Bilateral rearfoot asymmetry and anterior knee pain syndrome. *J Orthop Sports Phys Ther.* 2003;33(1):48–55.

60. Otsuki T, Nawata K, Okuno M. Quantitative analysis of gait patterns in patients with osteoarthrosis of the knee before and after total knee arthroplasty. Gait analysis using a pressure measuring system. *J Orthop Sci.* 1999;4(2):99–105.

61. Lafuente R, Belda JM, Sanchez-Lacuesta J, Soler C, Poveda R, Prat J. Quantitative assessment of gait deviation contribution to the objective measurement of disability. *Gait Posture.* 2000;11(3):191–198.

62. Cliborne AV, Wainner RS, Rhon DI, Judd CD, Fee TT. Clinical hip tests and a functional squat test in patients with knee osteoarthritis: reliability, prevalence of positive test findings, and short-term response to hip mobilization. *J Orthop Sports Phys Ther.* 2004;34(11):676–683.

63. Fitzgerald GK, Lephart SM, Hwang JH, Wainner RS. Hop tests as predictors of dynamic knee stability. *J Orthop Sports Phys Ther*. 2001;31(10):588–597.

64. Hayes W, Petersen C, Falconer J. An examination of Cyriax's passive motion tests with patients having osteoarthritis of the knee including commentary by Twomey LT, with author response. *Phys Ther*. 1994; 74:697–708.

65. Petersen C, Hayes K. Construct validity of Cyriax's selective tension examination: association of endfeels with pain at the knee and shoulder. *J Orthop Sports Phys Ther*. 2000;30:512–527.

66. Maitland G. *Peripheral manipulation*. 3rd ed. London; Butterworth-Heinemann: 1994.

67. Calmbach WL, Hutchens M. Evaluation of patients presenting with knee pain: Part I. History, physical examination, radiographs, and laboratory tests. *Am Fam Physician*. 2003;68(5):907–912.

68. Escolar DM, Henricson EK, Mayhew J, Florence J, Leshner R, Patel KM, Clemens PR. Clinical evaluator reliability for quantitative and manual muscle testing measures of strength in children. *Muscle Nerve*. 2001;24(6):787–793.

69. Roy MA, Doherty TJ. Reliability of hand-held dynamometry in assessment of knee extensor strength after hip fracture. *Am J Phys Med Rehabil*. 2004; 83(11):813–818.

70. Taylor NF, Dodd KJ, Graham HK. Test-retest reliability of hand-held dynamometric strength testing in young people with cerebral palsy. *Arch Phys Med Rehabil*. 2004;85(1):77–80.

71. Merlini L, Mazzone ES, Solari A, Morandi L. Reliability of hand-held dynamometry in spinal muscular atrophy. *Muscle Nerve*. 2002;26:64–70.

72. Ford-Smith CD, Wyman JF, Elswick RK Jr, Fernandez T. Reliability of stationary dynamometer muscle strength testing in community-dwelling older adults. *Arch Phys Med Rehabil*. 2001;82:1128–1132.

73. Agre JC, Magness JL, Hull SZ, Wright KC, Baxter TL, Patterson R, Stradel L. Strength testing with a portable dynamometer: reliability for upper and lower extremities. *Arch Phys Med Rehabil*. 1987;68 (7):454–458.

74. Munich H, Cipriani D, Hall C, Nelson D, Falkel J. The test-retest reliability of an inclined squat strength test protocol. *J Orthop Sports Phys Ther*. 1997;26(4): 209–213.

75. McMurray TP. The semilunar cartilage. *Br J Surg*. 1942;29:407–414.

76. Stratford PW, Binkley J. A review of the McMurray test: Definition, interpretation, and clinical usefulness. *J Orthop Sports Phys Ther*. 1995;22:116–120.

77. Tria AJ Jr. Clinical examination of the knee. In: Insall JN, Scott WN, editors. *Surgery of the knee*. Volume 1. 3rd ed. New York; Churchill Livingstone: 2001.

78. Hoppenfield S. *Physical examination of the spine and extremities*. Norwalk, CT; Appleton and Lange: 1976.

79. Malanga G, Andrus A, Nadler S, McLean J. Physical examination of the knee: A review of the original test description and scientific validity of common orthopedic tests. *Arch Phys Med Rehabil*. 2003;84: 592–603.

80. Torg JS, Conrad W, Kalen V. Clinical diagnosis of anterior cruciate ligament instability in the athlete. *Am J Sports Med*. 1976;4:84–93.

81. Laprade R, Wentorf F, Diagnosis and treatment of posterolateral knee injuries. *Clin Orthop*. 2002;402: 110–121.

82. Hughston JC, Andrews JR, Cross MJ, Moschi A. Classification of knee ligament instabilities. Part 1: The medial compartment and cruciate ligaments. *J Bone Joint Surg Am*. 1976;58:159–172.

83. Nils J, van Geel C, van der Auwera, van de Velde B. Diagnostic value of five clinical tests in patellofemoral pain syndrome. *Man Ther*. 2005 (in press)

84. Mivaguchi M, Kobayashi A, Kadoya Y, Ohashi H, Yamano Y, Takaoka K. Biochemical change in joint fluid after isometric quadriceps exercise for patients with osteoarthritis of the knee. *Osteoarthritis Cartilage*. 2003;11:252–259.

85. Noel G, Verbruggen LA, Barbaix E, Duquet W. Adding compression to mobilization in a rehabilitation program after knee surgery. A preliminary clinical observational study. *Man Ther*. 2000;5:102–107.

86. Bonner BP, Deivert RG, Gould TE. The relationship between isometric contraction durations during hold-relax stretching and improvement of hamstring flexibility. *J Sports Med Phys Fitness*. 2004;44: 258–261.

87. de Weijer VC, Gorniak GC, Shamus E. The effect of static stretch and warm-up exercise on hamstring length over the course of 24 hours. *J Orthop Sports Phys Ther*. 2003;33:727–733.

88. Roberts JM, Wilson K. Effect of stretching duration on active and passive range of motion in the lower extremity. *Br J Sports Med*. 1999;33:259–263.

89. Meyer JJ, Zachman ZJ, Keating JC, Traina AD. Effectiveness of chiropractic management for patellofemoral pain syndrome's symptomatic control phase: a single subject experiment. *J Manipulative Physiol Ther*. 1990;13:539–549.

90. Watson CJ, Leddy HM, Dynjan TD, Parham JL. Reliability of the lateral pull test and tilt test to assess patellar alignment in subjects with symptomatic knees: student raters. *J Orthop Sports Phys Ther*. 2001;31(7):368–374.

91. Watson CJ, Propps M, Gait W, Redding A, Dobbs, D. Reliability of McConnell's classification of patellar orientation in symptomatic and asymptomatic

subjects, including commentary by McConnell J and Dye SF with author responses. *J Orthop Sports Phys Ther.* 1999;29(7):379–393.

92. Powers CM, Mortenson S, Nishimoto D, Simon D. Criterion-related validity of a clinical measurement to determine the medial/lateral component of patellar orientation. *J Orthop Sports Phys Ther.* 1999;29 (7):372–377.

93. Herrington LC. The inter-tester reliability of a clinical measurement used to determine the medial/lateral orientation of the patella. *Man Ther.* 2002;7(3): 163–167.

94. Deyle GD, Henderson NE, Matekel RL, Ryder MG, Garber MB, Allison SC. Effectiveness of manual physical therapy and exercise in osteoarthritis of the knee. A randomized, controlled trial. *Ann Intern Med.* 2000;132(3):173–181.

95. Hinman RS, Crossley KM, McConnell J, Bennell KL. Efficacy of knee tape in the management of osteoarthritis of the knee: blinded randomised controlled trial. *BMJ.* 2003;327(7407):135.

96. Topp R, Woolley S, Hornyak J 3rd, Khuder S, Kahaleh B. The effect of dynamic versus isometric resistance training on pain and functioning among adults with osteoarthritis of the knee. *Arch Phys Med Rehabil.* 2002;83(9):1187–1195.

97. Fraser A, Fearon U, Reece R, Emery P, Veale DJ. Matrix metalloproteinase 9, apoptosis, and vascular morphology in early arthritis. *Arthritis Rheum.* 2001;44(9):2024–2028.

98. Hurley MV. The effects of joint damage on muscle function, proprioception and rehabilitation. *Man Ther.* 1997;2(1):11–17.

99. Deyle G, Allison S, Matekel R, Ryder M, Stang J, Gohdes D, Hutton J, Henderson N, Garber M. Physical therapy treatment effectiveness for osteoarthritis of the knee: A randomized comparison of supervised clinical exercise and manual therapy procedures versus a home exercise program. *Phys Ther.* 2005;85:1301–1317.

100. Crossley K, Bennell K, Green S, McConnell J. A systematic review of physical interventions for patellofemoral pain syndrome. *Clin J Sport Med.* 2001;11(2):103–110.

101. Crossley KM, Cowan SM, McConnell J, Bennell KL. Physical therapy improves knee flexion during stair ambulation in patellofemoral pain. *Med Sci Sports Exerc.* 2005;37(2):176–183.

102. Harris GR, Susman JL. Managing musculoskeletal complaints with rehabilitation therapy: summary of the Philadelphia Panel evidence-based clinical practice guidelines on musculoskeletal rehabilitation interventions. *J Fam Pract.* 2002;51(12):1042–1046.

103. Barry OCD, Smith H, McManus F, MacAuley P. Clinical assessment of suspected meniscal tears. *Ir J Med Sci.* 1983;152:149–151.

104. Noble J, Erat K. In defense of the meniscus: A prospective study of 200 meniscectomy patients. *J Bone Joint Surg.* 1980;62:7–11.

105. Fowler P, Lubliner J. The predictive value of five clinical signs in the evaluation of meniscal pathology. *Arthroscopy.* 1989;5:184–186.

106. Saengnipanthkul S, Sirichativapee W, Kowsuwon W, Rojviroj S. The effects of medial patellar plica on clinical diagnosis of medial meniscal lesion. *J Med Assoc Thai.* 1992;75(12):704–708.

107. Kurosaka M, Yagi M, Yoshiya S, Muratsu H, Mizuno K. Efficacy of the axially loaded pivot shift test for the diagnosis of a meniscal tear. *International Orthop.* 1999;23:271–274.

108. Anderson AF, Lipscomb AB. Preoperative instrumented testing of anterior and posterior knee laxity. *Am J Sports Med.* 1989;17(3):387–392.

109. Akseki D, Ozcan O, Boya H, Pinar H. A new weight-bearing meniscal test and a comparison with McMurray's test and joint line tenderness. *Arthroscopy.* 2004;20(9):951–958.

110. Karachalios T, Hantes M, Zibis AH, Zachos V, Karantanas AH, Malizos KN. Diagnostic accuracy of a new clinical test (the Thessaly test) for early detection of meniscal tears. *J Bone Joint Surg Am.* 2005;87(5):955–962.

111. Eren OT. The accuracy of joint line tenderness by physical examination in the diagnosis of meniscal tears. *Arthroscopy.* 2003;19(8):850–854.

112. Stiell IG. Clinical decision rules in the emergency department. *CMAJ.* 2000;163(11):1465–1466.

113. Richman PB. More on the Ottawa knee rules. *Ann Emerg Med.* 1999;33(4):476.

114. Emparanza JI, Aginaga JR; Estudio Multicentro en Urgencias de Osakidetza: Reglas de Ottawa (EMUORO) Group. Validation of the Ottawa Knee Rules. *Ann Emerg Med.* 2001;38(4):364–368.

115. Szucs PA, Richman PB, Mandell M. Triage nurse application of the Ottawa knee rule. *Acad Emerg Med.* 2001;8(2):112–116.

116. Stiell IG, Wells GA, McDowell I, Greenberg GH, McKnight RD, Cwinn AA, Quinn JV, Yeats A. Use of radiography in acute knee injuries: need for clinical decision rules. *Acad Emerg Med.* 1995;2(11): 966–973.

117. Ketelslegers E, Collard X, Vande Berg B, Danse E, El-Gariani A, Poilvache P, Maldague B. Validation of the Ottawa knee rules in an emergency teaching centre. *Eur Radiol.* 2002;12(5):1218–1220.

118. Seaberg DC, Yealy DM, Lukens T, Auble T, Mathias S. Multicenter comparison of two clinical decision rules for the use of radiography in acute, high-risk knee injuries. *Ann Emerg Med.* 1998;32(1):8–13.

119. Tigges S, Pitts S, Mukundan S Jr, Morrison D, Olson M, Shahriara A. External validation of the Ottawa knee rules in an urban trauma center in the

United States. *AJR Am J Roentgenol.* 1999;172(4): 1069–1071.

120. Khine H, Dorfman DH, Avner JR. Applicability of Ottawa knee rule for knee injury in children. *Pediatr Emerg Care.* 2001;17(6):401–404.

121. Evans P, Bell D, Frank C. Prospective evaluation of the McMurray test. *Am J Sports Med.* 1993;21: 604–608.

122. Grifka J, Richter J, Moraldo M. (abstract). Was kann die eniskussonographie? *Arthroskopie.* 1991;4:193–199

123. Hardaker WT Jr, Garrett WE Jr, Bassett FH 3rd. Evaluation of acute traumatic hemarthrosis of the knee joint. *South Med J.* 1990;83(6):640–4.

124. Tonino AJ, Huy J, Schaafsma J. The diagnostic accuracy of knee testing in the acutely injured knee. Initial examination versus examination under anesthesia with arthroscopy. *Acta Orthop Belg.* 1986;52 (4):479–487.

125. Boeree NR, Ackroyd CE. Assessment of the menisci and cruciate ligaments: an audit of clinical practice. *Injury.* 1991;22(4):291–294.

126. Richter J, David A, Pape HG, Ostermann PA, Muhr G. (abstract) Diagnosis of acute rupture of the anterior cruciate ligament. Value of ultrasonic in addition to clinical examination. *Unfallchirurg.* 1996;99 (2):124–129.

127. Steinbruck K, Wiehmann JC. (abstract). Examination of the knee joint. The value of clinical findings in arthroscopic control. *Z Orthop Ihre Grenzgeb.* 1988;126(3):289–295.

128. Sandberg R, Balkfors B, Henricson A, Westlin N. Stability tests in knee ligament injuries. *Arch Orthop Trauma Surg.* 1986;106(1):5–7.

129. Braunstein EM. Anterior cruciate ligament injuries: a comparison of arthrographic and physical diagnosis. *AJR Am J Roentgenol.* 1982;138(3):423–425.

130. DeHaven KE. Arthroscopy in the diagnosis and management of the anterior cruciate ligament deficient knee. *Clin Orthop.* 1983;172:52–56.

131. Donaldson WF, Warren RF, Wickiewicz T. A comparison of acute anterior cruciate ligament examinations. Initial versus examination under anesthesia. *Am J Sports Med.* 1985;13:5–10.

132. Jonsson T, Althoff B, Peterson L, Renstrom P. Clinical diagnosis of ruptures of the anterior drawer ligament: A comparative study of the Lachman test and the anterior drawer sign. *Am J Sports Med.* 1982;10: 100–102.

133. Lee JK, Yao L, Phelps CT, Wirth CR, Czajka J, Lozman J. Anterior cruciate ligament tears: MR imaging compared with arthroscopy and clinical tests. *Radiology.* 1988;166:861–864.

134. Lui SH, Osti L, Henry M, Bocchi L. The diagnosis of acute complete tears of the anterior cruciate ligament. Comparison of MRI, arthometry, and clinical examination. *J Bone Joint Surg Br.* 1995;77:586–588.

135. Mitsou A, Vallianatos P. Clinical diagnosis of ruptures of the anterior cruciate ligament: a comparison between the Lachman test and the anterior drawer sign. *Injury.* 1988;19(6):427–428.

136. Gurtler RA, Stine R, Torg JS. Lachman test evaluated. Quantification of a clinical observation. *Clin Orthop Relat Res.* 1987;(216):141–150.

137. Dahlstedt LJ, Dalen N. Knee laxity in cruciate ligament injury. Value of examination under anesthesia. *Acta Orthop Scand.* 1989;60(2):181–184.

138. Baker CL Jr, Norwood LA, Hughston JC. Acute combined posterior cruciate and posterolateral instability of the knee. *Am J Sports Med.* 1984;12(3): 204–208.

139. Loos WC, Fox JM, Blazina ME, Del Pizzo W, Friedman MJ. Acute posterior cruciate ligament injuries. *Am J Sports Med.* 1981;9(2):86–92.

140. Rubenstein RA, Shelbourne KD, McCarroll JR, van Meter CD, Rettig AC. The accuracy of the clinical examination in the setting of posterior cruciate ligament injuries. *Am J Sports Med.* 1994;22:550–557.

141. Daniel DM, Stone ML, Barnett P, Sachs R. use of the quadriceps active test to diagnose posterior cruciate-ligament disruption and measure posterior laxity of the knee. *J Bone Jnt Surg Am.* 1988;70; 386–391.

142. Harilainen A, Myllynen P, Rauste J, Silvennoinen E. Diagnosis of acute knee ligament injuries: the value of stress radiography compared with clinical examination, stability under anesthesia and arthroscopic or operative findings. *Ann Chir Gynaecol.* 1986;75(1): 37–43.

143. Garvin GJ, Munk PL, Vellet AD. Tears of the medial collateral ligament: magnetic resonance imaging findings and associated injuries. *Can Assoc Radiol J.* 1993;44(3):199–204.

144. Sallay PI, Poggi J, Speer KP, Garrett WE. Acute dislocation of the patella. A correlative pathoanatomic study. *Am J Sports Med.* 1996;24(1):52–60.

# 15

# Manual Therapy of the Foot and Ankle

KEN LEARMAN AND CHAD E. COOK

## Objectives

- Understand the incidence and prevalence of ankle and foot pathologies and potential risk factors that are associated with occurrence.
- Outline the pertinent clinically relevant anatomy of the foot and ankle.
- Understand the clinical examination of the foot and ankle.
- Outline an effective treatment program for various foot and ankle impairments.
- Identify the outcomes associated with orthopedic manual therapy to the foot and ankle.

## INCIDENCE

**Ankle foot complex** (AFC) injuries account for a significant number of all orthopedic injuries sustained in the country today.[1,2] Most injuries are activity related and are associated with a high degree of recurrence. AFC injuries such as ankle sprains and fractures are more common in younger individuals while degenerative disorders and tendon-based injuries are more frequent in older subjects.[3]

Sports such as soccer demonstrate a high degree of ankle injuries. The incidence rate of ankle sprains for male soccer players is .46 for every 1,000 hours of playing time and .86 for every 1,000 hours of playing time for those with no previous history and those with a previous history of an ankle sprain.[1] Tropp reported a 25% recurrence rate for ankle sprains during a 6-month period of playing soccer among competitive adults.[2] Other sports such as basketball are also plagued with ankle-related injuries. A previous history of ankle injury resulted in a recurrence rate of 5 times the normal sprain rate of 3.85 per 1,000 participants,[4] a problem that frequently affects professional and/or recreational athletes. Recreational basketball players at the United States Military Academy experienced an injury rate of 5.2 per 100 participants for players not wearing a protective brace.[5]

Gender differences have been noted in the incidence of lower extremity injury rates for the knee and the ankle. Hosea found that female basketball players experienced a higher incidence rate than males at a seasonal rate of 8.6%.[6] Female handball players have likewise demonstrated high rates of ankle sprains at 50 injuries per 100 in 1,000 hours of playing time.[7]

### Summary

- AFC injuries are commonly encountered by older and younger individuals.
- Younger subjects appear to be more predisposed to ankle sprains and fractures whereas older subjects appear to be predisposed to tendon injuries and degeneration.

## ANATOMY

The AFC is made up of numerous joints including the inferior tibiofibular, talocrural, subtalar, transverse tarsal, tarsal-metatarsal, metatarsal–phalangeal, and interphalangeal joints.[3] All of these joints will directly affect the ankle complex by transmitting forces up the kinematic chain.

## Osseous Structures

There are 26 bones in each foot (Figure 15.1). It is best to describe the osseous structures based on location for understanding of the contribution to structural function. Classically, the foot is divided into the **forefoot, midfoot,** and **hindfoot** (Figures 15.2 and 15.3).[3]

### Hindfoot Bones

There are two bones of the hindfoot, the calcaneus and the talus. The calcaneus is the largest tarsal bone, forms the heel of the foot, and provides significant structural integrity to the ankle foot complex.

The talus is the second largest tarsal bone and forms the articulation between the lower leg and the foot. The articulation site of the talus is complex and consists of a number of facets with both convex and concave features.

### Midfoot Bones

The five midfoot bones are bordered by the Lisfranc joint distally and the transverse tarsal joint (Chopart's joint) proximally. The bones of the midfoot include the three cuneiforms, the cuboid, and the navicular bone. The navicular is responsible for transmitting forces from the hindfoot to the forefoot and demonstrates numerous articulation facets. Otherwise, the majority of the midfoot bones articulate and function as a complex system that provides stability, transmits mobility, and adapts appropriately to ground surface changes.[8]

### Forefoot Bones

The forefoot boundaries include the distal-most phalanges and the tarsometatarsal joint (Lisfranc's joint). The

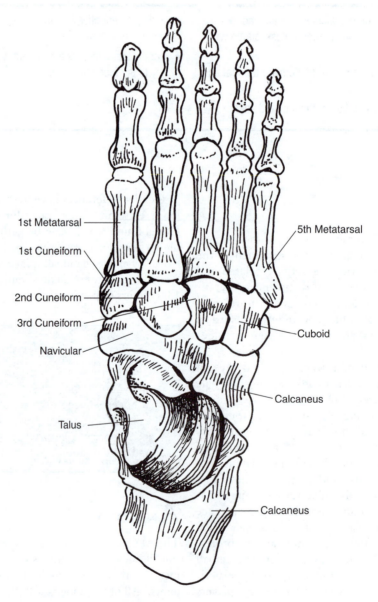

**Figure 15.1**  Dorsal View of the Osseous Structures of the Foot Including the Divisions of the Mid-, Fore-, and Hindfoot

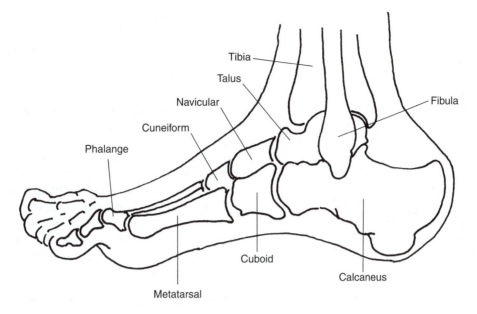

**Figure 15.2**    Lateral View of the Wholefoot

forefoot contains five metatarsals and 14 phalanges. The metatarsals are described by the medial to lateral position, therefore, the medial-most metacarpal is designated as digit 1, digit 2, digit 3, and so on. The articulation points of each metatarsal include medial and lateral articulations with other metatarsals and proximal articulations with the cuboid (4 and 5) and cuneiforms.[3] The metatarsals are unique as they are the only bone in the body that is weight bearing at a perpendicular axis.

Like the hand, there are two phalanges at digit 1 and three for digits 2 through 5. The digits serve as connection points for a number of muscles and are used primarily during propulsion. Occasionally, phalanges will be accom-

panied by sesamoid bones, which aid in providing an improved mechanical lever.[8]

## *Summary*

- There are 26 or more bones in the AFC.
- The osseous structures are generally divided into three primary groups: the hindfoot, midfoot, and forefoot.
- The calcaneus is the largest bone in the foot followed by the talus.

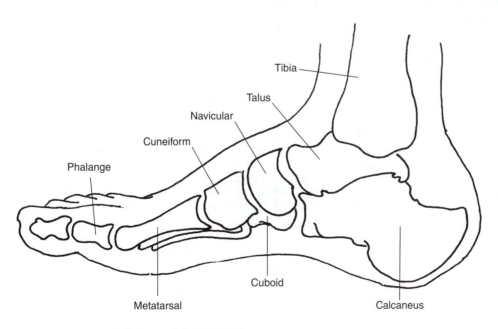

**Figure 15.3**    Medial View of the Wholefoot

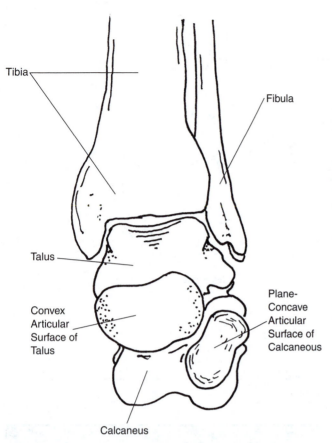

**Figure 15.4**   The Talocrural Articulation

## *Hindfoot Joints of Stabilizing Structures of the Ankle Foot Complex*

There are two primary joints of the hindfoot: the talocrural joint, which consists of the articulations of the

tibiotalar, tibiofibular, and fibulotalar structures and the subtalar joint, which consists of the articulations of the talus superiorly and the calcaneus inferiorly.

### *Talocrural Joint*

The distal tibiofibular joint is a syndesmotic joint connected by fibrous bands of tissue. The slightly concave tibial surface articulates with the plane[9] to convex,[9,10] the triangular-shaped distal end of the fibula. The structure of the mortise is represented by the tibia superiorly, the medial malleolus medially, and the lateral malleolus of the fibula laterally. The distal tibiofibular joint is stabilized by several ligaments including the anterior and posterior tibiofibular ligaments, the interosseus ligament, and the superior extensor retinaculum. The architecture of the tibia and fibula creates the mortise of the talocrural joint.

The mortise functions as a concave surface to accept the convex surface of the talus (Figure 15.4). The trochlea of the talus is up to 6 millimeters (mm) wider anteriorly than posteriorly, causing the talus to act as a wedge within the ankle mortise. The tibiotalar joint, fibulotalar joint, and the distal portion of the tibiofibular joint reside in the same joint capsule and make up the synovial hinge joint known as the talocrural.[10]

Displacement (distraction) of the joint can allow excess talar rotation within the talocrural joint. This excess rotation can cause the triplanar movement to occur out of the normal triplanar pattern, disrupting force translation in closed chain.

Ligaments supporting the talocrural joint include the anterior and posterior talofibular ligaments (ATFL and PTFL, respectively), the calcanealfibular ligament laterally and the deltoid ligament medially (Figures 15.5 and 15.6). The ATFL is frequently sprained during an uncontrolled inversion moment, typically from a plantarflexed position.[6]

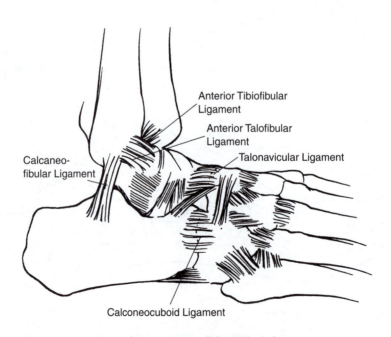

**Figure 15.5**   Lateral Ligaments of the Wholefoot

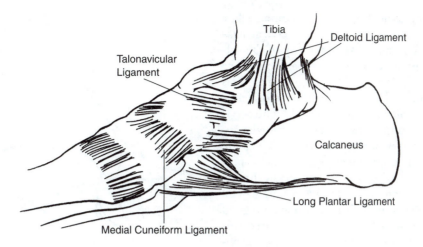

**Figure 15.6**   Medial Ligaments of the Wholefoot

When compared to other ligaments, ATFL sprains occur relatively easily secondary to low load to failure and high strain to failure.[11]

### Subtalar Joint

The subtalar joint is irregularly shaped and can be classified as a synovial bicondylar joint (Figure 15.7).[9] There are two articulating surfaces between the talus and the calcaneus. The anterior articulation is convex on the talus and concave on the calcaneus whereas the posterior articulation is concave on the talus and convex on the calcaneus. Between these two articulations is the interosseous membrane,

also referred to as the axial ligament, which assists in stabilization of an eversion movement.[12] With the anterior articulation lying medial to the posterior articulation and with the irregular joint surfaces, the subtalar joint will move in opposite directions during functional weight bearing.[9]

Ligaments are present to assist in maintaining integrity of the subtalar joint. They include the medial and lateral interosseous, the calcaneofibular (CFL), the deltoid (DL), and the lateral talocalcaneal ligaments (LTCL). The medial talocalcaneal interosseous ligament projects from the medial tubercle of the talus posteriorly to just behind the sustentaculum tali of the calcaneus and serves to prevent

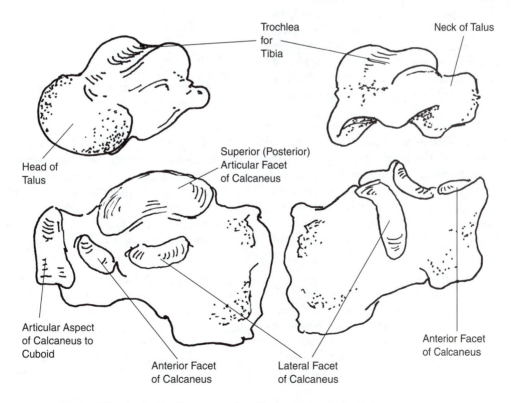

**Figure 15.7**   The Articular Processes that Form the Subtalar Joint

the talus from anterior translating on the calcaneus. The lateral talocalcaneal interosseous ligament (cervical ligament) projects from the sinus tarsi posteriorly to the calcaneus and serves to prevent the excess separation of the talus from the calcaneus during inversion moments. This ligament is typically injured when an excessive moment is applied in inversion coupled with dorsiflexion.[9] The cervical ligament is further fortified in preventing subtalar inversion by the deep fibers of the extensor retinaculum. Medially, the deltoid and calcaneonavicular ligaments prevent excessive eversion. Laxity of the ligaments in the lateral compartment is implicated frequently in lateral instability due to an excess of active and passive range of motion. Laxity in the medial compartment is predominantly less frequent but may be functionally more problematic since this type of sprain is associated with a higher incidence of cartilage damage and concomitant lateral ligamentous damage.[13]

## Midfoot Joints of Stabilizing Structures of the Ankle Foot Complex

Multiple joints make up the midfoot region. The proximal and distal boundaries include the proximal transverse tarsal joint and the distal Lisfranc joint. Between these boundaries are the talonavicular joint, the calcaneocuboid joint, the cuneonavicular joint, and the intermetatarsal joints.[8]

### Transverse Tarsal Joint (Chopart's Joint)

The transverse tarsal joint or "Chopart's joint" includes the articulations of the talus and navicular (talonavicular joint) and the calcaneus and the cuboid (calcaneocuboid joint) (Figure 15.8). The talonavicular joint is a ball and socket joint that allows triplanar movement. The anterior aspect of the talus is convex and articulates with the posterior concave aspect of the navicular. It is stabilized by the joint capsule, the dorsal talonavicular, and the medial portion of the bifurcate and the plantar calcaneonavicular (spring) ligaments.

The calcaneocuboid complex allows movement in both transverse and longitudinal planes. The anterior aspect of the calcaneus is convex in the horizontal plane and concave in the vertical plane articulating with the cuboid, which is concave in the horizontal plane and convex in the vertical plane,[14] making the joint a synovial modified sellar joint.[9] This joint is stabilized by the joint capsule, the spring ligament, the long plantar ligament, and dorsally by the bifurcate ligament.

### Cuneonavicular Joint

The convex surface of the navicular articulates with the combined concave surfaces of the three cuneiforms (medial, intermediate, and lateral) to form a compound synovial, modified sellar joint.[9] The three cuneiforms form the transverse arch. This arch is important for allowing room for neurovascular and musculotendinous structures

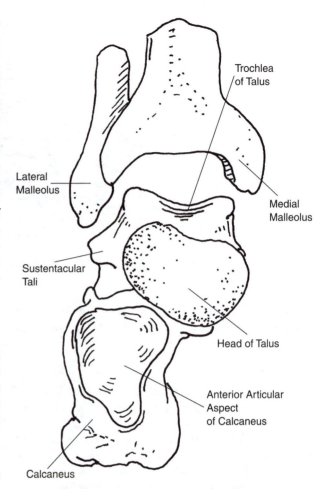

**Figure 15.8**    Anterior View of the Transverse Tarsal Joint

to pass through the plantar aspect of the foot.[9] The joint is stabilized by the joint capsule, the dorsal and plantar cuneonavicular ligaments. The transverse arch is stabilized and maintained by the peroneus longus muscle.

### Cubonavicular Joint

The cubonavicular joint is a plane joint and when synovial, is continuous with the cuneonavicular joint.[9] The cubonavicular joint is sometimes referred to as the cuboid-third cuneiform-navicular joint.[15] The joint is stabilized by the plantar cubonavicular ligament. The cuboid and the navicular bones tend to move together rather than on each other, allowing the forefoot to move as a unit on the hindfoot through the midtarsal joint.

### Tarsometatarsal Joints (Lisfranc's Joint)

The convex distal cuneiforms and cuboid bones articulate with the concave bases of the metatarsals to form plane synovial joints within three separate joint cavities (Figure 15.9).[10] The first joint cavity or medial tarsal-metatarsal joint consists of the medial cuneiform and the first metatarsal and is the most mobile. The intermediate tarsalmetatarsal joint consists of all three cuneiforms articulating with the second and third metatarsals and is the least mobile of the joint cavities. It is also important to note that the second metatarsal articulates with the intermediate cuneiform between the distal aspects of the larger medial and lateral cuneiforms to create a bony invagination to stabilize further this joint cavity, making the structure immobile. This fact may become clinically important in the second ray's ability to absorb stress since this region is frequently the site of stress fractures. The ligament of Lisfranc crosses from the medial cuneiform to the second metatarsal base to provide a strong, stabilizing mechanism that is important in keeping the first ray from separating from the second ray. If this ligament is torn, the medial forefoot becomes very mobile, acting independently of the rest of the forefoot. The final joint cavity consists of the articulations between the lateral cuneiform and the third metatarsal and the cuboid with the fourth and fifth metatarsals.[10]

## Forefoot Joints of Stabilizing Structures of the Ankle Foot Complex

### Metatarsal Phalangeal Joints (MTP)

Each of the metatarsals articulates with the proximal phalanx. The metatarsal is biconvex and the base of the phalanx is biconcave, making the metatarsalphalangeal joints both condyloid and synovial.[10] These joints are stabilized in part by the deep transverse metatarsal ligaments and the medial and lateral collateral ligaments, in addition to the plantar metatarsophalangeal ligaments and the dorsal extensor hood expansion.[16] The first MTP also receives stabilization from the expansion of the extensor hallucis tendon and ventrally from the plantar accessory ligament. Within the plantar accessory ligament lie the flexor hallucis tendon and the medial and lateral sesamoid bones.[9]

### Intermetatarsal Joints

The intermetatarsal joints are plane-type synovial joints that are considered extensions of the tarsometatarsal joints. The deep transverse metatarsal ligament and the interosseous ligaments, which assist in maintaining the transverse arch of the foot, stabilize them. The bases of the metatarsals glide both dorsally and plantarly and do not demonstrate much individual movement.[10]

### Interphalangeal Joints

Each of the phalanges has a base and a head described from proximal to distal.[10] The interphalangeal joints are synovial modified sellar joints that primarily move in flexion and extension. The convex phalangeal heads articulate with the concave bases of the phalanx just distal to it. It must be noted that a certain degree of freedom is also apparent in abduction, adduction, and rotation both medially and laterally.

The joints are stabilized by the joint capsule and collateral ligaments. There are two interphalangeal joints in the first ray and three interphalangeal joints in rays 2–5.

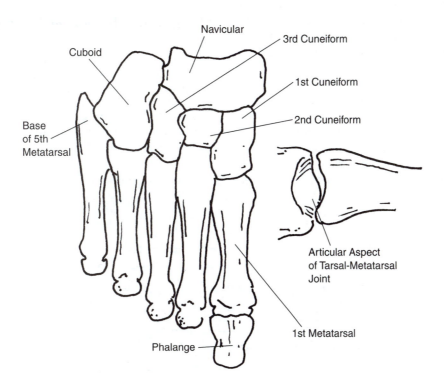

**Figure 15.9**    Tarsalmetatarsal Joints and the Joints of the Forefoot

## Summary

- The joints of the foot are further divided into the hindfoot joints, midfoot joints, and forefoot joints.
- Each joint system consists of numerous smaller joints.
- The majority of the stabilization associated with the joints in the AFC is primarily ligamentous supported.

## Pseudo-Joints (Longitudinal and Transverse Arches)

There are two major arches present in the mechanically normal foot, the transverse arch and the longitudinal arch. The longitudinal arch has two components, a medial and lateral arch. The medial arch, described from posterior to anterior, consists of the calcaneus, talus, navicular, three cuneiforms, and the first three metatarsals with the head of the talus acting as the keystone because it bears the direct pressure of the body's weight in a closed kinematic chain.[10]

The lateral arch consists of the calcaneus, cuboid, and lateral two metatarsals and lies on the ground during weight bearing. The difference in height between the medial and lateral longitudinal arches assists in the formation of the transverse arch, demonstrating the integration between the arches in the dispersion of forces during weight bearing. The medial longitudinal arch tends to be more important in function because it contributes to the positional mechanics of the mid and forefoot and helps determine the force transferal between the parts of the foot.

Numerous structures are required to maintain the arches of the foot including the plantar fascia (primarily), the central aponeurosis, the plantar ligaments and capsules, the congruency of bony anatomy, and tension within the tendons from their muscular action (Figure 15.10). Muscle action contributes the least since electromyographic analysis of the muscles of the foot has determined that very little muscle activity occurs until locomotion begins.[8] The plantar calcaneonavicular ligament (spring ligament) is the main structure responsible for maintaining the medial longitudinal arch. The long plantar ligament extends the length of the lateral longitudinal arch and is its main structure of support for the lateral arch.

The plantar aponeurosis supports the entire longitudinal arch with a fibrous band connecting the calcaneous to the tuberosity of the fifth metatarsal and the medial band attaching to the sesamoids under the first metatarsal. The plantar aponeurosis stabilizes the medial arch in toe standing. Finally, the plantar calcaneocuboid ligament, also known as the short plantar ligament, assists the spring and long plantar ligaments in supporting the longitudinal arches.[10] The plantar aponeurosis and plantar fascia in general frequently become the source of mechanical and chemical pain in dysfunction through apparent injuries involving repeated microtrauma.

## Summary

- Several pseudo-joints make up the AFC that provide the foot with an arch shape.
- The longitudinal arch has two components, a medial and lateral arch.
- The stabilization of the arches is from the combined efforts of passive and active stabilizers.

## Muscle of the Ankle Foot Complex

Like the joints of the AFC, the muscles are best divided into groups based on the compartments of the leg. However, division of compartments is generally described as lateral, medial, anterior, and posterior.

### Anterior Compartment

The tibialis anterior originates on the anterior proximal tibia and fibula and inserts on the first metatarsal and medial aspect of the medial cuneiform. Combined with the extensor digitorum longus, the tibialis anterior pro-

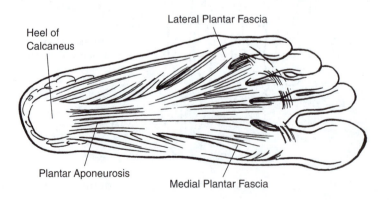

**Figure 15.10** The Plantar Aponeurosis of the Foot and Ankle

motes dorsiflexion of the ankle. The extensor digitorum longus originates from the upper two-thirds of the anterior border of the fibula, the lateral condyle of the tibia, and the interosseous membrane and inserts on the lateral four digits through the expansion hoods into the bases of the middle and distal phalanges affecting dorsiflexion and digit extension.

Less prominent muscles may assist in dorsiflexion. The peroneus tertious originates on the distal third of the anterior fibula and the interosseous membrane inserts on the dorsum of the fifth metatarsal and lateral aspect of the cuboid, which serves to dorsiflex and evert the foot. The extensor hallucis longus originates on the anterior fibula, inserts on the distal phalange of the first digit, and primarily extends the great toe and secondarily dorsiflexes the foot.

### Lateral Compartment

Muscles of the lateral compartment (Figure 15.11) are primarily responsible for eversion. The peroneus longus originates off the proximal half of the fibula on the lateral side, inserts on the plantar aspect of the first metatarsal and medial cuneiform, and is a strong evertor of the foot and a weak plantarflexor. The peroneus brevis originates on the distal lateral half of the fibula, inserts on the lateral base of the fifth metatarsal and cuboid, and functions to evert the foot, and is a weak plantarflexor.

### Posterior Compartment

The posterior compartment (Figure 15.12) is subdivided into the superficial posterior compartment and the deep posterior compartment. Within the superficial posterior compartment lie the triceps surae, which include the medial and lateral heads of the gastrocnemius and the soleus muscles. The gastrocnemius medial and lateral heads originate on the posterior femoral condyles and insert in the common calcaneal tendon in the posterior aspect of the calcaneus. This muscle is a strong plantarflexor and is used extensively for powerful movements. The soleus originates on the proximal third of the tibia and fibula and inserts on the common calcaneal tendon. The soleus plays a significant role in postural control. Lastly, the plantaris, which originates on the supracondylar ridge of the femur and inserts in to the posterior calcaneus through the calcaneal tendon, is also a weak plantarflexor of the foot and a knee flexor.

The deep posterior compartment includes the popliteus, the tibialis posterior, the flexor digitorum longus, and the flexor hallicus longus. The popliteus originates on the lateral epicondyle of the femur and inserts on the posterior proximal tibia above the origin of the soleus.[8] While the popliteus does not directly affect the foot and ankle, it is within the deep posterior compartment and can functionally influence the ankle by unlocking extension of the knee and allowing dorsiflexion of the ankle in closed-chain activity.

The tibialis posterior lies deep within the posterior compartment, originates on the posterior aspect of the tibia and fibula, and inserts on the navicular tubercle, the medial cuneiform, and the plantar aspect of the base of the lateral four metatarsals through fibrous attachments. It is important in maintaining the medial longitudinal arch of the foot as well as being a weak plantarflexor and invertor.

The flexor digitorum longus originates on the middle third of the posterior tibia just distal to the soleal line, inserts on the planar aspect of the bases of metatarsals 2–5, serves to flex the toes, inverts the foot, and assists in maintaining the medial longitudinal arch of the foot. The flexor hallucis longus originates on the distal two-thirds of the posterior fibula and inserts on the base of the distal phalanx of the first digit and acts as a flexor of the great toe and a plantarflexor of the foot.

### Dorsal Compartment of the Foot

The extensor digitorum brevis originates on the dorsal surface of the calcaneus and inserts onto the base of the proximal phalanx of digit 1 and into the tendons of EDL for digits 2–4 to extend the first four toes.

### Plantar Compartment of the Foot

There are four layers of muscle on the plantar aspect of the foot. Within the first layer lie the abductor hallicus, flexor digitorum, and the abductor digiti minimi. The abductor hallucis originates on the medial tuberosity of the calcaneus and from the flexor retinaculum and inserts on the medial aspect of the base of the proximal great toe, abducts, flexes the great toe in non–weight bearing, and braces medial longitudinal arch in weight bearing. The flexor digitorum brevis originates on the medial tuberosity of the calcaneus and the plantar aponeurosis and inserts on the medial and lateral aspects (tendon bifurcates at insertion) of the middle phalanges of the lateral four digits and serves to flex the metatarsal–phalangeal (MTP) and interphalangeal (PIP) joints. The abductor digiti minimi originates from the medial and lateral calcaneal tuberosities, inserts on the lateral base of the proximal fifth phalanx, abducts, flexes the fifth digit in non–weight bearing, and braces the lateral longitudinal arch in weight bearing.

The second layer consists of the lumbricals and the quadratus plantae. The lumbricals originates from the tendons of FDL, inserts on the extensor expansion base of proximal phalanges of digits 2–5 and the tendons of EDL, and serves to flex the MTP and extend the PIP joints. The quadratus plantae originates from the medial and lateral plantar surfaces of the calcaneus, inserts on the posterior aspect of the FDL tendon, and assists in the flexion of the lateral four DIP joints.

Within the third layer lie the muscles of the flexor hallicus brevis, the abductor hallucis, and the flexor digiti minimi. The flexor hallucis brevis originates from the cuboid and lateral cuneiform, inserts on the medial and lateral sides of the proximal great toe, and flexes the MTP of the first digit. The abductor hallucis has two heads: (1) the oblique, which originates from metatarsals 2–4, and (2) the transverse that originates from the plantar

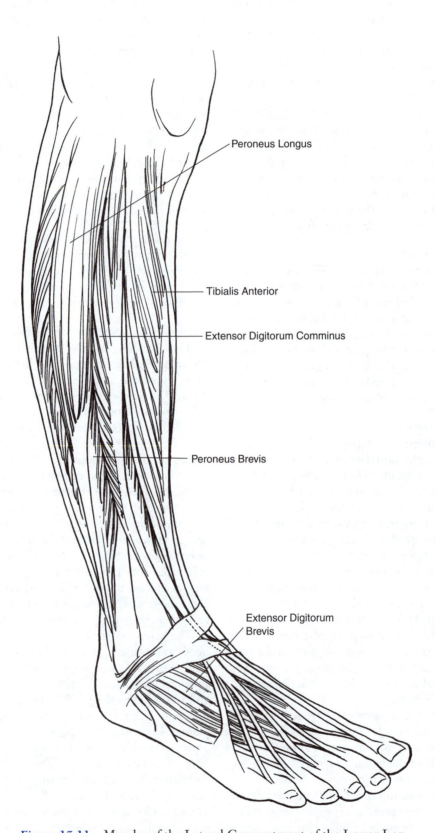

Peroneus Longus

Tibialis Anterior

Extensor Digitorum Comminus

Peroneus Brevis

Extensor Digitorum
Brevis

**Figure 15.11**    Muscles of the Lateral Compartment of the Lower Leg

Within the fourth layer lie the plantar interossei and the dorsal interossei. The plantar interossei originate on the plantar aspect of metatarsals 3–5 and insert on the medial planar surface of the base of the proximal phalanx of digits 3–5. The dorsal interossei originate on the medial aspect of one metatarsal and the lateral aspect of the adjacent metatarsal in all four intermetatarsal spaces. The lateral three dorsal interossei insert on the lateral plantar surface of the base of proximal phalanx on digits 2–4 and on the medial aspect of the base of the proximal phalanx of digit 2 (remember no plantar interosseus inserts here).[17]

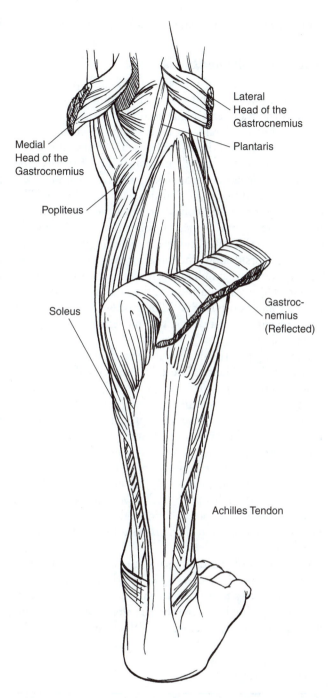

## Summary

- The muscles are best divided into lateral, medial, anterior, and posterior compartments.
- There are four layers of muscle on the plantar aspect of the foot.

# BIOMECHANICS

As in all joints, the ankle complex has two types of possible motion: translatory movement, also known as arthrokinematic motion and rotational movement, also known as osteokinematic motion. Osteokinematic movement incorporates translatory motion in order to stabilize the instantaneous axis of rotation. This is important to translate forces over a larger surface area within the joint as well as to prevent unnatural forces during end ranges, which may damage the passive structures of the joint.

The collective movement patterns and passive and active control of foot motion allows for transferal of force throughout the foot for confirmation to surfaces and propulsion during gait. This process involves the individual range of motions (ROM) provided at each articulation.

## Range of Motion

The talocrural joint demonstrates approximately 50 degrees of plantarflexion and 20 degrees of dorsiflexion. The subtalar joint is reported to have 40 degrees of inversion and 20 degrees of eversion. The tarsal joints are reported to have 10 degrees of pronation and 20 degrees of supination.[18] Extension of digits 2–5 includes 40 degrees of extension in the MTPs, 0 degrees of PIP extension, and 30 degrees of DIP extension. The first MTP has 70 degrees of extension and 0 degrees of IP extension. For flexion, the MTPs have 40 degrees, PIPs have 35 degrees, and the DIPs have 60 degrees. The great toe exhibits 45 degrees of flexion at the MTP and 90 degrees at the IP.

## Open- and Closed-Packed Positions

The terms open- and closed-packed positions of the ankle is in reference to the theoretical supposition that selected movements will increase the compression (closed-packed)

**Figure 15.12**   Muscles of the Posterior Compartment of the Lower Leg

ligaments of the lateral 4 MTPs and inserts on the lateral side of the base of the proximal phalanx of the first digit. The oblique head adducts and flexes the MTP of the great toe and the transverse head pulls all the metatarsals together, supports the transverse arch of the foot, and adducts the first digit. The flexor digiti minimi brevis originates off the base of the fifth metatarsal, inserts on the base of the proximal phalanx of digit 5, and serves to flex the fifth MTP joint.

Labels in figure:
Medial Head of the Gastrocnemius
Lateral Head of the Gastrocnemius
Plantaris
Popliteus
Soleus
Gastrocnemius (Reflected)
Achilles Tendon

or distraction (open-packed) position between the joints of the ankle. The articular reference of *closed-packed position* refers to a specific joint preposition when the articular surfaces are at the maximum point of congruency whereas *open-packed* is the opposite of this joint position. Unfortunately, no studies exist that support this assumption, thus the validity behind open and closed packed is essentially unknown.

Neumann suggests an alternative to the Cyriax-based definition of open- and closed-packed positions.[18] He reports that supination of the subtalar joint, the combined movement of inversion and adduction, increases the rigidity of the foot and should be considered the closed-pack position of the foot. Conversely, pronation of the subtalar joint (combined movement of abduction and eversion) is the loose-packed position of the foot and creates the most flexible environment for the mid and forefoot.

### Axis of Rotation/Movement

Axis of rotation refers to an imaginary line around which an object rotates. Rarely does the axis of rotation fall in a single plane. At the ankle, most motions are coupled and thus lead to complex multiplanar axes of rotations.[3] For example, pronation is a coupled movement pattern of dorsiflexion, abduction, and eversion. Supination is a coupled pattern of plantarflexion, adduction, and inversion.[18] The coupled movement allows greater confirmation between the ground reaction forces and the limb and allows alterations in the axis of rotation toward a more functional pattern.

The closed- and open-packed positions at the hindfoot work in concert with the axis of motion to create movement patterns in the lower extremity.[18] Subtalar supination assists in locking the midtarsal joints so the foot is rigid during push-off. Pronation at the subtalar joint unlocks the midtarsal joints, prompting a flexible foot when ambulating on unlevel surfaces. The axes of rotation allow the foot to further confirm and/or stabilize depending on the demands required. Table 15.1 outlines the axis of rota-tion for each of the movements available at the ankle foot complex.

### Articular Movements

The axis of rotation of the talocrural joint is primarily in the sagittal plane around a frontal axis but is 23 degrees lateral in the transverse plane secondary to external tibial torsion. The talocrural joint is also angled medially in the frontal plane around the sagittal axis, as the lateral malleolus is distal to the medial malleolus. The fact that the talocrural joint has components in all three planes makes dorsiflexion and plantarflexion triplanar movements. The talocrural joint can be considered to have 20 degrees of offset to the sagittal plane, causing motion in inversion/eversion and adduction/abduction accordingly.[19,20]

During dorsiflexion, the superior surface of the talus slides posteriorly simultaneously with anterior rotation (rolling). During plantarflexion, the talus slides anteriorly but also rotates posteriorly.[18] The motion, however, is not purely planar and may consist of movements of eversion and inversion.

The complex articulation of the subtalar joint is less easily described. Mantar[21] describes the axis of rotation as 42 degrees from the horizontal plane and 16 degrees from the sagittal plane, running in an anterior, medial, and superior direction. During subtalar pronation, the calcaneus moves in a curvilinear pattern around the axis of rotation. Thus, in pronation, the calcaneus moves into eversion and abduction and during supination, the calcaneus moves into inversion and adduction. During gait, when the calcaneus is fixed, the talus primarily moves on the calcaneus. This movement incorporates more adduction and abduction of the talus, controlled in part by rotation of the lower extremity.

Movements of the midtarsal joints occurs around two separate, independent axes.[22] The longitudinal axis occurs through the length of the foot in a cephalomedial direction and an oblique axis that occurs closer to the horizontal but is also cephalomedial.[21,22] When the subtalar joint

**TABLE 15.1** Axes of Rotation for the Ankle Foot Complex

| Movement | Primary Joint | Axis of Rotation |
|---|---|---|
| Pronation | Subtalar joint, Transverse tarsal | Combined axis of valgus, medial to lateral, and vertical |
| Supination | Subtalar joint, Transverse tarsal | Combined axis of varus, medial to lateral, and vertical |
| Abduction | Transverse tarsal, Metatarsophalangeal | Vertical |
| Adduction | Transverse tarsal, Metatarsophalangeal | Vertical |
| Inversion | Subtalar, talocrural, Transverse tarsal | Varus flare |
| Eversion | Subtalar, Talocrural, Transverse tarsal | Valgus flare |
| Dorsiflexion | Talocrural joint, First tarsometatarsal joint, Metatarsophalangeal, Interphalageal joint | Medial to lateral |
| Plantarflexion | Talocrural joint, First tarsometatarsal joint, Metatarsophalangeal, Interphalageal joint | Medial to lateral |

is pronated, the two axes become parallel to one another and maximum amount of motion is possible between the forefoot and hindfoot; but when the subtalar joint is supinated, the axes approach right angles to one another, providing little movement. This biomechanical variation allows the foot to adapt to uneven surfaces during the early stance phase of gait but then allows rigidity for an effective push-off during the terminal stance phase of gait.[20]

The Lisfranc joint primarily allows dorsiflexion and plantarflexion, mostly at the first tarsometatarsal joint.[18] Dorsiflexion of the first ray results in a superior migration of the metatarsal on the first cuneiform. Conversely, plantarflexion requires an inferior migration of the metatarsal on the first cuneiform. The movement patterns of the metatarsal phalangeal and interphalangeal joints are similar to those of the first metatarsal on the first cuneiform.

## Summary

- There is no evidence to support the theory of open- and closed-packed positions proposed by Cyriax.
- The axes of motion throughout the foot are reflective of the multiplanar movements of each joint.
- The articular movements of the joint involve complex movements reflective of convex on concave and variable axes of rotations during movements.

# ASSESSMENT AND DIAGNOSIS

## Differential or Contributory Diagnoses

Consequential foot and ankle disorders are common with conditions such as diabetes. These disorders may exist as stand-alone dysfunctions or primary pathologies. Peripheral vascular disease, a common comorbidity in patients with diabetes, may lead to skin breakdown, pain, burning symptoms, and secondary musculoskeletal disorders of the foot and ankle.[23]

Neurological conditions may mimic foot ankle dysfunction and require careful differentiation. Individuals with a history of alcoholism, diabetes, and vitamin deficiency are more likely to report radiculopathic-mimicking symptoms than those without these comorbidities.[3] A comprehensive lumbar examination may be required if the patient reports radiating or burning pain at the ankle.[3,24] Discomfort that exhibits radicular-like symptoms may be associated with a nerve root entrapment or radicular pain from the lumbar spine.[3,24] Conditions such as tarsal tunnel syndrome often result in pain patterns that are nonspecific.[3] In many cases, patients with tarsal tunnel syndrome report increased pain at night, often awakening the patient.[3]

## *Ottawa Ankle Rules*

The Ottawa Ankle Rules were developed in 1992 to reduce the necessity of radiographic imagery after the occurrence of an ankle sprain. Prior to the onset of these rules, nearly every ankle sprained was x-rayed, even though less than 15% of ankle sprains result in a fracture.[25,26] The rules dictate the need for an ankle radiograph if a patient demonstrates: (1) bone tenderness at the posterior edge or tip of the lateral malleolus, and/or (2) bone tenderness at the posterior edge or tip of the medial malleolus, and/or (3) inability to bear weight both immediately and in the emergency room. The rules also dictate the need for a foot radiograph if a patient demonstrates (1) bone tenderness at the base of the fifth metatarsal bone, and/or (2) bone tenderness at the navicular, and/or (3) inability to bear weight both immediately and in the emergency room (Figure 15.13). A summary of several studies has demonstrated that the negative presence of these factors is excellent at ruling out the presence of a fracture ($-LR = 0.07$; $CI = 0.03$ to $0.18$).[26]

## Summary

- A myriad of nonmechanical disorders exists for the foot. These disorders consist of neurological, referred pains, and vascular disorders.
- The Ottawa Ankle Rules are specific measurements designed to identify patients with a fracture after an ankle sprain.

## Subjective Considerations

Important history items collected during a subjective examination include the presence of comorbidities, any relevant past history of ankle disorders, a history of surgery, and occupational and avocation demands.[3] Ascertaining the mechanism of injury may assist in determining the likelihood of the presence of a fracture. High-impact injuries or profound ankle sprains should automatically initiate the assessment of the Ottawa Ankle Rules discussed earlier.[27]

The behavior of the symptoms may help outline the cause of the disorder. Locking disorders that exhibit an intermittent pattern may be indicative of osteochondritis dissecans (OD) of the talar dome.[27] Pain associated with OD should be queried to differentiate from anterior impingement at the joint line. Anterior impingement is consistently triggered during dorsiflexion at end range whereas OD may occur intermittently and during different planes of movement.

Lateral ankle pain associated with a sprain is the most common form of ankle injury and usually results from an inversion sprain.[28] Often, individuals report a previous injury that was similar in context. Some may report a "pop"

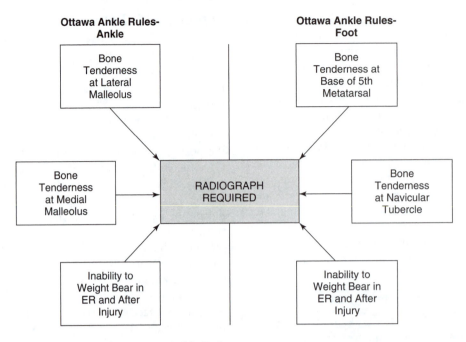

**Figure 15.13**   The Ottawa Ankle Rules

during the injury, which may represent a tear in the surrounding ligamentous structure.[28] A pop is also associated with Achilles tendon tears and should be differentiated using the appropriate physical examination methods.

Conditions such as plantar fasciitis are more common in middle-aged individuals and usually begin with a gradual onset of symptoms. Pain is typically isolated to the plantar aspect of the heel and is worsened during gait without shoe wear that stabilizes the foot. Plantar fasciitis differs from midfoot arthritis in etiology, but exhibits very similar characteristics. Patients will also complain of pain without supportive shoe wear, but will generally complain of pain in the arch or forefoot region, specifically at the Lisfranc joint.

Disability associated with AFC impairment is occasionally underreported. It has been stated that at least one-third of the time required for recovery is associated with the failure of appropriate measurement for ankle patients.[29] One reason may be associated with the relatively small loss of range of motion (ROM) noted in acute ankle sprains. Small losses of ROM can lead to significant reports of disability and adding activity limitation measures to the assessment may improve prediction of duration of disability and return to activity.[29]

Foot-ankle-specific outcome scales may function to identify the impact of disease on the ability to perform activities of daily life and are quickly becoming the standard evaluative tool in which legislators, insurers, consumers, and clinicians make informed decisions about the effectiveness and appropriateness of care.[1,4] While outcome measures are essential components of any clinical examination, foot disorders result in significant disability and functional limitations, hence clinicians must recognize the

need to use valid and responsive self-report measures to assist with determining the plan of care, documenting patient status and improvement, and justifying rehabilitative intervention to third-party payers with this patient population.[5–7,30]

Self-report measures appear to correlate well with laxity findings during a clinical examination. Fifty-one subjects with self-report of lateral ankle instability demonstrated AP laxity in the talocrural joint when compared to uninjured controls. This AP-related laxity was small (1.5 mm) but significant.[31] Because the accessory movements related to the ankle are often very small, the clinician must recognize the inherent relationship between subject report of dysfunction and the displacement of selected joints. Additionally, the relatively small displacements that are associated with ankle pain do not seem to be a deterrent in progression toward chronicity. Many patients develop functional ankle instability (FAI) that results in further injury, increased pain, and reduced participation in normal activities of daily living.

Recently the *Manchester Foot and Ankle Disability Scale*, a region-specific scale, was developed and validated in a group of over 1,000 patients with foot-related problems.[32] The questionnaire was initially 19 items, however, a principal component analysis revealed that two of the items did not apply to all patients with foot disorders and were eliminated from the final scale. The 17-item questionnaire exhibited high criterion validity and internal consistency. The *Manchester Foot and Ankle Disability Scale* is multidimensional, exhibiting two components of pain intensity, functional limitations, and tribulations associated with personal appearance.[31] Considering that the scale was developed and validated on a patient population with varying conditions, it was purported that the *Manchester Foot and Ankle Disability Scale* exhibits generalizability to the patient population with foot pain as a whole.

## Summary

- One essential element of the patient history during the examination of an AFC is the mechanism of injury.
- One of the reasons patients fail to recover is the inability to measure properly the disability associated with an AFC.
- The *Manchester Foot and Ankle Disability Scale* is a recently validated instrument that effectively measures AFC disability.

## Objective/Physical Examination

### Observation

Primarily, observational methods in detecting foot and ankle disorders are focused in three criteria. The first criterion involves inspection of the foot and ankle during standing. Abnormal alignment of the forefoot and hindfoot that is associated with a concordant pain (pain during stance) may require specific intervention such as orthotics or stabilization. The status of the longitudinal arch may provide the clinician with an understanding of the support mechanisms of the foot and the biomechanical consequences associated with important findings. For example, failure of the longitudinal arch may result in a phenomenon known as "too many toes" (Figure 15.14). This phenomenon when viewed posteriorly appears to demonstrate too many digits when in reality the fallen arch increases the amount of pronation during static stance.

The second criterion includes a gait evaluation. Patients should be asked to walk toward and then away from the examiner, walking forward and backward. If no abnor-

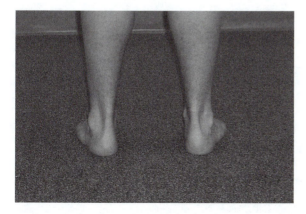

**Figure 15.14** Observation of Abnormal Ankle Biomechanics during Stance: Too Many Toes

mality is revealed by basic gait, then the subject could be asked to walk on toes both toward and away from the examiner followed by walking on heels in maximum dorsiflexion toward and away. If this is not provocative of symptoms and compensation, the subject could be asked to hop on toes and hop on heels to attempt to stimulate the concordant sign.[33]

The third criterion involves a skin and nails inspection. Trophic changes may be indicative of peripheral vascular disease. Pigmentation may be associated with venous insufficiency. Significant callus formation may be a consequence of abnormal gait or increased pressure during weight bearing. Toenail disorders may be a result of psoriasis, poor blood flow, and/or infection.[3]

## Summary

- Observational strategies during the examination of the AFC include biomechanical assessment of hindfoot and forefoot alignment.
- Often, a gait evaluation will identify a concordant abnormality in the AFC.
- Inspection of the skin and toenails may assist in identifying disorders such as vascular problems, psoriasis, and infections.

# CLINICAL EXAMINATION

## Active Physiological Movements

The focus of the active physiological examination is the reproduction of the concordant sign during activities.[27] Eliciting the concordant sign may require variations of physical activities, responses, or functional activities. By examining the activity performed during the concordant complaint the clinician may improve the likelihood of isolating the disorder.

A common method of elicitation of the concordant sign is the use of functional movements. Some of the movements such as stance and gait were discussed in the observation section of this chapter. Others, such as hopping, running, occupational-related activities, and additional static positions may further distill the underlying elements of the concordant pain. Because the quantities of functional movements that affect the ankle are of large quantity, it is impossible to represent these movements pictorially. However, functional activities such as single leg hopping, talar rotation during unilateral stance, and step-ups may be useful in eliciting the concordant sign (Figures 15.15 and 15.16). Lark et al.[34] reported that the elderly required necessary range of motion at the ankle, specifically controlled dorsiflexion, in order to ambulate using stairs. A step-down is a modification that may be useful to determine the availability of functional range of motion.

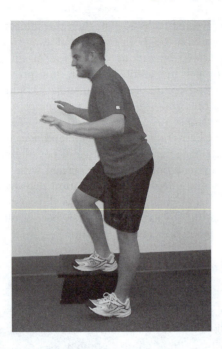

**Figure 15.15**    Step-Ups

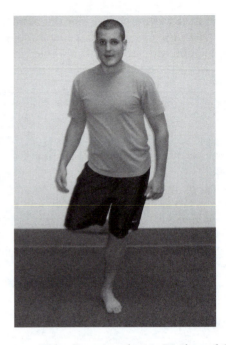

**Figure 15.16**    Talar Rotation during Unilateral Stance

The peroneus longus assists in propulsion of the foot during push-off. One method of assessing the ability of the peroneus longus to stabilize during this process is the

bilateral peroneus longus test. This test involves the simultaneous action of plantarflexion and eversion during weight bearing. Weakness or injury to the peroneus longus will result in the concordant reproduction of pain or inability to perform upon demand.

## Passive Movements

### *Passive Physiological Movements*

Although passive movements of the foot and ankle involve axes of movements that are multiplanar, it is easiest to define the movements by plane of motion. These planes include plantarflexion, dorsiflexion, abduction, adduction, and the combined planar movements of inversion and eversion.

## *Summary*

- The focus of the active physiological examination is the reproduction of the concordant sign during activities.
- Functional movements are best performed to outline the problems associated with the AFC.

## Plantarflexion

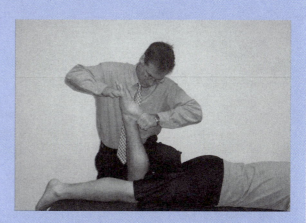

**Figure 15.17**    Plantarflexion of the Whole Foot

- Step One: The subject is placed in prone with the knee flexed and resting pain is assessed.
- Step Two: The examiner places the posterior hand on the postero-plantar calcaneus and the anterior hand on the dorsal forefoot.

- Step Three: The foot and ankle are then passively plantarflexed to the first point of concordant pain (if present). Repeated movements or sustained holds are applied to determine if the symptoms increase or decrease. The foot and ankle is then passively moved toward end range, allowing the same process of assessment for repeated movements and sustained holds.
- Step Four: Differentiation of whole foot and midfoot can be made with hand placement changes. The clinician stabilizes the hindfoot and passively applies a plantarflexion force on the midfoot. Pain and range–pain behavior is reassessed.

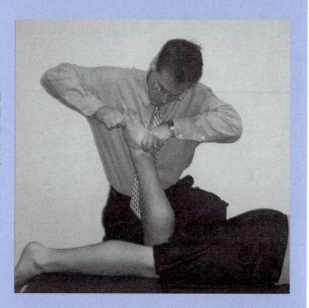

**Figure 15.18**    Plantarflexion of the Midfoot

- Step Five: The forefoot can be differentiated from the midfoot by stabilizing the midfoot and forcing the forefoot into plantarflexion. Pain and range–pain behavior is reassessed. A comparison of the subject's reaction to pain with the various positions implicates which anatomical region is the likely source of the pain.

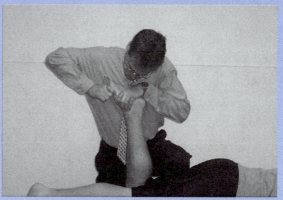

**Figure 15.19**    Forefoot Plantarflexion

## Dorsiflexion

- Step One: The subject is placed in prone with the knee flexed and resting pain is assessed.
- Step Two: The examiner places the posterior hand on the postero-dorsal calcaneous (over the calcaneal tendon) and the other hand on the palmar surface of the foot.
- Step Three: The foot and ankle are then passively dorsiflexed to the first point of concordant pain (if present). Repeated movements or sustained holds are applied to determine if the symptoms increase or decrease. The foot and ankle are then passively moved toward end range, allowing the same process of assessment for repeated movements and sustained holds.

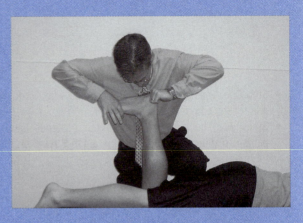

**Figure 15.20**    Dorsiflexion of the Whole Foot

- Step Four: Differentiation of hindfoot from the midfoot is made by stabilizing the hindfoot and promoting dorsiflexion of the midfoot. Pain and range–pain behavior is reassessed.

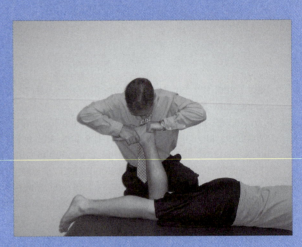

**Figure 15.21**    Dorsiflexion of the Midfoot from the Hindfoot

- Step Five: Differentiation of the forefoot from the midfoot is made by stabilizing the midfoot and applying a dorsiflexion force to the forefoot. Pain and range–pain behavior is reassessed.

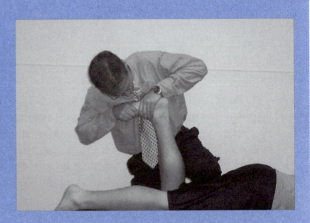

**Figure 15.22**    Dorsiflexion of the Forefoot

## Abduction

- Step One: The subject is placed in prone with the knee flexed and resting pain is assessed.
- Step Two: The examiner places the posterior hand on the postero-lateral calcaneus and the anterior hand on the medial forefoot.
- Step Three: The foot and ankle are then passively abducted to the first point of concordant pain (if present). Repeated movements or sustained holds are applied to determine if the symptoms increase or decrease. The foot and ankle are then passively moved toward end range, allowing the same process of assessment for repeated movements and sustained holds.

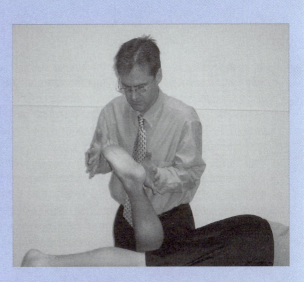

**Figure 15.23**    Abduction of the Whole Foot

- Step Four: Differentiation of hind, mid, and forefoot can be made with hand placement changes. The midfoot is differentiated by stabilizing the hindfoot and promoting abduction at the transversetarsal joint. Pain and range–pain behavior is reassessed.

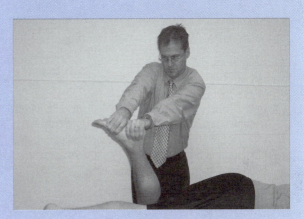

**Figure 15.24**    Abduction of the Midfoot in Relation to the Hindfoot

- Step Five: The forefoot and midfoot can be differentiated by stabilizing the midfoot with and abducting the forefoot. Pain and range–pain behavior is reassessed.

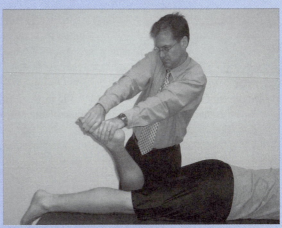

**Figure 15.25**    Abduction of the Forefoot on the Midfoot

## Adduction

- Step One: The subject is placed in prone with the knee flexed and resting pain is assessed.
- Step Two: The examiner places the posterior hand on the postero-medial calcaneus and the anterior hand on the lateral forefoot.
- Step Three: The foot and ankle are then passively abducted to the first point of concordant pain (if present). Repeated movements or sustained holds are applied to determine if the symptoms increase or decrease. The foot and ankle are then passively moved toward end range, allowing the same process of assessment for repeated movements and sustained holds.

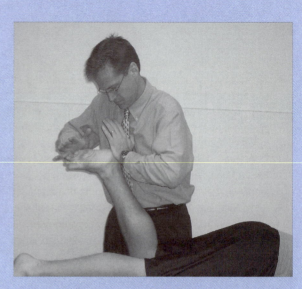

**Figure 15.26**    Adduction of the Whole Foot

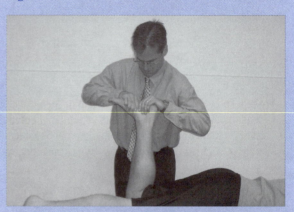

**Figure 15.27**    Adduction of the Midfoot Relative to the Hindfoot

- Step Four: Differentiation of hind, mid, and forefoot can be made with hand placement changes. Differentiation of the midfoot relative to the hindfoot is accomplished by stabilizing the hindfoot and promoting adduction at the transverse joint. Pain and range–pain behavior is established.

- Step Five: Differentiation of the forefoot from the midfoot is accomplished by stabilizing the midfoot and promoting adduction at the Lisfranc joint. Pain and range–pain behavior is reassessed. A comparison of the subject's reaction to pain with the various positions implicates which anatomical region is the likely source of the pain.

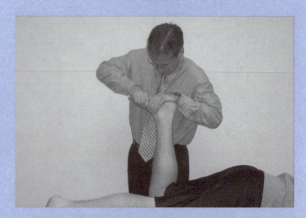

**Figure 15.28**    Adduction of the Forefoot Relative to the Midfoot

Combined passive physiological movements are useful in detection of articular or capsular structures. Inversion and eversion (see the following boxes) are considered combined movements.

## Inversion

- Step One: The subject is placed in prone with the knee flexed and resting pain is assessed.
- Step Two: The examiner places the posterior hand on the calcaneus (fingers medially and thumb laterally) and the anterior hand on the forefoot (fingers medially and thumb laterally).
- Step Three: The foot and ankle are then passively inverted as the clinician pulls the foot toward his or her body in a curvilinear fashion. This movement occurs to the first point of pain and the process is repeated at end range as well. Behavior with repeated movements or sustained holds is recorded.

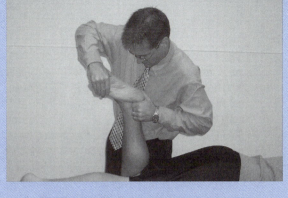

**Figure 15.29**   Inversion of the Wholefoot

- Step Four: Differentiation of hind, mid, and forefoot can be made with hand placement changes. The midfoot is differentiated from the hindfoot by blocking the hindfoot and promoting an inversion movement at the midfoot. Pain and range behavior is assessed.
- Step Five: The forefoot can be differentiated by stabilizing the midfoot and promoting inversion at the forefoot. Pain and range–pain behavior is reassessed. A comparison of the subject's reaction to pain with the various positions implicates which anatomical region is the likely source of the pain.

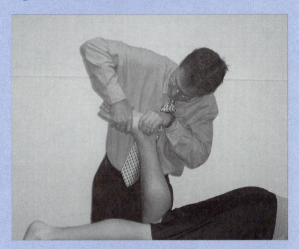

**Figure 15.30**   Inversion of the Midfoot with Respect to the Hindfoot

## Eversion

- Step One: The subject is placed in prone with the knee flexed and resting pain is assessed.
- Step Two: The examiner places the posterior hand on the calcaneus (fingers medially and thumb laterally) and the anterior hand on the forefoot (fingers medially and thumb laterally).
- Step Three: The foot and ankle are then passively inverted as the clinician pulls the foot toward his or her body in a curvilinear fashion. This movement occurs to the first point of pain and the process is repeated at end range as well. Behavior with repeated movements or sustained holds is recorded.

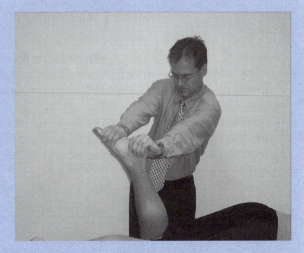

**Figure 15.31**   Eversion of the Wholefoot

(*continued*)

- Step Four: Differentiation of hind, mid, and forefoot can be made with hand placement changes. The midfoot is differentiated from the hindfoot by blocking the hindfoot and promoting an eversion movement at the midfoot. Pain and range–pain behavior is assessed.
- Step Five: The forefoot can be differentiated by stabilizing the midfoot and promoting eversion at the forefoot. Pain and range–pain behavior is reassessed. A comparison of the subject's reaction to pain with the various positions implicates which anatomical region is the likely source of the pain.

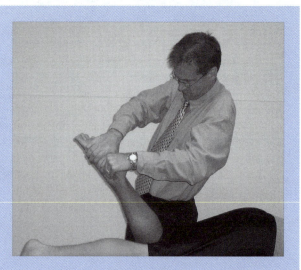

**Figure 15.32**    Eversion of the Midfoot with Respect to the Hindfoot

## Summary

- The purpose of passive physiological movements is to reproduce the concordant sign.
- Passive physiological movement further localizes AFC movements that contribute to concordant patient complaints.
- Passive physiological movements may be single plane or combined to engage the articular or surrounding structures.

## *Passive Accessory Movements*

The arthrokinematics at the multiple joints of the ankle foot complex are wrought with multiplanar movements, complicated rolling and gliding behaviors, and variable facet architecture. By addressing the pain provocation response the clinician is able to determine the concordant response and can cross the boundaries of complexities among the numerous joints.

### Antero-Posterior Glide of the Inferior Tibial–Fibular Joint

- Step One: The patient is sidelying with the medial border of the foot placed on a pillow for comfort. The clinician is standing in front of the patient facing the foot and resting symptom level is assessed.
- Step Two: The clinician places both thumbs on the anterior border of the distal fibula (the anterior border is oblique so care must be taken to stay on the bone) with the fingers resting across the posterior aspect of the heel and ankle.
- Step Three: The clinician performs a joint play movement by mobilizing the distal fibula directly posteriorly until the subject first reports concordant discomfort. The movement is repeated or sustained to assess the response of the movement.
- Step Four: The movement is then performed near end range. The movement is also repeated or sustained to assess the response of the movement on the concordant sign.

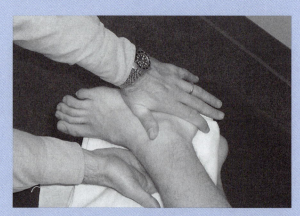

**Figure 15.33**    Anterior-Posterior Glide of the Inferior Tibial Fibular Joint

## Postero-Anterior Glide of the Inferior Tibial–Fibular Joint

- Step One: The patient is sidelying with the medial border of the foot placed on a pillow for comfort. The clinician is standing behind the patient facing the heel and resting symptom level is assessed.
- Step Two: The clinician places both thumbs on the posterior shelf of the distal fibula with the fingers resting across the posterior aspect of the heel and ankle.
- Step Three: The clinician performs a joint play movement by mobilizing the distal fibula directly anteriorly until the subject first reports concordant discomfort. The movement is repeated or sustained to assess the response of the movement.
- Step Four: The movement is then performed near end range. The movement is also repeated or sustained to assess the response of the movement on the concordant sign.

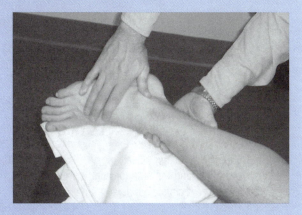

**Figure 15.34** Posterior Anterior Glide of the Inferior Tibial Fibular Joint

## Caudal Glide of the Inferior Tibial–Fibular Joint

- Step One: The patient is sidelying with the medial border of the foot placed on a pillow for comfort. The clinician stands cephalically to the foot of the patient.
- Step Two: The clinician takes the hindfoot in the distal hand with the thenar eminence stabilizing the foot just distal to the lateral malleolus and the proximal hand grasping the distal malleolus between the thumb and forefinger.
- Step Three: The clinician performs a caudal glide of the fibula by inverting the hindfoot until the subject reports concordant discomfort. The movement is sustained or repeated to assess the outcome of the technique.
- Step Four: The movement is then performed at end range to elicit a concordant sign. If concordant, repeated or sustained movements are performed.

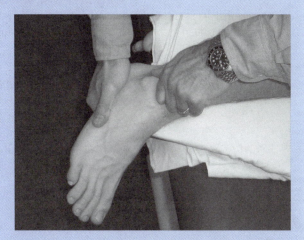

**Figure 15.35** Caudal Glide of the Inferior Tibial–Femoral Joint

## Cephalad Glide of the Tibial–Femoral Joint

- Step One: The patient is sidelying with the medial border of the foot placed on a pillow for comfort. The clinician stands caudally to the foot of the patient.
- Step Two: The clinician takes the hindfoot in the distal hand with the thenar eminence stabilizing the foot just distal to the lateral malleolus and the proximal hand grasping the distal malleolus between the thumb and forefinger.
- Step Three: The clinician performs a cephalad glide of the fibula by everting the hindfoot until the subject reports concordant discomfort. The movement is sustained or repeated to assess the outcome of the technique.
- Step Four: The movement is then performed at end range to elicit a concordant sign. If concordant, repeated or sustained movements are performed.

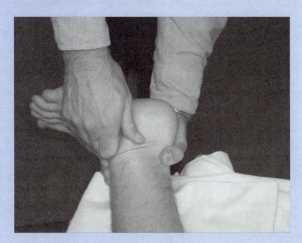

**Figure 15.36** Cephalic Glide of the Inferior Tibial–Femoral Joint

## Antero-Posterior Glide of the Talocrural Joint

During dorsiflexion, the superior surface of the talus slides posteriorly simultaneously with anterior rotation (rolling). An anterior-to-posterior glide of the talus should theoretically improve passive dorsiflexion.

- Step One: The subject is placed in prone with the knee flexed and resting pain is assessed.
- Step Two: The examiner places the posterior hand on the distal tibia and fibula and the anterior hand on the head of the talus with the elbows pointing out away from each other.
- Step Three: With the tibia and fibula stabilized, an anterior-to-posterior force is exerted on the talus until the subject reports concordant pain. If the pain reported is concordant, the movement is repeated or sustained to determine the effect of the technique.
- Step Four: The movement is then taken beyond the first point of pain toward end range. If the pain is concordant, the technique is repeated or sustained at end range. A reduction of symptoms associated with this technique may suggest that the procedure is a plausible treatment procedure.

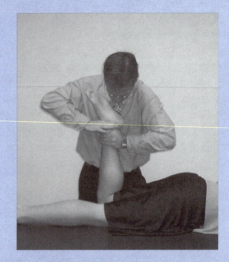

**Figure 15.37**    Antero-Posterior Glide of the Talocrural Joint

## Postero-Anterior Glide of the Talocrural Joint

During plantarflexion, the talus slides anteriorly but also rotates posteriorly (Neuman). A posterior-to-anterior glide of the talus on the calcaneus should theoretically improve passive plantarflexion.

- Step One: The subject is placed in prone with the knee flexed and resting pain is assessed.
- Step Two: The examiner places the posterior hand on the head of the talus and the anterior hand on the distal tibia and fibula with the elbows pointing out away from each other.
- Step Three: With the tibia and fibula stabilized, a posterior-to-anterior force is exerted on the talus until the subject reports concordant pain. If the pain reported is concordant, the movement is repeated or sustained to determine the effect of the technique.
- Step Four: The movement is then taken beyond the first point of pain toward end range. If the pain is concordant, the technique is repeated or sustained at end range. A reduction of symptoms associated with this technique may suggest that the procedure is a plausible treatment procedure.

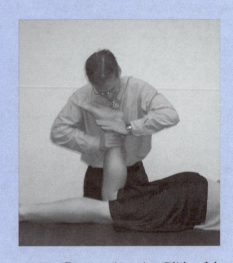

**Figure 15.38**    Postero-Anterior Glide of the Talocrural Joint

## Medial Rotation of the Talocrural Joint

- Step One: The subject is placed in prone with the knee flexed and resting pain is assessed.
- Step Two: The examiner places the posterior hand on the distal tibia and fibula and the anterior hand on the head of the talus with the elbows pointing out away from each other.
- Step Three: With the tibia and fibula stabilized, medial rotation of the talus is performed until the subject reports concordant pain. If the pain reported is concordant, the movement is repeated or sustained to determine the effect of the technique.
- Step Four: The movement is then taken beyond the first point of pain toward end range. If the pain is concordant, the technique is repeated or sustained at end range. A reduction of symptoms associated with this technique may suggest that the procedure is a plausible treatment procedure.

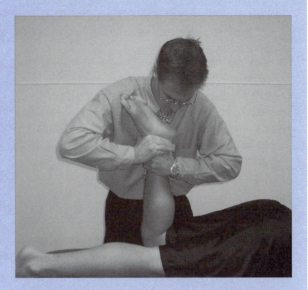

**Figure 15.39**    Medial Rotation of the Talocrural Joint

## Lateral Rotation of the Talocrural Joint

- Step One: The subject is placed in prone with the knee flexed and resting pain is assessed.
- Step Two: The examiner places the posterior hand on the distal tibia and fibula and the anterior hand on the head of the talus with the elbows pointing out away from each other.
- Step Three: With the tibia and fibula stabilized, lateral rotation of the talus is performed until the subject reports concordant pain. If the pain reported is concordant, the movement is repeated or sustained to determine the effect of the technique.
- Step Four: The movement is then taken beyond the first point of pain toward end range. If the pain is concordant, the technique is repeated or sustained at end range. A reduction of symptoms associated with this technique may suggest that the procedure is a plausible treatment procedure.

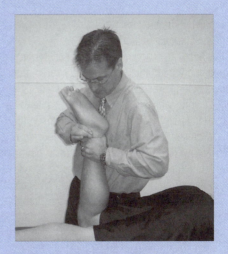

**Figure 15.40**    Lateral Rotation of the Talocrural Joint

## Longitudinal Distraction of the Talocrural Joint

- Step One: The subject is placed in prone with the foot hanging off the end of the mat table and resting symptoms are assessed.
- Step Two: The examiner places one hand under the foot, cupping the calcaneus, and the other hand on the dorsum of the foot with the fifth digit on the head of the talus.
- Step Three: With the feet placed in stride standing to stabilize the body, the clinician leans posteriorly to generate a longitudinal force to distract the talocrural joint until the subject reports concordant pain. If the pain reported is concordant, the movement is repeated or sustained to determine the effect of the technique.
- Step Four: The movement is then taken beyond the first point of pain toward end range. If the pain is concordant, the technique is repeated or sustained at end range. A reduction of symptoms associated with this technique may suggest that the procedure is a plausible treatment procedure.

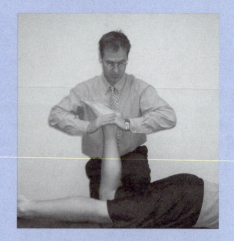

**Figure 15.41**    Longitudinal Distraction of the Talocrural Joint

## Postero-Anterior Movement of the Subtalar Joint

- Step One: The subject is placed in prone with the knee flexed and resting pain is assessed.
- Step Two: The examiner places the posterior hand on the calcaneus and the anterior hand on the head of the talus with the elbows pointing out away from each other.
- Step Three: With the talus stabilized (anteriorly), a posterior-to-anterior force is exerted on the calcaneus until the subject reports concordant pain. If the pain reported is concordant, the movement is repeated or sustained to determine the effect of the technique.
- Step Four: The movement is then taken beyond the first point of pain toward end range. If the pain is concordant, the technique is repeated or sustained at end range. A reduction of symptoms associated with this technique may suggest that the procedure is a plausible treatment procedure.

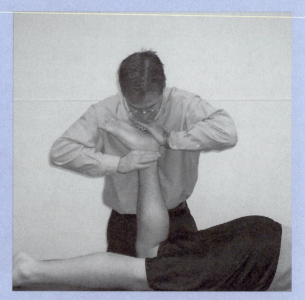

**Figure 15.42**    Postero-Anterior Movement of the Subtalar Joint

## Antero-Posterior Glide of the Subtalar Joint

- Step One: The subject is placed in prone with the knee flexed and resting pain is assessed.
- Step Two: The examiner stabilizes the talus posteriorly while gripping the calcaneus anteriorly.
- Step Three: An anterior to posterior glide is exerted on the calcaneus to the stabilized talus. If the pain reported is concordant, the movement is repeated or sustained to determine the effect of the technique.
- Step Four: The movement is then taken beyond the first point of pain toward end range. If the pain is concordant, the technique is repeated or sustained at end range. A reduction of symptoms associated with this technique may suggest that the procedure is a plausible treatment procedure.

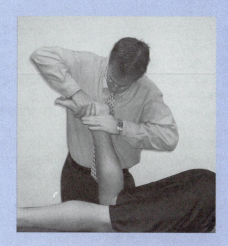

Figure 15.43    Antero-Posterior Glide of the Subtalar Joint

## Medial Rotation of the Subtalar Joint

- Step One: The subject is placed in prone with the knee flexed and resting pain is assessed.
- Step Two: The examiner places the posterior hand on the calcaneus and the anterior hand on the head of the talus with the elbows pointing out away from each other.
- Step Three: With the talus stabilized, medial rotation of the calcaneus (reference point is the heel not anatomical neutral) is performed until the subject reports concordant pain. If the pain reported is concordant, the movement is repeated or sustained to determine the effect of the technique.
- Step Four: The movement is then taken beyond the first point of pain toward end range. If the pain is concordant, the technique is repeated or sustained at end range. A reduction of symptoms associated with this technique may suggest that the procedure is a plausible treatment procedure.

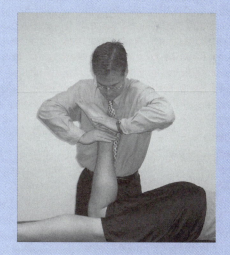

Figure 15.44    Medial Rotation of the Subtalar Joint

## Lateral Rotation of the Subtalar Joint

- Step One: The subject is placed in prone with the knee flexed and resting pain is assessed.
- Step Two: The examiner places the posterior hand on the calcaneus and the anterior hand on the head of the talus with the elbows pointing out away from each other.
- Step Three: With the talus stabilized, lateral rotation of the calcaneus is performed (reference point is the heel not anatomical neutral) until the subject reports concordant pain. If the pain reported is concordant, the movement is repeated or sustained to determine the effect of the technique.
- Step Four: The movement is then taken beyond the first point of pain toward end range. If the pain is concordant, the technique is repeated or sustained at end range. A reduction of symptoms associated with this technique may suggest that the procedure is a plausible treatment procedure.

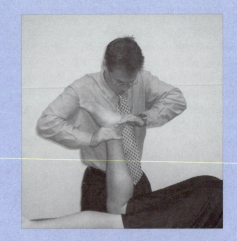

**Figure 15.45**    Lateral Rotation of the Subtalar Joint

## Medial Glide of the Subtalar Joint

- Step One: The patient is sidelying with the medial border of the leg placed on the clinician's forearm and the foot hanging off the mat. The clinician is standing behind the patient facing the foot and resting symptom level is assessed.
- Step Two: The clinician takes the hindfoot in the distal hand with the thenar eminence firmly placed against the lateral calcaneus and the proximal hand stabilizing the lower leg (from underneath) with the forefinger on the medial malleolus and talus.
- Step Three: The clinician performs a medial glide toward the floor while an eversion movement is provided to prevent the motion from becoming an inversion curvilinear movement rather than a medial glide of the calcaneus on the talus. The movement is provided until the subject reports concordant pain. If the pain reported is concordant, the movement is repeated or sustained to determine the effect of the technique.
- Step Four: The movement is then taken beyond the first point of pain toward end range. If the pain is concordant, the technique is repeated or sustained at end range. A reduction of symptoms associated with this technique may suggest that the procedure is a plausible treatment procedure.

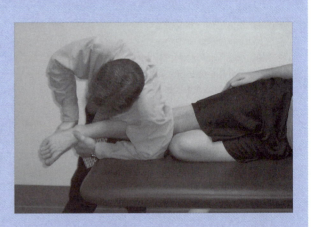

**Figure 15.46**    Medial Glide of the Subtalar Joint

## Lateral Glide of the Subtalar Joint

- Step One: The patient is sidelying with the lateral border of the leg placed on the clinician's forearm and the foot hanging off the mat. The clinician is standing behind the patient facing the foot and resting symptom level is assessed.
- Step Two: The clinician takes the hindfoot in the distal hand with the thenar eminence firmly placed against the medial calcaneus and the proximal hand stabilizing the lower leg (from underneath) with the forefinger on the lateral malleolus and talus.
- Step Three: The clinician performs a lateral glide toward the floor while an inversion movement is provided to prevent the motion from becoming an eversion curvilinear movement rather than a lateral glide of the calcaneus on the talus. The movement is provided until the subject reports concordant pain. If the pain reported is concordant, the movement is repeated or sustained to determine the effect of the technique.
- Step Four: The movement is then taken beyond the first point of pain toward end range. If the pain is concordant, the technique is repeated or sustained at end range. A reduction of symptoms associated with this technique may suggest that the procedure is a plausible treatment procedure.

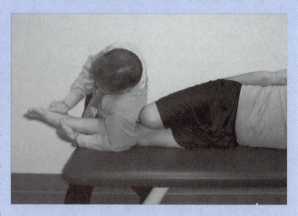

**Figure 15.47**   Lateral Glide of the Subtalar Joint

## Subtalar Inversion

- Step One: The patient is sidelying with the lateral border of the leg placed on the clinician's forearm and the foot hanging off the mat. The clinician is standing behind the patient facing the foot and resting symptom level is assessed.
- Step Two: The clinician takes the hindfoot in the distal hand with the thenar eminence placed against the lateral calcaneus and the proximal hand stabilizing the lower leg (from underneath) with the forefinger on the medial malleolus and talus.
- Step Three: The clinician performs an inversion moment (curvilinear movement) toward the floor of the calcaneus on the talus until the subject reports concordant pain. If the pain reported is concordant, the movement is repeated or sustained to determine the effect of the technique.
- Step Four: The movement is then taken beyond the first point of pain toward end range. If the pain is concordant, the technique is repeated or sustained at end range. A reduction of symptoms associated with this technique may suggest that the procedure is a plausible treatment procedure.

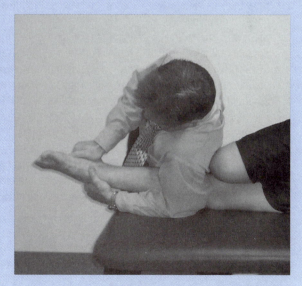

**Figure 15.48**   Subtalar Inversion

## Subtalar Eversion

- Step One: The patient is sidelying with the medial border of the leg placed on the clinician's forearm and the foot hanging off the mat. The clinician is standing behind the patient facing the foot and resting symptom level is assessed.
- Step Two: The clinician takes the hindfoot in the distal hand with the thenar eminence placed against the medial calcaneus and the proximal hand stabilizing the lower leg (from underneath) with the forefinger on the lateral malleolus and talus.
- Step Three: The clinician performs an eversion movement (curvilinear movement) toward the floor of the calcaneus on the talus until the subject reports concordant pain. If the pain reported is concordant, the movement is repeated or sustained to determine the effect of the technique.
- Step Four: The movement is then taken beyond the first point of pain toward end range. If the pain is concordant, the technique is repeated or sustained at end range. A reduction of symptoms associated with this technique may suggest that the procedure is a plausible treatment procedure.

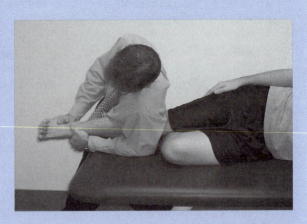

**Figure 15.49**    Subtalar Eversion

## Horizontal Flexion of the Forefoot

- Step One: The subject is placed in prone with the knee flexed and resting pain is assessed.
- Step Two: The examiner places both hands interlaced on the dorsum of the foot with both thumbs on the plantar surface.
- Step Three: The thumbs perform a mobilizing movement in a plantar to dorsal direction while the fingers draw the rays around the thumbs to increase the horizontal arch until the subject reports concordant pain. If the pain reported is concordant, the movement is repeated or sustained to determine the effect of the technique.
- Step Four: The movement is then taken beyond the first point of pain toward end range. If the pain is concordant, the technique is repeated or sustained at end range. A reduction of symptoms associated with this technique may suggest that the procedure is a plausible treatment procedure.

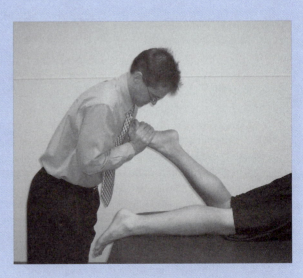

**Figure 15.50**    Horizontal Flexion of the Forefoot

## Horizontal Extension of the Forefoot

- Step One: The subject is placed in prone with the knee flexed and resting pain is assessed.
- Step Two: The examiner places both hands interlaced on the plantar surface of the foot with both thumbs on the dorsal surface.
- Step Three: The thumbs perform a mobilizing movement in a dorsal to plantar direction while the fingers draw the rays around the thumbs to decrease the horizontal arch until the subject reports concordant pain. If the pain reported is concordant, the movement is repeated or sustained to determine the effect of the technique.
- Step Four: The movement is then taken beyond the first point of pain toward end range. If the pain is concordant, the technique is repeated or sustained at end range. A reduction of symptoms associated with this technique may suggest that the procedure is a plausible treatment procedure.

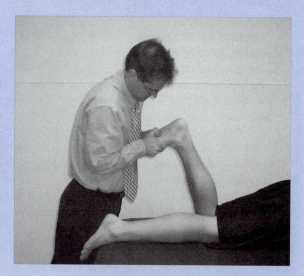

**Figure 15.51**    Horizontal Extension of the Forefoot

## PA Glide of the Metatarsal–Phalangeal and Interphalangeal Joints

- Step One: The subject is placed in prone with the knee flexed and resting pain is assessed.
- Step Two: The examiner stabilizes the proximal segment with one hand and grasps the distal segment of the joint that is to be assessed in the other hand.
- Step Three: Using the thumb to generate the mobilizing force, a PA (plantar to dorsal) shearing movement is performed until the subject reports concordant pain. If the pain reported is concordant, the movement is repeated or sustained to determine the effect of the technique.
- Step Four: The movement is then taken beyond the first point of pain toward end range. If the pain is concordant, the technique is repeated or sustained at end range. A reduction of symptoms associated with this technique may suggest that the procedure is a plausible treatment procedure.

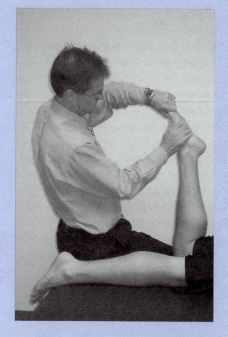

**Figure 15.52**    PA Glide of the MTP Joints

## AP Glide of the MTP Joints

- Step One: The subject is placed in prone with the knee flexed and resting pain is assessed.
- Step Two: The examiner stabilizes the proximal segment with one hand and grasps the distal segment of the joint that is to be assessed in the other hand.
- Step Three: Using the thumb to generate the mobilizing force, an A-P (dorsal to plantar) shearing movement is performed until the subject reports concordant pain. If the pain reported is concordant, the movement is repeated or sustained to determine the effect of the technique.
- Step Four: The movement is then taken beyond the first point of pain toward end range. If the pain is concordant, the technique is repeated or sustained at end range. A reduction of symptoms associated with this technique may suggest that the procedure is a plausible treatment procedure.

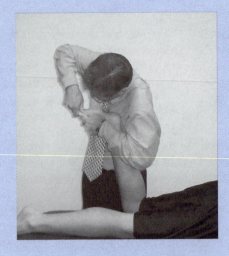

**Figure 15.53**    AP Glide of the MTP Joints

## Adduction of the MTP Joint

- Step One: The subject is placed in prone with the knee flexed and resting pain is assessed.
- Step Two: The examiner stabilizes the proximal segment with one hand and grasps the distal aspect of the tarsal bone in the other hand.
- Step Three: Using the thumb to generate the mobilizing force, an adduction (angular) movement is performed until the subject reports concordant pain. If the pain reported is concordant, the movement is repeated or sustained to determine the effect of the technique.
- Step Four: The movement is then taken beyond the first point of pain toward end range. If the pain is concordant, the technique is repeated or sustained at end range. A reduction of symptoms associated with this technique may suggest that the procedure is a plausible treatment procedure.

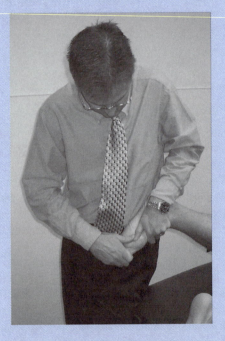

**Figure 15.54**    Adduction of the MTP Joints

## Abduction of the MTP Joints

- **Step One:** The subject is placed in prone with the knee flexed and resting pain is assessed.
- **Step Two:** The examiner stabilizes the proximal segment with one hand and grasps the distal segment of the joint that is to be assessed in the other hand.
- **Step Three:** Using the thumb to generate the mobilizing force, an abduction (angular) movement is performed until the subject reports concordant pain. If the pain reported is concordant, the movement is repeated or sustained to determine the effect of the technique.
- **Step Four:** The movement is then taken beyond the first point of pain toward end range. If the pain is concordant, the technique is repeated or sustained at end range. A reduction of symptoms associated with this technique may suggest that the procedure is a plausible treatment procedure.

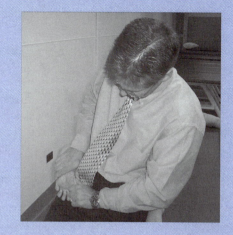

**Figure 15.55**    Abduction of the MTP Joints

## Medial Rotation of the Metatarsal–Phalangeal and Interphalangeal Joints

- **Step One:** The subject is placed in prone with the knee flexed and resting pain is assessed.
- **Step Two:** The examiner stabilizes the proximal segment with one hand and grasps the distal segment of the joint that is to be assessed in the other hand.
- **Step Three:** Using the thumb and forefinger to generate the mobilizing force, a medial rotational movement is performed until the subject reports concordant pain. If the pain reported is concordant, the movement is repeated or sustained to determine the effect of the technique.
- **Step Four:** The movement is then taken beyond the first point of pain toward end range. If the pain is concordant, the technique is repeated or sustained at end range. A reduction of symptoms associated with this technique may suggest that the procedure is a plausible treatment procedure.

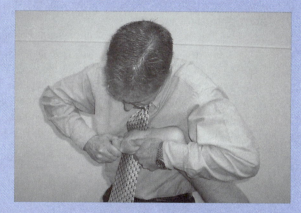

**Figure 15.56**    Medial Rotation Metatarsal–Phalangeal and Interphalangeal Joints

## Lateral Rotation of the Metatarsal–Phalangeal and Interphalangeal Joints

- Step One: The subject is placed in prone with the knee flexed and resting pain is assessed.
- Step Two: The examiner stabilizes the proximal segment with one hand and grasps the distal segment of the joint that is to be assessed in the other hand.
- Step Three: Using the thumb and forefinger to generate the mobilizing force, a lateral rotational movement is performed until the subject reports concordant pain. If the pain reported is concordant, the movement is repeated or sustained to determine the effect of the technique.
- Step Four: The movement is then taken beyond the first point of pain toward end range. If the pain is concordant, the technique is repeated or sustained at end range. A reduction of symptoms associated with this technique may suggest that the procedure is a plausible treatment procedure.

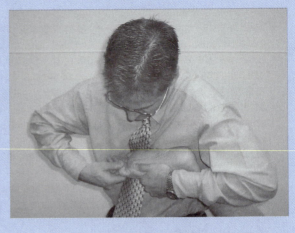

**Figure 15.57** Lateral Rotation of the MTP Joints

## Compression and Distraction of the MTP Joints

- Step One: The subject is placed in prone with the knee flexed and resting pain is assessed.
- Step Two: The examiner stabilizes the proximal segment with one hand and grasps the distal segment of the joint that is to be assessed in the other hand.
- Step Three: Using the thumb and forefinger to generate the mobilizing force, a compressive movement is performed until the subject reports concordant pain. If the pain reported is concordant, the movement is repeated or sustained to determine the effect of the technique.
- Step Four: The movement is then taken beyond the first point of pain toward end range. If the pain is concordant, the technique is repeated or sustained at end range. A reduction of symptoms associated with this technique may suggest that the procedure is a plausible treatment procedure.

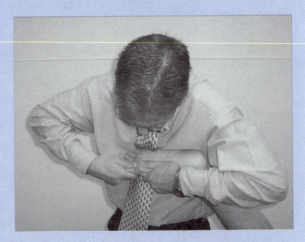

**Figure 15.58** Compression of the MTP Joints

## Distraction of the Metatarsal–Phalangeal and Interphalangeal Joints

- Step One: Using the thumb and forefinger to generate the mobilizing force, a distraction movement is performed until the subject reports concordant pain. If the pain reported is concordant, the movement is repeated or sustained to determine the effect of the technique.
- Step Two: The movement is then taken beyond the first point of pain toward end range. If the pain is concordant, the technique is repeated or sustained at end range. A reduction of symptoms associated with this technique may suggest that the procedure is a plausible treatment procedure.

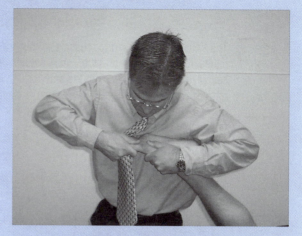

**Figure 15.59**    Distraction of the Metatarsal–Phalangeal and Interphalangeal Joints

## Summary

- The purpose of passive accessory movements is to reproduce the concordant sign.
- Passive accessory movements, when combined with elicitation of the concordant sign of the patient, are reliable and useful assessment tools.
- Passive accessory movement in absence of elicitation of the concordant sign demonstrates little usefulness or applicability to treatment.

## Clinical Special Tests

### Palpation

Palpation should be included in the objective examination to help the clinician determine which structures may be involved. The clinician must take care in determining whether the subjective complaints are consistent with the concordant sign.

### Clinical Special Tests for Ankle Sprains

## Anterior Drawer Test

The anterior drawer test is used to assess the integrity of the anterior talofibular ligament and the displacement within the ankle mortise.[27] A test is considered positive when displacements of 3–5 millimeters or more are noted in the affected side versus the nonaffected side.[27] Unfortunately, the interrater reliability of the anterior drawer test is poor,[35,36] thus findings are questionable of true pathology. When the anterior drawer test and the lateral stress tests are combined, the sensitivity for an ankle sprain increases to 68% but the specificity decreases to 71%.[35]

- Step One: The subject is placed in supine with the heel hanging off the end of the plinth.
- Step Two: The ankle mortise is stabilized against the plinth with one hand.
- Step Three: The ankle is plantarflexed approximately 20 degrees to place the ATFL perpendicular to the long axis of the leg.
- Step Four: The foot is drawn in a posterior-to-anterior direction to displace the talus anteriorly off the mortise.
- Step Five: Adding inversion and/or dorsiflexion can also add additional stress to the calcaneofibular ligament, testing its integrity.[37]

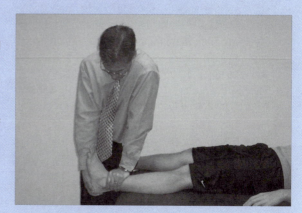

**Figure 15.60**    The Anterior Drawer Test for Ankle Sprains

## The Talar Tilt Test for an Inversion Sprain

The talar tilt test is used to measure angularity of inversion. The test measures the integrity of the calcanealfibular ligament and the anterior talofibular ligament during a varus force.[27,28] The test is more sensitive when combined with the anterior drawer test but also loses specificity when combined. The interrater reliability of the test in absence of pain provocation is poor.[35,36] It is suggested that clinicians may lack the discrimination to feel recommended 10 degrees or greater displacement when compared to the opposite side.[27,36]

- Step One: The patient assumes a sitting position. The clinician stabilizes the tibia distally and grasps the calcaneus at the plantar surface.
- Step Two: The clinician applies a talar tilt into inversion toward end range. The clinician must use care to ensure the movement is curvilinear in nature.
- Step Three: A positive test is considered excessive displacement as compared to the opposite side.

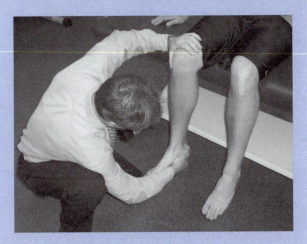

**Figure 15.61**    The Talar Tilt Test for Inversion

## The Talar Tilt Test for an Eversion Sprain

Although an injury associated with an eversion sprain is less common, a similar iteration of the talar tilt test is available for assessment. Because the force required to injure the medial ligamentous structures is so great, the patient generally exhibits concurrent syndesmosis injury.[35]

- Step One: The patient assumes a sitting position. The clinician stabilizes the tibia distally and grasps the calcaneus at the plantar surface.
- Step Two: The clinician applies a talar tilt into eversion toward end range. To increase the sensitivity of the test, the clinician may also apply an additional abduction force.
- Step Three: A positive test is considered excessive displacement as compared to the opposite side.

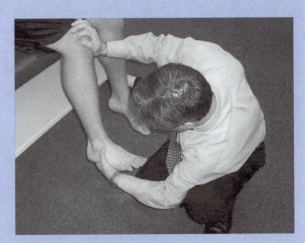

**Figure 15.62**    The Talar Tilt Test for Eversion

## *Clinical Special Tests for Pes Planus*

### Feiss Line Test

The **Feiss Line** test is performed to determine if the patient demonstrates a flatfoot and to grade the degree of flatfoot. There is evidence that suggests that navicular drop may not be a reliable indicator of foot flat posture[38,39] and may not be associated with excessive pronation, commonly found in pes planus. Subsequently, the value of this test is questionable.

- Step One: With the patient seated in a non-weight-bearing position, the clinician marks the patient's skin at the apex of the medial malleolus and the plantar surface of the first MTP.
- Step Two: The navicular tuberosity should be palpated to determine where it is in relationship to the line that joins the two points just marked.
- Step Three: The patient is then asked to stand with his or her feet 6 inches apart.
- Step Four: The points are rechecked to ensure that they still represent the points originally palpated.
- Step Five: The navicular tuberosity is again palpated to determine its relationship to the line between the points as performed previously.
- Step Six: The navicular tuberosity should be at or around the line between the malleolus and the first MTP. If it falls below that line, the degree of flatfoot is measured by (1) grade I—up to one-third of the distance between the line and the floor; (2) grade II—up to two-thirds of the distance to the floor; and (3) grade III—the navicular tuberosity is lying on the floor.

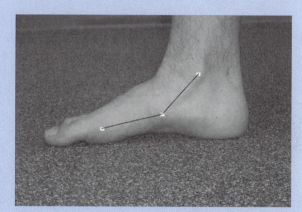

**Figure 15.63**    Feiss Line Test

### Navicular Drop Test

This test is used to determine the degree of flatfoot from the position of comfortable, relaxed standing. Reliability testing reveals an interrater ICC of .73 and an intrarater ICC of .78–.98 among four different studies.[40–43] A more recent study using a digital height gauge and repeated measures design determined that interrater and intrarater reliability were variable but good, ranging from .67 to .92 and .73 to .95, respectively.[44]

- Step One: The patient is placed in standing.
- Step Two: The clinician places the foot in subtalar joint neutral.
- Step Three: The height of the navicular tuberosity is measured from the floor using a paper guide.
- Step Four: The patient is asked to assume a comfortable standing position.
- Step Five: The navicular tuberosity height is remeasured with the paper guide.
- Step Six: The degree of functional pronation is the difference between the two measurements, but any drop greater than 10 mm is considered abnormal.

## Clinical Special Tests for Syndesmosis Injury

### Syndesmosis Squeeze Test

The **syndesmosis** squeeze test is used to implicate potential stress fracture in the ankle, fracture of the fibula, or damage to the syndesmosis of the fibula and tibia.[27,28,35] Additionally, the test is used to measure the presence of a high ankle sprain.[27] The test compresses the proximal fibula against the tibia and is best measured by using concordant pain response.[28,45]

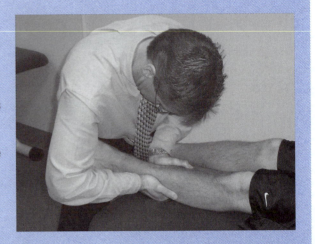

- Step One: The patient lies supine on a mat. The clinician grasps the lower leg at mid-calf with both hands.
- Step Two: The tibia and fibula are squeezed together.
- Step Three: If pain in the lower leg is elicited, it could indicate syndesmosis damage.

**Figure 15.64**   The Syndesmosis Squeeze Test

### The Dorsiflexion and External Rotation Test (DERT Test)

The movements associated with the DERT test are known causes of syndesmosis injury of the lower leg. During dorsiflexion, the talus spreads the mortise and places stress upon the syndesmosis. External rotation furthers the tension placed on the syndesmosis and may reproduce pain when passively performed.[35] Assessment of motion displacement is unreliable and is not an appropriate identifier for a syndesmosis injury.[45]

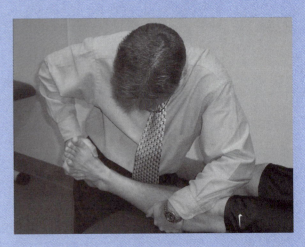

- Step One: The patient assumes a sitting position. The clinician stabilizes the tibia (midway between the knee and the ankle) with one hand and dorsiflexes the foot of the patient with the other.
- Step Two: The clinician maintains dorsiflexion then passively externally rotates the foot while stabilizing the tibia.
- Step Three: Reproduction of concordant symptoms is indicative of a syndesmosis injury.

**Figure 15.65**   The Dorsiflexion and External Rotation Stress Test

## Summary

- Typically, palpation and muscle strength assessment provide additional data whereas clinical tests provide diagnostic information.
- Three forms of clinical special tests are prevalent at the AFC. The primary areas include tests for ankle laxity, syndesmosis injury, and pes planus.

# TREATMENT TECHNIQUES

As stated throughout the textbook, the patient-response method endeavors to determine the behavior of the patient's pain and/or impairment by analyzing concordant movements and the response of the patient's pain to applied or repeated movements. The applied or repeated movements that positively or negatively alter the signs and symptoms of the patient deserve the highest priority for treatment selection and should be similar in construct to the concordant examination movements. Examination methods that fail to elicit the patient response may offer nominal or imprecise value, as do methods that focus solely on treatment decision making based on a single diagnostic label.

With the exception of manipulation, which is not an examination procedure, the majority of active and passive treatment techniques are nearly identical to the examination procedures. In all cases of manual therapy treatment, there should be a direct mechanical relationship between the examination and treatment techniques selected.

## Active Physiological Movements

Active physiological movements of the ankle are used effectively as gentle, early range-of-motion (ROM) activity. Active movements are particularly useful when implemented as a home exercise program used to maintain an increase in ROM following a more aggressive passive treatment. Strengthening programs for the foot and ankle can be isolated to a single leg or applied to both legs. A single leg strength program demonstrated carryover to the untrained leg, which indicates that it may be possible to start strengthening the involved leg through exercise of the uninvolved leg while following activity restriction orders (Figure 15.66).[46]

Patients with an ankle sprain appear to benefit from proprioception and balance training as well.[47] An injury such as an ankle sprain detrimentally affects postural stability and is retrained with postural exercise.

Active mobilization movements for self-stretching may also benefit the patient. If the patient's concordant movement is associated with tightness or capsular-based restrictions, active movements into the stiffness with the foot stabilized in weight bearing may be an effective self-mobilization (Figure 15.67).

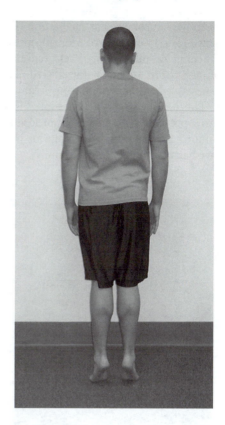

**Figure 15.66**    Heel Raises

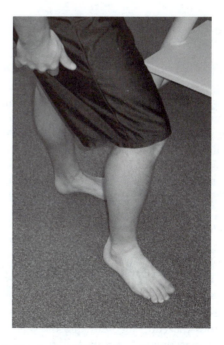

**Figure 15.67**    Isolated Rotations for Stretching

Proprioceptive neuromuscular facilitation (PNF) techniques (Figure 15.68) make use of proprioceptive stimulus for strengthening or inhibition of selected and targeted muscle groups.[48] Both are manually assisted methods and both have established benefit during manual therapy treatment. The benefit of PNF procedures is associated with the three-pronged outcome. PNF procedures are effective in improving strength and range of motion, and may improve balance and proprioception.[48]

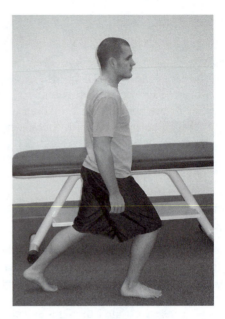

**Figure 15.69**    Repeated Movements into Dorsiflexion

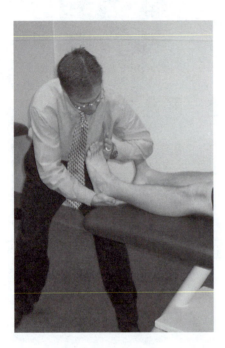

**Figure 15.68**    PNF Strengthening Exercises

## Passive Physiological Techniques

In lateral ankle sprains, dorsiflexion during weight-bearing activities is frequently lost and may contribute to an increased risk of a recurrent inversion sprain. Subsequently, passive stretching programs that incorporate physiological dorsiflexion stretching may be useful in targeting limitations of dorsiflexion in an acute phase.[27,49]

Dorsiflexion stretching by means of repeated self-mobilizations into dorsiflexion may also be useful for increasing range of motion in the acutely sprained ankle (Figure 15.69).[50] The procedure is performed with and without a tilt board and is considered a self-technique since the patient modulates the force of the stretch.

- Step One: The patient is instructed to weight bear on the targeted leg. The patient prepositions the foot into full dorsiflexion.
- Step Two: The patient is instructed to either rotate or glide into the end range dorsiflexion. The most concordant reproduction of pain during a specific motion should be targeted.

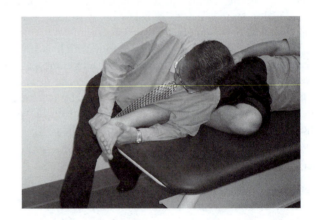

**Figure 15.70**    Passive Physiological Ankle Eversion

The curvilinear stretch into ankle eversion is often used to counter the hypermobility of the ankle into inversion (Figure 15.70). The technique is administered by the clinician or by the patient. The technique can be performed using oscillations or with a passive prolonged stretch.

The plantar splay stretch (Figure 15.71) is a technique used to stretch the plantar surface of the foot. The technique is generally considered beneficial for pain relief and may not actually increase gross range of motion.

- Step One: The patient assumes a prone or supine position. The clinician stands behind the patient to address the plantar surface of the foot.
- Step Two: The clinician applies a lateral load to each side of the foot in an attempt to splay the plantar tissue of the foot.

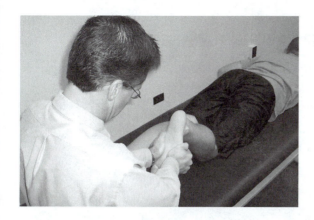

Figure 15.71    Plantar Splay Stretch

## Mobilization Techniques

The aforementioned examination methods double as treatment techniques for the foot and ankle. Each examination method should reproduce the concordant sign of the patient and should exhibit a reduction of pain with repeated movements or sustained holds. The following procedures demonstrate alterations in positioning from the examination and may be useful in isolating the targeted segment.

### Lateral Glide of the Subtalar Joint

- Step One: The patient lies in sidelying. The affected extremity is placed closest to the plinth.
- Step Two: The clinician cradles the lower leg in one arm. The fingers stabilize the talus by looping the first digit and thumb around the dome of the talus.
- Step Three: A lateral glide is performed using the nonstabilization hand. As with all mobilization techniques, repeated movements are performed at the first point of pain and at near end range, whichever elicits the most reduction of symptoms.

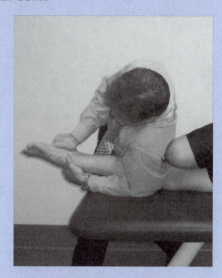

Figure 15.72    Lateral Glide of the Subtalar Joint

### Medial Glide of the Subtalar Joint

- Step One: The patient lies in sidelying. The affected extremity is placed furthermost from the plinth.
- Step Two: The clinician cradles the lower leg in one arm. The fingers stabilize the talus by looping the first digit and thumb around the dome of the talus.
- Step Three: A medial glide is performed using the nonstabilization hand. As with all mobilization techniques, repeated movements are performed at the first point of pain and at near end range, whichever elicits the most reduction of symptoms.

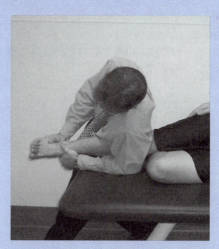

Figure 15.73    Medial Glide of the Subtalar Joint

## Posterior Glide of the Talus within the Talocrural Joint

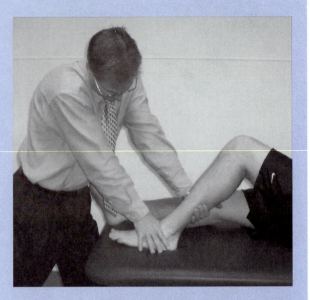

- Step One: The patient lies in supine or in a hooklying position. The clinician stabilizes the tibia by grasping the posterior aspect and stabilizing it to the plinth.
- Step Two: The clinician applies an AP force by using his or her web space to the anterior dome of the talus.
- Step Three: The glide is directed posteriorly. As with all mobilization techniques, repeated movements are performed at the first point of pain and at near end range, whichever elicits the most reduction of symptoms.

**Figure 15.74**    Anterior Posterior Glide at the Subtalar Joint

## Talocrural Distraction in Supine

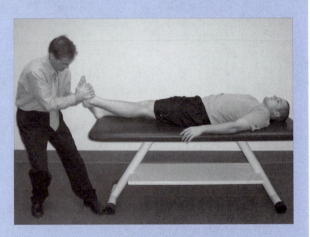

- Step One: The patient lies in supine. The clinician grasps the foot just distal to the talar dome.
- Step Two: The clinician applies a distraction force at the talocrural joint by shifting his or her weight away from the patient.
- Step Three: As with all mobilization techniques, repeated movements are performed at the first point of pain and at near end range, whichever elicits the most reduction of symptoms.

**Figure 15.75**    Distraction Based Mobilization of the Talocrural Joint

## Manipulation Techniques

Manipulation procedures have been reported in a number of studies.[51–56] The majority of studies used manipulation to improve dorsiflexion range-of-motion losses (see the boxes below).

---

### Talocrural Distraction Manipulation

- Step One: The patient lies in supine. The clinician grasps the foot just distal to the talar dome.
- Step Two: The clinician applies a distraction force at the talocrural joint by shifting his or her weight away from the patient. The movement is applied and a preload force is held at the end range of the distraction.
- Step Three: The manipulation is performed by applying a quick thrust at the end range. The thrust is targeted purely into distraction.

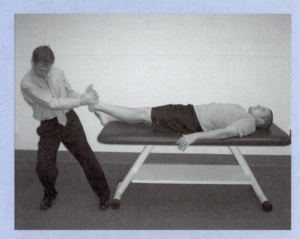

**Figure 15.76**    Distraction Based Manipulation

---

### Cuboid Whip Manipulation

Recently, Jennings and Davies[51] described a midfoot manipulation procedure designed for treatment of midfoot instability.

- Step One: The patient assumes a prone position. The clinician grasps the foot by stabilizing the medial and lateral sides of the foot within his or her web spaces. The thumbs of the clinician are placed on the cuboid on the plantar aspect of the foot.
- Step Two: The knee is flexed to approximately 70 degrees and the ankle is dorsiflexed to end range.
- Step Three: In a quick movement, the clinician moves the knee into extension, the ankle into plantarflexion and supination.
- Step Four: Concurrently with the physiological movements, the clinician also applies a plantar-to-dorsal thrust with his or her thumbs.
- Step Five: The procedure can be repeated if necessary.

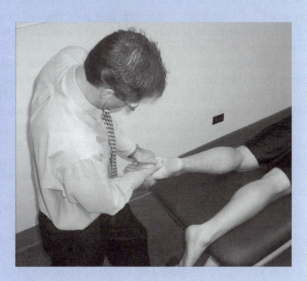

**Figure 15.77**    Cuboid Whip Manipulation

## Summary

- Strong association between examination and treatment should improve the outcome of a dedicated treatment program.
- Active physiological movements are beneficial in creating home exercise programs, working on abnormal posture, or strengthening the selected lower extremity musculature.
- Passive physiological and accessory techniques are reflective of the examination findings.
- Manipulation procedures are generally applicable in acute ankle sprains that do not exhibit detrimental laxity.

# TREATMENT OUTCOMES

## Exercise

One of the most effective treatment procedures includes the simple concept of early movement after injury. Early active movement results in improved outcomes versus immobilization and non-weight–bearing activities.[57,58] Generally, the active movements are included with forms of passive treatment such as mobilization and balance-related treatment.

## Proprioceptive Training

Proprioceptive training leads to improved joint position sense, decreased postural sway, and reduced muscle reaction times in the fibular muscles.[59] Furthermore, proprioception techniques reduce the risk of future inversion sprains[59] and may improve the strength of the lower extremity.[60] A four-week agility training program failed to show improvements in single leg stance over controls[61] but neither of these protocols was tested for an affect on recurrent sprain rates. Another study demonstrated that a supervised exercise program that consisted of balance-related activities demonstrated similar outcomes to an educational control program for postural sway, isometric ankle strength, and joint position sense.[62] However, the supervised program did result in reduced incidence of recurrent ankle sprains over the next 12 months.[62,63]

One study demonstrated that elderly individuals who regularly practiced Tai Chi had significantly better knee and ankle joint kinesthesia than their aged-matched sedentary counterparts, or swimmers and runners.[64] These changes were accompanied by improved sway characteristics that have been used to assess ankle proprioception in instability studies. The direct application of this study to lateral ankle instability treatment is questionable since the study did not directly assess the ankle, but the overlap of proprioception between joints and the contributions to proprioception through skin and other systemic inputs implies that the use of Tai Chi is a potential treatment option worth studying.

Training programs using a flexible disk that mimics an unstable surface to improve balance and proprioception have been demonstrated to decrease electromyographic (EMG) muscle reaction latency times[65] and have reduced the incidence of ankle injuries in female European handball players following a routine 10- to 15-minute training program performed for 10 months at each practice.[7] Wester et al. also found that training on a wobble board could reduce the incidence of recurrent ankle sprains but does not speed up the process of reduction of initial symptoms.[66]

## Mobilization

The majority of studies investigating the benefits of mobilization for the ankle foot complex are case reports or case series. Unfortunately, these studies demonstrated poor methodology with results that are not transferable to a pathologic population.[50] One of the best-designed studies[67] acknowledged that including mobilization in the treatment of acute inversion ankle sprains lead to decreased visits and quicker increases in range of motion.

A recent randomized controlled trial explored the use of a Mulligan technique, termed a mobilization with movement (MWM), on dorsiflexion in weight bearing and pressure pain threshold levels. Mulligan reports a 97% success rate with substantial improvement in active, pain-free dorsiflexion following treatment.[68] In another study, dorsiflexion range of motion did increase ($p < .002$), but pain pressure threshold level did not change, implying that ROM was increased by mechanical means rather than by reducing pain.[52]

## Manipulation

Manipulation has been thoroughly investigated as a treatment for ankle-related pathologies. The majority of studies have demonstrated improvements in patients who have received a manipulation procedure versus a benign control.[51,53–56] A variety of methods have demonstrated efficacy, the majority designed to reduce neurophysiologic reduction of pain more so than gains of range of motion.[56,69]

## Taping and Bracing Techniques

The primary benefit associated with taping to increase stiffness at the ankle is associated with the increase in the amplification ratio of proprioception through cutaneous mechanoreceptors, thereby increasing functional ankle stability while the tape remains tight.[70] A recent study demonstrated that a semi-rigid brace applied to the ankle could bring about a more favorable firing pattern to the muscles of the lower leg, allowing greater protection of the ankle from inversion sprains. This study suggests that previous concerns over brace usage causing a generalized weakening of muscles may be unfounded in clinical practice.[64,71–73] In subjects with no history of injury, a semi-rigid ankle brace enhanced excitability of the motor-neuron pool of the common fibular nerve innervating the fibularis longus muscle.[74] It seems reasonable that the mechanism of action is related to the stimulation of cutaneous afferents that alter the sensorimotor system in a positive manner. The use of a custom foot orthotic designed to correct abnormal talar alignment following ankle inversion sprain has been shown to reduce postural sway in single leg stance measured by force plate. This suggests that custom orthotics may be helpful in facilitating recovery following a lateral ankle sprain.[75]

## Summary

- Overall, there is limited empirical evidence and significant anecdotal evidence that a treatment approach consisting of some element of orthopedic manual therapy is associated with a positive outcome.
- There is a significant lack of controlled studies that have investigated the combinations of strengthening and mobilization or individualized treatment processes on patients with variations of AFC disorders.

# Chapter Questions

1. Describe the relationship of the soft and nonsoft tissues with the stabilization of the ankle.
2. Describe how compromised proprioception alters the functional stability of a patient during locomotion.
3. Outline the arthrological movements of the talocrural joint during dorsiflexion and plantarflexion.
4. Identify the variations associated with passive accessory examination of the AFC.
5. Describe the outcomes associated with mobilization and manipulation of the ankle.

# References

1. Surve I, Schwellnus MP, Noakes T, Lombard C. A fivefold reduction in the incidence of recurrent ankle sprains in soccer players using the sport-stirrup orthosis. *Am J Sports Med*. 1994;22:601–606.
2. Tropp H AC, Gillquist J. Prevention of ankle sprains. *Am J Sports Med*. 1985;13:259–261.
3. Thordarson D. *Orthopedic surgery essentials: Foot and ankle*. Philadelphia; Lippincott Williams & Wilkens: 2004.
4. McKay GD, Goldie PA, Payne WR, Oakes BW. Ankle injuries in basketball: Injury rate and risk factors. *Br J Sports Med*. 2001;35:103–108.
5. Sitler M, Ryan J, Wheeler B. The efficacy of a semi-rigid ankle stabilizer to reduce acute ankle injuries in basketball. A randomized clinical at West Point. *Am J Sports Med*. 1994;22:454–461.
6. Hosea TM, Carey CC, Harrer MF. Epidemiology of ankle injuries in athletes who participate in basketball. *Clin Orthop*. 2000;372:45–49.
7. Wedderkopp N, Kaltoft M, Lundgaard B, Rosendahl M, Froberg K. Prevention of injuries in young female players in European team handball. A prospective intervention study. *Scand J Med Science Sports*. 1999;9: 41–47.
8. Birrer R, Dellacorte M, Grisafi P. *Common foot problems in primary care*. 2nd ed. Philadelphia; Hanley and Belfus: 1998.
9. Dutton M. *Orthopaedic examination, evaluation and intervention*. New York; McGraw-Hill: 2004.
10. Moore K. *Clinically oriented anatomy*. Baltimore; Williams & Wilkens: 1985.
11. Attarian D. A biomechanical study of human lateral ankle ligaments and autogenous reconstructive grafts. *Am J Sports Med*. 1985;13:377–381.
12. Kapandji IA. *Physiology of the joints*, vol ii, the lower limb. London; Churchill Livingstone: 1970.
13. Hintermann B, Boss A, Schäfer D. Arthroscopic findings in patients with chronic ankle instability. *Am J Sports Med*. 2002;30:402–409.
14. Sarrafian SK. *Anatomy of the foot and ankle*. Philadelphia; JB Lippincott: 1983.
15. Kaltenborn FM. *Manual mobilization of the joints*. Oslo, Norway; Olaf Norlis Bokhandel: 2002.

16. Vogler HW BG. Contrast studies of the foot and ankle. In: Weissman SD, ed. *Radiology of the foot.* Baltimore: Williams and Wilkens; 1989:439–495.

17. Womble MD. Human gross anatomy for physical therapy: Part 3—the lower limb and deep back. Course handouts for Biology 869. 2005:59–76.

18. Neumann D. Kinesiology of the musculoskeletal system. *Foundations for physical rehabilitation.* St. Louis, MO; Mosby: 2002.

19. Singh AK, Starkweather KD, Hollister AM, Jatana S, Lupichuk AG. Kinematics of the ankle: A hinge axis model. *Foot Ankle.* 1992;13(8):439–446.

20. Donatelli RA. *The biomechanics of the foot and ankle.* Philadelphia; F. A. Davis: 1996.

21. Manter JT. Movements of the subtalar joint and transverse tarsal joints. *Anat Rec.* 1941;80:397–400.

22. Elftman H. The transverse tarsal joint and its control. *Clin Orthop Rel Res.* 1960;16:41–45.

23. Boyko EJ, Ahroni JH, Daviqnon D, Stensel V, Prigeon RL, Smith DG. Diagnostic utility of the history and physical examination for peripheral vascular disease among patients with diabetes mellitus. *J Clin Epidemiol.* 1997;50(6):659–668.

24. Meyer J, Kulig K, Landel R. Differential diagnosis and treatment of subcalcaneal heel pain: a case report. *J Orthop Sports Phys Ther.* 2002;32(3):114–122.

25. Sujitkumar P, Hadfield JM, Yates DW. Sprain or fracture? An analysis of 2000 ankle injuries. *Arch Emerg Med.* 1986;3(2):101–106.

26. Bachmann LM, Kolb E, Koller MT, Steurer J, ter Riet G. Accuracy of Ottawa ankle rules to exclude fractures of the ankle and mid-foot: systematic review. *BMJ.* 2003;326(7386):417.

27. Young B, Walker M, Strunce J, Boyles R. A combined treatment approach emphasizing impairment-based manual physical therapy for plantar heel pain: A case series. *J Orthop Sports Phys Ther.* 2004;34:725–733.

28. Rubin A, Sallis R. Evaluation and diagnosis of ankle injuries. *Am Fam Phys.* 1996;54:1609–1618.

29. Wilson RW, Gansneder BM. Measures of functional limitation as predictors of disablement in athletes with acute ankle sprains. *J Ortho Sports Phys Ther.* 2000;30:528–535.

30. Hubbard TJ, Kaminski TW, Vander Griend RA, Kovaleski JE. Quantitative assessment of mechanical laxity in the functionally unstable ankle. *Med Sci Sports and Exer.* 2004;36:760–766.

31. Bennet PJ, Patterson C, Wearing S, Baglioni T. Development and validation of a questionnaire designed to measure foot-health status. *J Am Podiatric Assoc.* 1998;88:419–428.

32. Garrow AP, Papageorgiou AC, Silman AJ, Thomas E, Jayson MI, MacFarlane GJ. Development and validation of a questionnaire to assess disabling foot pain. *Pain.* 2000;85:107–113.

33. Maitland GD. *Peripheral manipulation.* Oxford; Butterworth-Heinemann: 1991.

34. Lark SD, Buckley JG, Bennett S, Jones D, Sargeant AJ. Joint torques and dynamic joint stiffness in elderly and young men during stepping down. *Clin Biomech.* 2003;18(9):848–855.

35. Lynch S. Assessment of the injured ankle in the athlete. *J Athletic Train.* 2002;37:406–412.

36. Fujii T, Zong-Ping L, Kitaoka H, An KN. The manual stress test may not be sufficient to differentiate ankle ligament injuries. *Clin Biomech.* 2000;15:619–623.

37. Kjaersgaard-Anderson P, Frich LH, Madsen F, Helmig P, Sogard P, Sojbjerg JO. Instability of the hindfoot after lesion of the lateral ankle ligaments: Investigations of the anterior drawer and adduction maneuvers in autopsy specimens. *Clin Orthop.* 1991;266:170–179.

38. Vinicombe A, Raspovic A, Menz HB. Reliability of navicular displacement measurement as a clinical indicator of foot posture. *J Am Podiatr Med Assoc.* 2001;91:262–268.

39. Picciano AM, Rowlands MS, Worrell T. Reliability of open and closed kinematic chain subtalar joint neutral positions and navicular drop test. *J Orthop Sports Phys Ther.* 1993;18:553–558.

40. Mueller MJ, Host JV, Norton BJ. Navicular drop as a composite measure of excessive pronation. *J Am Pod Med Assoc.* 1993;83:198–202.

41. Sell KE, Verity TM, Worrell TW. Two measurement techniques for assessing subtalar joint position: A reliability study. *J Orthop Sports Phys Ther.* 1994;19(3):162–167.

42. McPoil TG, Cornwall MW. The relationship between static lower extremity measurements and hindfoot motion during walking. *J Orthop Sports Phys Ther.* 1996;24(5):309–314.

43. Allen MK, Glasoe WM. Metrecom measurement of navicular drop in subjects with anterior cruciate ligament injury. *J Athl Train.* 2000;35(4):403–406.

44. Shrader JA, Popovich JM, Gracey GC, Danoff JV. Navicular drop measurement in people with rheumatoid arthritis: Interrater and intrarater reliability. *Phys Ther.* 2005;85:656–664.

45. Beumer A, van Hemert WL, Swierstra BA, Jasper LE, Belkoff SM. A biomechanical evaluation of clinical stress tests for syndesmotic ankle instability. *Foot Ankle Int.* 2003;24:358–363.

46. Uh BS, Beynnon BD, Helie BV, Alosa DM, Renstrom PA. The benefit of a single-leg strength training program for the muscles around the untrained ankle: A prospective, randomized, controlled study. *Am J Sports Med.* 2000;28:568–573.

47. Goldie PA, Evans OM, Bach TM. Postural control following inversion injuries of the ankle. *Arch Phys Med Rehabil.* 1994;75(9):969–975.

48. Etnyre BR, Abraham LD. Gains in range of ankle dorsiflexion using three population stretching techniques. *Am J Phys Med.* 1986;65:189–1996.

49. Porter D, Barrill E, Oneacre K, May BD. The effects of duration and frequency of Achilles tendon stretching on dorsiflexion and outcome in painful hell syndrome: a randomized, blinded control study. *Foot Ankle Int.* 2002;23:619–624.

50. Whitman JM, Childs JD, Walker V. The use of manipulation in a patient with an ankle sprain injury not responding to conventional management: a case report. *Man Ther.* 2005;10:224–231.

51. Jennings J, Davies GJ. Treatment of cuboid syndrome secondary to lateral ankle sprains: A case series. *J Orthop Sports Phys Ther.* 2005;35:409–415.

52. Collins N, Teys P, Vicenzino B. The initial effects of a Mulligan's mobilization technique on dorsiflexion and pain in subacute ankle sprains. *Man Ther.* 2004;9:77–82.

53. Eisenhart AW, Gaeta TJ, Yeus DP. Osteopathic manipulative treatment in the emergency department for patients with acute ankle sprains. *J Am Ostepath Assoc.* 2003;103:417–421.

54. Fryer GA, Mudge JM, McLaughlin PA. The effect of talocrural joint manipulation on range of motion at the ankle. *J Manipulative Physiol Ther.* 2002;25(6):384–390.

55. Pellow JE, Brantingham JW. The efficacy of adjusting the ankle in the treatment of subacute and chronic grade I and grade II ankle inversion sprains. *J Manipulative Physiol Ther.* 2001;24:17–24.

56. Nield S, Davis K, Latimer J, Maher C, Adams R. The effect of manipulation on range of movement at the ankle joint. *Scand J Rehabil Med.* 1993;25:161–166.

57. Eiff MP, Smith AT, Smith GE. Early mobilization versus immobilization in the treatment of lateral ankle sprains. *Am J Sports Med.* 1994;22:83–88.

58. Karlsson J, Eriksson BI, Sward L. Early functional treatment for acute ligament injuries of the ankle joint. *Scand J Med Science Sports.* 1996;6:341–345.

59. De Carlo MS, Talbot RW. Evaluation of ankle joint proprioception following injection of the anterior talofibular ligament. *J Orthop Sports Phys Ther.* 1986;8:70–76.

60. Powers ME, Buckley BD, Kaminski TW, Hubbard TJ, Ortiz C. Six weeks of strength and proprioception training does not affect muscle fatigue and static balance in functional ankle instability. *J Sport Rehabil.* 2004;13:201–227.

61. Hess DM, Joyce CJ, Arnold BL, Gansneder BM. Effect of a 4-week agility-training program on postural sway in the functionally unstable ankle. *J Sport Rehabil.* 2001;10:24–35.

62. Holme E, Magnusson SP, Becher K, Bieler T, Aagaard B, Kjaer M. The effect of supervised rehabilitation on strength, postural sway, position sense and re-injury risk after acute ankle ligament sprain. *Scand J Med Science Sports.* 1999;9:104–109.

63. Verhagen E, Mechelen W, de Vente W. The effect of preventive measures on the incidence of ankle sprains. *Clin J Sport Med.* 2000;10:291–296.

64. Xu D HY, Li J, Chan K. Effect of tai chi exercise on proprioception on ankle and knee joints in old people. *Br J Sports Med.* 2004;38:50–54

65. Osborne MD CL, Laskowski ER, Smith J, Kaufman KR. The effect of ankle disk training on muscle reaction time in subjects with a history of ankle sprain. *Am J Sports Med.* 2001;29:627–632.

66. Wester JU, Jespersen SM, Nielsen KD, Neumann L. Wobble board training after partial sprains of the lateral ligaments of the ankle: A prospective randomized study. *J Orthop Sports Phys Ther.* 1996;23:332–336.

67. Green T, Refshauge K, Crosbie J, Adams R. A randomized controlled trial of a passive accessory joint mobilization on acute ankle inversion sprains. *Phys Ther.* 2001;81:984–994.

68. Mulligan BR. *Manual therapy "nags", "snags", "mwms" etc.* Wellington: Plane View Services Ltd; 1995.

69. Malisza KL, Gregorash L, Turner A, Foniok T, Stroman PW, Allman AA, Summers R, Wright A. Functional MRI involving painful stimulation of the ankle and the effect of physiotherapy joint mobilization. *Magn Reson Imaging.* 2003;21:489–496.

70. Lohrer H, Alt W, Gollhofer A. Neuromuscular properties and functional aspects of taped ankles. *Am J Sports Med.* 1999;27:69–75.

71. Conley K. The effects of selected modes of prophylactic support on reflex muscle firing following dynamic perturbation of the ankle. School of Health and Rehabilitation Science. Pittsburgh. 2005.

72. Cordova ML, Ingersoll CD. Peroneus longus stretch reflex amplitude increases after ankle brace application. *Br J Sports Med.* 2003;37:258–262.

73. Cordova ML, Cardona C, Ingersoll CD. Long-term ankle brace use does not affect peroneus longus muscle latency during sudden inversion in normal subjects. *J Athl Train.* 2000;35:407–411.

74. Nishikawa T, Grabiner MD. Peroneal motoneuron excitability increases immediately following application of a semirigid ankle brace. *J Orthop Sports Phys Ther.* 1999;29:168–173.

75. Guskiewicz KM, Perrin DH. Effect of orthotics on postural sway following inversion ankle sprain. *J Ortho Sports Phys Ther.* 1996;23:326–331.

# Glossary

**Absolute Contraindication to Manual Therapy:** Any situation in which the movement, stress, or compression placed on a particular body part involves a high risk of a deleterious consequence.

**Acromioclavicular Joint:** The articulation between the proximal aspect of the clavicle and the medial aspect of the acromion of the scapula.

**Active Movements:** Any form of physiological movements performed exclusively by the patient.

**Altman's Criteria for Osteoarthritis of the Hip:** Altman's criteria consist of limitations and pain of internal rotation, elevation of sedimentation rates, morning stiffness, and older age.

**Analgesia:** Associated with the capability of relieving pain.

**Ankle Foot Complex (AFC):** The AFC includes the inferior tibiofibular joint and all the osseous structures and joints of the foot and ankle.

**Annulus Fibrosis:** Outermost component of the intervertebral disc that consists primarily of fibrocartilage.

**Arthrokinematic:** Joint-related mechanical movement.

**Articular Disc:** The articular disc is a biconcave structure that separates the intraarticular region into an upper and a lower compartment.

**Auricular Canal:** The external auditory canal leading to the inner ear.

**Babinski Sign:** A consequence of an upper motor neuron sign associated with dorsiflexion and fanning of the toes during stimulus to the palmar aspect of the foot.

**Baseline:** The baseline is the base performance or pain indicator prior to the treatment intervention.

**Biomechanical Assessment Manual Therapy Model:** A manual therapy model that has evaluation methods and treatment techniques based on selected biomechanical theories.

**Black Flags:** Objective occupational or workplace factors that may initially lead to the onset of low back pain, and may promote disability once the acute episode has occurred.

**Blue Flags:** Perceived occupational factors believed by patients to impede their recovery include litigation, long-term worker's compensation, and a negative relationship with their supervisor.

**Canadian C-Spine Rules:** Guidelines designed to determine whether victims of a trauma should receive radiographic or MRI-based testing.

**Capsular Pattern Theory:** A theory advocated by James Cyriax that capsular dysfunction of the shoulder leads to consistent range-of-motion losses by ratios. His concept was that external rotation is limited more than abduction that is limited more than internal rotation proportionally.

**Catastrophisizing Behavior:** Fear of impending doom associated with a syndrome of problems and fear of movement.

**Central Facilitation of Pain:** Pain originating or facilitated by central (brain and spinal cord) related mechanisms.

**Centralization Phenomenon:** Within this textbook centralization is liberally defined as a movement, mobilization, or manipulation technique targeted to pain radiating or referring from the spine, which when applied abolishes or reduces the pain distally to proximally in a controlled, predictable pattern.

**Cervical Radiculopathy:** Radiculopathy originating from a cervical-based structure.

**Cervicogenic Headaches:** Headaches that originate from a cervical-based structure.

**Chamberlain X-ray:** A Chamberlain x-ray is performed while a patient assumes a unilateral standing (weight bearing) position. The x-ray is positive if a considerable amount of superior translation is noted between the two pubic bones at the pubic symphysis.

**Chin-Cradle Grip:** Hand placement technique designed to ensure maximum efficiency during treatment.

**Chronic Back Pain:** Long-term problems associated with low back pain. Typically associated with greater than 7 weeks of pain.

**Clinical Cervical Instability:** The failure of the active and passive structures of the neck to stabilize structures during static positions and dynamic movement.

**Clonus:** A consequence of an upper motor neuron lesion associated with repeated uncontrolled movements of a joint (typically the ankle) during an applied dorsiflexion force.

**Cock-Robin Posture:** Postural position generally associated with a C1-2 subluxation; consists of rotation, side flexion, and flexion to the same side.

**Combined Movements:** Movements of the vertebral column or periphery that occur in combination across planes rather than as pure movements in one plane.

**Comparable Sign:** A comparable joint or neural sign that refers to a combination of pain, stiffness, and spasm, which the examiner finds upon examination and considers comparable with the patient's symptoms.

**Concordant Sign:** The concordant familiar sign as the pain or other symptoms identified on a pain drawing, and verified by the patient as being the complaint that has prompted one to seek diagnosis and treatment.

**Convex–Concave Rule:** A concept developed by MaConail that suggests that selected arthrokinematic movements are determined by the physiological presence of a convex-on-concave congruency. The movement of initiation will dictate the direction of the motion.

**Costochondral Joint:** The costochondral joint consists of two factions: the sternal-chondral articulation and the costochondral articulation. A condition known as costochondritis, which mimics cardiac chest pain, may produce isolated pain directed at the two rib-sternal attachments.

**Costotransverse Joint:** The costotransverse joint yields two synovial capsules and is formed by articulation of the rib tubercle and thoracic vertebral transverse process.

**Costovertebral Joint:** The costovertebral joint is formed by a convex rib head with two adjacent vertebral bodies, superiorly and inferiorly. Although variable throughout the length of the thoracic spine, in the midthorax the concave inferior costal demi facet of the superior vertebral body and the concave superior costal construction of the inferior vertebral body provide a synovial attachment to the rib head.

**Counternutation:** Counternutation is analogous to anterior rotation of the innominate relative to the sacrum.

**Coupled Motion or Behavior:** Coupled motion is the rotation or translation of a vertebral body about or along one axis that is consistently associated with the main rotation or translation about another axis.

**Coupling Behavior:** The concept of corresponding movements during the initiation of a single plane movement.

**Cyriax's Selective Tension Testing Theory:** The theory that selected contractile tissues (muscle, tendon, and bony insertion) are painful during an applied isometric contraction and inert structures (capsule, ligaments, bursae) are painful during passive movement.

**Diagnostic Label:** The name provided to a disease process or pathology.

**Diagnostic Value:** Diagnostic value may consist of two methods: (1) to evaluate and form a hypothesis for labeling a specific pathology or (2) to classify a cluster of symptoms for selection of an intervention.

**Differentiation of Referred Pain:** The careful differential assessment and identification of the pain generator of referred pain.

**Directional Spine Coupling:** The theory that the vertebral spine will demonstrate predictable directional movement patterns during the initiation of motion.

**Discordant Sign:** A painful movement that is not the pain or other symptoms identified on a pain drawing, and verified by the patient as being the complaint that has prompted one to seek diagnosis and treatment.

**Dorsal Intercalated Segmental Instability:** A dorsal intercalated segmental instability results from a disruption between the scaphoid and the lunate, allowing the scaphoid to float into volar flexion.

**Double Injection Blocks:** Double injection blocks are anesthetic blocks used to obliterate pain that arises from the structure injected. Two blocks are used to ensure the location and appropriateness of the findings.

**End Feel:** Cyriax defines end feel as the extreme of each passive movement of the joint that transmits a specific sensation to the examiner's hands.

**Feiss Line:** The Feiss line is an imaginary line drawn from the medial malleolus to the midpoint of the medial first ray that bisects the navicular tubercle.

**Force Closure:** Force closure is in reference to the increase in SIJ stiffness attributed to muscular contraction.

**Forefoot:** The forefoot boundaries include the distalmost phalanges and the tarsometatarsal joint (Lisfranc's joint). The forefoot contains five metatarsals and 14 phalanges.

**Form Closure:** Form closure is in reference to the increase of SIJ stiffness attributed to the internal architecture of the joint.

**Functional Testing of the Hip:** Functional testing of the hip is more associated with functional movements during walking, pivoting, or standing than plane-based movements performed actively.

**General Inspection:** An observational analysis that examines visible static- and movement-related defects for analysis during the subjective (history) and objective (physical) examination.

**Generalized Manipulation:** A manipulative technique that involves less defined prepositioning methods, designed in such a manner as to provide the thrust to a dedicated region.

**Generic-Specific Questionnaires:**  Scales that measure activities of daily living, function, and general well-being across multiple bodily dimensions.

**Glenohumeral Joint:**  The glenohumeral joints consists of the articulation of the head of the humerus and the glenoid fossa of the scapula.

**Global Muscles:**  Muscles that are designed to provide movement, are poor stabilizers, and are generally not attached close to the segments.

**H Reflex:**  Excitability reflex modulated by spinal cord mechanisms.

**Hand Diagram:**  A hand diagram is an anatomical drawing that allows a patient to mechanically identify his or her area of discomfort.

**Hindfoot:**  There are two bones of the hindfoot (calcaneus and talus) and the boundaries include the Achilles tendon posteriorly and the midtarsal joint distally.

**Hip Labrum:**  The hip labrum is a cartilaginous addition to the acetabulum designed to increase the integrity of the hip joint.

**Hoffmann's Sign:**  A consequence of an upper motor neuron lesion associated with quick finger flexion during a provocative dorsal to palmar strumming of the middle finger.

**Hypertonicity:**  Increased tone.

**Hypomobility:**  A reduction in normal mobility. Movement that is demonstrably less than normal expectations.

**Impairment-Based Assessment Model:**  An assessment model that targets selective impairments versus an overall understanding of the label of pathology.

**In Vivo Analysis:**  An analysis performed on live subjects.

**Intertester Reliability:**  The measurement ability of multiple testers to score consistently during a clinical examination.

**Intraarticular Disorders:**  Any pathological condition of the knee in which the origin is located inside the knee capsule.

**Intraarticular Region of the TMJ:**  The intraarticular region is the space that occupies the synovial temporomandibular joint.

**Introspection:**  An internal analysis of the clinician that refers to the relationship of nonphysical findings with physical findings.

**Irritability:**  An evaluation of how petulant the patient's symptoms are based on three concepts: (1) What does the patient have to do to set this condition off? (2) Once set off, how long do the symptoms last? and (3) What does the patient have to do to calm the symptoms down?

**Kemp Test:**  A special clinical test designed to implicate lumbar radiculopathy.

**Kyphosis:**  Kyphosis corresponds to the degree of curvature within the sagittal plane of the spine. Within the thoracic spine, kyphosis may contribute to dysfunctions such as balance disturbance, pathologies such as insidious fractures, and impairments such as pain.

**Local Cervical Muscles:**  Muscles that are designed primarily for stability and originate and insert close to the spine segments.

**Localized Manipulative:**  A manipulation technique involved in the intent of applying a passive or assisted movement toward one specific functional region (i.e., spinal unit or single joint).

**Localized Mobilization:**  A specific technique that is directed to one segmental and/or joint region.

**Lower Quarter Screen:**  A comprehensive lower quarter assessment that is designed to assess movement, muscle strength, sensory condition, and reflexes.

**Manipulation:**  An accurately localized or globally applied; single, quick, and decisive movement of small amplitude, following a careful positioning of the patient.

**Manual Muscle Test:**  Examination method that endeavors to determine the raw strength of a selected muscle group.

**Manual Therapy Philosophical Approach:**  The education background of the manual therapist.

**Mechanoreceptors:**  A neural end organ (as a tactile receptor) that responds to a mechanical or chemical stimulus.

**Medical Screening:**  A comprehensive systems assessment that promotes awareness of comorbidities that may contribute or potentially harm a patient's recovery and/or function.

**Meniscectomy:**  Partial or total removal of the medial or lateral meniscus.

**Meniscofemoral Ligaments:**  Two different structures in the knee that are considered posterior stabilizers of the knee, specifically stabilizers in rotation.

**Meniscoid:**  A posterior fold of the zygopophyseal capsule that is designed to improve the joint congruency of the facet.

**Midfoot:**  There are five midfoot bones (navicular, cuboid, cuneiforms 1 through 3) and the section is bordered by the Lisfranc joint distally and the transverse tarsal joint (Chopart's joint) proximally.

**Mixed Manual Therapy Model:**  A manual therapy background that consists of a hybrid of selected philosophical approaches.

**Mobilization:**  Passive techniques designed to restore full painless joint function by rhythmic, repetitive passive movements to the patient's tolerance, in voluntary and/or accessory ranges.

**Moseley Criteria of Evidence:**  Classification system for research studies that divides studies in those that are Level I, very well designed randomized controlled trials; Level II, fairly well-designed randomized pragmatic controlled trials; and Level III, pseudo-randomized trials.

**Muscle Energy Technique:** A manually assisted method of stretching/mobilization where the patient actively uses their muscles, on request, while maintaining a targeted preposition, against a distinctly executed counterforce.

**Muscle Provocation Testing:** An examination method that endeavors to implicate a guilty muscle through provocation during contraction.

**Myelopathy:** Referred pain that originates from incursion or compression of the spinal cord.

**Myotome:** A set of muscles or muscle that it innervated by a selective nerve range.

**Neck Disability Index:** A functional scale designed to measure activity limitations due to neck pain and disability.

**Neck Pain and Disability Scale:** Functional scale designed to measure report of problems with neck movements, neck pain intensity, effect of neck pain on emotion and cognition, and the level of interference during life activities.

**Neurological Symptoms:** Symptoms resulting from myelopathy. Symptoms may include bilateral numbness and tingling and muscle weakness.

**Nucleus Pulposis:** Innermost aspect of the cervical intervertebral disc.

**Nutation:** Nutation is analogous to posterior rotation of the innominate relative to the sacrum.

**Observation:** Visual assessment.

**Ottawa Knee Rules:** A prospective set of clinical findings that are designed to assist in determining the use of a radiograph. There are five components to the Ottawa Knee Rules: (1) age > 55, (2) tenderness at the head of the fibula, (3) isolated tenderness of patella during palpation, (4) inability to flex knee to 90 degrees, and (5) inability to bear weight both immediately and in the emergency department.

**Overpressure:** Brief force applied at end range designed to further distill latent symptoms.

**Pain-Dominant Problems:** Impairments where the primary source of the disorder is inflammatory.

**Pain Maps:** Pain maps are self-report mechanisms designed to allow the patient to draw where his or her pain is most prevalent.

**Passive Accessory Intervertebral Movements:** Passive movement techniques designed to target individual arthrokinematic movements.

**Passive Movements:** Any planar or physiological motions that are performed exclusively by the clinician.

**Patellofemoral Pain Syndrome:** Multifactorial pathological condition that involves the movements and stability of the patellofemoral joint.

**Pathology-Based Assessment Models:** Assessment models that focus first on the pathology or diagnostic label then perform examination and treatment measures related to the pathology.

**Patient Response Manual Therapy Model:** An assessment model that guides treatment decision making and clinical reasoning based on the patient response to examination and treatment.

**Pelvic Girdle:** The pelvic girdle includes the articulations associated with the left and right sacroiliac joints and the pubic symphysis.

**Placebo:** The Placebo effect is the measurable or observable after-effect target to a person or group of participants that have been given some form of expectant care.

**Positioning Methods:** A postural method designed to provide a prolonged stretch in a selected position.

**Postural Syndromes:** Pain associated with maintenance of selected postures or positions.

**Proprioceptive Neuromuscular Facilitation:** Manually assisted movements where an active contraction by the subject is performed against passive application of a stress by the clinician, thus stimulating the proprioceptor system.

**Protrusion:** An anterior movement of the lower jaw within the transverse plane.

**Pubic Symphysis:** The pubic symphysis is a fibrocartilagenous joint with an articular disc that separates the two pubic rami.

**Quick Test:** Quick tests are synonymous with functional tests.

**Radiculopathy:** Referred pain that originates from either chemical irritation or nerve root compression.

**Red Flags:** Signs and symptoms that may tie a disorder to a serious pathology.

**Reflex Testing:** Deep tendon reflex testing is designed to determine if an impairment in the H reflex is present during clinical examination.

**Region-Specific Scales:** A scale designed to demonstrate physical, social, and mental changes, which demonstrates physiometric measures associated with a localized physiological region.

**Regional Mobilizations:** Mobilization methods that involve directed passive movement to more than one given area, segment, or physiological component.

**Relative Contraindication to Manual Therapy:** A situation that requires special care because an applied treatment runs a high risk of injury.

**Repeated Active Movements:** Repeated active physiological techniques performed exclusively by the patient.

**Retrodiscal Area:** The retrodiscal area lies within the intraarticular region and houses ligaments, connective tissue, and other sensitive receptors. This region provides and contributes to passive control of the articular disc during movements of the jaw.

**Retrusion:** A posterior movement of the lower jaw within the transverse plane.

**Scapulohumeral Rhythm:** The scapulohumeral rhythm is a three-dimensional movement of scapular and glenohumeral kinematics, which generally consist of two parts movement of glenohumeral joint to one part movement of the scapula.

**Scapulothoracic Joint:**   The scapulothoracic joint is the muscular articulation of the scapula and the thorax.

**Scoliosis:**   Scoliosis corresponds to the degree of curvature within the coronal plane of the spine. A small degree of scoliosis is considered common in the thoracic spine but can lead to functional impairments and pain when excessive.

**Screw Home Mechanism:**   Automatic rotation between the tibia and femur occurs automatically between full extension (0°) and 20° of knee flexion designed to increase the congruency of the knee.

**Sensation Testing:**   Comparative analysis between extremities of light touch, pain, vibration, and thermotesting (temperature) sensations.

**Shoulder Labrum:**   The shoulder labrum is a fibrocartilaginous structure that serves to deepen and increase the integrity of the glenohumeral joint.

**Sinister Disorders:**   Nonmechanically based disorders that are potentially life threatening.

**Slump Sit Test:**   A measure of neural tension designed to implicate the presence of a herniated disc.

**Somatic Referred Pain:**   Pain that originates from a structure other than a nerve root or organ.

**Special Clinical Test:**   Clinical tests designed to further provide information or diagnosis.

**Spurling's Compression Test:**   A cervical special clinical test designed to implicate cervical radiculopathy.

**Sternoclavicular Joint:**   The sternoclavicular joint is the articular of the medial aspect of the clavicle with the lateral aspect of the sternum.

**Stiffness:**   A linear concept of tissue extensibility.

**Straight Leg Raise:**   A measure of neural tension designed to implicate the presence of a herniated disc.

**Sympathetic Nervous System:**   Components of the sympathetic nervous system originate within the thoracic region and oppose the physiological effects of the parasympathetic nervous system. The system is considered an involuntary system because the responses are not consciously controlled nor implemented.

**Sympathoexcitatory Effect:**   A manual technique or procedure that results in an excitatory effect on sympathetic nervous system activity.

**Syndesmosis:**   The syndesmosis is the joint structure of the distal tibia and fibula.

**Temporomandibular Disorder (TMD):**   Pain that originates in the region of the temporomandibular joint manifested by one or more of the following: (1) joint sounds, (2) limitations of joint movements, (3) muscle tenderness, (4) joint tenderness, (5) pain just anterior to the ear.

**Tendonesis:**   Tendonesis is a chronic breakdown of the muscular–tendon junction leading to degeneration in the absence of an inflammatory process.

**Trendelenburg's Sign:**   A Trendelenburg's sign is the contralateral drop of the pelvis secondary to weakness or failure of the gluteus medius and minimus to stabilize the pelvis during unilateral weight bearing.

**Triangular Fibrocartilagenous Complex:**   The triangular fibrocartilagenous complex is the disc that lies between the ulna and the proximal carpal row. The disc provides a smooth and conformed gliding surface across the entire distal face of the ulna and proximal carpal row, allows flexion, extension, rotation, and translational movements, and cushions forces that are transmitted through this region thus reducing the risk of fracture.

**Uncinate Processes:**   Synovial joints within the cervical spine, which are saddle-like formations that increase the joint surface of the vertebral body of the above segment with the lower segment.

**Upper Limb Tension Test:**   An upper extremity neural tension test designed to implicate the presence of cervical radiculopathy.

**Upper Motor Neuron Lesion:**   An injury to the brain or spinal cord.

**Upper Quarter Screen:**   A comprehensive upper quarter assessment that is designed to assess movement, muscle strength, sensory condition, and reflexes.

**Vertebral Basilar Insufficiency:**   A localized or diffuse reduction in blood flow through the vertebral basilar arterial system, which results from selected positions of the head.

**Visceral Referred Pain:**   Pain that originates from a visceral organ.

**Volar Intercalated Segmental Instability:**   A volar intercalated segmental instability (VISI) results from a disruption between the trapezoid and lunate allowing volar drift of the lunate and problems during physiological flexion of the wrist.

**Whiplash:**   Pseudomechanistic term used to describe a traumatic incident to the cervical spine resulting in soft and deep tissue damage.

**Willingness to Move:**   The patient's willingness to move upon command. Often associated with the fear of movement exhibited by the patient.

**Y Ligament of Bigalow:**   The Y ligament of Bigalow is the integrated ligament and capsule of the hip and is the strongest ligament in the body.

**Yellow Flags:**   Potentially significant psychosocial risk factors for developing chronic low back pain that include sociodemographic, abnormal pain behavioral responses, compensation-related responses, and psychological elements.

**Zygopophyseal Joints:**   The facet joints of the spine are synovial joints that are located posteriorly at each lumbar level.

# Index

Illustrations of Photos are indicated by (f); Tables are indicated by (t).